THIRD EDITION

Developmental Care
of Newborns and Infants

A GUIDE FOR HEALTH PROFESSIONALS

THIRD EDITION

Developmental Care of Newborns and Infants

A GUIDE FOR HEALTH PROFESSIONALS

EDITED BY

Carole Kenner, PhD, RN, FAAN, FNAP, ANEF

Carol Kuser Loser Dean & Professor
The College of New Jersey
Ewing, New Jersey
Chief Executive Officer
Council of International Neonatal Nurses, Inc. (COINN)
Yardley, Pennsylvania

Jacqueline M. McGrath, PhD, RN, FNAP, FAAN

Thelma and Joe Crow Endowed Professor
Vice Dean for Faculty Excellence
School of Nursing
University of Texas Health Science Center San Antonio
San Antonio, Texas

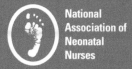

National
Association of
Neonatal
Nurses

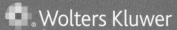

. Wolters Kluwer

Philadelphia · Baltimore · New York · London
Buenos Aires · Hong Kong · Sydney · Tokyo

Not authorised for sale in United States, Canada, Australia, New Zealand, Puerto Rico, and U.S. Virgin Islands.

Acquisitions Editor: Jamie Blum
Development Editor: Maria M. McAvey
Editorial Coordinators: Nancy Antony, Anju Radhakrishnan
Production Project Manager: Catherine Ott
Design Coordinator: Stephen Druding
Manufacturing Coordinator: Beth Welsh
Marketing Manager: Linda Wetmore
Prepress Vendor: TNQ Technologies

Third edition

9 8 7 6 5 4 3 2 1

Printed in Mexico

Library of Congress Cataloging-in-Publication Data

Names: Kenner, Carole, editor. | McGrath, Jacqueline M., editor. | National
Association of Neonatal Nurses, issuing body.
Title: Developmental care of newborns and infants : a guide for health
professionals / [edited by] Carole Kenner, Jacqueline M. McGrath.
Other titles: Developmental care of newborns & infants.
Description: Third edition. | Philadelphia : Wolters Kluwer, [2023] |
"National Association of Neonatal Nurses." | Includes bibliographical
references and index.
Identifiers: LCCN 2021048396 (print) | LCCN 2021048397 (ebook) | ISBN
9781975148393 (paperback) | ISBN 9781975148416 (epub) | ISBN
9781975148423 (epub)
Subjects: MESH: Intensive Care, Neonatal–methods | Infant, Newborn–growth
& development | Neonatal Nursing–methods | Family | Intensive Care
Units, Neonatal
Classification: LCC RJ254 (print) | LCC RJ254 (ebook) | NLM WS 421 | DDC
618.92/01–dc23/eng/20211005
LC record available at https://lccn.loc.gov/2021048396
LC ebook record available at https://lccn.loc.gov/2021048397

LWW.com

QUADM0722

Contributors

Heidelise Als, PhD

Professor of Psychology in the Department of Psychiatry
Harvard Medical School
Director, Neurobehavioral Infant and Child Studies
Boston Children's Hospital
Boston, Massachusetts

Leslie B. Altimier, RNC, DNP, MSN, BSN, NE-BC

Director of Clinical Innovation & Research
Institution Philips Healthcare
Cambridge, Massachusetts

Susan Tucker Blackburn, PhD, RN, FAAN

Professor Emerita
School of Nursing
University of Washington
Seattle, Washington

Marina Boykova, PhD, RN

Associate Professor
School of Nursing & Allied Health Professions
Holy Family University
Philadelphia, Pennsylvania

Maryann Bozzette, PhD, RN, CLC

Associate Professor
School of Nursing
Barnes Jewish College
St. Louis, Missouri

Joy V. Browne, PhD, PCNS, IMH-E (IV)

Clinical Professor of Pediatrics and Psychiatry
University of Colorado Anschutz Medical Campus
Aurora, Colorado

Nicole Cistone, MSN, RN, RNC-NIC

Pre-Doctoral Fellow
College of Nursing
The Ohio State University
Columbus, Ohio

Robin Clifton-Koeppel, DNP, RNC-NIC, CPNP, CNS

Neonatal Clinical Nurse Specialist
University of California
Irvine Medical Center
Orange, California

Mary Coughlin, MS, NNP, RNC-E

President and Founder Caring Essentials Collaborative, LLC.
Boston, Massachusetts

Ashley Darcy-Mahoney, PhD, NNP-BC, FAAN

Associate Professor & Neonatal Nurse Practitioner
The George Washington University School of Nursing
Director of Infant Research, Autism and Neurodevelopmental
    Disorder Institute
Washington, District of Columbia

Tara DeWolfe, PT, DPR, CNT, CLC

Certified Trauma Informed Professional
Certified to Reliability in NIDCAP
Faculty, Caring Essentials Collaborative Quantum Caring Institute
Pediatric Physical Therapist and Developmental Specialist, Way to
    Grow Pediatric
Therapy Peoria, Illinois

Kristy Fuller, OTR/L, CNT

Certified Trauma Informed Professional
Certified to Reliability in NIDCAP
Faculty, Caring Essentials Collaborative Quantum Caring Institute
President, Infant Feeding Strategies, LLC
Bettendorf, Iowa

Teresa Gutierrez, PT, MS, PCS, C/NDTA

Rocky Mountain University of Health Professions
Provo, Utah

Brenna Hogan, BSN, RN

Nursing Student, Marquette University, College of Nursing
Milwaukee, Wisconsin

Carol B. Jaeger, DNP, RN, NNP-BC

Adjunct Faculty, Advanced Practice Nursing Programs
The Ohio State University College of Nursing
Columbus, Ohio

Carole Kenner, PhD, RN, FAAN, FNAP, ANEF

Carol Kuser Loser Dean & Professor
The College of New Jersey
Ewing, New Jersey
Chief Executive Officer
Council of International Neonatal Nurses, Inc. (COINN)
Yardley, Pennsylvania

Kathleen S. S. Kolberg, PhD

Assistant Dean
College of Science
University of Notre Dame
Notre Dame, Indiana

Jan McElroy, PhD, PT, PCS

School of Health Professions
Physical Therapy Department
Columbia, Missouri

Kelly Sharmane McGlothen-Bell, PhD, RN, IBCLC

Assistant Professor
School of Nursing, Office for Faculty Excellence
University of Texas Health Science Center San Antonio
San Antonio, Texas

Jacqueline M. McGrath, PhD, RN, FNAP, FAAN

Thelma and Joe Crow Endowed Professor
Vice Dean for Faculty Excellence
School of Nursing
University of Texas Health Science Center San Antonio
San Antonio, Texas

Barbara Medoff-Cooper, PhD, RN, FAAN

Professor Emerita
University of Pennsylvania School of Nursing
Nurse Scientist
The Children's Hospital of Philadelphia
Philadelphia, Pennsylvania

Susan Orlando, DNS, APRN, NNP-BC, CNS

Associate Clinical Professor
Program Director, Neonatal Nurse Practitioner Program
Louisiana State University Health Sciences Center School of Nursing
New Orleans, Louisiana

Raylene M. Phillips, MD, FAAP, FABM, IBCLC

Medical Director, Neonatal Services
Pediatric, Department Chair
Loma Linda University Medical Center-Murrieta
Associate Professor, Pediatrics/Neonatology
Director, Breastfeeding/Lactation
Director, Neonatal Neurodevelopment
Loma Linda University School of Medicine
Loma Linda University Children's Hospital
Loma Linda, California

Rita H. Pickler, PhD, RN, FAAN

The FloAnn Sours Easton Professor of Child and Adolescent Health
Director, PhD & MS in Nursing Science Programs
Martha S. Pitzewr Center for Women, Children & Youth
The Ohio State University College of Nursing
Columbus, Ohio

Roberta Pineda, PhD, OTR/L, CNT

Assistant Professor
Chan Division of Occupational Science and Occupational Therapy
University of Southern California
Los Angeles, California

Jana Pressler, PhD, RN

Professor Emeritus
University of Nebraska Medical Center
College of Nursing
Lincoln, Nebraska

Barbara A. Reyna, PhD, RN, NNP-BC

Associate Professor, NNP Program Coordinator
University of Virginia
Charlottesville, Virginia
Neonatal Nurse Practitioner, VCU Health System
Richmond, Virginia

Christina Rigby-McCotter, BS, MS

Research Assistant, Children's Wisconsin, Department of Nursing Research
Milwaukee, Wisconsin

Amy L. Salisbury, PhD, RN, PMH-CNS, BC

Associate Dean for Research, Scholarship & Innovation
Professor
Virginia Commonwealth University
School of Nursing
Richmond, Virginia

Joan R. Smith, PhD, RN, NNP-BC, FAAN

Director of Quality, Safety & Practice Excellence
St. Louis Children's Hospital
St. Louis, Missouri

Tanya Sudia, PhD, RN, FAAN

Dean and Professor
College of Nursing
Augusta University
Augusta, Georgia

Jane K. Sweeney, PhD, PT, MS, PCS, FAPTA

Professor and Program Director
Pediatric Science Doctoral Programs
Rocky Mountain University of Health Professions
Provo, Utah

Annalyn Velasquez, MSN, NNP-BC, CPNP-PC

PhD Student
The George Washington University School of Nursing
Neonatal Nurse Practitioner
MEDNAX
Washington, District of Columbia

Dorothy Vittner, PhD, RN, CHPE, FAAN

Assistant Professor of Nursing
Marion Packham Egan School of Nursing & Health Studies
Fairfield University
Fairfield, Connecticut

Robert D. White, MD

Director, Regional Newborn Program
Beacon Children's Hospital
South Bend, Indiana

Rosemary White-Traut, PhD, RN, FAAN

Director, Nursing Research and Evidence Based Practice
Children's Wisconsin, Milwaukee, Wisconsin
Professor Emerita, University of Illinois at Chicago
Chicago, Illinois

Previous Edition Contributors

Heidelise Als, PhD

Diane D. Ballweg, MSN, RN, CNS

Susan Blackburn, PhD, RN, FAAN

Marina Boykova, MSc, RN

Maryann Bozzette, PhD, RN

Sharon Cone, PhD(c), NNP-BC

Mary Coughlin, MS, BSN, APN, CCRN

Ashley Darcy, MSN, RN, NNP-BC

Deborah Winders Davis, DNS

Juliette Dols, MS, RN

Gay Gale, MS, RNC-NIC

Sharyn Gibbins, PhD, RN

Teresa Gutierrez, MS, PT, PCS, C/NDT

Whitney Hardy, BSN, BS, RN

Mary Claire Heffron, PhD

Carole Helseth, BSN, RNC

Steven B. Hoath, MD

Jan Hunter, MA, OTR

Katherine M. Jorgensen, MBA, MSN, RNC, HonD

Carole Kenner, PhD, RNC-NIC, FAAN

Cheryl Ann King, MSN, CCRN

Jesse Kurtz, EdS

gretchen Lawhon, PhD, RN

Terrie Lockridge, MSN, RNC-NIC

Susan Ludington-Hoe, PhD, CNM, RN, FAAN

Jacqueline M. McGrath, PhD, RN, FNAP, FAAN

Barbara Medoff-Cooper, PhD, RN, PNP-BC, FAAN

Cheryl Milford, EdS

Ann E. Nepstad, MSN, RN-NIC

Susan Orlando, DNS, APRN, NNP-BC

Rita H. Pickler, PhD, RN, PNP

Ann Podruchny, MN, RNC-NIC

Jana Pressler, PhD, RN

Linda Rector, MS, CCLS

Barbara A. Reyna, MS, RN, NNP-BC

Dennis C. Stevens, MS, MD

Tanya Sudia-Robinson, PhD, RN

Jane K. Sweeney, PhD, PT

Lauren Thorngate, MS, RN, CCRN

Carol Spruill Turnage-Carrier, MSN, RN, CNS

Kathleen VandenBerg, PhD

Marlene Walden, PhD, APRN, NNP-BC, CCNS

Robert White, MD

Rosemary C. White-Traut, PhD, RN, FAAN

Barbara J. Zapalo, EdD

Foreword

Of all the remarkable advances in neonatal care over recent decades, perhaps the greatest has been our understanding of brain development in the preterm infant and the impact of the neonatal intensive care unit (NICU) environment on that development. We now know that negative environmental stimuli and policies that exclude families from care have lasting effects on developmental outcomes and parental attachment. However, we also know that care practices can be modified in such a way as to mitigate the adverse effects of the NICU environment and optimize brain development. Because of this, it is imperative that NICUs implement developmental care policies and protocols and integrate them into all aspects of care. Furthermore, we must begin to think beyond the walls of our NICUs and assure that developmental care practices continue after discharge. In many NICUs, this requires a shift in culture and a guidebook to assist with a transition to more comprehensive and developmentally appropriate care. *Developmental Care of Newborns and Infants*, third edition, is that guidebook. In this book, every aspect of newborn care is covered through a developmental care lens. Readers will learn new ways to touch, position, and feed babies. They will learn to provide care during painful procedures that minimizes a baby's response to that pain. And perhaps most importantly, they will better understand and value the integral role parents play in both recognizing the developmental needs of their baby and responding to those needs. This book is an essential resource for all nurseries. For those that have already developed a culture of development care, that culture will be strengthened. For those trying foster such a culture, there is no better place to start than with the information you will find here. But do not just read it and put in on a shelf. Read it, implement its contents, revisit it often, and build quality projects around it to assure you are creating lasting change in your nursery that will benefit every baby and every family you serve.

Robert C. Cicco, MD

Preface

Individualized family-centered developmental care (IFDC) is a framework for providing care that protects and enhances the neurodevelopment of the infant through interventions that support both the infant and the family. This foundation of caregiving requires collaboration among the healthcare team, and it views the family as an integral part of this team. Research has shown that developmental caregiving enhances the outcomes of high-risk infants—the small and sick newborns who require neonatal intensive care (NIC). Yet accurate and expedient implementation of evidence-based interventions has been difficult, given the existing intensive care environment and the medical priorities established by the needs of high-risk infants. Additionally, many existing "standard" procedures and caregiving practices as well as developmental interventions remain either untested or poorly tested within rigorous research designs and do not yet meet the test of being evidence based. These intervention strategies require continued study and cautious implementation. We made this statement in 2004 and certainly the evidence has grown, but there are still gaps and interventions that are now in practice are still not grounded in research findings.

To address the gaps in evidence to support IFDC, the National Association of Neonatal Nurses (NANN) initiated an interdisciplinary task force to develop a "*Core Curriculum*" that has evolved into NANN's *Developmental Care of Newborns and Infants* to serve as a cornerstone for education of and clinical practice by NICU professionals. This text, first published in 2004, the second in 2010, now in its third edition, provides evidence-based guidelines for the implementation of developmentally supportive care with infants and families served through the NICU and beyond. This text begins by reviewing the influence of prenatal and postnatal environments on development and stresses the need for an IFDC approach to care. Families are partners in this process, and this text represents an integrated, interdisciplinary approach.

The original NANN interdisciplinary task force developed the following philosophy statement:

> Developmental care is a philosophy that embraces the concepts of dynamic interaction between the infant, family, and surrounding environment. Developmentally supportive care provides a framework in which the environment of care and the process of delivering care are intentionally modified and structured to support the individualized needs of the developing newborn and family. This concept of care represents a continuum that begins antenatally, through the intrapartal period, at birth, throughout the hospitalization, discharge as the infant transitions home, and outcomes in infancy and later childhood. Links to care in the community are made prior to discharge.

What is developmental care? It is awareness—an intuitiveness to observe the infant and family and their interactions with the environment. It is a framework for providing care that protects and supports the neurobehavioral development of the infant. It involves a broad prevention orientation targeted to improve developmental processes and competence among infants at risk. It is a philosophy that is predicated on human needs and cues and not on administrative facility tasks and schedules. It is a willingness to look holistically at the infant, family, and environment and provide interdisciplinary care accordingly. It is not a type of intervention provided when an infant is stable; it is a method of care that promotes stability and reduces the prevalence of signs and symptoms of identifiable disorders by minimizing the ultimate impact upon normal functioning (how the care is provided). It is an approach to care that is, for the most part, infant driven. It requires collaboration among the healthcare team and views the family as an integral part of this team, inseparable from the needs of the infant. To accomplish this integration of care, all healthcare team members must be educated on the fundamental principles of developmental care.

Both the "macroenvironment" (the surrounding room lights and sounds, unit or home environment) and the "microenvironment" (the immediate infant, touch, positioning, sleep and arousal, feeding, pain and stress, skin-to-skin contact [SSC], as well as the family environment) are affected by alterations in either milieu. Most often these alterations within a developmental context are done to better match the environment surrounding the infant to the infant's maturation and/or the once-protective intrauterine environment in the extrauterine life. The process of care delivery is intentional and adjusted in response to communications from the infant, or behavioral cues. This care must be approached from a systems thinking perspective where all policies are developed and reviewed with infant- and family-centered developmental care (IFCDC) in mind. Procedural or medical care cannot be viewed as the priority with developmental care as secondary. For this caregiving to truly occur, developmental care becomes an aspect of how ALL care is delivered. The integration of developmental care with medical and nursing care must be truly interwoven and woven together to provide optimal care. The aim is to decrease associated stress and increase the potential of the available skills possessed by the infant as regulation and organization is attempted. Within the continuum, developmentally appropriate care also involves early screening to detect and abbreviate the course of action and extent of any behavioral disruptions before they develop into additional problems. This integration of caregiving depends on an interdisciplinary focus that is attuned to the unique characteristics of each infant and family.

Nurses; physicians; physical, occupational, and respiratory therapists; developmental specialists; infant mental health experts; and other ancillary personnel who touch or interact with the infant or family must be synchronized, familiar with, and practice the concepts of developmental care if it is to be interwoven into all practices in the neonatal care environment. Developmental care requires that each member of the health-care team, including the family, has a working knowledge of what developmental care is, how to "read" the behavioral cues, and what these significant cues have on an infant's growth and development. Families are an integral part of the team because family-centered care concepts support partnerships between the family and healthcare providers that facilitate the parental role as primary care provider. Infants and families must be viewed as inseparable, each affecting the other.

The clinical implications and future goals of the work represented in this text include holistic yet standardized implementation of evidence-based interventions with infants and families who are served by those in the NICU and support for further testing through clinical research of these interventions. It cannot be overstated that developmental caregiving is evolving; consequently, gaps as well as evidence to support this care must be acknowledged and changes in suggested practice will be expected to continue. To build on this process, NICU staff orientation and basic and advanced professional education programs must incorporate IFCDC into the routine curricula. NANN has implemented an examination leading the Neonatal Developmental Care Specialist designation to demonstrate competency in developmental care—that is how much the science has evolved since this text's first edition. Developmental care is an essential content for all neonatal care providers and it must be viewed as such to move developmental care to the next level of full implementation in the NICU and beyond. While in the NICU, the routine, standardized schedule of assessments, procedures, and tests often seemingly appear at odds with IFCDC. Yet, IFCDC interventions must be integrated into the NICU routine. This integration represents a blending of complementary agendas—the synchrony of caregivers with infants. They are the fluid performance of medical and nursing tasks. They are the gentle and calming baths to be given; the balancing of feeding with comforting; and the matching of awake periods to family times and kangaroo mother care (KMC) or SSC. For families and healthcare professionals, they are the moments to be treasured; the lesson to be learned; and the joys to be shared. These moments give meaning to our work and they are long lasting, going far beyond the walls of the NICU.

The basis of developmental care is the acknowledgment of the individual needs of the infant and family, but this cannot be done without standardized and essentially sound education and support of NICU professionals and families. As evidence grows, the importance of the infant as a competent interactor has shifted the framework to one that places the infant at the forefront. The framework now is referred to as IFCDC as developed by the Consensus Panel for Infant- and Family-Centered Developmental Care as described by Jaeger and in Chapter 1. The standards identified in this model are highlighted throughout the text. Several chapters represent the cornerstones of this model. They include sleep arousal, pain and stress, positioning, and touch.

This edition represents a thorough updating of each chapter. Quality indicators along with a description of a trauma-informed approach illustrates the recognition that an NICU stay results in "trauma" and stress for the infant, family, and professional staff. Use of the single-room NICU design has been updated to reflect the implementation on infants and families. The chapter "Beyond the NICU" illustrates that survival is improving, but thriving after discharge must be supported. Communication with families is a critical component of all this work, and at this time in our history, we recognize that health disparities and challenges exist for our families of color and that we must acknowledge structural racism and unconscious bias. As Brandon and McGrath (2021) suggest, we must "be an advocate for racial awareness and quality in your hospital and community" (p. 1).

The levels of evidence presented use the Melnyk and Fineout-Overholt model that identifies seven levels of evidence:

Level I: Evidence from a systematic review or meta-analysis of all relevant randomized controlled studies (RCTs), or evidence-based clinical practice guidelines, based on systematic reviews of RCTs.

Level II: Evidence obtained from at least one well-designed RCT.

Level III: Evidence obtained from well-designed controlled trials without randomization.

Level IV: Evidence from well-designed case-control and cohort studies.

Level V: Evidence from systematic reviews of descriptive and qualitative studies.

Level VI: Evidence from a single descriptive or qualitative study.

Level VII: Evidence from the opinion of authorities and/or reports of expert committees.

Used with permission from *Evidence-based practice in nursing & healthcare: A guide to best practice* (p. 10) by B. M. Melnyk & E. Fineout-Overholt, 2005.

The intended audience is the interdisciplinary team that takes care of the small and sick newborn in the NICU and beyond. It would be useful for students in the health professions and for families who have had an infant in the NICU.

Carole Kenner, PhD, RN, FAAN, FNAP, ANEF
Jaqueline M. McGrath, PhD, RN, FNAP, FAAN

REFERENCE

Brandon, D., & McGrath, J. M. (2021). Speaking up to address racism and health inequity. *Advances in Neonatal Care, 21*(4), 1–2

Acknowledgments

This project has had the support from many developmental care experts and families since its first edition in 2004. First, we would like to thank the National Association of Neonatal Nurses (NANN) for its foresight to bring together a team of interdisciplinary representatives to write this "core" individualized family-centered developmental care (IFDC) text. NANN entrusted us with this most-needed project, and we are grateful for having been a part of the process that will continue to make the concepts of IFDC growth in the NICU environment domestically and globally. We wish to thank Dr. Stanley Graven who gave the interdisciplinary team space to meet at the annual Gravens Conference on the Physical and Developmental Environment of the High-Risk Infant and guidance on how to bring an interdisciplinary focus to this text. Thank you too to the Wolters Kluwer team who assisted with the publication for this edition.

Carole Kenner, PhD, RN, FAAN, FNAP, ANEF
Jaqueline M. McGrath, PhD, RN, FNAP, FAAN

Contents

5   The Neonatal Intensive Care Unit Environment 85

Maryann Bozzette, Carole Kenner, Marina Boykova, Leslie B. Altimier, and Raylene M. Phillips

6   Single-Family Room Design in the Neonatal Intensive Care Unit 94

Leslie B. Altimier and Robert D. White

7   Infant Mental Health: Strategies for Optimal Social–Emotional Care of Infants and Families in the NICU 111

Jacqueline M. McGrath and Dorothy Vittner

13 Infant Sleep and Arousal. 213

Amy L. Salisbury and Kathleen S. S. Kolberg

14 Collaborative Therapeutic Positioning: Multisystem and Behavioral Implications. 231

Jane K. Sweeney and Jan McElroy

15 Oral Feeding and the High-Risk Infant 252

Jacqueline M. McGrath, Barbara Medoff-Cooper, Ashley Darcy-Mahoney, Kelly Sharmane McGlothen-Bell, and Annalyn Velasquez

16 Skin-to-Skin Contact Optimizes Outcomes for Infants and Families . . .284

Dorothy Vittner and Jacqueline M. McGrath

22 Developmental Care: Where Do We Go From Here? 365

Carole Kenner and Jacqueline M. McGrath

The Science

Carol B. Jaeger and Joy V. Browne

INTRODUCTION

Developmental care of newborns and infants has become a generic term. The term/concept is used in a multitude of ways, including but not limited to biophysiologic growth and development (Als, 2009; Als, et al., 2004); elements of care that promote neurologic and cognitive maturation (Als, et al., 2003, 2004; Liu, et al., 2007; Lubbe, 2012; Pineda, et al., 2014; Smith, et al., 2011; Vohr, 2014); use of devices and methods that support age-appropriate physiologic alignment (Monterosso, et al., 2003; Picheansathian, et al., 2009); environmental adjustments that promote neuroprotection and neurodevelopment (Almadhoob & Ohlsson, 2015; Lester, et al., 2014, 2016; Morag & Ohlsson, 2016; Pickler, et al., 2010; Ramm, et al., 2017; Roue, et al., 2017; White, 2020b); and provision of psychosocial support to strengthen nurturing and social engagement (Browne & Talmi, 2005; Lee, 2003; Pineda, et al., 2018; Ravn, et al., 2011; Roudebush, et al., 2006; Spence, 2016). Ongoing infant development is a complex integrative process supportive of the baby's biophysical, psychosocial, and emotional systems (Douglas, et al., 2011; Wilson, et al., 2001). Although affecting multiple systems and outcomes, developmental care interventions are often viewed as additive, providing comfort measures, rather than considered foundational to care provision, which integrates this caregiving framework into every aspect of practice.

The infant's primary developmental need is for biophysiologic regulation, essential to the baby's medical outcome as well as an attachment relationship with the parent(s)/family (Westrup, 2007). Nurturing and physical care provided by the parents is essential to all areas of development through the regulatory processes that they provide the baby (Feldman, 2007; Welch, et al., 2012). No parent chooses to relinquish nurturing and regulation of their baby to the healthcare system, yet circumstances of medical necessity often intervene. Parents want information and clear communication provided in a way that supports their integration into their baby's caregiving (Govindaswamy, et al., 2018; Guillaume, et al., 2013). They expect to be an essential member of the team, make decisions with the professionals, and share the accountability of disappointments and celebrations of outcomes (Bailey, et al., 2013; Cleveland, 2008; Johnson, 2016; Shaw, et al., 2016). Families do this best by knowing and trusting the professionals, learning with them, as well as observing and assessing their baby together (Ahlqvist-Bjorkroth, 2018; Johnson, et al., 2009).

Many developmental programs and resources promote theories, concepts, and practices of developmental care. Some are based on physiologic or psychosocial approaches that have strong quality of evidence; others are conceptual or procedural practices based on limited and/or weak evidence. The resulting scope of the terminology and meaning of developmental care and developmental care practice is not standardized and, in the essence of developmental care, individualized to the needs of the baby. Furthermore, the lack of science specificity has previously been considered an elusive element, a "fluff" addition, to our practice of neonatal care (Browne, et al., 2020).

HISTORY OF FAMILY-CENTERED CARE

Family-centered care (FCC) is a vital component of developmental care. FCC stresses the inclusivity of parents and family with the interprofessional team to collaborate and manage the individualized care of the baby and family consistent with evidence-based organizational policies (Johnson, 2000). The NICU views FCC as essential to meet the complex medical needs of sick infants and psychosocial dynamics of parents and family members (Johnson, et al., 2009). Cultural, social, and economic factors also influence the health environment of infants and families (Campinha-Bacote, 2011; Sigurdson, et al., 2019; Stevens, et al., 2010; Vance, et al., 2018).

FCC was a product of societal change in the 1960s—a time at which consumers (and women in particular) began to demand more control and involvement in their own healthcare (Galvin, et al., 2000). The advancement of person-centered care makes the patient the source of healthcare control. This is supported by the Institute of Medicine (IOM, 2001), professionals and professional organizations (Berwick, 2009; McCance, et al., 2011), and position statements advocating person-centered and FCC from the American Academy of Pediatrics (AAP, 2012) and the Institute for Patient and Family-Centered Care (IPFCC). The IOM's 2001 book, *Crossing the Quality Chasm: A New Health System for the 21st Century*, delineates six healthcare system improvement goals: safety, effectiveness, person-centeredness, timeliness, efficiency, and equity (IOM, 2001). Person-centeredness combined with FCC became a central tenet of health professional statements developed in partnership with families (McGrath, et al., 2011). The aim of equity in eliminating health disparities is closely related to the issue of person-centeredness/FCC, but more specifically addresses health disparities and cultural competency (Boghossian, et al., 2019; IOM, 2007; Orelus, 2012; Stevens, et al., 2010).

Advances in technology have increased the number of lives saved, but newborn infants may sustain biophysical and/or neurodevelopmental challenges. Over time, the parents of children with developmental and special healthcare needs have taken a more active role in their children's healthcare and in advocating individually, collectively, through legislative policy (Berman, et al., 2019; Bourque, et al., 2018; Loversidge & Zurmehly, 2019; Preyde & Ardal, 2003; Provenzi & Santoro, 2015; World Health Organization [WHO], 2015). The need to involve families in caregiving and decision-making has involved state and national policymakers (Johnson, et al., 2008). Critical components of this initiative include the medical home, uniform healthcare insurance coverage for all children, early and regular developmental screening, organization of healthcare services to identify needs, paid family leave to support parental engagement as primary caregivers for their child, and the provision of services for making the transition to adult healthcare services (Carver & Jessie, 2011; Jefferies, 2014; Murphy & Carbone, 2011; Nandi, et al., 2018; Petty, et al., 2018; Purdy, et al., 2015; Weber, et al., 2018). Cultural sensitivity and the involvement of cultural/religious leaders meaningful to the family also are of paramount importance in this program (Beck, et al., 2020; Brooks, et al., 2013; Huenink, 2017; Padula, et al., 2021; Stevens, et al., 2010; Thoma, et al., 2019).

EVOLUTION OF THE SCIENCE OF DEVELOPMENTAL CARE

The science of developmental care practice is young—approximately 40 years of evolutionary study since the first documentation of approaches that specifically address developmental care of the high-risk infant and family. Early systematic observational studies were initiated by Gesell and Amatruda (1945) when they observed preterm infant states and changes in states in response to environmental stimulation. Early on, considerations for protection of vulnerable preterm infants resulted in the development of separate intensive care units that provided protection from overwhelming sensory and social experiences (Gluck, 1970, 1992; Gluck, et al., 1976; Vohr, 2019). Later, emphasis was put on supplementary stimulation studies (Barnard & Bee, 1983; Chaze & Ludington-Hoe, 1984; Korner, et al., 1983; Scar-Salapatek & Williams, 1973; Thoman, et al., 1991; White & Labarba, 1976) to determine if the enrichment of babies' caregiving environments could lead to better outcomes. As

readily available physiologic monitoring became available, studies documented the impact of environmental stimulation on the infant's physiologic organization (Gottfried & Gaiter, 1985; Long, Lucey, et al., 1980; Long, Philip, et al., 1980). Graven and colleagues (Graven, 1997; Graven, et al., 1992a, 1992b) began gathering and promoting studies of the impact of the proximal and distal environment on infant outcomes and recognized the contributions of basic science findings that parallel animal and human research (Browne & White, 2011a, 2011b). In more recent years studies of a myriad of programs have studied environmental and caregiving interventions in intensive care, e.g., massage and music therapy (Bieleninik, et al., 2016; Juneau, et al., 2015; Picciolini, et al., 2014; Pineda, et al., 2017; Trivedi, 2015) with limited consensus regarding the impact on neurobehavioral developmental outcomes. Individualized, behavioral communication–based caregiver interventions have shown short- and long-term positive physiologic and developmental outcomes for infants in intensive care (Als, et al., 1996, 2004, 2011, 2012; McAnulty, et al., 2010, 2012; Mewes, et al., 2006). Parent education and support programs (Cheng, et al., 2019; Melnyk, et al., 2006; Mianaei, et al., 2014; O'Brien, et al., 2018; Toivonen, et al., 2020) and those that emphasize the parent–infant emotional connection show promise for enhancing both baby and parent outcomes (Porges, et al., 2019; Welch, et al., 2020). The goals of all programs have the objective of enhancing infant medical and developmental outcomes, parental coping/mental health, and optimizing the family's ability to support their baby.

Research design for developmental care practices is challenging in a medical field that is constantly changing with technology, pharmacology, and care practices emerging on a regular basis. Furthermore, the population of surviving babies is shifting to more of an understanding of a fetal-oriented approach. With the medical complexity and the importance of life-saving interventions, those that rely on survival and proven medical outcomes commonly take precedence even when one does not need to choose one to sacrifice the other. Often parents do not wish to engage in research of any kind as they will not choose to risk experimentation on their baby, even if the approaches appear benign or protective (Weiss, et al., 2021).

The research in developmental care has often been less rigorous in quality because the components of the research are often multimodal so that it is difficult to determine exactly which strategies or interventions are effective or deleterious. In addition, studies that focus on unimodal approaches do not address the complexity of development and/or developmental care practices, for the very immature baby. Randomized controlled trials are often retrospective, as opposed to experimental or quasi-experiment designed trials; longitudinal studies are limited so that long-term outcomes are not apparent; and appropriate evaluation measures and assessments do not capture the complexity of potential outcomes. Due to the complexity of implementing broad-based and continually enhanced approaches into intensive care units, integration of evidence-based developmental and family-centered care must be thoughtfully and systematically conceptualized and implemented. It is a well-planned journey rather than a quickly implemented "short trip," with consideration for all the detours, roadblocks, and missed turns that inevitably occur.

Previous editions of this book have articulated the scope of the science current to each printing, having been 10 years since the last printing. This edition describes the evolution of science since the previous edition as a base for standardizing practice, professional competence, and best practices integral to the baby's holistic system. Emerging brain and behavior science emphasize the need for neuroprotective and nurturing environments in intensive care, as well as support for the transition to home and continuing care. The understanding that families are central to their baby's well-being is a primary and integral approach in intensive care, which emphasizes the need for a shift in perspectives to dyadic interventions and practices.

SHARING THE JOURNEY: ADMINISTRATION, PROFESSIONAL STAFF, AND FAMILIES ON THE ROAD TOGETHER

How different it would be if intensive care vision, mission, policies and procedures, professional job descriptions, staff competence evaluations, collaborative team education, and simulation reflected the following values:

- Integration of the baby's unique behavioral communication and interaction in provision of care (Filippa, et al., 2017)
- Shared decision-making with the parent(s) (Craig, et al., 2015)
- A sense of cultural humility (Brooks, et al., 2013; Campinha-Bacote, 2011; Lake, et al., 2018)
- Changing the control of system management of the care of the baby through health professional dominance to a shared model of education/decision-making and caregiving with the baby and their families, necessary to impact quality of care through the baby's and family's lifespan (Johnson, 2016; Umberger, et al., 2018)
- Attention to the importance of nurturing relationships at all levels of care: leadership, professionals, families, and babies (Browne, 2021; Evans & Porter, 2009; Feldman, 2007, 2009; Feldman & Eidelman, 2007; Montirosso & McGlone, 2020; Neu, et al., 2014; Provenzi, et al., 2019)

GAPS IN PRACTICE

As noted previously, developmental care is typically not well defined and administered, and often seen as additional to care practices representing significant gaps in best practice. These gaps interfere with true integration of developmental care measures with procedural care and can affect short-term and long-term biophysical and psychosocial outcomes. Several of these gaps include:

- Provision of medical and surgical intensive care is often separate from integrated developmental care practices, both conceptually and practically (Smith, et al., 2011).
- Interprofessional healthcare roles are siloed by discipline (Melnyk, 2018).
- There is a lack of integration and collaboration among professionals in planning, executing, and evaluating care to the baby (Reeves, et al., 2017).
- The baby is not viewed or valued as a primary communicator and interactor in their own care (Als, 1982, 1986, 2009; Westrup, 2015).
- Parents and baby are not considered the focus of care practices with attention to the importance of the attachment relationship and mental health outcomes (Als, 1982, 1986, 2009; Westrup, 2015).
- Parents and family feel like visitors and are often referred to as visitors, within the in-patient culture and environment of the hospital professional milieu (Berwick, 2009; Cleveland, 2008; Tallon, et al., 2015; Thiele, et al., 2016; Wigert, et al., 2013).
- Parents are separated from their baby and feel fractured from their own family support, social connections, traditions, and intimacy of their home environment (Boykova, 2016a, 2016b; Choi, et al., 2020; Stuebe, 2020; Vetulani, 2013).
- Parents are confused, emotional, fearful, hurting, uninformed, lost, and floundering in a complex, unfamiliar maze of buildings, hallways, rooms, equipment, supplies, noise, lights, and people asking a multitude of questions (Gallagher, et al., 2018; Johnson & Abraham, 2020).
- Parents often are not adequately prepared to care for a growing but medically challenged baby in their transition home and after discharge due to the lack of referral to appropriate community supports (Boykova, 2016a, 2016b; Murphy & Carbone, 2011; Petty, et al., 2018; Purdy, et al., 2015).

Identified gaps are often not addressed and evidence to manage these gaps has not been systematically examined. Recent efforts have recognized and confronted many of these concerns and are identified in the following section.

SEARCH FOR EVIDENCE TO ADDRESS CURRENT GAPS

A consensus panel of international interprofessional experts and parents representing multiple professional organizations formed—to study the concept, practice, and outcome of developmental care in hospital units that provide intensive care to newborns and young babies and their families. The goal of the Consensus Panel for Infant and Family-Centered Developmental Care (IFCDC) was to organize, prioritize, and standardize evidence-based developmental practice. Standards, performance competencies, and best practices were developed by committee content experts and a consensus of the committee members endorsed the recommendations and recommended changes for inclusion in the document. See the Appendix for the process used by the panel to search and evaluate evidence for the IFCDC standards, competencies, and best practices.

INFANT AND FAMILY-CENTERED DEVELOPMENTAL CARE CONSIDERATIONS ADDRESSED BY THE PANEL

To address the previously identified issues and considerations of current developmental care practices, a common definition that includes the baby's and the family's experience in intensive care was proposed, and foundational evidence-based principles articulated. Infant and family-centered developmental care (IFCDC) is defined as a process of blending the natural unified growth of biologic and cognitive system organization and regulation of an infant with the continuous coordinated support of parent(s), family, and interprofessional health team. Several foundational principles describe the cornerstones of the process and are demonstrated in the conceptual model.

CONCEPT PRINCIPLES

The principles of IFCDC include individualized care, family involvement in all aspects of care, the baby as a competent interactor, environmental protection, neuroprotection of the developing brain, and infant mental health. Systems thinking in complex adaptive systems, as the overarching principle, is described first and foremost, because without integration of developmental care practices into system policies, procedures, and culture, successful implementation of developmental care will not be achieved.

The description of each principle is listed as follows:

Systems thinking within a complex adaptive system describes the integration of the principles of IFCDC that are strongly influenced by the process of systems thinking within a complex, dynamic, and continually evolving system. Systems thinking examines the components of a system—human or organization—from a holistic perspective considering each system component as interrelated, capable of influencing, and being influenced by each other (Douglas, et al., 2011; Plsek & Greenhalgh, 2001; Wilson, et al., 2001). Systems thinking is essential in the integration of all other components of the model and should be considered as the initial consideration in implementing IFCDC.

Baby as a competent interactor describes the importance of recognizing each baby's strengths and vulnerabilities by the behavior(s) facial expression(s) and physiologic changes they communicate that indicate distress, pain, comfort, and/or the need for interaction. Excellence in developmental caregiving can be characterized as modifying caregiving approaches according to the babies' communication style, medical history, and current medical status. Encouraging the baby's family to engage in nurturing interactions with their baby is essential in their understanding and optimization of the baby's performance as a competent interactor (Gonya, et al., 2018; Kolstad, 2013; Lavelli, et al., 2019; Levin, 1999; Westrup, 2007).

Individualized care focuses on the individual strengths, needs, and availability of each baby and family. For the baby, it is based on the identified behavioral communication, typically defined as approach and avoidance behavior, in the context of interactions perceived to be stressful or comforting. For the family, it is based on the voiced and inferred responses to physical or emotionally interpreted stressful events either for themselves or for their baby (Als, 1982, 2009; Browne & White, 2011a, 2011b; McCance, et al., 2011; Westrup, 2007).

Family integration identifies the essential nature of the family within the interprofessional team to provide developmental support of the baby (Thiele, et al., 2016; Trajkovski, et al., 2015; Van Riper, 2001). Family integration is assured through intensive care management regardless of social determinants that may influence perceptions of the family related to their caregiving approaches (Beck, et al., 2020; Boghossian, et al., 2019; DeSisto, et al., 2018; Epstein, et al., 2009; Hall, et al., 2020; Horbar, et al., 2019; Howell, et al., 2019; Louis-Jacques, et al., 2017; Padula, et al., 2021; Sigurdson, et al., 2019; Thoma, et al., 2019; Tucker, et al., 2003; Vance, et al., 2018). Compelling evidence of the physiologic, nutritional, and emotional regulation that is provided by the m/other[*] contributes to the baby's stability and makes a strong case for caring for the baby and m/other simultaneously (Craig, et al., 2015; Feldman & Eidelman, 2007; Hynan, et al., 2015; Thoyre, et al., 2013). Similarly, it is essential that the m/other's partner/significant other and close family members be available to support the m/other physically and emotionally throughout the ICU stay (Als, 2009; Hagen, et al., 2016; Hall, et al., 2016; Hynan, 2005).

Environmental protection relates to the field of applied neuroscience and provides evidence of distal (the physical, e.g., sound, light, and activity) and proximal (the bedding and caregiving) sensory environments that available data indicate can impact the baby's development. All procedures and caregiving should be conducted with attention to promotion of an environment that diminishes adverse responses from the infant and increases the opportunity for intimate interactions with their family

---

[*]M/other = describes the dyad and signifies the baby as an active interactor in the nurturing relationship with the mother (biologic or other), and with the interactive and integrated influence of the father/partner/significant other. Family members reinforce and enhance the supportive relationship.

(Bronfenbrenner, 1986; Bronfenbrenner & Ceci, 1994; Consensus Committee on Infant and Family Centered Developmental Care, 2020; Lester, et al., 2014, 2016; White, 2020a).

Neuroprotection of the developing brain stresses that optimal brain and body development should be an ultimate objective of every baby's plan of care. The baby's brain develops faster and is more vulnerable during the time around birth (regardless of the gestational age of the baby) than at any time in the baby's life. The baby's brain is also vulnerable to environmental input including stressful and painful procedures. Attention to neuroprotection by provision of individualized, sensitive caregiving, primarily through the m/other's regulatory influence of holding, feeding, and interacting is essential for optimal brain development (Gorzilio, et al., 2015; Graven & Browne, 2008; Lockridge, 2018; Porges, et al., 2019; Soleimani, et al., 2020).

Infant mental health offers intervention strategies that not only provide infant and family-driven individualized care and developmentally appropriate regulation of biophysiology, arousal and sleep, body movement, eating, and soothing, but also focus on enhancing the relationship between babies and their parents and primary caregivers. Essential to practice with babies and families is a reflective stance and a commitment to engage in ongoing reflective consultation and/or supervision to promote best practices and optimal mental health for families and professionals alike (Browne, 2021; Choi, et al., 2020; D'Agata, et al., 2016; Evans & Porter, 2009; Ishizaki, 2013).

In implementing IFCDC, babies, parents, and the family should be considered as partners in collaborative practice with professionals. This partnership will influence care and well-being through the active exchange of perspective, information, observation, and expectation of optimal outcomes.

CONCEPTUAL MODEL

The conceptual model of IFCDC is illustrated as a circle to show systems thinking as a dynamic process that integrates the principles underpinning the management and support of the baby. The m/other is the primary nurturer. M/other is the term used to describe the dyad and signifies the baby as an active interactor in the nurturing relationship with the mother (biologic or other), and with the interactive and integrated influence of the father/partner/significant other. Family members reinforce and enhance the supportive relationship (Fig. 1-1).

Sections of IFCDC Practice

Six sections of IFCDC practice were considered to exemplify the principles of the model and were strongly supported by evidence (Altimier & Phillips, 2013, 2016; Cardin, 2015; Coughlin, et al., 2009; Lopez-Maestro, et al., 2020; O'Brien, et al., 2018; Phillips, 2015; Roue, et al., 2017). They included:

- systems thinking in complex adaptive systems,
- positioning and touch for the newborn,
- sleep and arousal interventions for the newborn,
- skin-to-skin contact with intimate family members,
- reducing and managing pain and stress in newborns and families, and
- management of feeding, eating, and nutrition delivery.

Although other areas of clinical practice were identified, the levels of evidence were not considered to be strong enough to be included in the recommended standards, at this time. As evidence becomes available and components are included, additions to the current standards may be considered.

It is the recommendation of the consensus panel that the implementation of IFCDC practice include all sections that have evidence to make a positive difference in outcome for the baby, parents, and family. A recent study has indicated that practice settings are likely to prioritize implementation of one practice over another given the size of the unit, census, and resources (Lopez-Maestro, et al., 2020). Therefore, evaluation of implementation for effectiveness, satisfaction, and outcome should be considered to realize the value of the integrated practice sections of IFCDC.

Systems thinking is a separate but critical and overarching section that needs to be foremost in the implementation of any evidence-based developmental approach. Systems thinking is a series of linked processes of care essential interaction based on a vision, values, principles, communication, collaboration, education, and evaluation specific to IFCDC in intensive care. It is key to integrating the care practices of all the sections for the short-term and long-term benefit of the baby and the family in intensive care.

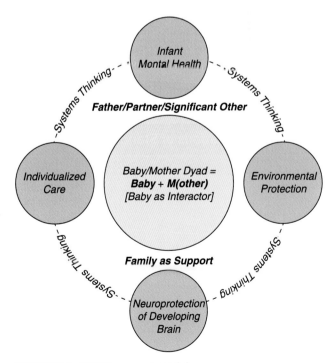

FIGURE 1-1. IFCDC concept model.

STANDARDS, COMPETENCIES, AND BEST PRACTICES

Using a systematic process, evidence-based practice guidelines should be standardized, disseminated, utilized, monitored, and compared in similar care settings to evaluate outcome, and to identify opportunities for continuing improvement with sustainable metrics. IFCDC implementation can be standardized through the application of standards, performance competencies, and best practices (Table 1-1).

The standards and competencies are written as objective measurable performance experiences to guide the standardization of IFCDC practice in the Intensive Care Unit (Committee) system by the interprofessional health team, parent(s), and family and that can guide evaluation of practice implementation.

The complete document, Report of the First Consensus Conference on Standards, Competencies, and Recommended Best Practices for Infant and Family Centered Developmental Care in the Intensive Care Unit, can be located on the University of Notre Dame world wide web at https://nicudesign.nd.edu/nicu-care-standards/ (Browne, et al., 2020; Consensus Committee on Infant and Family Centered Developmental Care, 2020). The IFCDC report is intentionally published with the Recommended Standards for Newborn ICU Design, ninth edition, on the website. The evidence to support environmental design in the intensive care unit is a part of the growing body of evidence that supports IFCDC practice. The environment, the practice, and the care providers/givers/family create a system to actively facilitate the continuing biophysical, psychosocial, cognitive maturation of the baby. The IFCDC standards are published in the subsequent chapter and highlighted through this edition with examples of implementation.

EVIDENCE-BASED PRACTICE MODELS

Since the IFCDC standards, competencies, and best practices serve as a framework with essential elements of care for sick and premature babies in the intensive care unit, other evidence-based neurodevelopmental and psychosocial program models may be implemented to augment infant and family-centered care practice. Many parent, professional, and interprofessional groups are establishing evidence-based neonatal practice guidelines or standards. Some are certification programs to standardize practice(s):

- NIDCAP Nursery Program, https://nidcap.org
- European Standards of Care for Newborn Health developed by the European Foundation for the Care of Newborn Infants (EFCNI, 2018; https://www.efcni.org/activities/projects-2/escnh/)
- Interdisciplinary Recommendations for the Psychosocial Support of NICU Parents, https://nature.com/articles/jp2015141
- Guidelines for Institutional Implementation of Developmental Care in the ICU—A Joint Positional Statement from CANN, CAPWHN, NANN, and COINN (Milette, et al., 2017a, 2017b)
- National Perinatal Association (NPA) Multidisciplinary Guidelines for the Care of Late Preterm Infants, https://www.nationalperinatal.org/Resources/Late, PretermGuidelinesNPA.pdf
- National Perinatal Association (NPA) Discharge Transition Planning (in development)
- Alliance for the Advancement of Infant Mental Health Competencies, https://www.allianceaimh.org/competency-guidelines
- Council of International Neonatal Nurses (COINN) International Neonatal Nursing Competency Framework (Jones & on behalf of the Council, 2019) (Table 1-2)

TABLE 1-1 Definitions of Standard and Competency

Component	Definition	Example
Standard	A safe evidence-based expectation, or measure, of best practice.	**Standard 4, Skin-to-Skin Contact (SSC):** Parents shall be provided information about the benefits of SSC that continue for babies and parents after discharge.
Competency	The action, or sequence of actions, that constitutes the performance of the standard.	**Competency 4.1:** Discharge planning with parents shall include information regarding the continued value of SSC, holding of babies, and encouragement for parents to continue SSC at home. **Competency 4.2:** Parents shall be supported in how to safely hold and carry their baby after discharge, including the use of a baby carrier if desired.

TABLE 1-2 Levels of Evidence (LOE)

Topic	Points	LOE	Evidence
Definition of developmental care (DC)	• Biophysiologic growth and development • Neurologic and cognitive maturation • Devices and methods of support • Environmental protection • Psychosocial support • Complex systems integration • Essential component of care	II II VI V IV IV V IV I I III III I VI III VI VII II VII VI II VII VII VI VII VI	Als et al., 2004; Als et al., 2003; Liu et al., 2007; Lubbe, 2012; Pineda et al., 2014; Smith et al., 2011; Vohr, 2014; Monterosso, Kristjanson, Cole, & Evans, 2003; Picheansathian, Woragidpoonpol, et al., 2009; Almadhoob & Ohlsson, 2015; Lester et al., 2014; Lester et al., 2016; Morag & Ohlsson, 2016; Pickler et al., 2010; Ramm, Mannix, Parry, & Gaffney, 2017; Roue et al., 2017; White, 2020b; Browne & Talmi, 2005; Lee, 2003; Pineda et al., 2018; Ravn et al., 2011; Roudebush, Kaufman, Johnson, et al., 2006; Spence, 2016; Douglas, Hill, & Brodribb, 2011; Wilson, Holt, & Greenhalgh, 2001; Browne, Jaeger, & Kenner, 2020
Regulation	• Attachment relationship • Nurturing and physical care	VI VI II	Björn Westrup, 2007; Feldman, 2007; Welch et al., 2012
Communication and shared decision-making	• Information and clear communication between parent and team • Parent(s) as essential member(s) of team • Trust	IV VI VI V VII VI VII VII	Govindaswamy et al., 2018; Guillaume et al., 2013; Bailey, Hendricks-Munoz, & Mally, 2013; Cleveland, 2008; Johnson, 2016; Shaw, Stokoe, Gallagher, et al., 2016; Ahlqvist-Bjorkroth, 2018; Johnson, Abraham, & Shelton, 2009
Family-centered care (FCC)	• Inclusion of parents and family • Individualized care • Essential to meet needs of baby • Integrate cultural, social, economic dynamics of family • Person-centered care • Quality of care includes safety, effectiveness, person-centeredness, timeliness, efficiency, equity	VII VII VI V VII VII VII VII V VII VII VII III VII VI	Johnson, 2000; Johnson et al., 2009; Campinha-Bacote, 2011; Sigurdson et al., 2019; Stevens, Helseth, & Kurtz, 2010; Vance, McGrath, & Brandon, 2018; Institute (IOM), 2001; Berwick, 2009; McCance, McCormack, & Dewing, 2011; American (AAP), 2012; IPFCC; McGrath, Samra, & Kenner, 2011; Boghossian et al., 2019; Institute (IOM), 2007; Orelus, 2012

(Continued)

TABLE 1-2 Levels of Evidence (LOE) (Continued)

Topic	Points	LOE	Evidence
FCC	• Advocacy of infant/child and policy development • Cultural humility/sensitivity	VII III V VII VI VII VII VI VII VII I VI VII VI VI IV VI IV VII VI	Loversidge & Zurmehly, 2019; Preyde & Ardal, 2003; Provenzi & Santoro, 2015; World Health Organization (WHO), 2015; Berman et al., 2019; Bourque et al., 2018; Johnson et al., 2008; Carver & Jessie, 2011; Jefferies, 2014; Murphy & Carbone, 2011; Nandi et al., 2018; Petty, Whiting, Green, & Fowler, 2018; Purdy, Craig, & Zeanah, 2015; Weber, Harrison, Steward, et al., 2018; Beck et al., 2020; Brooks, Holditch-Davis, & Landerman, 2013; Huenink, 2017; Padula et al., 2020; Stevens et al., 2010; Thoma et al., 2019
Evolution of DC	• Preterm infant states and changes in states • Environmental stimulation • Impact of environment on the baby's physiologic organization	VII VII VII VII III VI II VI III III VI VI III	Gesell & Amatruda, 1945; Gluck, 1970; Gluck, Wimmer, Mannino, DeLue, et al., 1976; Vohr, 2019; Barnard & Bee, 1983; Chaze & Ludington-Hoe, 1984; Korner, Schneider, & Forrest, 1983; Scar-Salapatek & Williams, 1973; Thoman, Ingersoll, & Acebo, 1991; White & Labarba, 1976; Gottfried & Gaiter, 1985; Long, Lucey, & Philip, 1980; Long, Philip, & Lucey, 1980
Evolution of DC	• Contributions of basic science to affect infant outcomes • Environmental and caregiving interventions • Individualized behavioral communication–based caregiving • Parent education and support programs to promote parent–infant emotional connection and improved outcome	VII VII VII I V IV V I II V II VII II II III I II III II VI II II	Graven, 1997; Graven et al., 1992a, 1992b; Browne & R.D. White, 2011; Bieleninik, Ghetti, & Gold, 2016; Juneau, Aita, & Héon, 2015; Picciolini et al., 2014; Pineda et al., 2017; Trivedi, 2015; Als et al., 2012; Als, Duffy, & McAnulty, 1996; Als et al., 2011; Als et al., 2004; McAnulty et al., 2012; McAnulty et al., 2010; Mewes et al., 2006; Cheng et al., 2019; Melnyk et al., 2006; Mianaei, Karahroudy, Rassouli, et al., 2014; O'Brien et al., 2018; Toivonen, Lehtonen, Löyttyniemi, et al., 2020; Porges et al., 2019; Welch et al., 2020

TABLE 1-2 Levels of Evidence (LOE) (Continued)

Topic	Points	LOE	Evidence
Risk of experimentation	• Parent hesitation to engage in research studies	VI	Weiss et al., 2021
Infant and family-centered developmental care (IFCDC)	• Integration of baby's unique behavioral communication and interaction in care • Share decision-making • Cultural humility • Share control of education/decision-making and caregiving among the baby, parent(s), family, and team members • Importance of nurturing relationships	V VII VI VI IV VII VI VI VI VI VI VII II III	Filippa et al., 2017; Craig et al., 2015; Brooks et al., 2013; Campinha-Bacote, 2011; Lake, Staiger, Edwards, Smith, et al., 2018; Johnson, 2016; Umberger, Canvasser, & Hall, 2018; Browne, 2020; Evans & Porter, 2009; Feldman, 2007, 2009; Feldman & Eidelman, 2007; Montirosso & McGlone, 2020; Neu, Hazel, Robinson, Schmiege, et al., 2014; Provenzi et al., 2019
Gaps	• Medical/surgical intensive care separate from DC • Interprofessional discipline silos • Lack of professional integration and collaboration • Baby overlooked as primary communicator/interactor in own care • Lack of attention to attachment relationship and mental health of baby/parents • Parents/family viewed as visitors • Parent/baby separation and parents fractured from family, friends, and home • Parent confusion, fear, lost, emotional in complex health environment • Parents not prepared to care for medically challenged/chronic baby	IV VII I VI VII VII V VI VII VI VI V VII VII VI VI VI VII VI VII	Smith et al., 2011; Melnyk, 2018; Reeves, Pelone, Harrison, et al., 2017; Als, 1982, 2009; Als, 1986; Westrup, 2015; Berwick, 2009; Cleveland, 2008; Tallon, Kendall, & Snider, 2015; Thiele, Knierim, & Mader, 2016; Wigert, Dellenmark, & Bry, 2013; Boykova, 2016a; Boykova, 2016b; Choi et al., 2020; Stuebe, 2020; Vetulani, 2013; Gallagher, Shaw, Aladangady, et al., 2018; Johnson & Abraham, 2020; Murphy & Carbone, 2011; Petty et al., 2018; Purdy et al., 2015
Systems thinking within a complex adaptive system	• Biologic and organizational systems are holistic with parts that interrelate to influence and be influenced by each other	VI VII VII	Douglas et al., 2011; Plsek, P.E. & Greenhalgh,T., 2001; Wilson et al., 2001
Baby as a competent interactor	• Recognize individual strengths/vulnerabilities of the baby through behaviors, facial expressions, and physiologic responses/movement/changes	IV VII VI VII VI	Gonya et al., 2018; Kolstad, 2013; Lavelli, Carra, Rossi, & Keller, 2019; Levin, 1999; Björn Westrup, 2007
Individualized care	• Management of individualized strengths, needs, and availability/receptiveness of the baby and family to stress, relaxation, and comfort	VI VII V VI	Als, 1982, 2009; Browne & White, 2011; McCance et al., 2011; Björn Westrup, 2007

(Continued)

TABLE 1-2 Levels of Evidence (LOE) (Continued)

Topic	Points	LOE	Evidence
Family integration	• Family integrated within interprofessional team to provide support of baby • Assure family integration regardless of perception/bias based on social determinants • Physiologic, nutritional, and emotional regulation between baby and m/other • Essential support of parent/partner and family to m/other through baby's ICU stay	VII VI VI VI III III VII VI IV VII VI IV V VI VI VII VII VI VII VI VI VI VII VI	Thiele et al., 2016; Trajkovski, Schmied, Vickers, & Jackson, 2015; Van Riper, 2001; Beck et al., 2020; Boghossian et al., 2019; DeSisto, Hirai, Collins, & Rankin, 2018; Epstein, Jimenez-Rubio, Smith, et al., 2009; Hall, Shahidullah, & Lassen, 2020; Horbar et al., 2019; Howell, Hebert, & Zeitlin, 2019; Louis-Jacques, Deubel, Taylor, et al., 2017; Padula et al., 2020; Sigurdson et al., 2019; Thoma et al., 2019; Tucker et al., 2003; Vance et al., 2018 Craig et al., 2015; Feldman & Eidelman, 2007; Hynan et al., 2015; Thoyre, Park, Pados, & Hubbard, 2013; Als, 2009; Hagen, Iversen, & Svindseth, 2016; Hall, Phillips, & Hynan, 2016; Hynan, 2005
Environmental protection	• Baby's development impacted by sensory stimuli such as the physical environment, contact/touch, and caregiving	V VI VII III III VII	Bronfenbrenner, 1986; Bronfenbrenner & Ceci, 1994; Committee [NICU Design], 2020; Lester et al., 2014; Lester et al., 2016; White, 2020a
Neuroprotection of the developing brain	• Neuroprotection of individualized sensitive caregiving through m/other's regulatory influence of holding, feeding, and interacting is essential for optimal brain growth	VI VI VI II I	Gorzilio, Garrido, Gaspardo, et al., 2015; Graven & Browne, 2008; Lockridge, 2018; Porges et al., 2019; Soleimani et al., 2020
Infant mental health	• Promote engagement through a focus on enhancing the relationship between babies, parents, and primary caregivers	VI VII VI VI VII	Browne, 2020; Choi et al., 2020; D'Agata, Young, Cong, Grasso, et al., 2016; Evans & Porter, 2009; Ishizaki, 2013
Principles of the components/sections of IFCDC	• Systems thinking • Positioning and touch • Sleep and arousal interventions • Skin-to-skin contact • Reducing and managing pain and stress • Management of feeding, eating, and nutrition delivery • Implementation of one component section over another	VI VII VI VI VI II VI VI	Altimier & Phillips, 2013; Leslie Altimier & Phillips, 2016; Cardin, 2015; Coughlin, Gibbins, & Hoath, 2009; Lopez-Maestro et al., 2020; O'Brien et al., 2018; Phillips, 2015; Roue et al., 2017
Standards, competencies, and best practices of IFCDC	• Systematic process using evidence-based practice guidelines to standardize, disseminate, utilize, monitor, and compare among similar units and demonstrate improved baby/parent/family outcomes for the short- and long-term of the lifespan • Evidence-based report of expert interprofessional committee	VI VII	Browne et al., 2020; Care [IFCDC], 2020

CONCLUSION

Although there is a beginning foundation of evidence to support integration of developmental care into all intensive care practices and procedures, there is a need for further study, evidence-based improvement, dissemination of improvement work, and continuing update of the recommendations. The IFCDC consensus panel will be expanding the evidence-based standards and competencies specific to infant and parent mental health, inclusion, diversity, and equity, and the effect of family separation due to the pandemic. It is important for all professionals to share IFCDC improvement work including development of clinical studies across similar level units to standardize practice and compare outcome metrics.

Intensive care professionals tend to see the baby and family only as they are during the time from birth to discharge. However, IFCDC guides a vision of the equitable holism in our care from admission through the baby's lifespan. The quality of care creates an opportunity for enhancing quality of life. Interprofessionals and parents working collaboratively make this possible.

IFCDC should be integrated with all the care provided to babies and families. Professionals should promote a spirit of inquiry and evaluate the culture of each unit and the developmental care that is provided in collaboration with parents. Measures of the care and the short-term and long-term outcomes of the baby should be examined routinely and often.

Potential Research Questions

- What can *you* do to promote IFCDC?
- What changes will you make to improve the care that you give? How will you sustain your progress?

REFERENCES

Ahlqvist-Bjorkroth, S. (2018). Communication between healthcare professionals and parents is a key factor in involving parents in neonatal intensive care. *Acta Paediatrica, 107*(1), 12–13. https://doi.org/10.1111/apa.14111

Almadhoob, A., & Ohlsson, A. (2015). Sound reduction management in the neonatal intensive care unit for preterm or very low birth weight infants. *Cochrane Database of Systematic Review, 1,* CD010333. https://doi.org/10.1002/14651858.CD010333.pub2

Als, H. (1982). Toward a synactive theory of development: Promise for the assessment and support of infant individuality. *Infant Mental Health Journal, 3*(4), 229–243.

Als, H. (1986). *A synactive model of neonatal behavioral organization: Framework for the assessment of neurobehavioral development in the premature infant and for support of infants and parents in the neonatal intensive care environment.* In *The high-risk neonate: Developmental therapy perspectives* (pp. 3–53). The Haworth Press.

Als, H. (2009). Newborn Individualized Developmental Care and Assessment Program (NIDCAP): New frontier for neonatal and perinatal medicine. *Journal of Neonatal-Perinatal Medicine, 2,* 135–147.

Als, H., Duffy, F. H., & McAnulty, G. B. (1996). Effectiveness of individualized neurodevelopmental care in the newborn intensive care unit (NICU).

Acta Paediatrica Supplement, 416, 21–30. https://doi.org/10.1111/j.1651-2227.1996.tb14273.x

Als, H., Duffy, F. H., McAnulty, G., Butler, S. C., Lightbody, L., Kosta, S., Weisenfeld, N. I., Robertson, R., Parad, R. B., Ringer, S. A., Blickman, J. G., Zurakowski, D., & Warfield, S. K. (2012). NIDCAP improves brain function and structure in preterm infants with severe intrauterine growth restriction. *Journal of Perinatology, 32*(10), 797–803. https://doi.org/10.1038/jp.2011.201

Als, H., Duffy, F. H., McAnulty, G. B., Fischer, C. B., Kosta, S., Butler, S. C., Parad, R. B., Blickman, J. G., Zurakowski, D., & Ringer, S. A. (2011). Is the Newborn Individualized Developmental Care and Assessment Program (NIDCAP) effective for preterm infants with intrauterine growth restriction? *Journal of Perinatology, 31*(2), 130–136. https://doi.org/10.1038/jp.2010.81

Als, H., Duffy, F. H., McAnulty, G. B., Rivkin, M. J., Vajapeyam, S., Mulkern, R. V., Warfield, S. K., Huppi, P. S., Butler, S. C., Conneman, N., Fischer, C., & Eichenwald, E. C. (2004). Early experience alters brain function and structure. *Pediatrics, 113*(4), 846–857. https://doi.org/10.1542/peds.113.4.846

Als, H., Gilkerson, L., Duffy, F. H., Mcanulty, G. B., Buehler, D. M., Vandenberg, K., Sweet, N., Sell, E., Parad, R. B., Ringer, S. A., Butler, S. C., Blickman, J. G., & Jones, K. J. (2003). A three-center, randomized, controlled trial of individualized developmental care for very low birth weight preterm infants: Medical, neurodevelopmental, parenting, and caregiving effects. *Journal of Developmental and Behavioral Pediatrics, 24*(6), 399–408.

Altimier, L., & Phillips, R. (2013). The neonatal integrative developmental care model: Seven neuroprotective core measures for family-centered developmental care. *Newborn and Infant Nursing Reviews, 13*(1), 9–22.

Altimier, L., & Phillips, R. (2016). The Neonatal Integrative Developmental Care Model: Advanced clinical applications of the seven core measures for neuroprotective family-centered developmental care. *Newborn and Infant Nursing Reviews, 16*(4), 230–244. https://doi.org/10.1053/j.nainr.2016.09.030

American Academy of Pediatrics (AAP). (2012). Patient-and family-centered care and the pediatrician's role. *Pediatrics, 129*(2), 394–404. https://doi.org/10.1542/peds.2011-3084

Bailey, S. M., Hendricks-Munoz, K. D., & Mally, P. (2013). Parental influence on clinical management during neonatal intensive care: A survey of US neonatologists. *The Journal of Maternal-Fetal & Neonatal Medicine, 26*(12), 1239–1244. https://doi.org/10.3109/14767058.2013.776531

Barnard, K. E., & Bee, H. L. (1983). The impact of temporally patterned stimulation on the development of preterm infants. *Child Development, 54*(5), 1156–1167.

Beck, A. F., Edwards, E. M., Horbar, J. D., Howell, E. A., McCormick, M. C., & Pursley, D. M. (2020). The color of health: How racism, segregation, and inequality affect the health and well-being of preterm infants and their families. *Pediatric Research, 87*(2), 227–234. https://doi.org/10.1038/s41390-019-0513-6

Berman, L., Raval, M. V., Ottosen, M., Mackow, A. K., Cho, M., & Goldin, A. B. (2019). Parent perspectives on readiness for discharge home after neonatal intensive care unit admission. *The Journal of Pediatrics, 205,* 98–104.e104. https://doi.org/10.1016/j.jpeds.2018.08.086

Berwick, D. M. (2009). What 'patient-centered' should mean: Confessions of an extremist. *Health Affairs, 28*(4), w555–w565. https://doi.org/10.1377/hlthaff.28.4.w555

Bieleninik, Ł., Ghetti, C., & Gold, C. (2016). Music therapy for preterm infants and their parents: A meta-analysis. *Pediatrics, 138*(3). https://doi.org/10.1542/peds.2016-0971

Boghossian, N. S., Geraci, M., Lorch, S. A., Phibbs, C. S., Edwards, E. M., & Horbar, J. D. (2019). Racial and ethnic differences over time in outcomes of infants born less than 30 weeks' gestation. *Pediatrics, 144*(3), e20191106. https://doi.org/10.1542/peds.2019-1106

Bourque, C. J., Dahan, S., Mantha, G., Robson, K., Reichherzer, M., & Janvier, A. (2018). Improving neonatal care with the help of veteran resource parents: An overview of current practices. *Seminars in Fetal and Neonatal Medicine, 23*(1), 44–51. https://doi.org/10.1016/j.siny.2017.10.005

Boykova, M. (2016a). Life after discharge: What parents of preterm infants say about their transition to home. *Newborn and Infant Nursing Reviews, 16*(2), 58–65. https://doi.org/10.1053/j.nainr.2016.03.002

Boykova, M. (2016b). Transition from hospital to home in parents of preterm infants: A literature review. *The Journal of Perinatal & Neonatal Nursing, 30*(4), 327–348. https://doi.org/10.1097/jpn.0000000000000211

Bronfenbrenner, U. (1986). Ecology of the family as a context for human development: Research perspectives. *Developmental Psychology, 22,* 723–742. https://doi.org/10.1037/0012-1649.22.6.723

Bronfenbrenner, U., & Ceci, S. J. (1994). Nature-nurture reconceptualized in developmental perspective: A bioecological model. *Psychological Review, 101*(4), 568–586. https://doi.org/10.1037/0033-295x.101.4.568

Brooks, J. L., Holditch-Davis, D., & Landerman, L. R. (2013). Interactive behaviors of ethnic minority mothers and their premature infants. *Journal of Obstetric, Gynecologic & Neonatal Nursing, 42*(3), 357–368. https://doi.org/10.1111/1552-6909.12037

Browne, J. V. (2021). Infant mental health in intensive care: Laying a foundation for social, emotional and mental health outcomes through regulation, relationships and reflection. *Journal of Neonatal Nursing, 27*(1), 33–39. https://doi.org/ 10.1016/j.jnn.2020.11.011

Browne, J. V., Jaeger, C. B., & Kenner, C. (2020). Executive summary: Standards, competencies, and recommended best practices for infant-and family-centered developmental care in the intensive care unit. *Journal of Perinatology, 40*(Suppl. 1), 5–10. https://doi.org/10.1038/s41372-020-0767-1

Browne, J. V., & Talmi, A. (2005). Family-based intervention to enhance infant-parent relationships in the neonatal intensive care unit. *The Journal of Pediatrics Psychology, 30*(8), 667–677. https://doi.org/10.1093/jpepsy/jsi053

Browne, J. V., & White, R. D. (2011a). Developmental care for high-risk newborns: Emerging science, clinical application, and continuity from newborn intensive care unit to community. *Clinics in Perinatology, 38*(4), 719–729. https://doi.org/10.1016/j.clp.2011.08.003

Browne, J. V., & White, R. D. (2011b). Foundations of developmental care. *Clinics in Perinatology, 38*(4), xv–xvii. https://doi.org/10.1016/j.clp.2011.09.001

Campinha-Bacote, J. (2011). Delivering patient-centered care in the midst of a cultural conflict: The role of cultural competence. *OJIN: The Online Journal of Issues in Nursing, 16*(2, Manuscript 5), 5. https://doi.org/10.3912/OJIN.Vol16No02Man05

Cardin, A. D. (2015). Neuroprotective core measures 1–7: A developmental care journey. Transformations in NICU design and caregiving attitudes. *Newborn and Infant Nursing Reviews, 15*(3), 132–141.

Carver, M. C., & Jessie, A. (2011). Patient-centered care in a medical home. *OJIN: The Online Journal of Issues in Nursing, 16*(2, Manuscript 4), 4. https://doi.org/10.3912/OJIN.Vol16No02Man04

Centre for Evidenced-Based Medicine (CEBM). (2009). *Oxford centre for evidence-based medicine-levels of evidence.* https://www.cebm.net/2009/06/oxford-centre-evidence-based-medicine-levels-evidence-march-2009/

Chaze, B. A., & Ludington-Hoe, S. M. (1984). Sensory stimulation in the NICU. *American Journal of Nursing, 84*(1), 68–71.

Cheng, C., Franck, L. S., Ye, X. Y., Hutingson, S. A., Lee, S. K., O'Brienon, K., & behalf of the FICare Study Group and FICare Parent. (2019). Evaluating the effect of family integrated care on maternal stress and anxiety in neonatal intensive care units. *Journal of Reproductive and Infant Psychology, 10,* 1–14.

Choi, K. R., Records, K., Low, L. K., Alhusen, J. L., Kenner, C., Bloch, J. R., Premji, S. S., Hannan, J., Anderson, C. M., Yeo, S., & Cynthia Logsdon, M. (2020). Promotion of maternal–infant mental health and trauma-informed care during the COVID-19 Pandemic. *Journal of Obstetric, Gynecologic & Neonatal Nursing, 49*(5), 409–415. https://doi.org/10.1016/j.jogn.2020.07.004

Cleveland, L. M. (2008). Parenting in the neonatal intensive care unit. *Journal of Obstetric, Gynecologic & Neonatal Nursing, 37*(6), 666–691. https://doi.org/10.1111/j.1552-6909.2008.00288.x

Committee to Establish Recommended Standards for Newborn ICU Design. (2020). *Recommended standards for newborn ICU design* (9th ed.). https://nicudesign.nd.edu/nicu-standards/

Consensus Committee on Infant and Family Centered Developmental Care. (2020). *Report of the first consensus conference on standards, competencies and best practices for infant and family centered developmental care in the intensive care unit.* https://nicudesign.nd.edu/nicu-care-standards/:

Coughlin, M., Gibbins, S., & Hoath, S. (2009). Core measures for developmentally supportive care in neonatal intensive care units: Theory, precedence and practice. *Journal of Advanced Nursing, 65*(10), 2239–2248. https://doi.org/10.1111/j.1365-2648.2009.05052.x

Craig, J. W., Glick, C., Phillips, R., Hall, S. L., Smith, J., & Browne, J. (2015). Recommendations for involving the family in developmental care of the NICU baby. *Journal of Perinatology, 35,* S5–S8. https://doi.org/10.1038/jp.2015.142

D'Agata, A. L., Young, E. E., Cong, X., Grasso, D. J., & McGrath, J. M. (2016). Infant medical trauma in the neonatal intensive care unit (IMTN): A proposed concept for science and practice. *Advances in Neonatal Care, 16*(4), 289–297. https://doi.org/10.1097/ANC.0000000000000309

DeSisto, C. L., Hirai, A. H., Collins, J. W., & Rankin, K. M. (2018). Deconstructing a disparity: Explaining excess preterm birth among U.S.-born black women. *Annals of Epidemiology, 28*(4), 225–230. https://doi.org/10.1016/j.annepidem.2018.01.012

Douglas, P. S., Hill, P. S., & Brodribb, W. (2011). The unsettled baby: How complexity science helps. *Archives of Disease in Childhood, 96*(9), 793–797. https://doi.org/10.1136/adc.2010.199190

(EFCNI), European Foundation for the Care of Newborn Infants. (2018). *European standards of care for newborn health project report.* https://newborn-health-standards.org/

Epstein, D., Jimenez-Rubio, D., Smith, P. C., & Suhrcke, M. (2009). Social determinants of health: An economic perspective. *Health Economics, 18*(5), 495–502. https://doi.org/10.1002/hec.1490

Evans, C. A., & Porter, C. L. (2009). The emergence of mother-infant co-regulation during the first year: Links to infants' developmental status and attachment. *Infant Behavior and Development, 32*(2), 147–158. https://doi.org/10.1016/j.infbeh.2008.12.005

Feldman, R. (2007). Parent-infant synchrony and the construction of shared timing; physiological precursors, developmental outcomes, and risk conditions. *The Journal of Child Psychology and Psychiatry, 48*(3-4), 329–354. https://doi.org/10.1111/j.1469-7610.2006.01701.x

Feldman, R. (2009). The development of regulatory functions from birth to 5 years: Insights from premature infants. *Child Development, 80*(2), 544–561. https://doi.org/10.1111/j.1467-8624.2009.01278.x

Feldman, R., & Eidelman, A. I. (2007). Maternal postpartum behavior and the emergence of infant-mother and infant-father synchrony in preterm and full-term infants: The role of neonatal vagal tone. *Developmental Psychobiology, 49*(3), 290–302. https://doi.org/10.1002/dev.20220

Filippa, M., Panza, C., Ferrari, F., Frassoldati, R., Kuhn, P., Balduzzi, S., & D'Amico, R. (2017). Systematic review of maternal voice interventions demonstrates increased stability in preterm infants. *Acta Paediatrica, 106*(8), 1220–1229. https://doi.org/10.1111/apa.13832

Gallagher, K., Shaw, C., Aladangady, N., & Marlow, N. (2018). Parental experience of interaction with healthcare professionals during their infant's stay in the neonatal intensive care unit. *Archives of Disease in Childhood — Fetal and Neonatal Edition, 103*(4), F343–F348. https://doi.org/10.1136/archdischild-2016-312278

Galvin, E., Boyers, L., Schwartz, P. K., Jones, M. W., Mooney, P., Warwick, J., & Davis, J. (2000). Challenging the precepts of family-centered care: Testing a philosophy. *Journal of Pediatric Nursing, 26*(6), 625–632.

Gesell, A., & Amatruda, C. S. (1945). *The embryology of behavior: The beginnings of the human mind.* Harper and Brothers.

Gluck, L. (1985, October 1992). *Conceptualization and initiation of a neonatal intensive care nursery in 1960.* Paper presented at the Paper presented at the Neonatal Intensive Care History of Excellence: A Symposium Commemorating Child Health Day.

Gluck, L. (1970). Design of a perinatal center. *Pediatric Clinics of North America, 17*(4), 777–791. https://doi.org/10.1016/s0031-3955(16)32480-4

Gluck, L., Wimmer, J., Mannino, F., DeLue, N., & Feldman, B. (1976). Neonatal intensive care in community hospitals and remote areas. The problems and a possible solution. *Clinics in Perinatology, 3*(2), 297–306.

Gonya, J., Feldman, K., Brown, K., Stein, M., Keim, S., Boone, K., Rumpf, W., Ray, W., Chawla, N., & Butter, E. (2018). Human interaction in the NICU and its association with outcomes on the Brief Infant-Toddler Social and Emotional Assessment (BITSEA). *Early Human Development, 127*, 6–14. https://doi.org/10.1016/j.earlhumdev.2018.08.010

Gorzilio, D. M., Garrido, E., Gaspardo, C. M., Martinez, F. E., & Linhares, M. B. (2015). Neurobehavioral development prior to term-age of preterm infants and acute stressful events during neonatal hospitalization. *Early Human Development, 91*(12), 769–765. https://doi.org/10.1016/j.earlhumdev.2015.09.003

Gottfried, A. W., & Gaiter, J. L. (1985). *Infant stress under intensive care.* University Park Press.

Govindaswamy, P., Laing, S., Waters, D., Walker, K., Spence, K., & Badawi, N. (2018). Needs of parents in a surgical neonatal intensive care unit. *The Journal of Paediatrics and Child Health, 55*(5), 567–573. https://doi.org/10.1111/jpc.14249

Graven, S. N. (1997). Clinical research data illuminating the relationship between the physical environment & patient medical outcomes. *Journal of Healthcare Design, 9*, 15–19, discussion 21–14.

Graven, S. N., Bowen, F. W., Jr., Brooten, D., Eaton, A., Graven, M. N., Hack, M., Hall, L. A., Hansen, N., Hurt, H., & Kavalhuna, R. (1992a). The high-risk infant environment. Part 1. The role of the neonatal intensive care unit in the outcome of high-risk infants. *Journal of Perinatology, 12*(2), 164–172.

Graven, S. N., Bowen, F. W., Jr., Brooten, D., Eaton, A., Graven, M. N., Hack, M., Hall, L. A., Hansen, N., Hurt, H., & Kavalhuna, R. (1992b). The high-risk infant environment. Part 2. The role of caregiving and the social environment. *Journal of Perinatology, 12*(3), 267–275.

Graven, S. N., & Browne, J. V. (2008). Sleep and brain development: The critical role of sleep in fetal and early neonatal brain development. *Newborn and Infant Nursing Reviews, 8*(4), 173–179. http://dx.doi.org/10.1053/j.nainr.2008.10.008

Guillaume, S., Michelin, N., Amrani, E., Benier, B., Durrmeyer, X., Lescure, S., Bony, C., Danan, C., Baud, O., Jarreau, P.-H., Zana-Taïeb, E., & Caeymaex, L. (2013). Parents' expectations of staff in the early bonding process with their premature babies in the intensive care setting: A qualitative multicenter study with 60 parents. *BMC Pediatrics, 13*, 18. https://doi.org/10.1186/1471-2431-13-18

Hagen, I. H., Iversen, V. C., & Svindseth, M. F. (2016). Differences and similarities between mothers and fathers of premature children: A qualitative study of parents' coping experiences in a neonatal intensive care unit. *BMC Pediatrics, 16*, 92. https://doi.org/10.1186/s12887-016-0631-9

Hall, S. L., Phillips, R., & Hynan, M. (2016). Transforming NICU care to provide comprehensive family support. *Newborn and Infant Nursing Reviews, 16*, 69–73.

Hall, E. M., Shahidullah, J. D., & Lassen, S. R. (2020). Development of postpartum depression interventions for mothers of premature infants: A call to target low-SES NICU families. *Journal of Perinatology, 40*(1), 1–9. https://doi.org/10.1038/s41372-019-0473-z

Horbar, J. D., Edwards, E. M., Greenberg, L. T., Profit, J., Draper, D., Helkey, D., Lorch, S. A., Lee, H. C., Phibbs, C. S., Rogowski, J., Gould, J. B., & Firebaugh, G. (2019). Racial segregation and inequality in the neonatal intensive care unit for very low-birth-weight and very preterm infants. *JAMA Pediatrics, 173*(5), 455–461. https://doi.org/10.1001/jamapediatrics.2019.0241

Howell, E. A., Hebert, P. L., & Zeitlin, J. (2019). Racial segregation and inequality of care in neonatal intensive care units is unacceptable. *JAMA Pediatrics, 173*(5), 420–421. https://doi.org/10.1001/jamapediatrics.2019.0240

Huenink, E. (2017). Parent support programs and coping mechanisms in NICU parents. *Advances in Neonatal Care, 17*(2), E10–E18. https://doi.org/10.1097/ANC.0000000000000359

Hynan, M. T. (2005). Supporting fathers during stressful times in the nursery: An evidence-based review. *Newborn and Infant Nursing Reviews, 5*(2), 87–92.

Hynan, M. T., Steinberg, Z., Baker, L., Cicco, R., Geller, P. A., Lassen, S., Milford, C., Mounts, K. O., & Patterson, C., Saxton, S., Segre, L., Stuebe, A. (2015). Recommendations for mental health professionals in the NICU. *Journal of Perinatology, 35*(Suppl. 1), S14–S18. https://doi.org/10.1038/jp.2015.144

Institute of Medicine (IOM). (2007). *Preterm birth: Causes, consequences, and prevention.* The National Academies Press.

Institute of Medicine (IOM). (2001). *Crossing the quality chasm: A new health system for the 21st century.* The National Academies Press.

Institute for Patient-and Family-Centered Care (IPFCC). (2019). www.ipfcc.org

Ishizaki, Y. (2013). Mental health of mothers and their premature infants for the prevention of child abuse and maltreatment. *Health, 5*(3), 612–616.

Jefferies, A. L. (2014). Going home: Facilitating discharge of the preterm infant. *Paediatrics and Child Health, 19*(1), 31–42.

Johnson, B. H. (2000). Family-centered care: Four decades of progress. *Families, Systems, & Health, 18*(2), 137–156. https://doi.org/10.1037/h0091843

Johnson, B. H. (2016). Promoting patient-and family-centered care through personal stories. *Academic Medicine, 91*(3), 297–300. https://doi.org/10.1097/acm.0000000000001086

Johnson, B. H., & Abraham, M. R. (2020). Reinforcing the essential role of families through first impressions of the physical environment. *Journal of Perinatology, 40*(Suppl. 1), 11–15. https://doi.org/10.1038/s41372-020-0747-5

Johnson, B., Abraham, M., Conway, J., Simmons, L., Edgman-Levitan, S., Sodomka, P., Schlucter, J., & Ford, D. (2008). *Partnering with patients and families to design a patient-and family-centered health care system: Recommendations and promising practices.* www.ipfcc.org

Johnson, B. H., Abraham, M. R., & Shelton, T. L. (2009). Patient-and family-centered care: Partnerships for quality and safety. *North Carolina Medical Journal, 70*(2), 125–130.

Jones, T., & on behalf of the Council of International Neonatal Nurses, Inc. (COINN) Working Group. (2019). International neonatal nursing competency framework. *Journal of Neonatal Nursing, 25*, 258–264. https://doi.org/10.1016/j.jnn.2019.07.007

Juneau, A. L., Aita, M., & Héon, M. (2015). Review and critical analysis of massage studies for term and preterm infants. *Neonatal Network, 34*(3), 165–177. https://doi.org/10.1891/0730-0832.34.3.165

Kolstad, A. (2013). The nature-nurture problem revisited. Some epistemological topics in contemporary human sciences. *Open Journal of Philosophy, 3*(4), 517–521. http://dx.doi.org/10.4236/ojpp.2013.34074

Korner, A. F., Schneider, P., & Forrest, T. (1983). Effects of vestibular-proprioceptive stimulation on the neurobehavioral development of preterm infants: A pilot study. *Neuropediatrics, 14*(3), 170–175. https://doi.org/10.1055/s-2008-1059573

Lake, E. T., Staiger, D., Edwards, E. M., Smith, J. G., & Rogowski, J. A. (2018). Nursing care disparities in neonatal intensive care units. *Health Services Research, 53*(Suppl. 1), 3007–3026. https://doi.org/10.1111/1475-6773.12762

Lavelli, M., Carra, C., Rossi, G., & Keller, H. (2019). Culture-specific development of early mother-infant emotional co-regulation: Italian, Cameroonian, and West African immigrant dyads. *Developmental Psychology, 55*(9), 1850–1867. https://doi.org/10.1037/dev0000696

Lee, C. (2003). Bonding. *Pediatrics in Review, 24*(8), 289–290.

Lester, B. M., Hawes, K., Abar, B., Sullivan, M., Miller, R., Bigsby, R., Laptook, A., Salisbury, A., Taub, M., Lagasse, L. L., & Padbury, J. F. (2014). Single-family room care and neurobehavioral and medical outcomes in preterm infants. *Pediatrics, 134*(4), 754–760. https://doi.org/10.1542/peds.2013-4252

Lester, B. M., Salisbury, A. L., Hawes, K., Dansereau, L. M., Bigsby, R., Laptook, A., Taub, M., Lagasse, L. L., Vohr, B. R., & Padbury, J. F. (2016). 18-month follow-up of infants cared for in a single-family room neonatal intensive care unit. *The Journal of Pediatrics, 177*, 84–89. https://doi.org/10.1016/j.jpeds.2016.06.069

Levin, A. (1999). Humane neonatal care initiative. *Acta Paediatrica, 88*(4), 353–355. https://doi.org/10.1080/08035259950169657

Liu, W. F., Laudert, S., Perkins, B., MacMillan-York, E., Martin, S., Graven, S., & the NIC/Q 2005 Physical Environment Exploratory Group. (2007). The development of potentially better practices to support the neurodevelopment of infants in the NICU. *Journal of Perinatology, 27*, S48–S74. https://doi.org/10.1038/sj.jp.7211844

Lockridge, T. (2018). Neonatal neuroprotection: Bringing best practice to the bedside in the NICU. *MCN: The American Journal of Maternal/Child Nursing, 43*(2), 66–76. https://doi.org/10.1097/nmc.0000000000000411

Long, J. G., Lucey, J. F., & Philip, A. G. (1980). Noise and hypoxemia in the intensive care nursery. *Pediatrics, 65*(1), 143–145.

Long, J. G., Philip, A. G., & Lucey, J. F. (1980). Excessive handling as a cause of hypoxemia. *Pediatrics, 65*(2), 203–207.

Lopez-Maestro, M., De la Cruz, J., Perapoch-Lopez, J., Gimeno-Navarro, A., Vazquez-Roman, S., Alonso-Diaz, C., Muñoz-Amat, B., Morales-Betancourt, C., Soriano-Ramos, M., & Pallas-Alonso, C. (2020). Eight principles for newborn care in neonatal units: Findings from a national survey. *Acta Paediatrica, 109* (1651–2227 (Electronic)), 1361–1368. https://doi.org/10.1111/apa.15121

Louis-Jacques, A., Deubel, T. F., Taylor, M., & Stuebe, A. M. (2017). Racial and ethnic disparities in U.S. breastfeeding and implications for maternal and child health outcomes. *Seminars in Perinatology, 41*(5), 299–307. https://doi.org/10.1053/j.semperi.2017.04.007

Loversidge, J., & Zurmehly, J. (2019). *Evidence-informed health policy: using EBP to transform policy in nursing and healthcare.* Sigma Theta Tau, International.

Lubbe, W. (2012). Integrative literature review defining evidence-based neurodevelopmental supportive care of the preterm infant. *The Journal of Perinatal & Neonatal Nursing, 26*(3), 251–259. https://doi.org/10.1097/JPN.0b013e3182650b7e

McAnulty, G., Duffy, F., Kosta, S., Butler, S., Bernstein, J., Als, H., Weisenfeld, N., Warfield, S., & Zurakowski, D. (2012). School age effects of the newborn individualized developmental care and assessment program for medically low-risk preterm infants: Preliminary findings. *Journal of Clinical Neonatology, 1*(4), 184–194. https://doi.org/10.4103/2249-4847.105982

McAnulty, G. B., Duffy, F. H., Butler, S. C., Bernstein, J. H., Zurakowski, D., & Als, H. (2010). Effects of the Newborn Individualized Developmental Care and Assessment Program (NIDCAP) at age 8 years: Preliminary data. *Clinical Pediatrics, 49*(3), 258–270. https://doi.org/10.1177/0009922809335668

McCance, T., McCormack, B., & Dewing, J. (2011). An exploration of person-centredness in practice. *OJIN: The Online Journal of Issues in Nursing, 16*(2, Manuscript 1). https://doi.org/10.3912/OJIN.Vol16No02Man01

McGrath, J., Samra, H., & Kenner, C. (2011). Family-centered developmental care practices and research: What will the next century bring? *The Journal of Perinatal & Neonatal Nursing, 25*, 165–170.

Melnyk, B. M. (2018). Breaking down silos and making use of the evidence-based practice competencies in healthcare and academic programs: An urgent call to action. *Worldviews on Evidence-Based Nursing, 15*(1), 3–4. https://doi.org/10.1111/wvn.12271

Melnyk, B. M., Feinstein, N. F., Alpert-Gillis, L., Fairbanks, E., Crean, H. F., Sinkin, R. A., Stone, P. W., Small, L., Tu, X., & Gross, S. J. (2006). Reducing premature infants' length of stay and improving parents' mental health outcomes with the Creating Opportunities for Parent Empowerment (COPE) neonatal intensive care unit program: A randomized, controlled trial. *Pediatrics, 118*(5), e1414–e1427.

Melnyk, B. M., & Fineout-Overholt, E. (2019). *Evidenced-based practice in nursing & healthcare: A guide to best practice* (4th ed.). Wolters Kluwer | Lippincott Williams & Wilkins.

Mewes, A. U. J., Hüppi, P. S., Als, H., Rybicki, F. J., Inder, T. E., McAnulty, G. B., Mulkern, R. V., Robertson, R. L., Rivkin, M. J., & Warfield, S. K. (2006). Regional brain development in serial magnetic resonance imaging of low-risk preterm infants. *Pediatrics, 118*(1), 23–33. https://doi.org/10.1542/peds.2005-2675

Mianaei, S. J., Karahroudy, F. A., Rassouli, M., & Tafreshi, M. Z. (2014). The effect of Creating Opportunities for Parent Empowerment program on maternal stress, anxiety, and participation in NICU wards in Iran. *Iranian Journal of Nursing and Midwifery Research, 19*(1), 94–100.

Milette, I., Marte, M., da Silva, M. R., & McNeil, M. C. (2017a). Guidelines for the institutional implementation of developmental neuroprotective care in the neonatal intensive care unit. Part A: Background and rationale. A joint position statement from the CANN, CAPWHN, NANN, and COINN. *Canadian Journal of Nursing Research, 49*(2), 18. https://doi.org/10.1177/0844562117706882

Milette, I., Martel, M., da Silva, M. R., & McNeil, M. C. (2017b). Guidelines for the institutional implementation of developmental neuroprotective care in the NICU. Part B: Recommendations and justification. A joint position statement from the CANN, CAPWHN, NANN, and COINN. *Canadian Journal of Nursing Research, 49*(2), 12. https://doi.org/10.1177/0844562117708126

Monterosso, L., Kristjanson, L. J., Cole, J., & Evans, S. F. (2003). Effect of postural supports on neuromotor function in very preterm infants to term equivalent age. *The Journal of Paediatrics and Child Health, 39*(3), 197–205.

Montirosso, R., & McGlone, F. (2020). The body comes first. Embodied reparation and the co-creation of infant bodily-self. *Neuroscience & Biobehavioral Reviews, 113*, 77–87. https://doi.org/10.1016/j.neubiorev.2020.03.003

Morag, I., & Ohlsson, A. (2016). Cycled light in the intensive care unit for preterm and low birth weight infants. *Cochrane Database of Systematic Review,* (8), CD006982. https://doi.org/10.1002/14651858.CD006982.pub4

Murphy, N. A., & Carbone, P. S. (2011). Parent-provider-community partnerships: Optimizing outcomes for children with disabilities. *Pediatrics, 128*(4), 795–802. https://doi.org/10.1542/peds.2011-1467

Nandi, A., Jahagirdar, D., Dimitris, M. C., Labrecque, J. A., Strumpf, E. C., Kaufman, J. S., Vincent, I., Atabay, E., Harper, S., Earle, A., & Heymann, S. J. (2018). The impact of parental and medical leave policies on socioeconomic and health outcomes in OECD countries: A systematic review of the empirical literature. *Milbank Quarterly, 96*(3), 434–471. https://doi.org/10.1111/1468-0009.12340

Neu, M., Hazel, N. A., Robinson, J., Schmiege, S. J., & Laudenslager, M. (2014). Effect of holding on co-regulation in preterm infants: A randomized controlled trial. *Early Human Development, 90*(3), 141–147. https://doi.org/10.1016/j.earlhumdev.2014.01.008

O'Brien, K., Robson, K., Bracht, M., Cruz, M., Lui, K., Alvaro, R., da Silva, O., Monterrosa, L., Narvey, M., Ng, E., Soraisham, A., Ye, X. Y., Mirea, L., Tarnow-Mordi, W., & Lee, S. K. (2018). Effectiveness of Family Integrated Care in neonatal intensive care units on infant and parent outcomes: A multicentre, multinational, cluster-randomised controlled trial. *The Lancet Child & Adolescent Health, 2*(4), 245–254. https://doi.org/10.1016/s2352-4642(18)30039-7

Orelus, P. W. (2012). Being black and brown in the 21st century: Challenges and pedagogical possibilities. *SAGE Open, 2*(4), 8. https://doi.org/10.1177/2158244012464979

Padula, A. M., Shariff-Marco, S., Yang, J., Jain, J., Liu, J., Conroy, S. M., Carmichael, S. L., Gomez, S. L., Phibbs, C., Oehlert, J., Gould, J. B., & Profit, J. (2021). Multilevel social factors and NICU quality of care in California. *Journal of Perinatology, 41*, 404–412. https://doi.org/10.1038/s41372-020-0647-8

Petty, J., Whiting, L., Green, J., & Fowler, C. (2018). Parents' views on preparation to care for extremely premature infants at home. *Nursing Children and Young People, 30*(4), 22–27. https://doi.org/10.7748/ncyp.2018.e1084

Phillips, R. (2015). Seven core measures of neuroprotective family-centered developmental care: Creating an infrastructure for implementation. *Newborn and Infant Nursing Reviews, 15*, 87–90.

Picciolini, O., Porro, M., Meazza, A., Gianni, M. L., Rivoli, C., Lucco, G., Barretta, F., Bonzini, M., & Mosca, F. (2014). Early exposure to maternal voice: Effects on preterm infants development. *Early Human Development, 90*(6), 287–292. https://doi.org/10.1016/j.earlhumdev.2014.03.003

Picheansathian, W., Woragidpoonpol, P., & Baosoung, C. (2009). Positioning of preterm infants for optimal physiological development: A systematic review. *JBI Library of Systematic Reviews, 7*(7), 224–259.

Pickler, R. H., McGrath, J. M., Reyna, B. A., McCain, N., Lewis, M., Cone, S., Wetzel, P., & Best, A. (2010). A model of neurodevelopmental risk and protection for preterm infants. *The Journal of Perinatal & Neonatal Nursing, 24*(4), 356–365. https://doi.org/10.1097/JPN.0b013e3181fb1e70

Pineda, R., Bender, J., Hall, B., Shabosky, L., Annecca, A., & Smith, J. (2018). Parent participation in the neonatal intensive care unit: Predictors and relationships to neurobehavior and developmental outcomes. *Early Human Development, 117*, 32–38. https://doi.org/10.1016/j.earlhumdev.2017.12.008

Pineda, R., Guth, R., Herring, A., Reynolds, L., Oberle, S., & Smith, J. (2017). Enhancing sensory experiences for very preterm infants in the NICU: An integrative review. *Journal of Perinatology, 37*(4), 323–332. https://doi.org/10.1038/jp.2016.179

Pineda, R. G., Neil, J., Dierker, D., Smyser, C. D., Wallendorf, M., Kidokoro, H., Reynolds, L. C., Walker, S., Rogers, C., Mathur, A. M., Van Essen, D. C., & Inder, T. (2014). Alterations in brain structure and neurodevelopmental outcome in preterm infants hospitalized in different neonatal intensive care unit environments. *The Journal of Pediatrics, 164*(1), 52–60.e2. https://doi.org/10.1016/j.jpeds.2013.08.047

Plsek, P. E., & Greenhalgh, T. (2001). The challenge of complexity in health care. *British Medical Journal, 323*, 625–628.

Porges, S. W., Davila, M. I., Lewis, G. F., Kolacz, J., Okonmah-Obazee, S., Hane, A. A., Kwon, K. Y., Ludwig, R. J., Myers, M. M., & Welch, M. G. (2019). Autonomic regulation of preterm infants is enhanced by Family Nurture Intervention. *Developmental Psychobiology, 61*(6), 942–952. https://doi.org/10.1002/dev.21841

Preyde, M., & Ardal, F. (2003). Effectiveness of a parent "buddy" program for mothers of very preterm infants in a neonatal intensive care unit. *Canadian Medical Association Journal, 168*, 969–973.

Provenzi, L., Giusti, L., Fumagalli, M., Frigerio, S., Morandi, F., Borgatti, R., Mosca, F., & Montirosso, R. (2019). The dual nature of hypothalamic-pituitary-adrenal axis regulation in dyads of very preterm infants and their mothers. *Psychoneuroendocrinology, 100*, 172–179. https://doi.org/10.1016/j.psyneuen.2018.10.007

Provenzi, L., & Santoro, E. (2015). The lived experience of fathers of preterm infants in the Neonatal Intensive Care Unit: A systematic review of qualitative studies. *Journal of Clinical Nursing, 24*(13–14), 1784–1794.

Purdy, I. B., Craig, J. W., & Zeanah, P. (2015). NICU discharge planning and beyond: Recommendations for parent psychosocial support. *Journal of Perinatology, 35*(Suppl. 1), S24–S28. https://doi.org/10.1038/jp.2015.146

Ramm, K., Mannix, T., Parry, Y., & Gaffney, M. P. (2017). A comparison of sound levels in open plan versus pods in a Neonatal Intensive Care Unit. *Health Environments Research & Design Journal, 10*(3), 30–39.

Ravn, I. H., Smith, L., Lindemann, R., Smeby, N. A., Kyno, N. M., Bunch, E. H., & Sandvick, I. (2011). Effect of early intervention on social interaction between mothers and preterm infants at 12 months of age: A randomized controlled trial. *Infant Behavior and Development, 34*, 215–225.

Reeves, S., Pelone, F., Harrison, R., Goldman, J., & Zwarenstein, M. (2017). Interprofessional collaboration to improve professional practice and healthcare outcomes. *Cochrane Database of Systematic Review, 6*, CD000072. https://doi.org/10.1002/14651858.CD000072.pub3

Roudebush, J. R., Kaufman, J., Johnson, B. H., Abraham, M. R., & Clayton, S. P. (2006). Patient-and family-centered perinatal care: Partnerships with childbearing women and families. *The Journal of Perinatal & Neonatal Nursing, 20*(3), 201–209.

Roue, J. M., Kuhn, P., Lopez Maestro, M., Maastrup, R. A., Mitanchez, D., Westrup, B., & Sizun, J. (2017). Eight principles for patient-centred and family-centred care for newborns in the Neonatal Intensive Care Unit. *Archives of Disease in Childhood - Fetal and Neonatal Edition, 102*(4), F364–F368. https://doi.org/10.1136/archdischild-2016-312180

Scar-Salapatek, S., & Williams, M. L. (1973). Early stimulation based on a deprivation construct. *Child Development, 44*(1), 94–101. https://doi.org/10.2307/1127684

Shaw, C., Stokoe, E., Gallagher, K., Aladangady, N., & Marlow, N. (2016). Parental involvement in neonatal critical care decision-making. *Sociology of Health and Illness, 38*(8), 1217–1242. https://doi.org/10.1111/1467-9566.12455

Sigurdson, K., Mitchell, B., Liu, J., Morton, C., Gould, J. B., Lee, H. C., Capdarest-Arest, N., & Profit, J. (2019). Racial/ethnic disparities in neonatal intensive care: A systematic review. *Pediatrics, 144*(2), e20183114. https://doi.org/10.1542/peds.2018-3114

Smith, G. C., Gutovich, J., Smyser, C., Pineda, R., Newnham, C., Tjoeng, T. H., Vavasseur, C., Wallendorf, M., Neil, J., & Inder, T. (2011). Neonatal intensive care unit stress is associated with brain development in preterm infants. *Annals of Neurology, 70*(4), 541–549. https://doi.org/10.1002/ana.22545

Soleimani, F., Azari, N., Ghiasvand, H., Shahrokhi, A., Rahmani, N., & Fatollahierad, S. (2020). Do NICU developmental care improve cognitive and motor outcomes for preterm infants? A systematic review and meta-analysis. *BMC Pediatrics, 20*(1), 67. https://doi.org/10.1186/s12887-020-1953-1

Spence, K. (2016). Historical trends in neonatal nursing: Developmental care and NIDCAP. *Journal of Perinatal and Neonatal Nursing, 30*(3), 273–276.

Stevens, D. C., Helseth, C. C., & Kurtz, J. C. (2010). *Achieving success in supporting parents and families in the neonatal intensive care unit.* In *Developmental care of newborns & infants: A guide for health professionals* (2nd ed., pp. 161–190). National Association of Neonatal Nurses (NANN).

Stuebe, A. (2020). Should infants be separated from mothers with COVID-19? First, do no harm. *Breastfeeding Medicine, 15*(5), 351–352. https://doi.org/10.1089/bfm.2020.29153.ams

Tallon, M. M., Kendall, G. E., & Snider, P. D. (2015). Rethinking family-centred care for the child and family in hospital. *Journal of Clinical Nursing, 24*(9–10), 1426–1435. https://doi.org/10.1111/jocn.12799

Thiele, N., Knierim, N., & Mader, S. (2016). Parents as partners in care: Seven guiding principles to ease the collaboration. *Newborn and Infant Nursing Reviews, 16*, 66–68.

Thoma, M. E., Drew, L. B., Hirai, A. H., Kim, T. Y., Fenelon, A., & Shenassa, E. D. (2019). Black-white disparities in preterm birth: Geographic, social, and health determinants. *American Journal of Preventive Medicine, 57*(5), 675–686. https://doi.org/10.1016/j.amepre.2019.07.007

Thoman, E. B., Ingersoll, E. W., & Acebo, C. (1991). Premature infants seek rhythmic stimulation, and the experience facilitates neurobehavioral development. *Journal of Developmental and Behavioral Pediatrics, 12*(1), 11–18.

Thoyre, S., Park, J., Pados, B., & Hubbard, C. (2013). Developing a co-regulated, cue-based feeding practice: The critical role of assessment and reflection. *Journal of Neonatal Nursing, 19*(4), 139–148. https://doi.org/10.1016/j.jnn.2013.01.002

Toivonen, M., Lehtonen, L., Löyttyniemi, E., Ahlqvist-Björkroth, S., & Axelin, A. (2020). Close collaboration with parents intervention improves family-centered care in different neonatal unit contexts: A pre-post study. *Pediatric Research, 88*(3), 421–428. https://doi.org/10.1038/s41390-020-0934-2

Trajkovski, S., Schmied, V., Vickers, M., & Jackson, D. (2015). Using appreciative inquiry to bring neonatal nurses and parents together to enhance family-centred care: A collaborative workshop. *Journal of Child Health Care, 19*(2), 239–253. https://doi.org/10.1177/1367493513508059

Trivedi, D. (2015). Cochrane Review Summary: Massage for promoting mental and physical health in typically developing infants under the age of six months. *Primary Health Care Research & Development, 16*(1), 3–4. https://doi.org/10.1017/s1463423614000462

Tucker, C. M., Herman, K. C., Pedersen, T. R., Higley, B., Montrichard, M., & Ivery, P. (2003). Cultural sensitivity in physician-patient relationships: Perspectives of an ethnically diverse sample of low-income primary care patients. *Medical Care, 41*(7), 859–870. https://doi.org/10.1097/00005650-200307000-00010

Umberger, E., Canvasser, J., & Hall, S. L. (2018). Enhancing NICU parent engagement and empowerment. *Seminars in Pediatric Surgery, 27*(1), 19–24. https://doi.org/10.1053/j.sempedsurg.2017.11.004

Van Riper, M. (2001). Family-provider relationships and well-being in families with preterm infants in the NICU. *Heart & Lung, 30*(1), 74–84. https://doi.org/10.1067/mhl.2001.110625

Vance, A. J., McGrath, J. M., & Brandon, D. (2018). Where you are born really does matter: Why birth hospital and quality of care contribute to racial/ethnic disparities. *Advances in Neonatal Care, 18*(2), 81–82. https://doi.org/10.1097/anc.0000000000000480

Vetulani, J. (2013). Early maternal separation: A rodent model of depression and a prevailing human condition. *Pharmacological Reports, 65*(6), 1451–1461.

Vohr, B. R. (2014). Neurodevelopmental outcomes of extremely preterm infants. *Clinics in Perinatology, 41*(1), 241–255. https://doi.org/10.1016/j.clp.2013.09.003

Vohr, B. R. (2019). The importance of parent presence and involvement in the single-family room and open-bay NICU. *Acta Paediatrica, 108*(6), 986–988. https://doi.org/10.1111/apa.14783

Weber, A., Harrison, T. M., Steward, D., & Ludington-Hoe, S. (2018). Paid family leave to enhance the health outcomes of preterm infants. *Policy, Politics, & Nursing Practice, 19*(1-2), 11–28. https://doi.org/10.1177/1527154418791821

Weiss, E. M., Olszewski, A. E., Guttmann, K. F., Magnus, B. E., Li, S., Shah, A. R., Juul, S. E., Wu, Y. W., Ahmad, K. A., Bendel-Stenzel, E., Isaza, N. A., Lampland, A. L., Mathur, A. M., Rao, R., Riley, D., Russell, D. G., Salih, Z. N. I., Torr, C. B., Weitkamp, J.-H, … Shah, S. K. (2021). Parental factors associated with the decision to participate in a neonatal clinical trial. *JAMA Network Open, 4*(1), e2032106. https://doi.org/10.1001/jamanetworkopen.2020.32106

Welch, M. G., Barone, J. L., Porges, S. W., Hane, A. A., Kwon, K. Y., Ludwig, R. J., Stark, R. I., Surman, A. L., Kolacz, J., & Myers, M. M. (2020). Family nurture intervention in the NICU increases autonomic regulation in mothers and children at 4-5 years of age: Follow-up results from a randomized controlled trial. *PLoS One, 15*(8), e0236930. https://doi.org/10.1371/journal.pone.0236930

Welch, M. G., Hofer, M. A., Brunelli, S. A., Stark, R. I., Andrews, H. F., Austin, J., & Myers, M. M. (2012). Family nurture intervention (FNI): Methods and treatment protocol of a randomized controlled trial in the NICU. *BMC Pediatrics, 12*, 14. https://doi.org/10.1186/1471-2431-12-14

Westrup, B. (2007). Newborn Individualized Developmental Care and Assessment Program (NIDCAP)—Family-centered developmentally supportive care. *Early Human Development, 83*(7), 443–449. https://doi.org/10.1016/j.earlhumdev.2007.03.006

Westrup, B. (2015). Family-centered developmentally supportive care: The Swedish example. *Archives de Pediatrie, 22*(10), 1086–1091. https://doi.org/10.1016/j.arcped.2015.07.005

White, J. L., & Labarba, R. C. (1976). The effects of tactile and kinesthetic stimulation on neonatal development in the premature infant. *Developmental Psychobiology, 9*(6), 569–577. https://doi.org/10.1002/dev.420090610

White, R. D. (2020a). Recommended standards for newborn ICU design, 9th edition. *Journal of Perinatology, 40*(Suppl. 1), 2–4. https://doi.org/10.1038/s41372-020-0766-2

White, R. D. (2020b). Right lighting the NICU. *Acta Paediatrica, 109*(7), 1288–1289. https://doi.org/10.1111/apa.15193

White, R. D., Smith, J. A., & Shepley, M. M. (2013). Recommended standards for newborn ICU design, eighth edition. *Journal of Perinatology, 33*(Suppl. 1), S2–S16. https://doi.org/10.1038/jp.2013.10

Wigert, H., Dellenmark, M. B., & Bry, K. (2013). Strengths and weaknesses of parent-staff communication in the NICU: A survey assessment. *BMC Pediatrics, 13*, 71.

Wilson, T., Holt, T., & Greenhalgh, T. (2001). Complexity science: Complexity and clinical care. *British Medical Journal, 323*(7314), 685–688.

World Health Organization (WHO). (2015). *The global strategy for women's, children's and adolescents' health (2016-2030): Survive, thrive, transform.* Every Woman Every Child [EWEC].

CHAPTER 1 APPENDIX

Panel's Foundational Process Decisions

Concepts and terms were identified and defined based on evidence and group consensus. The committee elected to:

- Reference the "baby," rather than "infant," through the document as the term "baby" is more familiar to parents, families, and staff, thus making this content more relevant.
- Use "parents" and "family members" interchangeably to denote the primary caregiver.
- Refer to intensive care, consistent with the definition of newborn *intensive care* used by White and Colleagues.[a]
- Refer to intermediate care as less intensive observation/monitoring by professional staff.
- Include subspecialty intensive care units managed by neonatal, cardiac, neuro, and/or pediatric services where babies are cared for.

Recommend that interprofessional teams collaborate to provide standardized IFCDC, regardless of the unit location or specialty service.

Scientific Process for the Infant and Family-Centered Developmental Care (IFCDC) Consensus Panel

A consensus panel of international interprofessional experts and parents representing multiple professional organizations formed to:

- Study the concept, practice, and outcomes of developmental care.
- Discuss essential principles that needed to be addressed.
- Articulate essential principles and develop a model for IFCDC.
- Conduct systematic review of Medline, CINAHL, Cochrane Databases, and Web of Science studies.
- Identify and search with initial search terms pertinent to IFCDC.[b]
- Integrate six resulting essential evidence-based practice exemplars into aspects of the model.
- Expand search terms resulting from the initial search findings.[c]

Evaluation of the Evidence

- Collect and review over 1,200 articles, policy statements, and professional websites.
- Create and utilize a consensus process to assess quality and strength of collected evidence.
- Select 900 appropriate articles resulting in 450 cited in the report.
- Evaluate quality of evidence depending on the quality designated in the category which ranged from I to VII (Melnyk & Fineout-Overholt, 2019).
  - Shared website library used to review, level, and assess the evidence.
  - Much of selected evidence was descriptive, qualitative studies and reports (low to moderate grade).
  - Identified research was retrospective analyses using standardized procedural guidelines and clinical evaluation data.
- Exclude developmental practices with insufficient credible evidence and/or weak evidence.
- Determine strength of resulting evidence through committee consensus. Consensus was that evidence was strong (Centre, 2009).
- Prepare an integrative literature review for each concept, principle, term definition, subtopic area, and applicable best practice.
- Present process and content at the Gravens Conference for review, comment, and assessment of applicability to practice in the intensive care unit.
- Gather responses from over 250 international interprofessional and parent attendees over four years and make revisions based on responses.
- Obtain review from national and international external content experts from their respective professional fields.
- Assess each comment, recommendation, edit suggestion, and change; and revise as appropriate with regard to the evidence.
- Prepare and distribute the resulting IFCDC Standards, Competencies and Best Practice Guidelines on the web platform https://nicudesign.nd.edu/nicu-care-standards/.
- Publish an Executive Summary of the committee's work and conclusions (Browne, et al., 2020).

[a]*"care for medically unstable or critically ill newborns requiring constant nursing, complicated surgical procedures, continual respiratory support or other intensive interventions"* (White, et al., 2013, p. S5).

[b]**Initial search terms** developmental care, neonate, and infant.

[c]**Expanded search terms** based practice, neuroprotection, brain development, systems, systems thinking, intensive care, interprofessional collaboration, emotional intelligence, transition to home, discharge, continuing care, infant-centered, family-centered, parenting, infant mental health, mother–infant dyad, NICU design, infant positioning, infant touch, infant sleep, sleep states, activity states, infant arousal, skin-to-skin contact, kangaroo care, kangaroo mother care, neonatal pain, neonatal pain therapeutics, nonpharmacologic pain management, stress management, communication, posttraumatic stress disorder, psychosocial management, feeding, breast-feeding, nutrition delivery, health disparity, COVID-19.

The Infant and Family-Centered Developmental Care Standards for Babies in Intensive Care and Their Families

Carol B. Jaeger and Joy V. Browne

INTRODUCTION

The Infant and Family-Centered Developmental Care (IFCDC) Consensus Committee utilized credible evidence to identify standards and measurable competencies for each of six sections of practice—systems thinking in complex adaptive systems; positioning and touch for the newborn; sleep and arousal interventions for the newborn; skin-to-skin contact (SSC) with intimate family members; reducing and managing pain and stress in newborns and families; and feeding, eating, and nutrition delivery—the evidence and process outlined in the previous chapter (Care, 2020). The standards of each practice section are articulated in this chapter followed by a descriptive summary along with specific benefits and risks for each section of cited evidence-based practice. Both standards and related competencies can be found at the website https://nicudesign.nd.edu/nicu-care-standards/.

Checklists have been created using points to consider when implementing each practice section. These checklists can be found in the appendix along with suggestions of opportunities for reflection on an intensive care unit's (ICU's) current practice regarding the IFCDC evidence-based standards (Consensus Committee on Infant and Family Centered Developmental Care, 2020). The checklists can be used to regularly chart progress toward greater integration of developmental care practices as well as to consider where more growth is needed and what opportunities there are to focus the work in a particular setting. The remaining chapters of this edition provide evidence and implementation opportunities for each appropriate standard. We purposely "choose" to use "baby" instead of infant or neonate throughout this chapter and others to refocus this work such that the parents and family are central to the delivery of developmental care.

IFCDC STANDARDS IN COMPLEX ADAPTIVE SYSTEMS

Standard 1: The ICU shall exhibit an infrastructure of leadership, mission, and a governance framework to guide the performance of the collaborative practice of IFCDC.

Standard 2: The ICU shall provide a professionally competent interprofessional collaborative practice team to support the baby, parent, and family's holistic physical, developmental, and psychosocial needs from birth through the transition of hospital discharge to home and assure continuity to follow-up care.

Standard 3: The practice of IFCDC in the ICU shall be based on evidence that is ethical, safe, timely, quality driven, efficient, equitable, and cost-effective.

Standard 4: The ICU practice and outcomes will provide evidence that demonstrates the continuous monitoring of information relative to IFCDC practice.

Standard 5: The interprofessional collaborative practice team shall be transparent regarding the access and use of medical equipment, devices, and products; medications and vaccines; and technologies related to the IFCDC care in an in-patient setting, home, and the community.

Standard 6: The interprofessional collaborative team should provide IFCDC through transition to home and continuing care for the baby and family to support the optimal physiologic and psychosocial health needs of the baby and family (Kenner & Jaeger, 2020).

The system vision, culture, and practice should reflect the seamless integration of the values of IFCDC—systems thinking, individualized care, baby as a competent communicator and interactor, family involvement, environmental protection, neuroprotection of the developing brain, and infant mental health. In 2005, Westrup stated "We believe that focusing on *respect* for the very tiny and often fragile *human being* and his or her *family* not only is *essential* for the further *improvement of medical care* and *developmental outcome*…but is *important* from a *humane point of view*" (Westrup, 2005, 2007). The "humane point of view" is a perspective that must not be lost in our quest for hard evidence (Levin, 1999).

The evidence has demonstrated clear benefits and risks of implementing developmental care in the ICU. The baby, family and ICU unit are holistic systems that interact with each other (Douglas et al., 2011; Wilson et al., 2001). Without use of these systems standards and competencies, the benefits will not be realized and the risks will be amplified.

When the baby or family is negatively influenced, and the communication is lacking, there can be delays in healing (Berman et al., 2019). The result can be an increase in the hospital length of stay and/or a less-than-positive short-term or long-term outcome (Berman et al., 2019). The parent presence with the baby in the ICU is essential to nurture and provide care (Govindaswamy et al., 2018); otherwise, the parents are ill-prepared to manage the baby and their family (Boykova, 2016; Guillaume et al., 2013). The interprofessional team needs an open collaborative relationship with the family to learn together, build trust, and maintain a realistic perspective of the baby's outcome (Archer et al., 2012; Cleveland, 2008; Coughlin et al., 2009). Shared decision-making between the team and the parents strengthens the confidence in their ability to care for their baby at home (Craig et al., 2015; Johnson, 2016; Umberger et al., 2018).

Cultural humility and inclusivity within the ICU are vital to better understand the needs of babies and their families (Brooks et al., 2013). Without it there is a likelihood of bias, limited communication, increased staff ratios, and missed care. Lake and colleagues report higher staff ratios (Lake et al., 2018), Louis-Jacques describes inadequate breastfeeding support (Louis-Jacques et al., 2017), and Sigurdson and Beck identify disparities disadvantaging African American babies (Beck et al., 2020; Sigurdson et al., 2019). Much more work is needed to best support cultural inequities and decrease disparities in these populations.

The baby communicates his or her individualized needs through expressions and behavior, and age-appropriate developmental core competencies should be performed in response to the baby's needs by a nurturing caregiver. Variation in time, application, and caregiver can disrupt the healing process for the baby in the context of the family (Table 2-1).

Section Summary: The ICU system is the sum of its component parts, and systems thinking is an overarching process when implementing developmental family-centered care. Systems thinking is the critical process used collaboratively by interprofessional staff and parents to engage in the care planning, decision-making, and caregiving of the baby. It is a framework from which to build a dynamic culture that integrates the vision, values, policies and procedures, education,

TABLE 2-1 Benefit and Risk of Implementing Systems Standards

Benefit	Risk
• Holistic–positive influence of baby and family system. • Parent presence. • Collaboration. • Shared decision-making. • Culture of humility and inclusivity.	• Delayed response/failure to interpret baby and family needs leading to increased length of stay (LOS) or lesser outcome. • Unprepared for nurturing and managing baby within the family system at home. • Lack of trust and knowledge and depression. • Poor communication, stress, and self-doubt. • Bias, high staff ratios, and missed care.

performance competencies, and collaborative team of the ICU to implement developmental care.

Given the overarching nature of systems thinking, the application of this process to the following five (Liu et al., 2007) evidence-based IFCDC practice standards and competencies is articulated in each respective section.

IFCDC STANDARDS FOR POSITIONING AND TOUCH FOR THE NEWBORN

Standard 1: Babies in intensive care settings shall be positioned to support musculoskeletal, physiological, and behavioral stability.

Standard 2: Collaborative efforts among parents and ICU interprofessionals shall support optimal cranial shaping and prevent torticollis and skull deformity.

Standard 3: Body position shall be used as an ICU intervention for infants with gastrointestinal symptoms.

Standard 4: Babies in ICU settings shall experience human touch by family and caregivers (Sweeney & McElroy, 2020).

Picheansathian and Romantsik caution about the risk of cranial misshaping, torticollis, poor sleep, intraventricular hemorrhaging, and gastroesophageal reflux when babies are not positioned appropriately to support healing and maturation (Picheansathian et al., 2009; Romantsik et al., 2017). Hartley and Pillai Riddell identify that gentle touch assists with pain management during some medical procedures, such as endotracheal suctioning (Hartley et al., 2015; Pillai Riddell et al., 2015). The calming effects of touch decreases heart rate and increases rapid eye movement sleep (Smith, 2012). The risk of overstimulation with touch, especially with low-gestational-age babies, can be bradycardia and oxygen desaturation (Cone et al., 2013) (Table 2-2).

TABLE 2-2 Benefit and Risk of Implementing Positioning and Touch Standards	
Benefit	Risk
• Musculoskeletal, physiologic, and behavioral stability. • Experience human touch–synchronize with baby's physiological and behavioral patterns.	• Cranial misshaping, torticollis, poor sleep, intraventricular hemorrhaging, gastroesophageal. • Increased stress and poor self-regulation of behavior during procedures.

TABLE 2-3 Benefit and Risk of Implementing Sleep and Arousal Interventions	
Benefit	Risk
• CNS plasticity and neuronal circuitry. • Cortical and subcortical brain activation patterns. • Regulation of sleep and wake states and arousal from sleep to wake.	• Poor neurodevelopment associated with hypoxic–ischemic encephalopathy, congenital heart disease, neonatal abstinence syndrome, inborn errors of metabolism, chronic lung disease.

Systems thinking is used to monitor and document observations of behavior indicating readiness for positional change and gentle touch. It is used to educate the parents about positional guidance and system maturation.

Section Summary: The practice of positioning and touch for the baby includes significant benefits and potential risks. Varied body positions are indicated for postural alignment, extremity movement, and physiological stability with repositioning at 3- to 4-hour intervals (Madlinger-Lewis et al., 2014; Vaivre-Douret et al., 2004; Zahed et al., 2015).

IFCDC STANDARDS OF SLEEP AND AROUSAL INTERVENTIONS FOR THE NEWBORN

Standard 1: ICUs shall promote developmentally appropriate sleep and arousal states and sleep–wake cycles.

Standard 2: The ICU shall provide modifications to the physical environment and to caregiving routines that are specifically focused on optimization of sleep and arousal of ICU babies.

Standard 3: The ICU shall encourage family presence at the baby's bedside and family participation in the care of their baby.

Standard 4: Interprofessional team members shall review trends in documented arousal and sleep as part of routine data presented on rounds, within the context of feeding and weight gain/energy conservation and parent involvement in care.

Standard 5: Families shall be provided multiple opportunities to observe and interpret their baby's states of arousal and sleep and to practice safe sleep positioning, to support successful parent–infant participation in care routines during the transition home (Bigsby & Salisbury, 2020).

Sleep and arousal intervention for the newborn is essential for healing. Interpreting the communication and behavior of the baby helps assist the baby to achieve the quantity and quality of sleep needed to grow and develop. From preterm to term, the baby will establish predictable age-related patterns of sleep and arousal. These changes reflect maturation in the central nervous system (CNS) as well as coordination of the peripheral nervous system. Sleep may facilitate the CNS plasticity through enhanced production of the structures involved in building the neuronal circuitry (Bennet et al., 2018; Yang & Gan, 2012). Sleep-state organization is the ability to transition smoothly between states of sleep and wakefulness and to regulate the transition between states of alertness (Bueno & Menna-Barreto, 2016; Takenouchi et al., 2011; Weisman et al., 2011). These capabilities reflect maturation, including predictable cortical and subcortical brain activation patterns (Anders & Keener, 1985; Chu et al., 2014). Shellhaas and Barbeau report that poor neurodevelopment can be associated with hypoxic-ischemic encephalopathy, congenital heart disease, neonatal abstinence syndrome, inborn errors of metabolism, and chronic lung disease (Barbeau & Weiss, 2017; Shellhaas et al., 2018) (Table 2-3).

Systems thinking is used to minimize environmental distractions, cycle light consistent with age-appropriateness, and adjust the physical space for the comfort of the parent. Observe, assess, and document the baby's behavior and response. Engage the parents in nurturing and care.

Section Summary: Sleep and gentle arousal provide healing benefits to the baby. However, disrupting the baby's natural process causes biophysical and neurodevelopmental consequences.

IFCDC STANDARDS FOR SKIN-TO-SKIN CONTACT WITH INTIMATE FAMILY MEMBERS

Standard 1: Parents shall be encouraged and supported in early, frequent, and prolonged SSC with their babies.

Standard 2: Education and policies in support of SSC between parents and their baby shall be developed, implemented, monitored, and evaluated by an interprofessional collaborative team.

Standard 3: Babies shall be evaluated to (a) determine their readiness for transfer to Kangaroo Care (KC); (b) assess stability during transfer from bed to parent's chest; (c) assess baby's response to SSC (KC or Hand Containment); and (d) assess their stability during and after transfer back to the bed.

Standard 4: Parents shall be provided information about the benefits of SSC that continue for babies and parents after discharge (Phillips & Smith, 2020).

Parents should be encouraged to have early, frequent, and prolonged SSC with their baby whenever possible. They may need support to engage with their baby and instruction to position the baby in proper alignment. Simulation learning with a mannequin may be helpful prior to holding the baby. The staff can be helpful teaching the therapeutic benefits of SSC, such as brain and neurodevelopment (Head, 2014), increased physiologic stability (Chi Luong et al., 2016), less stress and feeling of pain (Johnston et al., 2017; Vittner et al., 2018), better feeding tolerance and growth (Evereklian & Posmontier, 2017; Gianni et al., 2016), and early and longer duration of breastfeeding (Boundy et al., 2016; Casper et al., 2018). In addition, staff will want to show parents the behavior their baby exhibits when relaxed and stressed to learn the communication and behavior of their baby. Studies by Conde-Agudelo and Boundy have demonstrated a decreased incidence of sepsis and mortality in babies experiencing SSC (Boundy et al., 2016; Conde-Agudelo & Diaz-Rosselio, 2016).

The risks of the parent and baby not engaging in SSC include separation anxiety for lack of the nurturing experience for the baby and mother (Vittner et al., 2018), poor parent–infant attachment (Feldman et al., 2014; Neu & Robinson, 2010; Tessier et al., 1998), and a decrease in oxytocin and prolactin levels in mothers resulting in decreased milk production (Cong et al., 2015; Sriraman, 2017). Parents want the sensation of natural closeness with their baby to feel like a parent (Table 2-4).

Systems thinking is used during the implementation of SSC. Creating an environment of privacy, physical comfort, and minimized distractions is important. Preparing the parent for the experience and demonstrating handling and positioning of the baby prompt engagement and empower the parent as a caregiver and decision maker. The experience is

a powerful symbiotic example of biologic, physiologic, and environmental interaction.

Section Summary: Holding/touching the baby is essential to the process of attachment for the m/other and parent partner. The benefits are compelling. Likewise, the risk of separation or interruption to this process can be disastrous for the baby and the parent.

IFCDC STANDARDS FOR REDUCING AND MANAGING PAIN AND STRESS IN NEWBORNS AND FAMILIES

Standard 1: The interprofessional team shall document increased parental/caregiver well-being and decreased emotional distress during the intensive care hospital (Consensus Committee on Infant and Family Centered Developmental Care, 2020) stay. Distress levels of baby's siblings and extended family should also be considered.

Standard 2: The interprofessional collaborative team shall develop care practices that prioritize multiple methods to optimize baby outcomes by minimizing the impact of stressful and painful stimuli (Hynan et al., 2020).

Reducing pain and stress in families and babies is essential to healing and well-being. Realizing that the baby and the parents are stressed with worry and fear in a foreign environment, the staff should be mindful to assess parents for symptoms of poor adjustment, attachment, and nurturing (Craig et al., 2015; Hall et al., 2017; Hynan et al., 2015; Lester et al., 2016; O'Brien et al., 2013). A lack of confidence interacting with the baby in an ICU setting is not unnatural at first, but withdrawal from relationships and a loss of self-confidence in daily interactions suggest the need for a mental health assessment and intervention (Aftyka et al., 2017). The collaborative team should have interprofessionals readily available to manage psychosocial situations with parents and families, to include economic concerns. Systems thinking involves realizing the impact of multiple factors influencing the ability of the parent and family to manage the stressful event of a hospitalization and potential long-term management of chronic concerns.

Babies do demonstrate responses of stress and pain. It is important that staff share with parents the unique responses of their baby so that they can actively participate in the assessment, caregiving, and decision-making for their baby. Managing stress and pain in a premature or sick baby is crucial to the baby's biophysiologic, neurodevelopmental, and psychosocial healing and maturation (Anand et al., 2006; Carbajal et al., 2008, 2015). Nonpharmacologic measures of management are preferable to pharmacologic therapeutics (Johnston et al., 2017; Pillai Riddell et al., 2011, 2015; Shah et al., 2012; Yin et al., 2015). Vinall and Grunau, Doesburg, and Hermann describe adverse responses to pain and stress that can negatively impact the short-term and long-term outcomes of the baby (Doesburg et al., 2013; Hermann et al., 2006; Johnston et al., 2014; Pillai Riddell et al., 2011, 2015; Shah et al., 2012;

TABLE 2-4 Benefit and Risk of Implementing Skin-to-Skin Contact With Intimate Family Members

Benefit	Risk
• Brain and neurodevelopment. • Reduced mortality. • Increased physiologic stability. • Less stress/pain. • Greater feeding tolerance. • Increased growth. • Early and longer duration of breastfeeding. • Reduced incidence of sepsis.	• Separation causing increased stress for m/other and baby. • Poor parent–infant attachment. • Decreased oxytocin and prolactin levels in mothers resulting in reduced milk production.

TABLE 2-5 Benefit and Risk of Implementing Interventions to Reduce and Manage Pain and Stress

Benefit	Risk
• Parent/family well-being–assessment, support, and intervention. • Nonpharmacologic measures to decrease baby's stress/pain, i.e., nonnutritive sucking opportunities, skin-to-skin contact. • Enhanced parent–baby relationships.	• Increased stress and anxiety, i.e., poor adjustment, self-doubt, and poor attachment and nurturing. • Adverse response to pain and stress and poor outcome. • Parental stress and mental health affect social and emotional development.

Vinall & Grunau, 2014; Yin et al., 2015). Some nonpharmacologic measures that can decrease pain and stress in the baby are nonnutritive sucking opportunities and SSC with the parent (Johnston et al., 2014; Pillai Riddell et al., 2011, 2015; Shah et al., 2012; Yin et al., 2015) (Table 2-5).

Systems thinking guides the process to strengthen parent and baby relationships by engaging parents in the caregiving (Hynan & Hall, 2015; Pineda et al., 2018) and manage parent stress and mental health (Feldman & Eidelman, 2007). The baby and parents are the sustaining family unit that the team must teach and support.

Section Summary: The promotion of healing is best served through comfort and calm. Pain, stress, and anxiety can be disruptive to the biophysical, neurodevelopmental, and psychosocial short-term and long-term outcomes of the baby and the family.

IFCDC STANDARDS FOR FEEDING, EATING, AND NUTRITION DELIVERY

Standard 1: Feeding experiences in the ICU (Consensus Committee on Infant and Family Centered Developmental Care, 2020) shall be behavior based and baby led. Baby-led principles are similar whether applied to enteral-, breast-, or bottle-feeding experience.

Standard 2: Every mother shall be encouraged and supported to breastfeed and/or provide human milk for her baby.

Standard 3: Nutrition shall be optimized during the ICU period.

Standard 4: M/others shall be supported to be the primary feeders of their baby.

Standard 5: Caregiving activities shall consider baby's response to input, especially around face/mouth, and aversive non-critical care oral experiences shall be minimized.

Standard 6: Professional staff shall consider smell and taste experiences that are biologically expected.

Standard 7: Support of baby's self-regulation shall be encouraged, especially as it relates to sucking for comfort.

Standard 8: Environments shall be supportive of an attuned feeding for both the feeder and the baby.

Standard 9: Feeding management shall focus on establishing safe oral feedings that are comfortable and enjoyable.

Standard 10: ICUs shall include interprofessional perspectives to provide best feeding management.

Standard 11: Feeding management shall consider short- and long-term growth and feeding outcomes (Ross et al., 2020).

The primary tenet of infant and family-centered developmental care is the importance of recognizing and responding to the communication and behavior of the baby. Caregiving that responds to these behaviors has been shown by Als and others to result in improved baby outcomes (Als, 1986; Als et al., 2003). The risk of not responding to the messaging of the baby is poor feeding and growth, decreased weight, anxiety, and poor neurodevelopmental maturation (Horta et al., 2015; Lennon, 2011).

Meier, Ellsbury, Kumar, and Gregory emphasize the protective benefits of breastmilk or human milk and the psychosocial support of the mother's nurturing during the feeding (Ellsbury et al., 2016; Gregory et al., 2016; Kumar et al., 2017; Meier et al., 2010). The mother's role as the primary feeder should be encouraged and supported. Her experience should be comfortable, calm, and free of distraction to promote a sense of competence (Brown & Pickler, 2013; Deloian, 1998). Padovani reports that distractions and lack of positive support for the mother and baby can lead to poor short-term and long-term outcomes (Padovani et al., 2011). The baby may exhibit instability and decreased efficiency and endurance, leading to consuming less volume (Thoyre & Brown, 2004; Thoyre et al., 2012; Thoyre et al., 2016). The feeding plan should be mother-driven and developed in collaboration with the parents (Jadcherla et al., 2012, 2015). The relationship between the interprofessional team and the parents should be built on trust, respect, and open communication (Table 2-6).

TABLE 2-6 Benefit and Risk of Implementing Interventions to Manage Feeding, Eating, and Nutrition Delivery

Benefit	Risk
• Behavior based and baby led. • Breastmilk (BM) or human milk (HM). • M/other competence as the primary feeder in a comfortable, calm, distraction-free environment. • Feeding plan developed collaboratively with parents and team.	• Poor feeding, growth, neurodevelopmental outcomes. • Lack of BM/HM protective benefits and psychosocial support. • Decreased weight of baby, anxiety and stress. • Distracted m/other and/or baby with poor outcome. • Baby instability, inefficiency, less endurance, reduced volume.

The use of systems thinking in managing the eating, feeding, and nutrition delivery process for the baby and parent stresses the importance of communicating, planning, interacting, and evaluating outcomes with the interprofessional team. Simulation learning may be helpful to parents as they manage the feeding experience with their baby. Adapting to the changing condition and maturation of the baby is important to the psychological well-being of the parents and family.

Section Summary: Feeding is a nurturing process that is often interrupted during the care of sick and premature babies. The risk of disruption is significant to the growth and well-being of the baby, and the psychosocial attachment process and well-being of the m/other and partner.

CONCLUSION

The benefits of implementing evidence-based IFCDC standards are well substantiated, and the risk of not implementing these standards is also well documented. Evidence-based infant and family-centered developmental care is ESSENTIAL to the short-term and long-term physical, mental, and social well-being of the baby and family, and without attention to the systematic implementation of these standards, outcomes can be compromised. Developmental care makes a positive DIFFERENCE to the baby, parents, and family from birth through the baby's lifespan. Developmental care needs to be INTEGRATED with medical protocols/guidelines. Developmental care cannot be discounted. Influencers and distractors must be effectively managed using current credible evidence to maintain the value of developmental care.

REFERENCES

Aftyka, A., Rybojad, B., Rosa, W., Wrobel, A., & Karakula-Juchnowicz, H. (2017). Risk factors for the development of posttraumatic stress disorder and coping strategies in mothers and fathers following infant hospitalization in the neonatal intensive care unit. *Journal of Clinical Nursing, 26,* 338–347.

Als, H. (1986). *A synactive model of neonatal behavioral organization: Framework for the assessment of neurobehavioral development in the premature infant and for support of infants and parents in the neonatal intensive care environment.* In *The high-risk neonate: Developmental therapy perspectives* (pp. 3–53). The Haworth Press.

Als, H., Gilkerson, L., Duffy, F., Mc Anulty, G., Buehler, D., Vandenberg, K., Sweet, N., Sell, E., Parad, R. B., Ringer, S. A., Butler, S. C., Blickman, J. G., & Jones, K. J. (2003). A three-center, randomized, controlled trial of individualized developmental care for very low birth weight preterm infants: Medical, neurodevelopmental, parenting, and caregiving effects. *Journal of Developmental Behavioral Pediatrics, 24*(6), 399–408.

Anand, K. J., Aranda, J. V., Berde, C. B., Buckman, S., Capparelli, E. V., Carlo, W., Hummel, P., Johnston, C. C., Lantos, J., Tutag-Lehr, V., Lynn, A. M., Maxwell, L. G., Oberlander, T. F., Raju, T. N., Soriano, S. G., Taddio, A., & Walco, G. A. (2006). Summary proceedings from the neonatal pain-control group. *Pediatrics, 117*(3 pt 2), S9–S22. https://doi.org/10.1542/peds.2005-0620C

Anders, T. F., & Keener, M. (1985). Developmental course of nighttime sleep-wake patterns in full-term and premature infants during the first year of life. I. *Sleep, 8*(3), 173–192.

Archer, J., Bower, P., Gilbody, S., Lovell, K., Richards, D., Gask, L., Dickens, D., & Coventry, P. (2012). Collaborative care for depression and anxiety problems. *Cochrane Database of Systematic Reviews,* (10), CD006525. https://doi.org/10.1002/14651858.CD006525.pub2

Barbeau, D. Y., & Weiss, M. D. (2017). Sleep disturbances in newborns. *Children, 4*(10), 90. https://doi.org/10.3390/children4100090

Beck, A. F., Edwards, E. M., Horbar, J. D., Howell, E. A., McCormick, M. C., & Pursley, D. M. (2020). The color of health: How racism, segregation, and inequality affect the health and well-being of preterm infants and their families. *Pediatric Research, 87*(2), 227–234. https://doi.org/10.1038/s41390-019-0513-6

Bennet, L., Walker, D. W., & Horne, R. S. C. (2018). Waking up too early - the consequences of preterm birth on sleep development. *Journal of Physiology, 596*(23), 5687–5708. https://doi.org/10.1113/JP274950

Berman, L., Raval, M. V., Ottosen, M., Mackow, A. K., Cho, M., & Goldin, A. B. (2019). Parent perspectives on readiness for discharge home after neonatal intensive care unit admission. *The Journal of Pediatrics, 205,* 98–104. e4. http://doi.org/10.1016/j.jpeds.2018.08.086

Bigsby, R., & Salisbury, A. (2020). IFCDC recommendations for best practices to support sleep and arousal. In Consensus Committee on Infant and Family Centered Developmental Care, (Ed.), *Report of the first Consensus Conference on standards, competencies and best practices for infant and family centered developmental care in the intensive care unit.* https://nicu-design.nd.edu/nicu-care-standards/

Boundy, E. O., Dastjerdi, R., Spiegelman, D., Fawzi, W. W., Missmer, S. A., Lieberman, E., Kajeepeta, S., Wall, S., & Chan, G. J. (2016). Kangaroo mother care and neonatal outcomes: A meta-analysis. *Pediatrics, 137*(1), e20152238. https://doi.org/10.1542/peds.2015-2238

Boykova, M. (2016). Transition from hospital to home in parents of preterm infants: A literature review. *Journal of Perinatal and Neonatal Nursing, 30*(4), 327–348. https://doi.org/10.1097/jpn.0000000000000211

Brooks, J. L., Holditch-Davis, D., & Landerman, L. R. (2013). Interactive behaviors of ethnic minority mothers and their premature infants. *Journal of Obstetric, Gynecologic, and Neonatal Nursing, 42*(3), 357–368. http://doi.org/10.1111/1552-6909.12037

Brown, L. F., & Pickler, R. (2013). A guided feeding intervention for mothers of preterm infants: Two case studies. *Journal for Specialists in Pediatric Nursing, 18*(2), 98–108. https://doi.org/10.1111/jspn.12020

Bueno, C., & Menna-Barreto, L. (2016). Development of sleep/wake, activity and temperature rhythms in newborns maintained in a neonatal intensive care unit and the impact of feeding schedules. *Infant Behavior and Development, 44,* 21–28. http://doi.org/10.1016/j.infbeh.2016.05.004

Carbajal, R., Eriksson, M., Courtois, E., Boyle, E., Avila-Alvarez, A., Andersen, R. D., Sarafidis, K., Polkki, T., Matos, C., Lago, P., Papadouri, T., Montalto, S. A., Ilmoja, M. L., Simons, S., Tameliene, R., van Overmeire, B., Berger, A., Dobrzanska, A., Schroth, M., Bergqvist, L., ... Anand, K. J. S., & EUROPAIN Survey Working Group. (2015). Sedation and analgesia practices in neonatal intensive care units (EUROPAIN): Results from a prospective cohort study. *Lancet Respiratory Medicine, 3*(10), 796–812. https://doi.org/10.1016/S2213-2600(15)00331-8

Carbajal, R., Rousset, A., Danan, C., Coquery, S., Nolent, P., Ducrocq, S., Saizou, C., Lapillonne, A., Granier, M., Durand, P., Lenclen, R., Coursol, A., Hubert, P., de Saint Blanquat, L., Boëlle, P. Y., Annequin, D., Cimerman, P., Anand, K. J., & Breart, G. (2008). Epidemiology and treatment of painful procedures in neonates in intensive care units. *Journal of American Medical Association, 300*(1), 60–70. https://doi.org/10.1001/jama.300.1.60

Casper, C., Sarauk, I., & Paylyshyn, H. (2018). Regular and prolonged skin-to-skin contact improves short-term outcomes for very preterm infants: A dose-dependent intervention. *Archives Pediatrics, 25*(3), 469–475.

Chi Luong, K., Long, N. T., Huong Huynh Thi, D., Carrara, H. P. O., & Bergman, N. J. (2016). Newly born low birthweight infants stabilize better in skin-to-skin contact than when separated from their mothers: A randomized controlled trial. *Acta Paediatrica, 105*(4), 381–390.

Chu, C. J., Leahy, J., Pathmanathan, J., Kramer, M. A., & Cash, S. S. (2014). The maturation of cortical sleep rhythms and networks over early development. *Clinical Neurophysiology, 125*(7), 1360–1370. https://doi.org/10.1016/j.clinph.2013.11.028

Cleveland, L. M. (2008). Parenting in the neonatal intensive care unit. *Journal of Obstetric, Gynecologic, and Neonatal Nursing, 37*(6), 666–691. http://doi.org/10.1111/j.1552-6909.2008.00288.x

Committee to Establish Recommended Standards for Newborn ICU Design. (2020). *Recommended standards for newborn ICU design* (9th ed.). https://nicudesign.nd.edu/nicu-standards/

Conde-Agudelo, A., & Diaz-Rosselio, J. L. (2016). Kangaroo mother care to reduce morbidity and mortality in low birthweight infants. *Cochrane Database of Systematic Reviews, 2006*(8), CD002771.

Cone, S., Pickler, R. H., Grap, M. J., McGrath, J., & Wiley, P. M. (2013). Endotracheal suctioning in preterm infants using four-handed versus routine care. *Journal of Obstetric, Gynecologic, and Neonatal Nursing, 42*(1), 92–104. https://doi.org/10.1111/1552-6909.12004

Cong, X., Ludington-Hoe, S. M., Hussain, N., Cusson, R. M., Walsh, S., Vazquez, V., Briere, C-E., & Vittner, D. (2015). Parental oxytocin responses during skin-to-skin contact in pre-term infants. *Early Human Development, 91*(7), 401–406. https://doi.org/10.1016/j.earlhumdev.2015.04.012

Consensus Committee on Infant and Family Centered Developmental Care (2020). *Report of the first Consensus Conference on standards, competencies and best practices for infant and family centered developmental care in the intensive care unit.* https://nicudesign.nd.edu/nicu-care-standards/

Coughlin, M., Gibbins, S., & Hoath, S. (2009). Core measures for developmentally supportive care in neonatal intensive care units: Theory, precedence and practice. *Journal of Advanced Nursing, 65*(10), 2239–2248. https://doi.org/10.1111/j.1365-2648.2009.05052.x

Craig, J. W., Glick, C., Phillips, R., Hall, S. L., Smith, J., & Browne, J. (2015). Recommendations for involving the family in developmental care of the NICU baby. *Journal of Perinatology, 35*(suppl 1), S5–S8. https://doi.org/10.1038/jp.2015.142

Deloian, B. (1998). *Caring connections: Nursing support transitioning premature infants and their families home from the hospital.* University of Colorado Health Sciences Center, School of Nursing.

Doesburg, S. M., Chau, C. M., Cheung, T. P., Moiseev, A., Ribary, U., Herdman, A. T., Miller, S. P., Cepeda, I. L., Synnes, A., & Grunau, R. E. (2013). Neonatal pain-related stress, functional cortical activity and visual-perceptual abilities in school-age children born at extremely low gestational age. *Pain, 154*(10), 1946–1952. https://doi.org/10.1016/j.pain.2013.04.009

Douglas, P. S., Hill, P. S., & Brodribb, W. (2011). The unsettled baby: How complexity science helps. *Archives of Disease in Childhood, 96*(9), 793–797. https://doi.org/10.1136/adc.2010.199190

Ellsbury, D. L., Clark, R. H., Ursprung, R., Handler, D. L., Dodd, E. D., & Spitzer, A. R. (2016). A multifaceted approach to improving outcomes in the NICU: The pediatrix 100 000 babies campaign. *Pediatrics, 137*(4), e20150389. https://doi.org/10.1542/peds.2015-0389

Evereklian, M., & Posmontier, B. (2017). The impact of kangaroo care on premature infant weight gain. *Journal of Pediatric Nursing, 34*, e10–e16.

Feldman, R., & Eidelman, A. I. (2007). Maternal postpartum behavior and the emergence of infant-mother and infant-father synchrony in preterm and full-term infants: The role of neonatal vagal tone. *Developmental Psychobiology, 49*(3), 290–302. https://doi.org/10.1002/dev.20220

Feldman, R., Rosenthal, Z., & Eidelman, A. I. (2014). Maternal-preterm skin-to-skin contact enhances child physiologic organization and cognitive control across the first 10 years of life. *Biological Psychiatry, 75*(1), 56–64. https://doi.org/10.1016/j.biopsych.2013.08.012

Gianni, M. L., Sannino, P., Bezze, E., Comito, C., Plevani, L., Roggero, P., Agosti, M., & Mosca, F. (2016). Does parental involvement affect the development of feeding skills in preterm infants? A prospective study. *Early Human Development, 103*, 123–128. https://doi.org/10.1016/j.earlhumdev.2016.08.006

Govindaswamy, P., Laing, S., Waters, D., Walker, K., Spence, K., & Badawi, N. (2018). Needs of parents in a surgical neonatal intensive care unit. *Journal Paediatrics and Child Health. 55*, 567–573. https://doi.org/10.1111/jpc.14249

Gregory, K. E., Samuel, B. S., Houghteling, P., Shan, G., Ausubel, F. M., Sadreyev, R. I., & Walker, W. A. (2016). Influence of maternal breast milk ingestion on acquisition of the intestinal microbiome in preterm infants. *Microbiome, 4*(1), 68. https://doi.org/10.1186/s40168-016-0214-x

Guillaume, S., Michelin, N., Amrani, E., Benier, B., Durrmeyer, X., Lescure, S., Bony, C., Danan, C., Baud, O., Jarreau, P-H., Zana-Taïeb, E., & Caeymaex, L. (2013). Parents' expectations of staff in the early bonding process with their premature babies in the intensive care setting: A qualitative multicenter study with 60 parents. *BMC Pediatrics, 13*, 18. doi:10.1186/1471-2431-13-18

Hall, S. L., Hynan, M. T., Phillips, R., Lassen, S., Craig, J. W., Goyer, E., Hatfield, R. F., & Cohen, H. (2017). The neonatal intensive parenting unit: An introduction. *Journal of Perinatology, 37*(12), 1259–1264. https://doi.org/10.1038/jp.2017.108

Hartley, K. A., Miller, C. S., & Gephart, S. M. (2015). Facilitated tucking to reduce pain in neonates: Evidence for best practice. *Advances in Neonatal Care, 15*(3), 201–208. https://doi.org/10.1097/ANC.0000000000000193

Head, L. M. (2014). The effect of kangaroo care on neurodevelopmental outcomes in preterm infants. *Journal of Perinatal and Neonatal Nursing, 28*(4), 290–299.

Hermann, C., Hohmeister, J., Demirakca, S., Zohsel, K., & Flor, H. (2006). Long-term alteration of pain sensitivity in school-aged children with early pain experiences. *Pain, 125*(3), 278–285. https://doi.org/10.1016/j.pain.2006.08.026

Horta, B. L., Loret de Mola, C., & Victora, C. G. (2015). Breastfeeding and intelligence: A systematic review and meta-analysis. *Acta Paediatrics, 104*(467), 14–19. https://doi.org/10.1111/apa.13139

Hynan, M., Cicco, R., & Hatfield, B. (2020). IFCDC recommendations for best practice reducing and managing pain and stress in newborns and families. In Consensus Committee on Infant and Family Centered Developmental Care, (Ed.), *Report of the first Consensus Conference on standards, competencies and best practices for infant and family centered developmental care in the intensive care unit.* https://nicudesign.nd.edu/nicu-care-standards/

Hynan, M. T., & Hall, S. L. (2015). Psychosocial program standards for NICU parents. *Jouranl Perinatology, 35*(suppl 1), S1–S4. https://doi.org/10.1038/jp.2015.141

Hynan, M. T., Steinberg, Z., Baker, L., Cicco, R., Geller, P. A., Lassen, S., Milford, C., Mounts, K. O., Patterson, C., Saxton, S., Segre, L., & Stuebe, A. (2015). Recommendations for mental health professionals in the NICU. *Journal of Perinatology, 35*(suppl 1), S14–S18. https://doi.org/10.1038/jp.2015.144

Jadcherla, S. R., Dail, J., Malkar, M. B., McClead, R., Kelleher, K., & Nelin, L. (2015). Impact of process optimization and quality improvement measures on neonatal feeding outcomes at an all-referral neonatal intensive care unit. *J Parenteral and Enteral Nutrition, 40*(5), 646–655. https://doi.org/10.1177/0148607115571667

Jadcherla, S. R., Peng, J., Moore, R., Saavedra, J., Shepherd, E., Fernandez, S., Erdman, S. H., & DiLorenzo, C. (2012). Impact of personalized feeding program in 100 NICU infants: Pathophysiology-based approach for better outcomes. *Journal of Pediatric Gastroenterology and Nutrition, 54*(1), 62–70. https://doi.org/10.1097/MPG.0b013e3182288766

Johnson, B. H. (2016). Promoting patient-and family-centered care through personal stories. *Academic Medicine, 91*(3), 297–300. https://doi.org/10.1097/acm.0000000000001086

Johnston, C., Campbell-Yeo, M., Disher, T., Benoit, B., Fernandes, A., Streiner, D., Inglis, D., & Zee, R. (2017). Skin-to-skin care for procedural pain in neonates. *Cochrane Database of Systematic Review, 2*, Cd008435. https://doi.org/10.1002/14651858.CD008435.pub3

Johnston, C., Campbell-Yeo, M., Fernandes, A., Inglis, D., Streiner, D., & Zee, R. (2014). Skin-to-skin care for procedural pain in neonates. *Cochrane Database of Systematic Review,* (1), Cd008435. https://doi.org/10.1002/14651858.CD008435.pub2

Kenner, C., & Jaeger, C. B. (2020). IFCDC recommendations for best practices in systems thinking. In Consensus Committee on Infant and Family Centered Developmental Care, (Ed.), *Report of the first Consensus Conference on standards, competencies and best practices for infant and family centered developmental care in the intensive care unit.* https://nicudesign.nd.edu/nicu-care-standards/

Kumar, R. K., Singhal, A., Vaidya, U., Banerjee, S., Anwar, F., & Rao, S. (2017). Optimizing nutrition in preterm low birth weight infants-consensus summary. *Frontiers Nutrition, 4,* 20. https://doi.org/10.3389/fnut.2017. 00020

Lake, E. T., Staiger, D., Edwards, E. M., Smith, J. G., & Rogowski, J. A. (2018). Nursing care disparities in neonatal intensive care units. *Health Services Research, 53*(suppl 1), 3007–3026. https://doi. org/10.1111/1475-6773.12762

Lennon, M. (2011). Improving in-hospital breastfeeding management for the late preterm infant. *Neonatal Intensive Care, 24*(1), 18–21.

Lester, B. M., Salisbury, A. L., Hawes, K., Dansereau, L. M., Bigsby, R., Laptook, A., Taub, M., Lagasse, L. L., Vohr, B. R., & Padbury, J. F. (2016). 18-Month follow-up of infants cared for in a single-family room neonatal intensive care unit. *Journal of Pediatrics, 177,* 84–89. https://doi. org/10.1016/j.jpeds.2016.06.069

Levin, A. (1999). Humane neonatal care initiative. *Acta Paediatrics, 88*(4), 353–355. https://doi.org/10.1080/08035259950169657

Liu, W. F., Laudert, S., Perkins, B., MacMillan-York, E., Martin, S., Graven, S., & the NIC/Q 2005 Physical Environment Exploratory Group. (2007). The development of potentially better practices to support the neurodevelopment of infants in the NICU. *Journal of Perinatology, 27,* S48–S74. https://doi.org/10.1038/sj.jp.7211844

Louis-Jacques, A., Deubel, T. F., Taylor, M., & Stuebe, A. M. (2017). Racial and ethnic disparities in U.S. breastfeeding and implications for maternal and child health outcomes. *Seminars in Perinatology, 41*(5), 299–307. https://doi.org/10.1053/j.semperi.2017.04.007

Madlinger-Lewis, L., Reynolds, L., Zarem, C., Crapnell, T., Inder, T., & Pineda, R. (2014). The effects of alternative positioning on preterm infants in the neonatal intensive care unit: A randomized clinical trial. *Research in Developmental Disabilities, 35*(2), 490–497. https://doi.org/10.1016/j. ridd.2013.11.019

Meier, P. P., Engstrom, J. L., Patel, A. L., Jegier, B. J., & Bruns, N. E. (2010). Improving the use of human milk during and after the NICU stay. *Clinics in Perinatology, 37*(1), 217–245. https://doi.org/10.1016/j.clp.2010.01.013

Neu, M., & Robinson, J. (2010). Maternal holding of preterm infants during the early weeks after birth and dyad interaction at six months. *Journal of Obstetric, Gynecologic and Neonatal and Nursing, 39*(4), 401–414. https:// doi.org/10.1111/j.1552-6909.2010.01152.x

O'Brien, K., Bracht, M., Macdonell, K., McBride, T., Robson, K., O'Leary, L., Christie, K., Galarza, M., Dicky, T., Levin, A., & Lee, S. K. (2013). A pilot cohort analytic study of Family Integrated Care in a Canadian neonatal intensive care unit. *BMC Pregnancy and Childbirth, 13*(suppl 1), S12.

Padovani, F. H., Duarte, G., Martinez, F. E., & Linhares, M. B. (2011). Perceptions of breastfeeding in mothers of babies born preterm in comparison to mothers of full-term babies. *The Spanish Journal of Psychology, 14*(2), 884–898.

Phillips, R., & Smith, K. (2020). IFCDC recommendations for skin-to-skin contact with intimate family members. In Consensus Committee on Infant and Family Centered Developmental Care, (Ed.), *Report of the first Consensus Conference on standards, competencies and best practices for infant and family centered developmental care in the intensive care unit.* https://nicudesign.nd.edu/nicu-care-standards/

Picheansathian, W., Woragidpoonpol, P., & Baosoung, C. (2009). Positioning of preterm infants for optimal physiological development: A systematic review. *JBI Library Systematic Reviews, 7*(7), 224–259.

Pillai Riddell, R. R., Racine, N. M., Gennis, H. G., Turcotte, K., Uman, L. S., Horton, R. E., Ahola Kohut, S., Hillgrove Stuart, J., Stevens, B., & Lisi, D. M. (2015). Non-pharmacological management of infant and young child procedural pain. *Cochrane Database of Systematic Reviews,* (12), CD006275. https://doi.org/10.1002/14651858.CD006275.pub3

Pillai Riddell, R., Racine, N. M., Turcotte, K., Uman, L., Horton, R., Din Osmun, L., Kohut, S. A., Stuart, J. H., Stevens, B., & Lisi, D. (2011). Nonpharmacological management of procedural pain in infants and young children: An abridged Cochrane review. *Pain Research and Management, 16*(5), 321–330.

Pineda, R., Bender, J., Hall, B., Shabosky, L., Annecca, A., & Smith, J. (2018). Parent participation in the neonatal intensive care unit: Predictors and relationships to neurobehavior and developmental outcomes.

Early Human Development, 117, 32–38. https://doi.org/10.1016/j. earlhumdev.2017.12.008

Romantsik, O., Calevo, M. G., & Bruschettini, M. (2017). Head midline position for preventing the occurrence or extension of germinal matrix-intraventricular hemorrhage in preterm infants. *Cochrane Database of Systematic Reviews, 7,* CD012362. https://doi.org/10.1002/14651858. CD012362.pub2

Ross, E., Arvedson, J. C., & McGrath, J. (2020). IFCDC recommendations for best practices for feeding, eating and nutrition delivery. In Consensus Committee on Infant and Family Centered Developmental Care, (Ed.), *Report of the first Consensus Conference on standards, competencies and best practices for infant and family centered developmental care in the intensive care unit.* https://nicudesign.nd.edu/nicu-care-standards/

Shah, P. S., Herbozo, C., Aliwalas, L. L., & Shah, V. S. (2012). Breastfeeding or breast milk for procedural pain in neonates. *Cochrane Database of Systematic Reviews, 12,* Cd004950. https://doi.org/10.1002/14651858. CD004950.pub3

Shellhaas, R. A., Kenia, P. V., Hassan, F., Barks, J. D. E., Kaciroti, N., & Chervin, R. D. (2018). Sleep-disordered breathing among newborns with myelomeningocele. *Journal of Pediatrics, 194,* 244–247.e1. https://doi. org/10.1016/j.jpeds.2017.10.070

Sigurdson, K., Mitchell, B., Liu, J., Morton, C., Gould, J. B., Lee, H. C., Capdarest-Arest, N., & Profit, J. (2019). Racial/Ethnic disparities in neonatal intensive care: A systematic review. *Pediatrics, 144*(2), e20183114. https://doi.org/10.1542/peds.2018-3114

Smith, J. R. (2012). Comforting touch in the very preterm hospitalized infant: An integrative review. *Advances in Neonatal Care, 12,* 349–365.

Sriraman, N. K. (2017). The nuts and bolts of breastfeeding: Anatomy and physiology of lactation. *Current Problems Pediatric and Adolescent Health Care, 47*(12), 305–310. https://doi.org/10.1016/j.cppeds.2017.10.001

Sweeney, J., & McElroy, J. (2020). IFCDC recommendations for best practice for positioning and touch. In Consensus Committee on Infant and Family Centered Developmental Care, (Ed.), *Report of the first Consensus Committee on standards, competencies and best practices for infant and family centered developmental care in the intensive care unit.* https://nicudesign.nd.edu/nicu-care-standards/

Takenouchi, T., Rubens, E. O., Yap, V. L., Ross, G., Engel, M., & Perlman, J. M. (2011). Delayed onset of sleep-wake cycling with favorable outcome in hypothermic-treated neonates with encephalopathy. *The Journal of Pediatrics, 159*(2), 232–237. https://doi.org/10.1016/j.jpeds.2011.01.006

Tessier, R., Cristo, M., Velez, S., Giron, M., de Calume, Z. F., Ruiz-Palaez, J. G., Charpak, Y., & Charpak, N. (1998). Kangaroo mother care and the bonding hypothesis. *Pediatrics, 102*(2), e17.

Thoyre, S. M., & Brown, R. L. (2004). Factors contributing to preterm infant engagement during bottle-feeding. *Nursing Research, 53*(5), 304–313.

Thoyre, S. M., Holditch-Davis, D., Schwartz, T. A., Melendez Roman, C. R., & Nix, W. (2012). Coregulated approach to feeding preterm infants with lung disease: Effects during feeding. *Nursing Research, 61*(4), 242–251. https://doi.org/10.1097/NNR.0b013e31824b02ad

Thoyre, S. M., Hubbard, C., Park, J., Pridham, K., & McKechnie, A. (2016). Implementing Co-regulated feeding with mothers of preterm infants. *MCN The American Journal of Maternal Child Nursing, 41*(4), 204–211. https://doi.org/10.1097/NMC.0000000000000245

Umberger, E., Canvasser, J., & Hall, S. L. (2018). Enhancing NICU parent engagement and empowerment. *Seminars in Pediatric Surgery, 27*(1), 19–24. https://doi.org/10.1053/j.sempedsurg.2017.11.004

Vaivre-Douret, L., Ennouri, K., Jrad, I., Garrec, C., & Papiernik, E. (2004). Effect of positioning on the incidence of abnormalities of muscle tone in low-risk, preterm infants. *European Journal of Paediatric Neurology, 8,* 21–34. https://doi.org/10.1016/j.ejpn.2003.10.001

Vinall, J., & Grunau, R. E. (2014). Impact of repeated procedural pain-related stress in infants born very preterm. *Pediatrics Research, 75*(5), 584–587. https://doi.org/10.1038/pr.2014.16

Vittner, D., McGrath, J., Robinson, J., Lawhon, G., Cusson, R., Eisenfeld, L., Walsh, S., Young, E., & Cong, X. (2018). Increase in oxytocin from skin-to-skin contact enhances development of parent-infant relationship. *Biological Research Nursing, 20*(1), 54–62. https://doi.org/10.1177/1099800417735633

Weisman, O., Magori-Cohen, R., Louzoun, Y., Eidelman, A. I., & Feldman, R. (2011). Sleep-wake transitions in premature neonates predict early development. *Pediatrics, 128*(4), 706–714. https://doi.org/10.1542/peds.2011-0047

Westrup, B. (2005). Newborn individualized developmental care and assessment program (NIDCAP): Family-centered developmentally supportive care. *Neoreviews, 6*, e115.

Westrup, B. (2007). Newborn individualized developmental care and assessment program (NIDCAP)—family-centered developmentally supportive care. *Early Human Development, 83*(7), 443–449. https://doi.org/10.1016/j.earlhumdev.2007.03.006

Wilson, T., Holt, T., & Greenhalgh, T. (2001). Complexity science: Complexity and clinical care. *British Medical Journal, 323*(7314), 685–688.

Yang, G., & Gan, W. B. (2012). Sleep contributes to dendritic spine formation and elimination in the developing mouse somatosensory cortex. *Developmental Neurobiology, 72*(11), 1391–1398. https://doi.org/10.1002/dneu.20996

Yin, T., Yang, L., Lee, T. Y., Li, C. C., Hua, Y. M., & Liaw, J. J. (2015). Development of atraumatic heel-stick procedures by combined treatment with non-nutritive sucking, oral sucrose, and facilitated tucking: A randomized controlled trial. *International Journal of Nursing Studies, 52*(8), 1288–1289.

Zahed, M., Berbis, J., Brevaut-Malaty, V., Busuttil, M., Tosello, B., & Gire, C. (2015). Posture and movement in very preterm infants at term age in and outside the nest. *Childs Nervous System, 31*(12), 2333–2340.

CHAPTER 2 APPENDIX

Infant Family Centered Developmental Care (IFCDC)
Considerations for Implementation[1]
Authors: Consensus Committee on Recommended Standards, Competencies and Best Practices for Infant and Family Centered Developmental Care in the Intensive Care Unit.
January 2020.
Please consider where you are in implementing competency-based IFCDC standards of practice in your intensive care unit by an interprofessional collaborative team:

Please indicate "NOT YET" **if you have not implemented the competency in your unit or need to improve the application of this competency.**

Please indicate "SOME" **if you do address this competency sometimes but are not consistent in application of this competency.**

Please indicate "YES" **if you and your unit always or almost always meet the competency criteria.**

Please include comments and/or indicators of what you are currently doing.

STANDARDS: SYSTEMS THINKING IN COMPLEX ADAPTIVE SYSTEMS

Competency	NOT YET	SOME	YES	Comments/Indicators
Are the baby and the family central to the mission, values, environment, practice, and care delivery?				
Do you work as an interdisciplinary team with representatives from all disciplines?				
Does your team welcome the integration and interaction of the family?				
Does your team, including parents and family, educate and train together?				
Is the team competence regularly evaluated, as well as the competence of the individual professional?				
Is performance competence evaluated at least annually?				
Is the team, and the professional, held accountable for performance improvement?				
Does your ICU culture encourage open communication, relationship building, respect, and value for all individuals, and creative thinking?				
Do you have strategies and evaluative metrics that you use to accomplish open communication, relationship building, respect, value, and creative thinking for all individuals?				
Does the unit have the infrastructure to practice IFCDC? What are your strategies and metrics used to improve or sustain the infrastructure?				
Do you support families to feel confident as a nurturing caregiver of their baby and competent decision-maker in managing current and anticipatory health requirements?				
Is there consistency in information and care delivery along the continuum from inpatient to home and follow-up? How is this demonstrated and evaluated?				

[Continued]

---

[1]Developed by J. Browne from the IFCDC Consensus Committee "Questions to Consider," https://nicudesign.nd.edu/nicu-care-standards/.

STANDARDS: SYSTEMS THINKING IN COMPLEX ADAPTIVE SYSTEMS (Continued)

Competency	NOT YET	SOME	YES	Comments/Indicators
Are you aware of the information and data that can tell you about the operation, infrastructure, outcome, education and training, practice performance, and improvement implementation of the unit(s) of your institution?				
Is improvement continuous and is there a designated person assigned to the unit who is qualified to extract, program, manage, and report data?				
Do you collect articulated metrics monitor, evaluate, and compare with standardized outcomes?				
Is there transparency in the dissemination of information and data? Can you articulate a cost-to-benefit ratio to justify, or identify, opportunities for developmental care? How is this accomplished?				
Strategies are used to provide a continuum of care from admission to transition to home and follow-up care in the community.				
The information and data are shared between in-patient and primary care teams to improve the continuum of education and care management from in-patient through primary care.				

What are your ICU's strengths in the Systems Thinking in complex adaptive systems?

What are your ICU's challenges with Systems Thinking in complex adaptive systems?

What might be your next steps toward meeting the standards/competencies in Systems Thinking in complex adaptive systems?

Infant Family Centered Developmental Care (IFCDC)
Considerations for Implementation[2]
Authors: Consensus Committee on Recommended Standards, Competencies and Best Practices for Infant and Family Centered Developmental Care in the Intensive Care Unit.
January 2020.
Please consider where you are in implementing competency-based IFCDC standards of practice in your intensive care unit by an interprofessional collaborative team:

Please indicate "NOT YET" if you have not implemented the competency in your unit yet or need to improve the application of this competency.

Please indicate "SOME" if you do address this competency sometimes but are not consistent in application of this competency.

Please indicate "YES" if you and your unit always or almost always meet the competency criteria.

Please include comments and/or indicators of what you are currently doing.

STANDARDS OF PRACTICE: POSITIONING AND TOUCH FOR THE NEWBORN

Competency	NOT YET	SOME	YES	Comments/Indicators
Is there standardized education to guide the performance of team members, including families, to support the musculoskeletal, physiologic, and behavioral stability of the baby?				
Does the unit have a written evidence-based guideline to support the value and implementation of individualized developmentally appropriate position and touch management?				
Is positioning therapeutic and individualized to the baby given the care situation and support (equipment) modalities?				
Is body positioning used as an appropriate intervention for cranial shaping, prevention of torticollis and skull deformity, gastrointestinal symptoms, and safe sleep?				
Is the assessment and intervention of positioning consistently documented?				
Can you confidently describe the "voice," or behavioral communication, of the baby, and is this documented?				
Is the assessment and plan for touch individualized to the baby—frequency, duration, for comfort, physiologic regulation, and quiet sleep?				
Is the documentation of positioning and touch evaluated by the team and changed consistent with the needs of the baby?				
Does the family demonstrate confidence in managing the baby's positioning during daily life activity?				

What are your ICU's strengths in <u>positioning and touch for the newborn?</u>

What are your ICU's challenges with <u>positioning and touch for the newborn?</u>

What might be your next steps toward meeting the standards/competencies in <u>positioning and touch for the newborn?</u>

---

[2]Developed by J. Browne from the IFCDC Consensus Committee "Questions to Consider," https://nicudesign.nd.edu/nicu-care-standards/.

Infant Family Centered Developmental Care (IFCDC)
Considerations for Implementation[3]
Authors: Consensus Committee on Recommended Standards, Competencies and Best Practices for Infant and Family Centered Developmental Care in the Intensive Care Unit.
January 2020.
Please consider where you are in implementing competency-based IFCDC standards of practice in your intensive care unit by an interprofessional collaborative team:

Please indicate "NOT YET" if you have not implemented the competency in your unit yet or[3] need to improve the application of this competency.

Please indicate "SOME" if you do address this competency sometimes but are not consistent in application of this competency.

Please indicate "YES" if you and your unit always or almost always meet the competency criteria.

Please include comments and/or indicators of what you are currently doing.

STANDARDS FOR PRACTICE: SLEEP AND AROUSAL INTERVENTION FOR THE NEWBORN

Competency	NOT YET	SOME	YES	Comments/Indicators
Are the environment and the furnishings conducive to optimizing developmentally appropriate sleep for the baby?				
Does the unit have a written guideline to support the value and implementation of individualized developmentally appropriate sleep and arousal management?				
Is there standardized evidence-based education to guide the performance of team members, including families, to assess, support, and evaluate individualized age-appropriate quality and quantity of sleep?				
Can you, and the family, confidently describe the "voice," or behavioral communication, of the baby?				
Is the assessment of the baby's cyclical rest and activity pattern, and response, documented?				
Does the individualized plan of care reflect modifications to optimize sleep and arousal?				
Are the rest and sleep periods of the baby protected in the plan of care?				
Do the team professionals encourage family presence, engage individualized interaction with their baby, strengthen their confidence to evaluate response, and foster developmentally appropriate behavior modification?				
Is the documentation, individually and population, regularly evaluated for improvement opportunities in education, interaction, and performance?				

What are your ICU's strengths in supporting <u>sleep and arousal interventions for the newborn?</u>

What are your ICU's challenges with supporting <u>sleep and arousal interventions for the newborn?</u>

What might be your next steps toward meeting the standards/competencies in <u>sleep and arousal interventions for the newborn?</u>

---

[3]Developed by J. Browne from the IFCDC Consensus Committee "Questions to Consider," https://nicudesign.nd.edu/nicu-care-standards/.

Infant Family Centered Developmental Care (IFCDC)
Considerations for Implementation[4]
Authors: Consensus Committee on Recommended Standards, Competencies and Best Practices for Infant and Family Centered Developmental Care in the Intensive Care Unit.
January 2020.
Please consider where you are in implementing competency-based IFCDC standards of practice in your intensive care unit by an interprofessional collaborative team:

Please indicate "NOT YET" if you have not implemented the competency in your unit yet or need to improve the application of this competency.

Please indicate "SOME" if you do address this competency sometimes but are not consistent in application of this competency.

Please indicate "YES" if you and your unit always or almost always meet the competency criteria.

Please include comments and/or indicators of what you are currently doing.

STANDARDS OF PRACTICE: SKIN-TO-SKIN CONTACT WITH INTIMATE FAMILY MEMBERS

Competencies	NOT YET	SOME	YES	Comments/Indicators
Is there an evidence-based policy, guideline, education and training, and competencies to standardize the performance of skin-to-skin contact for the team, parents, and family members?				
Are the parents and families included in the learning process and practice?				
Is the education and performance demonstration mandatory?				
Is the practice of skin-to-skin contact individualized to the baby and family?				
Are the parents, and family members, physically and psychologically comfortable during skin-to-skin contact? How do you know?				
Can you, and the family, confidently describe the "voice," or behavioral communication, of the baby's readiness, stability, engagement, response, and monitoring data, through the process of skin-to-skin contact?				
Do the parents, and family members, interact with the baby to calm, soothe, and connect?				
Are improvements continuously implemented based on credible evidence, data, and evaluation?				
Does the team provide anticipatory guidance, safety measures, and support for continuing contact with the baby transitioning to home, and home care?				

What are your ICU's strengths in supporting skin-to-skin contact with intimate family members?

What are your ICU's challenges with supporting skin-to-skin contact with intimate family members?

What might be your next steps toward meeting the standards/competencies in supporting skin-to-skin contact with intimate family members?

---

[4]Developed by J. Browne from the IFCDC Consensus Committee "Questions to Consider," https://nicudesign.nd.edu/nicu-care-standards/.

Infant Family Centered Developmental Care (IFCDC)
Considerations for Implementation[5]
Authors: Consensus Committee on Recommended Standards, Competencies and Best Practices for Infant and Family Centered Developmental Care in the Intensive Care Unit.
January 2020.
Please consider where you are in implementing competency-based IFCDC standards of practice in your intensive care unit by an interprofessional collaborative team:

Please indicate "NOT YET" if you have not implemented the competency in your unit yet or need to improve the application of this competency.

Please indicate "SOME" if you do address this competency sometimes but are not consistent in application of this competency.

Please indicate "YES" if you and your unit always or almost always meet the competency criteria.

Please include comments and/or indicators of what you are currently doing.

STANDARDS OF PRACTICE: REDUCING AND MANAGING PAIN AND STRESS IN FAMILIES

Competency	NOT YET	SOME	YES	Comments/Indicators
Are there sufficient specialty professionals to support the psychiatric, psychological, social, cultural, and spiritual needs of parents, families, and staff?				
Do parents and families have access to peer-to-peer and psychoeducational group support while in the hospital and following the transition to home?				
Are there routine educational sessions for staff, including (a) recognizing symptoms of emotional distress in parents and family members, (b) communication skills emphasizing reflective listening and nonjudgmental feedback, (c) available resources for family members in distress, and (d) self-care and avoiding burnout?				
Does your team assess and document well-being and the emotional distress of staff, parents, and families?				
Do the ICU mental health professionals have dedicated time to informally communicate with all parents at the bedside on a routine basis?				
What strategies are implemented to assist staff, parents, and families who experience a lack of well-being or emotional distress to cope in a healthy manner?				
Is information about parental well-being and distress communicated with follow-up providers?				
Do you have sufficient resources to support the psychosocial needs of staff, parents, and families through hospitalization and following the transition to home?				

What are your ICU's strengths in <u>reducing and managing pain and stress in families?</u>

What are your ICU's challenges with <u>reducing and managing pain and stress in families?</u>

What might be your next steps toward meeting the standards/competencies in <u>reducing and managing pain and stress in families?</u>

---

[5]Developed by J. Browne from the IFCDC Consensus Committee "Questions to Consider," https://nicudesign.nd.edu/nicu-care-standards/.

Infant Family Centered Developmental Care (IFCDC)
Considerations for Implementation[6]
Authors: Consensus Committee on Recommended Standards, Competencies and Best Practices for Infant and Family Centered Developmental Care in the Intensive Care Unit.
January 2020.

Please consider where you are in implementing competency-based IFCDC standards of practice in your intensive care unit[6] by an interprofessional collaborative team:

Please indicate "NOT YET" if you have not implemented the competency in your unit yet or need to improve the application of this competency.

Please indicate "SOME" if you do address this competency sometimes but are not consistent in application of this competency.

Please indicate "YES" if you and your unit always or almost always meet the competency criteria.

Please include comments and/or indicators of what you are currently doing.

STANDARDS OF PRACTICE: REDUCING AND MANAGING PAIN AND STRESS IN BABIES

Competency	NOT YET	SOME	YES	Comments/Indicators
Are parents encouraged and supported to engage and interact as members of the interprofessional collaborative team?				
Do parents have unlimited opportunities to be with their baby?				
Can you confidently describe the "voice," or behavioral communication, of the baby?				
Do you support parents and family members to understand the communication of the baby?				
Do you have written evidence-based policies, guidelines, education and training programs, and performance measures to guide the use of pharmacologic and nonpharmacologic measures to manage the baby's stress, discomfort, and pain?				
Does the team regularly assess, monitor, and evaluate the baby's stress, discomfort, and pain?				
Are parents supported to be present during stressful procedures to provide nonpharmacologic support for the baby?				
Are pharmacologic interventions used routinely for babies who are being mechanically ventilated?				
Are nonpharmacologic interventions routinely utilized to supplement the use of pharmacologic therapies?				

What are your ICU's strengths in <u>reducing and managing pain and stress in babies?</u>

What are your ICU's challenges with <u>reducing and managing pain and stress in babies?</u>

What might be your next steps toward meeting the standards/competencies in <u>reducing and managing pain and stress in babies?</u>

---

[6]Developed by J. Browne from the IFCDC Consensus Committee "Questions to Consider," https://nicudesign.nd.edu/nicu-care-standards/.

Infant Family Centered Developmental Care (IFCDC)
Considerations for Implementation[7]
Authors: Consensus Committee on Recommended Standards, Competencies and Best Practices for Infant and Family Centered Developmental Care in the Intensive Care Unit.
January 2020.
Please consider where you are in implementing competency-based IFCDC standards of practice in your intensive care unit[7] by an interprofessional collaborative team:

Please indicate "NOT YET" if you have not implemented the competency in your unit yet or need to improve the application of this competency.

Please indicate "SOME" if you do address this competency sometimes but are not consistent in application of this competency.

Please indicate "YES" if you and your unit always or almost always meet the competency criteria.

Please include comments and/or indicators of what you are currently doing.

STANDARDS OF PRACTICE: MANAGEMENT OF FEEDING, EATING, AND NUTRITION DELIVERY

Competency	NOT YET	SOME	YES	Comments/Indicators
Do you provide education on behaviors and physiologic parameters of the baby that indicates age-appropriate feeding readiness, engagement, and the need to stop?				
Are staff, parents, and families included in the educational offering?				
Is the desire of the m/other central to the feeding plan designed by the team? Is this consistently reflected in the documentation?				
Do you provide continuing education and evidence-based interventions that are safe and individualized to the baby and the feeding technique used—enteral, breast, or bottle?				
Are team members/staff regularly evaluated on performance competencies of individualized feeding?				
Is variability in the skill of feeding the baby minimized?				
Is discomfort or distress recognized and managed? Does the baby exhibit a comfortable and enjoyable response?				
Is nutritional/growth outcome monitored?				
Is suctioning and oral care performed so that stress to the baby is minimized? Is human milk considered for oral care?				
Are there sufficient team/staff professionals to guide and support caregivers, parents, and family members as needed during feeding?				
Is breastfeeding by the mother encouraged and supported?				
Is early breastfeeding, or feeding with breastmilk, promoted? Do you have a way of monitoring how the information is disseminated?				
Does the feeding management plan demonstrate a feeding and nutrition continuum from in-hospital care through the transition to home and home care? Are parents and family members informed of feeding and nutrition resources available to them when at home?				

What are your ICU's strengths in the <u>management of feeding, eating, and nutrition delivery?</u>

What are your ICU's challenges with <u>management of feeding, eating, and nutrition delivery?</u>

What might be your next steps toward meeting the standards/competencies in <u>management of feeding, eating, and nutrition delivery?</u>

---

[7]Developed by J. Browne from the IFCDC Consensus Committee "Questions to Consider," https://nicudesign.nd.edu/nicu-care-standards/.

CHAPTER 3

Theoretical Perspective for Developmentally Supportive Care

Heidelise Als

Developmental Care Standards for Infants in Intensive Care

Standard 1: Systems thinking

- The intensive care unit shall exhibit an infrastructure of leadership, mission, and a governance framework to guide the performance of the collaborative practice of Infant Family-Centered Developmental Care Standards and Competencies (IFCDC).

Standard 2: Positioning and touch

- Babies in intensive care settings shall be positioned to support musculoskeletal, physiological, and behavioral stability.

Standard 3: Sleep and arousal

- Intensive care units (ICUs) shall promote developmentally appropriate sleep and arousal states and sleep–wake cycles.

Standard 4: Skin-to-skin contact

- Parents shall be encouraged and supported in early, frequent, and prolonged skin-to-skin contact with their babies.

Standard 5: Pain and stress, families

- The interprofessional team shall document increased parental/caregiver well-being and decreased emotional distress during the intensive care hospital (ICU) stay. Distress levels of baby's siblings and extended family should also be considered.

Standard 6: Feeding

- Feeding experiences in the ICU shall be behavior based and baby led. Baby-led principles are similar whether applied to enteral, breast, or bottle-feeding experience.

*This list only represents the first standard in each section of the framework and none of the associated competencies. For a complete list please see https://nicudesign.nd.edu/nicu-care-standards/

INTRODUCTION

The purpose of this chapter is to provide a theoretical perspective for developmentally supportive care for newborns. Appreciation of the evolution of newborn development within a neurobiological neurosocial context leads to an understanding of the newborn's behavior that then guides the parents' and the professional caregivers' approach (Als, 1977). Because behavior is the newborn and very young infants' main channel of communication, it is of paramount importance that parent and professional caregivers appreciate the importance of understanding the meaning of behavior. This requires sensitivity and education in recognizing and appreciating infants' subtle, nuanced cues while responding to them in adapting necessary interventions in a developmentally supportive manner (Franck & Lawhon, 2000). Through trust in the meaningfulness of all infant behavior, the traditional task-oriented care model of care is transformed into a collaborative relationship-based model that understands infants as active participants in their care and as the caregivers' guide (Als, 1977; Als & Gilkerson, 1997).

Supportive research findings that test this theoretical perspective in the clinical arena are reviewed. Finally, the Newborn Individualized Developmental Care and Assessment Program (NIDCAP; **NIDCAP® is a registered**

trademark of the NFI, Inc.) (Boston, MA) guidelines for provision of individualized developmentally supportive family-centered care are summarized.

All standards and competencies as spelled out in the Graven Infant Family-Centered Developmental Care Standards and Competencies (IFCDC) (Browne et al., 2020) will be addressed in this chapter. The chapter focusses on the underlying principles and the "how" of activities more than the specific activities themselves.

Advances in newborn intensive care have led to significant changes in survival rates of preterm infants. According to the National Center for Health Statistics (US Department of Health and Human Services, 2019), the premature birth rate in the United States rose to 10.02% in 2018, a 1% rise from 2017 (9.93%), and the fourth straight year of increases in this rate (9.57% in 2014). The March of Dimes (2019) has recognized another growing group, "late-preterm" infants, who are born at 34 to 36 weeks. These infants are at increased risk for certain health problems when compared with full-term newborns. Some of these infants seem healthy at first and typically are significantly larger than very premature infants. However, they often have breathing problems, jaundice, feeding difficulties, low blood sugar, unstable body temperatures, and/or other medical conditions. Late-preterm infants account for about two-thirds of all infants born prematurely. Between 1990 and 2003, the late-preterm birth rate increased by more than 20% in the United States. This increase has focused needed research on understanding the risks and effects of being born early for this group of preterm infants (March of Dimes, 2016). These infants more closely resemble their premature rather than their full-term born peers.

They have all the morbidities and mortalities associated with other premature births. Beyond the newborn period, preterm and late-preterm infants experience a disproportionate amount of morbidity and requirement for medical services (Gouyon et al., 2012). Even if these infants escape major medical complications, very-low-birth-weight (VLBW) infants represent a larger proportion of children with learning problems and developmental limitations, especially in visual-perceptual-motor skills, and emotional regulation disorders. These deficits in neurobehavioral outcome are particularly pronounced in extremely and very preterm and/or extremely low-birthweight and VLBW children, for whom moderate-to-severe deficits in academic achievement, attention problems, internalization, as well as executive function have been documented. Increasingly, follow-up into early adulthood indicates that these problems often persist (Boyle et al., 2012; Madzwamuse et al., 2015; Ment et al., 2003).

There is growing effort to reduce these sequelae by reducing stress involved in requiring newborn intensive care and building on the infants' strengths from earliest on, thus encouraging and facilitating infants' emerging competence.

Brain Development

In full-term infants, the post-neuronal migratory phase of brain organization, i.e., axonal and dendritic proliferation as well as synapse formation, is the most rapid phase of brain development in the course of the human life span. The associated increase in cortical tissue volume leads to the brain's highly complex gyri and sulci formation (Cowan, 1979). This rapid brain development occurs in the womb, which provides the evolutionarily assured stimulus barrier, of which Freud speaks, as quoted by Eagle (Eagle, 2000). Nutrition, temperature control, and numerous regulating systems provide chronobiologic rhythms in the womb (Reppert & Rivkees, 1989). The finite space and lack of gravity in the amniotic sac assures reliable return to flexion as well as movement development and self-initiated neuronal feedback loop establishment by touching mouth, face, and head; sucking on own hand; grasping the umbilical cord; bracing feet to the amniotic sac wall; the gradual development of cross midline reach; and many others (Hepper & Shahidullah, 1992; Hepper et al., 2005; Hepper, 2013).

These protections are replaced for preterm infants with stimuli from the quite differently organized newborn intensive care unit (NICU). The NICU environment stands in stark sensory mismatch to the developing nervous system's growth requirements (Freud, 1991; Wolke, 1987) as has been documented extensively in the literature (Anderson et al., 1983; Long, Lucey, & Philip, 1980; Long, Philip, & Lucey, 1980; Martin, Herrell, Rubin, & Fanaroff, 1979; Martin, Okken, & Rubin, 1979; Murdoch & Darlow, 1984; Norris et al., 1982). Estimating the effects on preterm infants' nervous systems when they move from intrauterine aquatic environments to extrauterine terrestrial NICU environments (Alberts & Cramer, 1988), identifying the infants' strengths and vulnerabilities in the NICU's alien environment, and estimating costs incurred and ways to reduce costs and enhance strengths (Als, 2010) will be discussed in this chapter.

Developmental Theory

The principle of phylogenetic and ontogenetic adaptation concerns the individual organism as an evolving member of a species. The construct of adaptation (Babson, 1970; Jones, 1972, 1974, 1976) suggests that an organism at any stage of development has evolved to implement a level of adaptation that is not only species appropriate but also species parsimonious and specific for the organism in its particular eco niche. The process of selection takes place at the behavioral level and over generations. Species repertoire essentials may become hard-wired (Lettvin et al., 1959), and the longer an environment remains stable, the more species specific and effective the organism–environment fit will become at the level of the organism's central nervous system (CNS). The simpler an organism's CNS, the more likely it is that behavior sequences will be hard-wired on a simple level. If an organism's CNS is more complex, the behavioral repertoire that is necessary to ensure the species' survival will be more complex and flexible, the sensory association cortical areas will be larger in proportion to the primary sensory cortical areas, and the response repertoire that is soft-wired will be more differentiated. Flexibility and complexity of behavioral response systems are the landmarks of such soft-wired flexible and complex nervous systems (Als, 1982a, 1992a, 1999; Als & Brazelton, 1981; Als et al., 1982b).

Ethological studies of the interaction between human newborns and caregivers have identified the importance, complexity, and subtlety of parent–infant interactions. Although the human newborn has evolved to count on the ventroventral primate Tragling (being carried) configuration (Hassenstein, 1973), human newborns depend on their parents' active physical support to be carried successfully. Positive elicitors that engage caregivers to perform such carrying are required early on to keep human parents socially and affectively close to their infants. Infants are motorically incapable of maintaining physical closeness, although it is necessary for their survival. Immediately after birth, the connections between newborn eye opening and attention and parents' affectionate behavior demonstrate complex homeostatic regulation patterns (Als, 1975, 1977; Grossman, 1978; Minde et al., 1980; Robson, 1967) that function as mutual releasers. These patterns launch both infant and parent on their path to complex affective and cognitive interchanges and mutually potentiated competence that extends well beyond the removal of pain and discomfort, provision of shelter, and alleviation of hunger and thirst. The principle of adaptedness emphasizes the importance of recognizing behaviors as species adapted at each stage of ontogenetic development. The principle identifies the human newborn as a socially competent and active partner in a feedback system with the caregiver, who elicits physiologic, motor, state, and attention interactive coregulation from the environment to support self-actualization (Als, 1999; Beeghly et al., 2016).

Beginning at birth, human newborns are structured to actively elicit the emotional and affective/cognitive support and input that launches and fuels their own increasing behavioral differentiation and organization (Als, 1977). Human newborns actively shape their own development. Adult humans in turn place a high value on their offspring's early interactive attention; this is in keeping with their species-specific human adaption and predisposition for affective closeness that facilitates physical closeness.

Applying principles of organism–environment transaction to the study of human newborns has led to identification of the interplay of various behaviorally expressed subsystems of functioning. These subsystems are the infants' physiologic or autonomic, motor, and state organization systems. Within the state system is the evolving attention system and the self-regulatory system, which ensure the reintegration of the other subsystems as they interact with the caregiving environment. The infant's adaptive task is to achieve synchronization among the periodicities of these different subsystems, as well as synchronization between the internal subsystem events and the external environmental events (Sander, 1975; Sander, 1980; Sander et al., 1979). Stimuli that are poorly timed may disrupt all subsystems, whereas appropriately timed stimuli will maintain and enhance functional integration and support development. The caregiver's task lies in identifying synchronous, cohesive, well-integrated, and harmonious subsystem functioning and recognizing the thresholds to disruption before they are reached and passed.

According to Denny-Brown (Denny-Brown, 1962, 1966), a motor system physiologist, the tension between two basic response antagonists underlies an organism's development toward smooth functioning. The two basic response antagonists are the exploratory and avoiding responses; in other words, the "toward" and the "away" responses or the approaching or reaching out response and the withdrawing or defending response. These two response antagonists are released together at times when they conflict with one another. When a threshold of organism-appropriate stimulation is surpassed, one response antagonist may abruptly switch into the other. These two antagonistic poles of behavior are biologically very basic, as is demonstrated by the existence of single cells in the somatosensory cortex of the primate that are programmed to produce total body-toward movements upon stimulation, whereas other single cells produce total body-avoidance movements (Duffy & Burchfiel, 1971). The same basic principle has been demonstrated in the behavioral development of a number of other nonprimate species (Rosenblatt, 1976; Schneirla, 1959, 1965; Schneirla & Rosenblatt, 1961, 1963).

The principles as outlined are all relevant to the understanding of preterm newborns, who find themselves in the extrauterine environment of the NICU. The principle of dual-antagonist integration is helpful in understanding preterm infants' behavioral patterns that indicate thresholds from integration to disorganization. When behavior is well integrated, the toward and away antagonists modulate one another and bring about an adaptive response. If an input is compelling to the infant, the infant will approach the input, interact with it, seek it out, and become receptive to it. If the input exceeds the infant's capacity to respond, they actively will avoid the input and withdraw from it. One response modulates the other. For example, a full-term newborn is drawn to the animated face of an interacting caregiver. As the infant's attention intensifies, the infant's eyes will widen, eyebrows rise, and the mouth will shape toward the interactor (Als, 1975, 1977). However, when the dampening systems are immature as in the preterm infant, responses may be generalized, for instance, the infant's whole head may move forward, arms and legs may thrust forward, and fingers and toes may extend toward the interactor. The response, early on, may involve the entire body in an undifferentiated way and only gradually become increasingly confined to the face alone (Als, 1979). The differentiation process appears to be regulated by homeostatic infant behaviors such as gaze-aversion yawning, sneezing, or hiccoughing. Or it may be regulated by the caregiver who through kissing, nuzzling, or moving the infant close-in will reduce the intensity of attention–interaction and reset its cycle (Als, 1975, 1977). When neither of these regulatory processes is brought into play or when the initial input is too strong, an infant may turn away, grimace, extend arms to the side, arch the trunk, splay fingers and toes, cry, hiccough, spit up, stop breathing, or defecate. In short, an infant may call up and respond with clear avoidance behaviors at the various behavioral subsystem levels of functioning. Consequently, very early behavioral functioning may be conceptualized as the continuous negotiation of balancing avoidance and approach behaviors in continuation of the intrauterine fetal developmental progression (Als, 1978, 1979, 1982a, 1982b, 1983; Brazelton & Als, 1979).

The initial challenge for premature human newborns is stabilization and integration of autonomic functioning such as breathing, heart rate, temperature control, and digestive function, for which technologic supports such as respirators,

incubators, and intravenous and/or tube feedings typically are required. The premature infant's motor system is the competent fetus' motor system at the gestational stage at which the preterm infant is born. This motor system is capable of initiating and maintaining flexion, rotation, bringing hands to the mouth, sucking, grasping, and so on.

State organization and other periodicities that in the womb used to be regulated by maternal sleep–wake and rest–activity cycles and maternal hormonal and nutritional cycles now are at the mercy of the rhythms of the NICU environment. The synactive model of subsystem differentiation (Als, 1982a) highlights the simultaneity of all subsystems in their interaction with one another and with the environment (Fig. 3-1).

It brings to the forefront the unexpected discrepancy between the experience outside the womb and the biologically expected intrauterine experience. The preterm infant's autonomic system typically requires technological support, which presents a significant continuous challenge and cost to the motor and state systems.

MODEL OF THE SYNACTIVE
ORGANIZATION OF BEHAVIORAL DEVELOPMENT

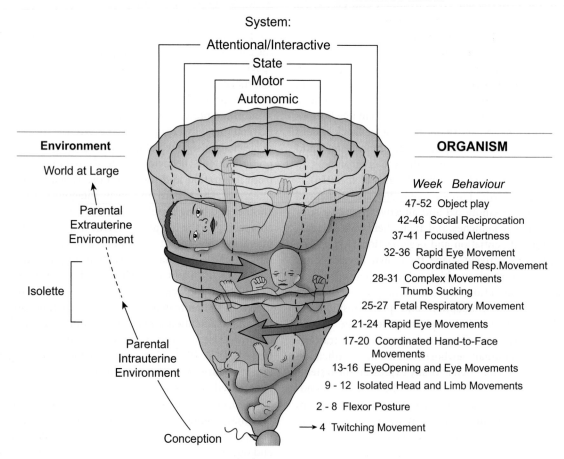

FIGURE 3-1. The synactive theory model of development.

The process of development entails subsystem stabilization and integration to promote continued differentiation and emergence of next capabilities. Each newly integrated accomplishment in turn engenders a reopening of the established balance and a new level of disorganization and disequilibrium as the next developmental goal pushes into the foreground and is conquered. This ontogenetic drive to differentiate and reintegrate is a lifelong process that begins in the womb. It aims for ever higher levels of differentiation and reintegration of the overall system, e.g., from kicking one's legs to crawling, standing, walking, ice-skating, and ice-dancing. In this model, the entire system continually reopens and progresses to new, further levels of more differentiated integration from which the next emerging subsystem differentiation and reorganization occurs (Als, 1979, 1982a, 1982b, 1983; Als et al., 1982a; Als et al., 1982b). To paraphrase Erikson (Erikson, 1962), self-actualization is participation with the world and interaction with another with a "minimum of defensive maneuvers and a maximum of activation, a minimum of idiosyncratic distortion and a maximum of joint validation" (p. 463).

UNDERSTANDING NEWBORN BEHAVIOR

Taking into consideration the anatomic and functional development of the brain, this model of development hypothesizes that, by observing infant behavior, it is feasible to estimate the expectation of the fetal infant's brain for input as well as infer the infant's developmental goals for coregulatory support. The approach postulates that an infant's behavior provides the best information from which to estimate his or her current capabilities and infer the goals the infant attempts to accomplish and the processes involved to achieve each next level of differentiation. With such information, practitioners should be in a position to predict the supports that may further the infant's competencies toward achieving the infant's goals and support overall neurobehavioral organization in the face of necessary medical and nursing procedures. Because infants are seen as continuously and actively self-constructing (Fischer & Rose, 1994; Ford, 1987) living systems, the task of care becomes a task of collaborating with infants. Observation and the design of subsequent support for premature infants conceptually is based on a combination of knowledge about the fetal brain, behavioral developmental progression, and the demand characteristics of newborn intensive care and environments. The developmental functioning of full-term infants provides a biologic blueprint that is modified by the altered environment–fetus transaction and by each infant's individual characteristics and expectations. Accurate interpretation of infant behavior makes construction and implementation of individually appropriate environments and care not only feasible but also an obligation and responsibility (Als, 1982a).

It has been shown that even the earliest-born and most fragile infants display reliably observable behaviors that take the form of autonomic and visceral responses such as respiration patterns, color fluctuations, spitting, gagging, hiccoughing, and straining. Other behaviors include movement patterns, postures, truncal tone, and tone of extremities and face, reflected as finger splaying, arching, and grimacing, among others. Other parameters to consider are levels of awareness, referred to as "states," such as sleeping, wakefulness, and aroused upset, and their respective characteristics (Als, 1983, 1984; Als et al., 1982b).

The infant's behavioral repertoire has been identified along the lines of three main subsystems: the autonomic system, the motor system, and the state system. Infants' communication with the environment along these subsystems is readily accessible for observation, even without instrumentation, and will indicate if the activity currently going on around or within the infant supports the infant's functioning or is taxing, demanding, or potentially stressful (Als, 1982a; Als et al., 1986). The autonomic system's functioning is observable in an infant's breathing patterns, color fluctuation, and visceral stability or instability. Examples of autonomic systems responses include respiratory regularities or irregularities, color changes such as cyanosis or pallor, and visceral stability reflected in hiccoughing, gagging, or spitting up. Observe an infant's body tone, postural repertoire, and movement patterns to assess the effects of motor-system integrity and functioning. Examples of these effects are reflected in facial and trunk tone; tone of the extremities; in the extensor and flexor postures; and movements of the face, trunk, and limbs. State organization is observable in an infant's range of available states, the robustness and modulation of the states, and the patterns of transition from state to state. Some infants show the full continuum of states, from deep sleep, to light sleep, to drowsy, to quiet alert, to active awake and aroused, to upset and crying (Brazelton, 1973). Alternately, during interactions some infants move from sleep to aroused states and immediately back to sleep again, skipping the alert state. State stability and the smooth transition from state to state reflect intact state organization and CNS control, whereas the opposite would reflect CNS disorganization.

Newborn Individualized Developmental Care and Assessment Program (Boston, MA)

NIDCAP has created a clinically usable paper-and-pen methodology to record detailed observations of an infant's naturally occurring behaviors in the NICU and to document infant communication. The observer stands near the bedside and watches and records the infant's behavior and vital signs as well as the caregiver's action sequence. To understand an infant's current functioning and thresholds of stability of the autonomic, motor, and state organizational systems, it is useful to observe an infant for at least 60 to 90 minutes. This period includes approximately 10 minutes of observation before a caregiving interaction is initiated, followed by the duration of the caregiving interaction itself, be it taking of vital signs, suctioning, diaper change, and feeding, and subsequent to the care interaction approximately 10 minutes of observation or until the infant has returned to a recognizable pattern of behavior. Such an observation, especially if repeated on a weekly basis or more frequently, yields specific information regarding an infant's relative robustness and fragility as well as highlights the care situations and/or actions in which the infant thrives or which the infant experiences as stressful (Als, 1981 rev. 1995; Als et al., 1986, 1994). These observations then, are utilized to infer the infant's own goals for next steps of development and to formulate for caregiving suggestions and modifications in environmental structuring that are hypothesized to be supportive of the infant's own goal achievements. Implementation of the recommendations and the resulting infant behavior and functioning is the proof of the aptness or inaptness of the recommendations made.

The detailed behavioral recordings serve the opportunities to support and educate the reader, be it the professional or the parent caregiver, in understanding the infant's language and communication. Professional staff typically lack the time to stand at a bedside for an hour or longer and simply observe. The NIDCAP observer therefore provides the caregiver with a narrative translation of the infant's story as gleaned from the observation. In integrating the infant's observed behavioral communication into a descriptive narrative, the caregiver is afforded the opportunity to see the infants with the NIDCAP Professionals eyes and learn about the effects of their care from the infant's perspective. The narrative provides the caregiver with a shortcut to feel and live the care experience as the infant did. First, the environment is described in terms of light, sound, and activity. The behavioral picture derived from the observation period preceding the caregiving interaction then is described in its relationship to heart rate (HR), respiratory rate (RR), and blood oxygen levels. The caregiving actions and their effect on the infant are then documented, with specific infant behaviors observed, again in conjunction with the HR, RR, and oxygen levels and their changes. The infant's efforts to integrate the effects of the interaction and the caregiver's efforts are described. It is important to stay cognizant of the fact that infants have strategies and mechanisms available to move away from and avoid environmental demands or configurations that are inappropriate in complexity, intensity, and/or timing. Infants also have strategies and mechanisms available to seek out and move toward inputs that are at the level of their current intake and processing capabilities. Avoidance behaviors reflect stress. Approach behaviors reflect well-being and/or the striving toward well-being via self-regulatory efforts. Approach and self-regulatory behaviors, when exceeded by the current stimulus, may shift into stress behaviors; similarly, stress behaviors, when the current stimulus is reduced, may transform into self-regulatory strategies and/or well-being behaviors.

In this model, extension behaviors largely are thought to reflect stress and flexion behaviors are thought to reflect self-regulatory efforts and competence. Diffuse behaviors are thought to reflect stress, and well-defined robust behaviors to reflect self-regulatory balance. Self-regulatory balance is reflected in regular, smooth breathing, which is neither too fast nor too slow and is free of pauses. Heart rates between 120 and 160 beats a minute, breathing rates of between 40 and 60 breaths a minute, and oxygen saturation in the blood between 92% and 98% as measured with pulse oximetry typically are interpreted as effective self-regulation indices. Other evidence of balance is the presence of pink color; the absence of tremors, startles, and twitches; the absence of visceral signs such as gagging, hiccoughing, vomiting, flatulence, and bowel evacuations; the absence of flaccidity; the presence of smooth, softly flexed arm, leg, and trunk positions; smooth movements of arms, legs, and trunk; and efforts and successes at tucking trunk and limbs together as well as modulated smooth tone throughout face and body. Other signs are searching to suck on something and actively sucking, hand and foot clasping, hand-to-mouth efforts, grasping and holding on, the presence of robust states, raising of eyebrows (face opening), frowning, forward shaping of the mouth (ooh face) and face (frowning), looking, cooing, and speech-like mouth and lip movements. Stress and low thresholds to react, reflecting greater sensitivity, are thought to be reflected by uneven breathing patterns (overly slow or fast and/or pausing) and color other than pink such as pale, mottled, red, dusky, or blue.

Other evidence indicating stress is the presence of tremors, startles, and twitches and visceral signs as described above including spitting up; gagging; hiccoughs; grunting; and bowel movement straining, sounds, gasps, and sighs. Motor signs of stress include flaccidity of the face, arms, legs, and trunk; frequent extensor movements of the arms and legs; stretching and drowning-like behavior; squirming; arching; tongue extensions; grimacing; specific finger, arm, and leg extensions (splaying, airplaneing, saluting, and sitting on air); fisting, fussing, yawning, and sneezing; floating eye movements; and visual averting. A heart rate lower than 120 or higher than 160 beats a minute, a breathing rate lower than 40 or higher than 60 breaths a minute, and blood oxygenation saturation levels lower than 92% or higher than 98% also are considered likely the signs of stress. A picture emerges from such a description as to the level of support with which the infant will thrive and the relative intensity of sensory input at which the infant will move from self-regulatory balance to stress. The behavioral report that articulates the infant's behavioral regulation is written in a language understandable to parents as well as professionals alike. The report's purpose (Box "NIDCAP® Report Example–Behavioral Observation [Verbatim]") is to avail caregivers to hear and understand the infant, that is to educate and support caregivers in understanding each infant's individual behavioral functioning and threshold to stress. The report describes and highlights the infant as an active structurer and participant in their own development (Als, 1999).

NIDCAP® Report Example–Behavioral Observation (Verbatim)

Introduction

The observation of Robert took place at the Newborn Intensive Care Nursery at St. L. Hospital in the context of a teaching session, scheduled for March 1, 1995, 8:12 to 8:52 a.m. Robert's nurse Nancy cared for Robert at the time of the observation. Four observers participated in the teaching session.

Observation

1. Nursery Environment
   Robert lived in an incubator, in Room 3, a large rectangular care room with big windows along one of the long and one of the short walls of the room. Eleven beds stood along the two long walls of the room; 10 of them provided care spaces for infants. Several of the infants lay in incubators, two in open cribs, and the infant immediately next to Robert received care on an open warming table, a special high-frequency breathing machine, which made continuous loud sounds, supported that infant's breathing. Robert's incubator stood directly under one of the large windows and immediately across the open room door leading to the hallway.

   Bright sunlight streamed through the windows. Staff members quietly walked back and forth; several shielded their eyes from the sun with their hands. Blinds partly drawn reduced the sunlight from a few of the windows. In addition to the sunlight full overhead ceiling lights further added to the room's brightness. At times up to 10 staff members and several parents engaged in various care activities in the room. Support staff members emptied refuse bins. Alarms sounded. A telephone rang repeatedly. Voice levels rose and fell repeatedly. At the foot of the incubators and cribs stood large wooden cabinets painted white. They further narrowed the passage between the incubators and cribs so that only one person at a time could pass along the center aisle of the room. Soft quilts covered some of the incubators; hospital blankets covered others. At some of the bedsides stood straight chairs. Overall, the room appeared bright and full of sound and activity; space appeared tight, although relatively well organized.

2. Robert's Bedspace and Bedding
   Robert lay quietly in his incubator, bedded on his tummy on a soft sheepskin-covered mattress. A blanket roll supported his feet and curled along his sides and head. He faced to his left, his eyes shielded with a mask to protect him from the special bright lights (bilirubin lights) above him used to treat the yellowness of his skin (jaundice), caused by bilirubin, a yellow substance that is made up of the left-over parts of used-up red blood cells, and that Robert's still immature liver finds difficult to break down further and get rid of. He held his buttocks tucked up; his knees lay turned out beside his hips and his ankles and feet pointed outward into the blanket roll. He wore a diaper, which appeared big for him. Robert held his right arm tucked up close to his right shoulder, his hand tightly fisted. A thin line, that brought fluid from a pump above him, went into a blood vessel on the underside of Robert's left wrist (intravenous line, IV). Robert held his left arm stretched out straight as if the line was perhaps hurting him. He fisted his left hand tightly. Leads to keep track of his heart rate, breathing rate, the oxygen level in his blood stream, and his body temperature were fastened to his chest, back, and his left foot. The lines attached to him draped neatly alongside him.

3. Robert's Behavior Before Caregiving Interaction
   Robert appeared to be asleep under his eye mask. He lay there very quietly. The fisting of his left hand at times became tighter. As he paled more, he appeared to be increasingly yellow; his legs and feet stayed very dark and dusky. He breathed with fluttering breaths, at times quite shallow and labored, at other times fast and unsteady; he took approximately 30 to 40 breaths a minute. His heart beat quite steadily about 130 to 140 times a minute. The oxygen level in his blood stream stayed steady much of the time at about 99%, with only one dip to 76% after his breathing had become quite unsteady for a period. As he squirmed and adjusted his position, he recovered his oxygen level quickly.

4. Robert's Behavior During Caregiving Interaction
   As Robert's nurse Nancy stepped to his bedside, she first arranged the necessary materials for the planned caregiving interaction. She then quietly observed Robert for a minute and counted his breathing rate. Then she turned off the bilirubin light above him and moved it away from the bedside, quietly opened the portholes of the incubator, and gently placed a thermometer under Robert's left arm. Robert immediately became dark and dusky and quickly pulled his arms closer in, fisted even more tightly and pulled his legs up. The oxygen level in his blood stream dropped to 88%, and he held his

breath for a number of seconds. His nurse Nancy turned him quickly onto his back, one hand under his buttocks and one under his shoulders; Robert's arms and hands flew out to the sides, his fingers fully extended. He attempted to bring his arms back in and tuck his legs and feet in, turned his ankles outward into the bedding and grasped the bedding with his toes and fingers. His nurse Nancy now immediately listened to his chest and belly and took his pulse with a stethoscope. She then quite quickly pulled her hands out of the incubator and attended to another staff member, who had come to her with a question. Robert continued to breathe quite unsteadily. He continued to make efforts to tuck his arms closer in and grasp and reached with his hands and feet at his bedding. His face puckered up and his forehead furrowed, and he appeared to cry. The oxygen level in his blood was at 89% as his heart rate rose to 162 beats a minute. He became increasingly dark and dusky all over; his feet became deep purple. His nurse Nancy gathered Robert up, briefly held him in, and then turned him quickly onto his tummy so he faced now to his right. His head lay now elevated on a folded diaper, his neck and shoulders sank off the diaper. All the while the eye shield continued to cover Robert's eyes. Robert's nurse Nancy then adjusted the blanket rolls around him and fastened several straps across his back; the straps seemed to hold the nest's edges together. Nancy then closed the incubator doors matter-of-factly and moved the bilirubin lights back into position and turned them on above Robert. Robert attempted to settle and tucked his arms close up to his chest, with his knees and ankles turned out. The inside of his feet pressed into his bedding. His whole body looked very dark and dusky; he breathed unsteadily and appeared to be restless and awake. He raised his eyebrows repeatedly above the bilirubin mask and opened and closed his mouth as if searching for something to suck on.

5. Robert's Behavior Following Caregiving Interaction
   For the next 6 minutes Robert squirmed and attempted to tuck together more; he twitched and searched with his mouth. He brought his left hand closer up to his mouth, and one finger touched his lips. He raised his eyebrows and forehead several more times, and he probably stayed awake under his mask for quite some time. During the course of his efforts to settle, the oxygen level in Robert's bloodstream repeatedly dropped below 85%. Each time he recovered with further squirming. Gradually his face appeared to lose energy more and more and

he eventually became very still. His shoulders sank more into the bedding. His left hand stayed close to his mouth and occasionally his mouth opened and closed slightly. He continued to stay quite dark and purple; his heart rate ranged between 130 and 145 beats a minute. His breathing fluttered and at times appeared quite labored with an overall rate between 30 and 46 breaths a minute. The oxygen level in his blood stream now remained relatively steady at 95%. He appeared to be very exhausted.

Summary

Robert was born at the 29th week of pregnancy of his 31-year-old mother, Mrs. A., who has two other children. Mrs. A's pregnancy was complicated by high blood pressure. At 28 weeks, she began to show some vaginal bleeding and contractions. Her doctor admitted her to the hospital for 4 days and gave her medication (dexamethasone) in support of Robert's lung maturation and medication (terbutaline) to help prevent Robert's premature delivery. Mrs. A continued the terbutaline treatment at home for four more days, when her labor began. On her way to the regional maternity hospital, St. L., Robert's father stopped at a hospital nearer to the parents' home, since Robert was ready to be born, feet first. He was somewhat limp at birth with poor color, as reflected in his score of well-being (Apgar Score) of 5 at 1 minute, 10 being the best score. He recovered quickly, and by 5 minutes he received a score of 7, by 10 minutes a score of 9. The Apgar Score is named after a Newborn Infant Doctor (neonatologist) Virginia Apgar. It measures the infant's well-being right after birth by measuring breathing, color, heart rate, reactivity, and muscle tone, each on a scale from 0 to 2. An infant at best may be scored 2 on all five categories measured and thus receives a total score of 10. Robert did very well with a score of 9 by 10 minutes after delivery. He received oxygen and was transported together with his mother to St. L. Hospital. At birth, Robert weighed 2 lbs, 15 oz (1340 g; 50 %ile, which means that he weighed more than 50 out of 100 boys born at his age), measured 15 inches (38 cm; 50 %ile), and had ahead circumference of 11 inches (28 cm; 75 %ile). This shows that Robert had grown appropriately in his mother's womb. Once in the intensive care nursery, Robert received special support for his breathing with extra oxygen for less than a day. Since then he breathed room air on his own, supported only with some medication (caffeine). A vessel in his heart that was open in the womb continues to be open (patent ductus arteriosus; PDA). To support its closing, Robert currently receives steroid medication (Indocin). In order to protect his intestines from bleeding, his feeding has been stopped for the time being and he receives fluids by IV. Robert is now 4 days old since birth and has developed jaundice, which is treated with special light therapy (phototherapy; bilirubin lights).

From the observation today, Robert appeared to be a competent and very sensitive child. He made repeated efforts to adjust his position in the incubator and sought to be more comfortable. When cared for, he made strong efforts to tuck himself together and to settle. Despite the mask that continuously covered his eyes, he made great efforts to look. He also attempted to find something to suck on. He brought his hands to his mouth quite readily and several times. His sensitivity showed itself in his color changes, his shallow and labored breathing, the occasional drops in oxygen level in his blood, and his increasing exhaustion by the end of the caregiving interaction and the end of the observation.

Robert's Current Goals

From today's observation Robert appears to be working toward:

1. Becoming increasingly more robust and steady in his breathing and oxygen levels when resting and when interacted with.
2. Becoming increasingly successful in pulling himself into a more tucked restful position, bringing his hands to his mouth and bracing his legs into his bedding.
3. Awakening and looking, as well as sucking.

Recommendations

In support of Robert's goal strivings, the following suggestions may be helpful:

1. Nursery Environment
   a. Consider exploration of opportunities to reduce the sound generated by staff voices, alarms, the respirator at the next bedside, telephones, etc.
   b. In support of a calmer environment, consider reduction of the light levels in the room, perhaps drawing the blinds when the sunlight is bright and reducing overhead lighting.
   c. Consider provision of a darkened environment throughout the day for Robert in support of his alertness and sleep development; consider the use of a specialized light therapy blanket (biliblanket), which will free up his eyes from the need to be patched.
   d. Consider rearrangement of the cabinets at the foot of the beds in order to reduce the congestion in the room.
   e. Consider keeping the room door closed in order to reduce sound from the hallway.

2. Bedspace and Bedding
   a. Consider development of an inviting atmosphere around Robert's bedspace for his parents, brother, and sister to be with him for extended periods as well as in support of the comfort of his professional caregivers.
   b. Consider a recliner chair supportive of Robert's parents and professional caregivers when they hold Robert wrapped in a bilirubin blanket without eye patches; they would thereby facilitate his strengths, energy, and opportunity to look.
   c. Consider providing Robert with a soft, well-aligned nest, perhaps bedding him on his side and giving him the opportunity to tuck into a contained restful position.
   d. Consider the use of very small diapers for Robert in support of more well-aligned positions for his legs.
   e. Consider bedding Robert with a long soft pillow to hug with his arms and legs; this might bring his knees and ankles together when he lies on his side.

3. Caregiving Interaction
   a. Consider Robert as an active partner in his care and as a competent child who makes strong efforts to be restful and tuck himself together.
   b. Consider using your observation of Robert's breathing at the beginning of your caregiving interaction as an opportunity to let Robert tell you what he is attempting to accomplish.
   c. Consider as soon as you have turned off the bilirubin light above Robert, removal of Robert's eye patches before you care for him and while you care for and interact with him; observe his reaction and give him an opportunity to relax and recover from the periods of eye patching; give him the opportunity to experience and enjoy the social interchange with you.
   d. Consider introduction of your hands to Robert first; first learn how he responds to you and assist him in accomplishing the position and actions he aims for, before you engage in specific caregiving tasks.
   e. Consider supporting Robert gently into lying on his side; encourage him to hold onto your hands and offer him opportunities to suck. Contain him while taking his vital signs and changing his diaper.
   f. Consider containing and holding Robert when you interact with him; give him the opportunity to experience smooth movements of his arms and legs.

g. Consider involving a physical or occupational therapist in Robert's care in order to evaluate his leg and foot positions, as well as to consult to you about the best ways to support his leg position and movement.

h. Consider seeking developmental guidance in caring for Robert and in supporting your caregiving interactions to become increasingly collaborative with Robert. Enjoy his competence and your facilitation of his efforts.

i. Consider multiple thoughtful invitations to Robert's parents to be there as much and for as long as possible, in order to care for and hold Robert in soothing and growth promoting skin-to-skin contact (kangaroo care) as this may help him in preserving energy and regaining it quickly after more stressful necessary procedures.

[Used with permission from Pearls of Wisdom Task Group, NIDCAP Federation Int'l. 2020.]

RESEARCH TO TEST THE EFFICACY OF NIDCAP

Very-Early-Born High-Risk Infants Born Below 29 Weeks' Gestation

The NIDCAP approach to individualized environmental and care support based on reading preterm infants' behavioral cues increasingly is advocated for preterm infants at the highest risk for later disability (Becker et al., 1993; Grunwald & Becker, 1990; Lawhon, 1986; Lawhon & Melzar, 1991; VandenBerg, 1990a, 1990b; VandenBerg & Franck, 1990; Wolke, 1987) among others. In the past 35 years, this approach has been tested in numerous studies. Als, Lawhon, and colleagues (1986) found improved medical outcomes of VLBW ventilated preterm infants as evidenced by shorter stays on the respirator and a decrease in the need for supplemental oxygen as well as gavage feedings. Improved neurobehavioral outcomes at 2 weeks corrected age, as assessed with the Assessment of Preterm Infants' Behavior (APIB) (Als et al., 1982a; 1982b), and at 9 months using the Bayley Scales of Infant Development, again were found. Furthermore, there was improved behavioral regulation and planning was evident as assessed by using a videotaped play paradigm (the Kangaroo Box Paradigm) (Als & Berger, 1986). Becker and colleagues (Becker et al., 1991; Grunwald & Becker, 1990) found significantly lower scores of morbidity in the first 4 weeks of hospitalization as measured with the Minde Daily Morbidity Scale (Minde et al., 1983). The researchers documented significantly earlier onset of oral feedings, better average daily weight gain, shorter hospital stays, and improved overall behavioral functioning at discharge as measured with the Neonatal Behavioral Assessment Scale (Brazelton, 1984). Longer-term outcomes assessed for the study by Als et al. (1994) at 18 months and 3 years continued to show a consistent developmental advantage of the experimental group over the control group (McAnulty et al., 2010). The preliminary results from the longitudinal data available show much improved performance of the experimental group at 8 years on several neuropsychological measures (McAnulty et al., 2009). A study by Als et al. (1994) used random assignment

of infants weighing less than 1,251 g born before 30 weeks' gestational age, intubated within the first 3 hours after delivery, and requiring mechanical ventilation for at least 24 of the first 48 hours. A total of 18 control and 20 experimental group infants met these criteria. For this study, a group of nurses were educated and trained in the behaviorally based approach of individualized caregiving. Staffing was structured in such a way that, for the experimental group infants, a nurse, educated in the behavioral approach, cared for an infant and family during at least one shift in every 24-hour cycle. Formal behavioral observations were conducted by a psychologist in collaboration with a developmental clinical nurse specialist. The observations were initiated within the first 24 hours and were repeated every 10th day until the infant's discharge from the nursery. The observations provided the basis of support to the primary care teams for individualization of care for the experimental group infants and their families. The control group infants were identified to the NICU staff within 2 weeks before discharge so that staffing and care remained unbiased. The control and experimental groups were comparable on all background variables including birth weight, gestational age at birth, Apgar scores at 1 and 5 minutes, mean and maximum fractions of inspired oxygen in the first 48 hours and the first 10 days, incidence of patent ductus arteriosus, maternal age, social class, Obstetric Complication Scale Scores (Littman & Parmelee, 1974), gender, ethnicity, birth order, and the use of prenatal corticosteroids. The experimental group infants showed significant reduction in the length of hospitalization, were younger at discharge, had reduced hospital charges, and improved weight gain to 2 weeks after their due date. They had a significantly reduced rate of intraventricular hemorrhage (IVH) and reduced severity of chronic lung disease. They also showed improved developmental outcome at 2 weeks corrected age as measured with the APIB (Als et al., 1982b), with much better functioning in terms of autonomic regulation, motor system performance, and self-regulation. Systematic electrophysiological group differences by quantified electroencephalography (qEEG) with topographic mapping (Duffy et al., 1979) also were found at 2 weeks post term, suggesting differences in function in a large frontocentral region of the brain and in an extensive portion of the right occipital hemisphere, two left parietal, a right parietal, and an additional right occipital region. The right hemisphere is known to develop with greater velocity in the last 12 weeks' gestation in comparison with the left hemisphere. This appears to make the right hemisphere more vulnerable to external experiences as compared with the left hemisphere (Kasprian et al., 2011).

By 9 months after the expected date of confinement (EDC) on assessment with the Bayley Scales of Infant Development, the experimental group, as compared with the control group, showed a significantly higher Mental Developmental Index (118.30 ± 17.35 vs. 94.38 ± 23.31; $F = 12.47$; $df = 1,34$; $p \leq .001$) and Psychomotor Developmental Index (100.60 ± 20.19 vs. 83.56 ± 17.97; $F = 6.97$; $df = 1,34$; $p \leq .01$). Furthermore, of 20 infant variables measured in the 6-minutes Kangaroo Box Paradigm play episode, 16 showed differences favoring the experimental group. They ranged in significance level from less than 0.03 to less than 0.0001. The largest differences were found in gross and fine motor modulation, overflow postures and associated movements, the complexity and modulation of combining object and social play, the ability to stay engaged in a task, and the degree of facilitation necessary to accomplish a task. In the 6-minute Still-Face episode, 12 of 19 infant parameters showed significant group differences ($p < .04$ to < 0.0001), again favoring the experimental group infants. None of the 14 parent variables assessed showed a significant group difference, yet all three interaction variables (turn taking, overall synchrony of the interaction, and overall quality of the interaction variables ($p < .0004$) favored the experimental group. Consequently, infants in the experimental group appeared significantly better organized, better differentiated, and better modulated than the control group infants. Canonical correlation between the factors derived from the APIB variables and the Kangaroo Box variables was statistically significant. This indicates a strong relationship between overall behavioral regulation at 2 weeks, as measured with the APIB, and overall regulation at 9 months, as measured with the Kangaroo Box Paradigm.

Neither IVH nor bronchopulmonary dysplasia (BPD) had significant indirect effects on any of the medical outcome variables. In terms of electrophysiological outcome, IVH had a significant indirect effect on only one variable. However, even for this variable, the direct intervention effect was stronger. The presence of BPD had no indirect effect on any of the electrophysiological findings. Neither IVH nor BPD had any significant indirect effects on any of the APIB or Bayley outcome measures. Furthermore, only 2 of the 32 Kangaroo Box measures showed significant indirect IVH effects, namely, symmetry of motor performance in the Play and in the Still-Face episode. None showed indirect BPD effects. Consequently, the direct effects of the intervention on outcome appear to go beyond the indirect contribution from reduction in IVH and BPD.

In a longitudinal study recalling the 38 infants in the 1994 study by Als and colleagues (Als et al., 1994), a total of 19 children at 8 years of age (9 control and 10 experimental) were fully evaluated for neuropsychological and neurophysiological functioning (McAnulty et al., 2010). The children who had been in the NIDCAP (experimental) group in the NICU demonstrated significantly better spatial visualization and mental control than those who had received standard (control) care. The neurobehavioral (APIB) and neurophysiological (EEG coherence) measures in the newborn period were better predictors of neuropsychological functioning at 8 years than the medical outcome variables from the NICU. Two studies from other centers (Fleisher et al., 1995; Westrup et al., 2000) focused on the same high-risk populations and were conducted after the introduction of surfactant in the NICUs. The studies found significant positive medical results and, in the study testing behavioral outcome, positive APIB results, although the NIDCAP intervention in both studies only involved in-service orientations to the nursing staff and relied on an experienced NIDCAP-trained professional and leader in each of the two NICUs to provide daily support to those caring for the experimental group infants. The study conducted in Sweden (Westrup et al., 2000) also reported long-term, significantly improved neurodevelopmental outcome for the experimental group children at 1, 3, and 5 years of age (Kleberg et al., 2000; Kleberg et al., 2002; Westrup et al., 2003).

In another study (McAnulty et al., 2009), the integration of this individualized approach into the NICU was tested by assignment of experimental group high-risk infants to specially trained care teams supported on an ongoing basis by two developmental specialists yet without conducting serial behavioral observations. Analysis of outcome again showed a reduction in the number of days on a ventilator and reduced days for gavage-tube feedings, decreased lengths of hospitalization, and improved weight gain, as well as improved developmental outcome at 2 weeks and 9 months after the EDC. However, the incidence of IVH and severity of chronic lung disease were comparable between the two groups. IVH effects may depend on developmental support in the acute first few hours of admission when systematic feedback might be productive differentially.

A recent, multicenter study tested the NIDCAP approach simultaneously in three different NICUs (Als et al., 2003). This randomized clinical (multicenter) trial focused on ventilator-dependent, very-high-risk preterm infants born at 28 weeks' gestation or earlier. The study involved an inborn as well as two transport NICUs. Two of the NICUs used primary care nursing, and one of the transport nurseries used conventionally scheduled nursing. Results validated the effectiveness of the developmental care model based on significant improvement in terms of weight gain and growth parameters and reduced length of hospital stay and hospital costs. Developmental outcome, as measured with the APIB, also showed significant improvement. Analysis of the assessment of family functioning showed that the experimental group parents were significantly less stressed (Abidin, 1995) and more effective in understanding their infants as individuals and themselves as parents (O'Donnell, 1986). Furthermore, the consistency of NIDCAP care implementation for the experimental groups was found to be significantly higher than for the control group in all parameters that involved care aspects under the direction of individual caregivers at the bedside (Als et al., 1990, 1995. Rev. 1997). The three NICU-wide parameters of light, sound, and activity level were found to be comparable between control and experimental group infants. This was interpreted to mean that NIDCAP care involves more than light, sound, and activity control and seems to include the quality of individually sensitive caregiving interaction with infants that relies on each infant's cues to guide the timing, intensity, and duration of all action sequences and subcomponents.

A randomized controlled NIDCAP trial involving similarly early-born high-risk preterm infants in Alberta, Canada, showed significant reduction in ventilation support requirements and significant reduction in severe disability at 24 months corrected age (Peters et al., 2009).

Infants Born Between 28 and 33 Weeks of Gestation

To test the efficacy of the NIDCAP approach to caregiving in supporting brain development, a sample of healthy, low-risk, preterm infants, free of known focal and suspected brain or lung lesions, was studied (Buehler et al., 1995). Twenty-four consecutively inborn preterm singleton infants cared for in a 16-bed, level II special care nursery (SCN) were randomly assigned to experimental and control groups. They were younger than 34 weeks' gestational age at birth, appropriate weight for gestational age, had uneventful labor and delivery histories, required mechanical ventilation for less than 24 hours, were genetically and neurologically intact, and had healthy mothers. The experimental group infants were formally observed within the first 24 hours after birth and every seventh day thereafter. A psychologist in collaboration with a developmentally trained nurse clinician provided the group with ongoing individualized developmental care observations and recommendations to the healthcare team and the parents. The control group infants received the standard of care practiced throughout the SCN. A group of 12 healthy, full-term infants was studied as a comparison group. All infants were assessed at 42 weeks post menstrual age, i.e., two weeks post term corrected age, by trained examiners blind to the infants group status. Although the preterm experimental group infants showed no differences in terms of medical outcome compared with the preterm control group or the full-term group, significant differences among the three groups were found on two behavioral outcome measures, namely, the APIB (Als et al., 1982a) and the *Neurological Examination of the Full Term Infant: A Manual for Clinical Use* (Prechtl, 1977).

Four of the six APIB subsystem scores showed significant group differences. As the post hoc pair-wise comparisons indicated, the preterm control group displayed the least well-organized behavioral performance, whereas the preterm experimental and full-term groups were behaviorally comparable. The preterm control group was significantly less well organized than the preterm experimental group on autonomic, motor, and attention parameters. The preterm control group differed even more significantly from the full-term comparison group on measures of autonomic, motor, and regulatory organization. The preterm control group was the least well modulated, the preterm experimental group the second best modulated, and the full-term group the most well-modulated group of infants.

Measures of electrophysiological function (qEEG with significance probability mapping—qEEG with statistical probability mapping) also showed significant advantages for the preterm intervention group as compared with the preterm control group. Thirteen significant correlations were found between the frontal lobe features and APIB variables measuring attention control and state organization. An additional nine features representing the temporal, parietal, and central regions also correlated significantly with APIB measures of attention. The remaining six correlations indicated significant relationships with measures of autonomic and motor organization. Consequently, medically healthy preterm infants, who received individualized developmental care, were better adjusted autonomically and motorically, especially in terms of state regulation and attention functioning than preterm infants who received standard care. Furthermore, they were comparable with the healthy full-term infants with respect to these functions. The neurophysiologic differences were seen despite the fact that there were no medical differences between the groups at the time of the qEEG study. The frontal region demonstrated significant correlation with behavioral indices of attention control and state organization and appeared to show differential vulnerability in the preterm control group. This is not surprising given that, as pointed out earlier, neuronal organization of this region occurs relatively late in the developmental sequence (Huttenlocher, 1984; Schade & van Groenigen, 1961; Yakovlev & Lecours, 1967).

Previous studies of prematurity have indicated the frontal region's differential vulnerability (Arnsten, 2009; Duffy et al., 1990; Hodel, 2018; Padilla et al., 2014). It appears that the NIDCAP intervention supports a more full-term-like, more mature differentiation of brain function for these healthy preterm infants and that it might protect frontal lobe functioning especially.

A second study (Als et al., 2004) of medically low-risk, preterm infants born at 28 to 33 weeks' gestational age and appropriate in growth for age found similarly encouraging behavioral and electrophysiological results and further identified for the first time brain structural effects of NIDCAP care. Total cerebral tissue volumes of subcortical gray matter, as measured by three-dimensional magnetic resonance (MR) imaging tissue segmentation techniques, was significantly increased, as was white matter fiber tract development in frontal lobes and internal capsule (corticospinal tract) as measured by MR diffusion tensor imaging. On follow-up at school age, it was found that the group differences persisted despite different home and school experiences. The experimental group children performed significantly better on executive function capacities, i.e., frontal lobe function, as assessed with the Rey-Osterrieth Complex Figure Test (Bernstein & Waber, 1996; Holmes Bernstein & Waber, 2007; Rey, 1941), as well as on EEG-based, unrestricted spectral coherence measures with significantly better frontal and prefrontal cortex engagement and long-distance bihemispheric connectivities between the occipital and wide regions of frontal and prefrontal cortex, as well as occipital to right and left temporal lobe connections. Brain structural findings as assessed with magnetic resonance imaging (MRI) using fiber tract cartography and mean diffusivity as indicator showed that the NIDCAP group school-aged children had significantly lower mean diffusivity scores; e.g., they were significantly more mature in corticospinal tract fiber development than the control group.

Aside from the study of medically low-risk preterm infants, a randomized (NIDCAP vs. Control) group of in utero severely growth restricted (IUGR) preterm infants comparable in gestational age at birth with the low-risk well-grown preterm infants studied were also assessed in the newborn period (Als et al., 2012) and at 8 to 10 years corrected age, i.e., at school age (McAnulty et al., 2013).

The infants were selected to be below the fifth percentile in birthweight and head circumference and free of all chromosomal and/or genetic or congenital abnormalities; their mothers were free of major medical conditions as well as of nicotine or any other addition including alcohol. All infants had absent, intermittent, or reversed umbilical artery blood flow issues as diagnosed by Doppler ultrasound, and all were delivered because of their severe growth restriction in utero. The study attempted to answer the question of NIDCAP effectiveness in ameliorating existing brain compromise due to intrauterine growth restriction. It is known that preterm infants with severe IUGR are doubly jeopardized given their status as preterm infants and their compromised brains. NIDCAP significantly improved outcome at 42 weeks post menstrual age, i.e., at 2 weeks post term corrected age and at school age. At 2 weeks after term due date the NIDCAP group showed significantly better autonomic, motor, state, and self-regulatory function as assessed with the APIB. They also showed a series of more mature EEG-based connectivities and improved brain structure, i.e., corticospinal tract development as measured by mean diffusivity. Thus, again improvement was documented for the NIDCAP group in all three domains, namely, behavior, EEG, and MRI. At school age the study tested NIDCAP effectiveness regarding executive function, electrophysiology (EEG), and neurostructure (MRI). Of the original 30 infants, 23 (14 control, 9 experimental) school-aged, former growth-restricted preterm infants, randomized at birth to standard care or NIDCAP, were assessed with standardized measures of cognition, achievement, and executive function; electroencephalography, and MRI. The participating children were comparable with those lost to follow-up, and the control

group to the experimental, in terms of newborn background health and demographics. Control and experimental group children were comparable in age at testing, anthropometric and health parameters, and in cognitive and achievement scores. Experimental group children scored better in executive function, spectral coherence, and cerebellar volumes. Furthermore, executive function, spectral coherence, and brain structural measures discriminated the control from the experimental group children. Executive function correlated with EEG spectral coherence and brain structure measures and with newborn-period neurobehavioral assessment.

It appears that the NIDCAP intervention in the intensive care nursery when employed in the care of well-grown low-risk as well as of poorly grown (IUGR) high-risk infants between 28 and 33 weeks' gestational age significantly improved executive function as well as spectral coherence between the occipital and frontal as well as parietal regions. In addition, the IUGR infants, when at school age, showed significantly larger, more well-grown right and left cerebellar cortices than the controls. The cerebellar cortex receives information from most parts of the body and from many other regions of the brain. The cerebellum integrates this information and sends signals back to the rest of the brain, thereby potentiating accurate and well-coordinated movements as well as emotion regulation (Bernard et al., 2012).

The results of the studies reviewed above point to the long-term improvement of health and brain development in well-grown as well as in intrauterine growth–compromised preterm infants when individualized intervention in the NIDCAP model begins with admission to the NICU and extends throughout the hospital stay. The studies clearly document effectiveness of developmental care in the NIDCAP model for very early-born, very high-risk preterm infants. They suggest that differences in experience during the last 16 weeks of gestation differentially influence infants' brain structure and neurodevelopmental functioning. These differences are measurable at 2 weeks and 9 months post term and continue to be significant at preschool and into school age.

NIDCAP GUIDELINES FOR COLLABORATIVE CARE

The clinical framework of NIDCAP developmental care, derived from the conceptual and empirical work outlined, has been developed into a quality-assured replicable training program for multidisciplinary professionals in intensive care and other hospital settings for high-risk newborns and young infants. The NIDCAP Federation International, founded in 2001, a not-for-profit charitable international membership organization, assures the quality of training and certification. In order to integrate effectively individualized developmentally supportive, family-centered care in the NIDCAP framework into hospital settings, guidelines are provided for the individualized structuring of an infant's 24-hour day, enhancement of the physical environment, and caregiving team collaboration. These guidelines were derived from and reflect the experiences of NIDCAP research and clinical teams over many years and must be individualized to the meet the expectations of each infant and family (Als & Gilkerson, 1997; Als & McAnulty, 1998; Gilkerson & Als, 1995; Holmes, Sheldon, & Als, 1995; Vento & Feinberg, 1998).

Structuring the Infant's 24-Hour Day

The primary care team coordinates all interventions across several 24-hour time epochs into individually appropriate clusters timed in accordance with each infant's sleep–wake cycles, state of alertness, medical care requirements, and feeding competence (IFSDS Standard 6). All interventions are evaluated for their necessity and appropriateness in timing for each respective infant. The goal is to provide restfulness and to support growth. Infants' caregiving schedules are coordinated with family schedules in order to support the integration of the infant into the family and the family into the healthcare setting. The goal is to foster family involvement and competence in nurturing and caring for their child. For care delivery, caregivers approach the infant and family in a calm, attentive manner. Caregivers are encouraged to observe the infant first in order to understand their current state of well-being and their ways to communicate this. Caregivers explain the goals and approximate sequence of planned care components to the family. They then introduce themselves to the infant with a soft voice and gentle touch (IFCDC Standard 2). Depending on the infant's location, be it on the parents' chest or in an incubator or crib, etc., they think through the most supportive and stable way for the infant to experience the care sequence deemed indicated. Should it be the parent's body as is often the case, caregivers calmly support family and infant to move into the most supportive situation appropriate. Most medical and nursing care procedure lend themselves well to be performed most supportively while the parent holds the infant skin-to-skin (IFCDC Standard 4). This includes extubation, suctioning, eye examination, central line check, diaper change, blood pressure and other vital sign assessments, and heel sticks. In many NIDCAP-engaged nurseries these approaches are practiced successfully.

Caregivers provide periods of rest and recovery between care actions and contain the infant in a gentle embrace with their hands and preferentially encourage the parents to do so. Hand embrace of the infant, sucking on a pacifier or finger, hand holding, and hand-to-mouth exploration are ways to support the dialogue between infant and caregiver and to foster the infant and parent's overall competence. During transition periods between caregiving components, caregivers must continue to direct careful attention to the infant's behavior. Typically, increased support is indicated when an infant awakens spontaneously, makes efforts to come to alertness, and then returns to sleep. This especially is the case for very prematurely born infants and for those with dysmature or impaired nervous systems, such as infants who experienced birth asphyxia, intrauterine growth restriction, and

narcotic or cocaine exposure. Such infants typically demonstrate lower thresholds to disorganization. During alert periods, caregivers attempt to balance sensory input they provide and that are inherent in the environment with the infant's current level of alertness and competence. Caregiver interactions are guided by the infant behavioral cues toward support of robust wakefulness, increasingly well-focused alertness, and well-modulated social interaction. Caregivers should support softly flexed, comfortably aligned positions during sleep, routine care, feeding, bathing, and special procedures. Aids such as blanket rolls, nests, gentle swaddling, special buntings, and hands-on containment may be helpful. Dressing an infant in soft cotton garments appropriate in size and covering the infant with a soft cotton or silk blanket have been found to facilitate restfulness and comfort. The use of support is adapted to the infant's competence; support is increased or decreased depending on the infant's autonomous maintenance of vital sign stability, tone, and well-adjusted positions and movements, as well as robustness or fragility of state organization.

Feeding method and frequency also are individualized and based on infant competence. The goal is to progress toward infant-initiated and infant-controlled breast feeding. The more time the infant spends in skin-to-skin holding with the mother the sooner the infant will progress from nuzzling and licking the breast to suckling from the breast, even when for a while the milk is given simultaneously by nasal feeding tube. Should the professional caregiver feed the infant, which should be the exception, the caregiver should aim to decrease environmental stimulation and securely cradle the infant in semi upright soft flexion, with hands in midline, free to grasp and hold on, and with legs and feet contained. Feeding success foremost is judged by an infant's overall energy levels and autonomic, motor, and state functioning and less by the amount of intake. More frequent shorter feedings are less energy consuming and biologically more compatible with the human newborn who is a continuous feeder. Feeding must be conceptualized as a pleasurable and nurturing experience (IFSDS Standard 6).

Suctioning and pulmonary care should be performed only when clinically indicated, and always by a two-person team. Routine suctioning and chest physical therapy for premature infants have been shown to lead to abrupt changes in blood flow velocity that have been associated with IVH and cerebral infarction and must be avoided. When indicated, such a procedure must be performed gently, supported by a second caregiver who, whenever possible, should be the parent. Containment and stabilization of the infant throughout the procedure lessens potential risks and increases support for the infant.

Opportunities for skin-to-skin holding must be available at all times and to families of all NICU infants, including infants requiring ventilator support. Reclining chaise lounges with foot and head rests that are large enough to accommodate two parents should be available at each bedside. Staff must be specially trained in the care and comfort of postpartum parents and of infants for the provision of skin-to-skin nurturing. The parent's body has been shown to provide warmth and maintain the infant's stable body temperature. The infant has been shown to experience increased respiratory stability with decreased incidence of apnea, bradycardia, and oxygen desaturation. Such physical contact appears to result in more restful sleep in the infant and a sense of calm and fulfillment in parents. Mothers, who hold their infant skin-to-skin experience increased milk production and success and enjoyment in breastfeeding. Fathers report similar enjoyment and feelings of closeness with and protectiveness of their infant (Abdulghani et al., 2018; Deng et al., 2018; Karimi et al., 2019; Moore et al., 2012; Svensson et al., 2013; UNICEF, 2021).

All infants with intact skin should be bathed with full immersion to the shoulder and neck level in suitably sized tubs filled with warm water. The infant should be supported and placed in a deep warm water bath while loosely swaddled. Providing hands-on containment will further support the infant's relaxation and temperature stability. As soon and as frequently as possible, parents are the caregivers of choice to bathe their infant. Infants are weighed, softly swaddled in a blanket or bunting, with gentle movement from bed to scale and back, unless the bed simultaneously provides a scale. All special examination and assessment procedures, including physical examinations, ultrasound examinations of the head, chest radiographs (Blickman et al., 1990), EEGs, eye examinations (Kleberg et al., 2008), and neurologic examinations, are performed collaboratively by the respective specialist, assisted by the infant's nurse and facilitated by the parent's skin-to-skin holding, when possible, to support infant comfort and well-being in the course of required position changes, palpations, auscultations, and the like (Patricia et al., 2003).

The infant's face should be shielded from direct illumination at all times. At all times, the size and quality of equipment, materials, and devices required are apportioned to the size and strength of the infant's limbs and skin to ensure maximal comfort and physiologically appropriate alignment and movement of head, trunk, limbs, and joints. Intravenous boards, whenever possible, must support elbow flexion and finger grasp. The tape that is used is expected to be skin friendly. When bilirubin lights and eye patches are necessary, rest periods with bilirubin lights turned off and eye covers removed must be provided with each caregiving interaction. Infants may rest in skin-to-skin holding with the parent while receiving bilirubin light therapy with eye protection for infant and parent, or if sufficient, they may be wrapped in biliblankets (Goudarzvand et al., 2019).

Supportive Enhancement of the Physical Environment

Lighting should be adjusted to support each infant's and family's best sleep and awake organization and to deliver care without impinging on the development, comfort, and care of other infants. Individualized bedside-controlled lighting with dimmer capacity should be available. General nursery lighting should be indirect and readily adjusted in terms of brightness. Furthermore, nurseries should be quiet, soothing places. Suggestions for sound containment include creating a space within the nursery for admissions and special procedures; educating staff about preterm infant responses to various sound levels as part of staff training; moving daily rounds and conversations away from infant and family bed spaces; dampening sounds from equipment, such as telephones, waste receptacles, monitor alarms, sinks, doors, and movable equipment; eliminating radios, overhead pagers, and all other unnecessary sounds; transferring infants from warming tables to incubators with quiet motors as soon after admission as possible; covering incubators with thick blankets fitted with sound-shielding material; choosing wall covering with sound-absorbent materials and architecturally structuring walls for maximal sound absorption; and carpeting all care areas.

Caregivers should avoid the use of perfumes, colognes, and scented hair sprays as infants are sensitive to these odors. The odor of tobacco on caregiver bodies and clothing as well as the odors of dry cleaning chemicals should be avoided. Alcohol or sulfa-based chemicals should be used only when infants are away from the care area. Care should be taken to allow cleaning fluids to dry and vapors to evaporate before bedding the infant back in the incubator. While parents are holding their infant skin-to-skin, a soft cloth placed across the infant and their own breasts or chests or a mother's breast pads should be used to enhance and extend the infant's comfort in the recognition of the parents' scent when the infant is returned to the incubator or crib and tucked in with the parent-scented cloth or pad.

NICU environments should be structured so that infants are cared for in collaboration with their families. This is aligned with Standard 1 Systems Thinking at the beginning of the chapter. Specific aids such as soft bedding, buntings, water mattresses, and size-appropriate pacifiers should be used to lessen the impact of necessary medical procedures and equipment. Homelike, individualized spaces or coves for infants and families within the NICU; secure, attractive cabinets to store belongings; communal space equipped with kitchen facilities; a library with computers and written and audiovisual materials; washer and dryer facilities; rooms for sleeping; and bathroom and shower facilities for family members should be available. Twin and multiple infants should be cared for in one family area and in one bed or incubator as possible. Parents are encouraged to consider their infants' care spaces as their space. They are encouraged to arrange the space to their aesthetic liking. Bedside telephones for family members are of great importance for all families, especially when mobile phone use is restricted. It is suggested that NICUs be structured for the 24-hour comfort of parents as well as siblings and other family members. Family participation should be facilitated by readily available, trained child care for siblings. Siblings, who pass a screen for exposure to varicella and the presence of respiratory or other communicable illnesses present little risk to infants. Because the infant's medical and nursing record (chart) are their parents' property, parents should be guided and encouraged to read the chart regularly and should be encouraged to enter their own observations and comments on a regular basis. This facilitates communication, builds mutual trust, and enhances the success of collaborative care. Individual private infant–family care rooms with private showers, etc. increasingly are becoming the model of choice for renovated or newly built nurseries. Staffing adaptations and support are important as this architectural model reduces staff peer-to-peer support possible in open bay nurseries. These strategies support IFCDC Standard 4.

Care Provider Collaboration

Implementation of developmental care in the NICU requires a multidisciplinary, collaborative approach. Each infant should have a primary care team, which includes the family and representatives from nursing, medicine, respiratory therapy, and social work. This team should be identified within the first 24 hours of admission. The primary team works collaboratively to develop an individualized plan of care. The care plan, which must include the parents' input, is reviewed daily with the parents and healthcare team during rounds. Regular team meetings are scheduled at the convenience of the family to ensure their continued observations and input.

Specially NIDCAP-trained and certified developmental professionals should be available full-time as an integral part of the staff in each NICU. These professionals are expected to have knowledge of high-risk newborn and family development, as well as infant, parent, and professional mental health. They support the primary teams in developmental care planning and implementation. They serve as resources and catalysts in developmental care collaboration. A multidisciplinary developmental care committee should support the unit-wide implementation of developmental care. This committee focuses on coordinating unit-based developmental rounds, initiates quality improvement projects that focus on appropriate sound and light environments, organize case presentations, develop a parent support group, and support developmental leadership in each of the nursery's disciplines. A formal parent council with multicultural representation also is suggested.

As the nursery moves to becoming a family-integrated care environment, the nursery staff's need for private space must be considered carefully. Resources and opportunities for personal and professional growth, such as regular meetings with a psychiatrist, licensed clinical social worker, psychologist, psychiatric clinical nurse specialist or other mental health professional for the supportive discussion and reflection of family–staff and staff–staff issues must be provided for medical and nursing professionals and all other disciplines including secretarial and housekeeping staff alike. Ongoing collaboration with families in support of their appreciation of and pride in their infants' strengths and individuality prepares families for their infant's discharge home from the NICU. Formal behavioral observation using the NIDCAP approach in conjunction with formal assessment with the APIB before an infant's NICU discharge or transfer to a community hospital is recommended in order to support parent and staff understanding of the infant's current behavioral functioning and to guide referrals to community services and early intervention programs (Avery & First, 1994).

Box "Development Care Guidelines for Use in the NICU" shows NIDCAP Federation International (NFI)-recommended NIDCAP Care Guidelines for staff in summary table format. These may be printed out and distributed to the staff to keep with them for easy reference during work hours, and/or be kept at the bedside for reference by parents and staff, or reformatted into Rolodex cards kept on a ring and chain attached to the incubator or crib as is practice in a number of nurseries.

Developmental Care Guidelines for Use in the NICU

A. Infant's Bedspace and Bedding

• Design of Bedspace

Arrange all equipment aesthetically and assure ready access to the infant at all times. Make available two comfortable chairs, at least one of which is a reclining chair, with bedding for kangaroo care, extended naps, and overnight stays of the parent. Invite and encourage the family to personalize and decorate their infant's bedspace with items brought from home (incubator cover, photos, stuffed animals, etc.). Make drawer or shelf space available for the family's personal belongings.

• Light

Assure darkness for the infant during sleep, and maintain low, muted light levels at all other times in order to support alertness. Make sure that all lighting that falls on the infant's face is indirect. Make use of window shades and screens as indicated. In caring for an infant who requires phototherapy and protective eye patches, be sure to first turn off the therapy light, gently speak to the infant and introduce your hands to the infant, cradling them around the infant softly until you feel the infant's body tone relax. Gently remove the eye patches and help the infant recover from the intense light exposure. Only then begin the formal caregiving interaction. After your caregiving interaction, and once you have helped the infant be restful again, gently replace the eye patches, help the infant settle, turn the light back on and stay with the infant until the infant has settled under the light. Be aware of the high amount of energy that is required from the infant when exposed to intense light. Consider exploring appropriate ways for the infant to be held by the parent while receiving phototherapy. Shield other bedsides from the phototherapy light used.

• **Sound**

Speak with a soft voice at all times and walk softly. Wear quiet shoes only. Move softly and gently. Always close incubator portholes and cupboard doors gently and quietly; move all equipment quietly. Encourage staff to speak softly. Remove all radios from the area. Set monitors and telephones to the lowest settings and softest rings. Be sure that rounds occur away from the bedside. Maintain a peaceful and quiet care area for the infant. Think of it as the bedroom of a very sensitive infant.

• **Activity Level**

Maintain a very calm, quiet, and soothing atmosphere at all times. Handle emergency situations in a calm and quiet manner. Help others involved in the infant's care feel calm and welcome in the infant care area. Be helpful to them in their respective roles in caring for the infant. Assist them by helping the infant stay calm and restful in the course of needed procedures and interventions. Move all staff interactions away from the bedside unless they are directly relevant to the infant.

• **Visual Array Inside or Near the Incubator and Crib**

Choose with care the objects that are in the infant's visual field in or near the incubator and crib. Ask yourself whether they are soothing or arousing. Familiarity with a soothing object makes it comforting over time. Save stimulating toys and pictures with contrasts and bright colors for the time when the infant will be strong enough to enjoy them. Your and the parents' soft familiar faces are often what the infant values most. Always maintain a gentle warm facial expression. Stay with the infant for assurance when others interact with the infant who is not familiar to the infant. Always introduce a new visual stimulus gradually and only when the infant is ready for it. Soften and remove animating visual stimuli from the infant's visual field when the infant becomes drowsy, hyper alert, upset, or averts the gaze. Disorganized eye

movements, averted gaze, hyper alertness, and worried or panicked facial expressions are signs that the infant is overstimulated.

• **Olfactory Inputs**

Remove all noxious and unfamiliar odors (e.g., perfume, hair spray, nicotine on your clothing) from the infant's immediate care area; provide a familial, comforting olfactory environment for the infant in the incubator or crib and when the infant is held by a caregiver. Invite the parents to provide a soft, small blanket, little pillow, silk cloth, or soft piece of clothing the mother or father have worn or held on their body. Have several of these available at all times so that the infant may count on them for comfort. The consistent familial olfactory environment of the parents' body is soothing and comforting and is reinforced when the parent cares for and holds the infant in skin-to-skin contact.

• **Bedding and Clothing**

Individualize bedding and clothing in keeping with the infant's preferences and needs. This may include providing a water pillow, sheepskin, boundaries, "nesting," clothing with soft one-piece suits appropriate for the infant's size, a soft hat, gentle swaddling, soft and small diapers, and a soft, long "hugging pillow." Since the parent is the infant's most posturally supportive bed and affective nurturer, encourage extended periods of skin-to-skin contact for infant and parents. In order to help relax the parents' upper body, make sure the parents' legs are elevated and well supported. Encourage "rooming-in" at the bedside with the infant.

• **Specific Regulatory Supports**

Use regulatory supports consistently, including holding, bedding, foot rolls, and buntings. Gently cradle the infant in your hands and help the infant contain disorganized and agitated movements when the infant becomes aroused and upset. Gentle cradling also helps an infant when becoming exhausted and when losing body tone. During and between procedures, use your finger or a small pacifier and give the infant the opportunity to suck; do so also during gavage feedings. Offer the infant your finger to hold onto during manipulations. Encourage the parents to support their infant to feel soothed and comforted. Skin-to-skin holding during procedures and caregiving is especially assuring to the infant. When the parent is not in a position to be with the infant, encourage another familiar caregiver entrusted by the parent with the infant's care to be there in support of the infant.

- **Adjustment of Medical Equipment**

Adjust all medically necessary equipment that is in direct contact with the infant's body to provide maximum comfort for the infant. Assure comfortable adjustment of all breathing equipment including a large enough oxyhood that reaches to the infant's waist, in order to support the infant in bringing the hands up close to the face. Make sure that IV boards are small, softly padded, and securely held in place. Use soft, skin-friendly eye patches, soft probe wrappings, and soft, small diapers. Avoid all Velcro, plastic, and other rough materials.

B. Specific Aspects of Direct Infant Care

- **Approaching the Infant**

When you approach the infant's bedside always position yourself so that you may see the infant's face. The infant's facial expression will help you be aware of how the infant may be feeling, whether the infant is unsettled or comfortable and restful. Ask yourself when the infant last saw you and felt the touch of your hands. Is the infant likely to recognize you as familiar, or should you introduce or reintroduce your hands and face slowly so the infant may realize that you are now with the infant and there to support the infant.

- **Position Support**

Consistently support and facilitate physiologically well-aligned positions whether the infant is on the back, tummy, or side. Be aware of the infant's position during daily and specialized procedures, between interventions, when holding the infant, and when bedding the infant on the parent or in the incubator or crib. When moving the infant or changing the infant's position, always support the infant's arms and legs into soft, relaxed flexion. Place your hand softly around the back of the infant's head, reaching from behind and cradling the infant's head gently in your hand; simultaneously align your arm alongside the infant's back and with your other arm support the infant along the front, helping the infant's head rest in midline, hands tucked up toward the face. Once the infant's whole body has settled into the secure cradling provided by the womb nest of your arms and hands, gently and slowly change the infant's position and/or lift the infant up in this secure fashion. Before returning the infant to the bed or moving the infant onto the scale to be weighed or onto another surface always prepare the surface first. Cover it with soft padding and have a soft blanket or bunting ready and available to receive the infant. Always gently and slowly lower the infant onto the surface cradled in a securely enveloping fashion. Make sure that the infant's head stays well aligned at all times with respect to the infant's spine. Once the infant is securely lowered onto the surface, first maintain your arms and hands securely cradled around the infant as you gently swaddle the infant in the blanket or bunting you have prepared in advance. Support the infant with gentle swaddling when you move the infant, especially when you weigh the infant. Once the infant has settled into the blanket or bunting in the nest of your cradling arms, very gradually remove your hands and arms one at a time; assure yourself of the infant's continued restfulness as you very gradually decrease your direct support. Continue to assure yourself of the infant's restfulness once you no longer physically support the infant with your hands and arms. Whenever the infant begins to stir and become unsettled gently support the infant again so that the infant may be restful or sleep peacefully.

- **Feeding**

From early on time the infant's feeding to be supportive of the infant's sleep and wake cycles so that the infant may learn to recognize feelings of hunger and satiation. Support the parent to breastfeed the infant. Should the infant not yet be strong enough to nurse on the mother's breast, support the mother to pump her breast. Make arrangements so that she may comfortably do so at her infant's bedside. This may help lessen the stress of pumping, assure her of its value, and make her feel close to her infant. Create a nurturant feeding environment, which is calm, warm, and muted in lighting. Throughout any gavage feeding hold the infant in a well-supported and comfortable position. Securely snuggle the infant against your chest. Be sure that the infant's hands are free to grasp onto you as you help the infant bring the hands close to the mouth. Offer your finger or pacifier to the infant to suck on while you gavage feed the infant. Control appropriately the flow of the milk to be slow enough for the infant's comfort. As indicated, provide rests during the feeding. Whenever possible bed the infant on the parent's chest in skin-to-skin contact to nuzzle against the parent's chest and breast for all gavage feedings. Continue to support the infant after feeding, in order to assure comfortable return to sleep. Encourage the parent from the beginning in their role as the infant's most important nurturer and provider of nutrition.

- **Burping**

Facilitate burping by gently positioning the infant against your chest or shoulder in response to the infant's cues. Move softly and slowly; relaxation is the goal. Should the infant continue to appear uncomfortable while cradled upright against you, move your body slowly in an up and down motion in the rhythm of gentle walking. This will likely promote a burp. Continue to hold the infant in an upright position snuggled against you after a burp before gradually moving the infant into a feeding or resting position.

• Diaper Changing and Skin Care

Make all arrangements needed and gather all necessary supplies for diaper changes and skin care in advance of approaching the infant. Be sure the room is warm. Be mindful of the infant's state and position. Begin the care procedures once the infant is bedded comfortably in flexion, best lying on the side. Gently contain and support the infant. Use materials that are soft, comfortable, and appropriate in size, texture, and shape. To clean the infant, keep the infant's ankles close to the bedding and gently lift the infant's upper leg slightly while keeping both legs tucked. Avoid changing the infant's diaper in supine and lifting the infant's legs by the ankles off the bed; this suddenly alters blood flow to the infant's head and makes breathing difficult. Encourage and assist the parent to become skilled in changing the infant's diaper and providing skin care in a gentle and containing manner.

• Bathing

Assure that the infant is restful and has enough energy to be bathed. Assure that the care space is calm, soothingly lighted, and warm. Cradle the infant gently in your hands and use a blanket for containment. As indicated by the infant's movements, a hooded bathing blanket may be helpful to wrap the infant in as the infant is lowered into the bathtub. Be sure the bath water is warm and deep enough for immersion as soon as the infant is stable enough for full bathing. Use a specialized bathtub at the bedside in order to decrease unnecessary movement and temperature fluctuation from the warm incubator or crib into the bath water and back. After bathing continue to hold the infant supportively to make sure the infant is comfortable and restful. Determine the frequency and timing of bathing by the infant's level of energy and the infant's sleep, wake, and feeding cycles in order to enhance restfulness and effective digestion.

• Timing and Sequencing of Caregiving Interactions

When timing caregiving, consider the infant's sleep-wake cycle and the infant's energy for feeding and for quiet-awake periods. When possible, consider these also when timing interventions by specialists and consultants, such as ophthalmology, neurology, ultrasound, and X-ray. Support the specialists and consultants in assuring the infant's comfort before, during, and after such interventions.

• Transition Facilitation During Procedures

Position the infant supportively and help the infant be restful during all care procedures, including IV line placements and blood drawing. Provide the infant with calm, gentle containment and comfort during all procedures. Continue support afterward in order to ensure the infant's return to restful calmness. Plan and make use of assistance from a second caregiver as needed in order to assure effective facilitation for the infant. Include the parent as the infant's most nurturing comforter.

• Comforting and Caregiving

Whenever the infant appears to be uncomfortable, i.e., the infant squirms or fusses, respond promptly and reliably. Always comfort an upset or crying infant. Stay emotionally available and attentive to the infant's feelings so that you may be attuned to the ways the infant is experiencing the care and environment that you provide for the infant. Earn and warrant the trust the infant and parent place in you, their caregiver, during this vulnerable time in the NICU.

• Organization of Alertness

Be aware at all times that you are the infant's regulator and supporter. When the infant awakens, look at the infant gently with a soft facial expression; always speak slowly with a very soft voice. At times the infant may enjoy your soft singing or humming. When the infant looks at you with shiny focused eyes and softly animated face, this usually indicates enjoyment of the interaction. Gently return the infant's gaze. The infant's averted eyes, discoordinated eye movements, strained facial expressions, wide-eyedness, paling, coughing, yawning, sneezing, or gradually draining face usually signal that the infant is exhausted or overstimulated. Always respect these signals by quietly holding the infant against you to remove all stimuli; always assure that the infant feels restful, supported, and nurtured at all times.

Special Notes for the Care of _____

_____

Infant's Name
Please date and sign each entry. Use additional pages as indicated.
Heidelise Als, PhD, and Gloria McAnulty, PhD, 1998, 2000
©NIDCAP Federation International, 2014.
NIDCAP® is a registered trademark of the NFI, Inc.

[Used with permission from Pearls of Wisdom Task Group, NIDCAP Federation Int'l. 2020.]

Supportive Guidelines for Parents

Parents often report feeling helpless and confused as to their role in the care of their infant in the medical intensive care environment. In support of parents in the nursery a series of encouragements has been developed in the form of Ten Pearls of NIDCAP Wisdom for Parents of Hospitalized Babies (Pearls of Wisdom Task Group, NIDCAP Federation. 2020).

These are presented in Box "Ten Pearls of NIDCAP Wisdom for Parents of Hospitalized Babies," with permission of the NFI.

Parents have found these suggestions helpful and supportive.

Ten Pearls of NIDCAP Wisdom for Parents of Hospitalized Babies

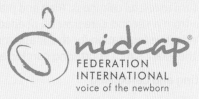

Ten Pearls of NIDCAP Wisdom for Parents of Hospitalized Babies

Pearls signify confidence, strength and peacefulness in facing life's challenges. They represent wisdom gained through experience.

The evidence-based Newborn Individualized Developmental Care and Assessment Program [NIDCAP] is a comprehensive model and approach to care. It provides guidance in support of the earliest development of the most vulnerable newborns and their families in newborn and other intensive care settings.

– D. Buehler, PhD, President, NIDCAP Federation International

Premature and medically high-risk birth may impede the earliest experiences between newborns and their parents and have a lifelong impact on the family, the baby's future development and overall health, as well as the parents' well-being. Parents might worry that their relationship with their hospitalized newborn feels so different from what they had hoped. There are many ways parents get to know their babies to improve their well-being. Babies rely on their parents to be strong supporters and advocates.

These NIDCAP-based considerations are for parents with hospitalized babies in the intensive care nursery. They were developed to support parents and their babies to get to know one another and build close and trusting relationships. Babies feel and experience their parents and the world around them through all of their senses. The baby's behavior guides the parent. How parents interact with their infant is much more important than what they do. The parents' gentle caresses and soft smiles and the tone of their voice provide comfort and assurance. A parent's presence and love provides invaluable healing medicine for their baby.

1. Plan Time and Be Present

Organize your time to be with your baby for as long and as often as possible. Seek ways to delegate your other responsibilities to family members and friends. This is an important time to accept help and support from others to care for your family and your home. At this time, more than at any other time in your baby's life, your baby will benefit from the consistency and familiarity of your assuring presence and love. Collaborate with your baby's healthcare team to plan whom you wish to be with your baby when you must be away from your baby. Provide your baby's healthcare team with a 24-hour rotation list that includes members of your family or close friends whom you trust to be with your baby in your absence. This might include grandmother, grandfather, older sibling, or a close friend who would be available reliably throughout your baby's time in the nursery. A small reliable group of such persons may be wonderful and consistent parents' extenders for your baby. They could hold your baby skin-to-skin and become skilled participants in your baby's care; they could feed and diaper your baby and speak and sing to your baby and provide the familiar nurturing presence your baby seeks throughout day and night. Advise the healthcare team of you and your extenders' calendar and availability for the coming week, and ensure that you and they are included in all aspects of the care of your baby.

2. Participate as the Primary Caregiver(s)

Inform your baby's healthcare team that you wish to be an active participant in all of your baby's care. Ask about how your baby has been since you last were with your baby. Articulate and communicate your questions, concerns, and expectations, as you are your baby's strongest supporter and advocate. Discuss with the team how you can take part in your baby's specific daily care practices. Every interaction with your baby is an opportunity to build trust and nurturance. Observe your baby's behavior to learn how best to respond to your baby's cues. Take care of your baby together with the professional healthcare team; collaborate and partner with the healthcare team to identify more and more ways to support your baby. You will gradually feel more secure and independent in being with your baby and providing your baby's care. This will create a strong bond between you and your baby and will help you gain the practice and confidence.

3. Seek Information Actively

Ask the healthcare team about your baby's feelings of well-being, medical status, progress, and challenges. Request updates about your baby's sleep, comfort, preferences, behaviors, personality, condition, medications, weight, how well your baby takes the milk offered, as well as about new developmental steps and achievements. Consider these topics part of your everyday dialogue with the healthcare team who care for your baby. Make sure you meet frequently with the multidisciplinary healthcare team, who participate in your baby's care, for example, the attending physician, bedside nurses, nurse practitioner, developmental specialist, physical therapist, occupational therapist, speech therapist, social worker, and psychologist. Ask for their guidance and insights. Share your impressions of your baby with the healthcare team. Also share the progress you observe in your baby, how your baby may have changed and appears different. Share your concerns and how you have learned to read your baby's behavior.

4. Shape the Environment

Keep your baby's surroundings in the nursery as calm and nurturing as possible. This will help your baby hear and respond with joy to your voice, experience fully your touch, and delight in the sight of your face. When your baby rests on your chest, or, when necessary, in the incubator or crib, make sure that your baby's face is protected at all times from direct bright light and loud sounds. Inquire from your baby's healthcare team whether you may bring in personal belongings such as soft blankets, soft well-fitting clothes, soft sheets on which to lie, or other belongings that provide you with a sense of familiarity and comfort at your baby's bed space. Consider wearing a soft cloth close to your body to place near your baby's face so your baby can smell your unique familiar scent when you must be away from your baby.

5. Provide Slow and Responsive Care and Interactions

Your baby's brain is still immature and processes the world more slowly than you. Slowing down all of your actions will support your baby's brain development. Your presence makes it easier for your baby to process each experience, all motions and changes in position, as well as each touch and sound and all that your baby sees. You help your baby to take in all experiences calmly and comfortably. Observe your baby's behavior to learn how best to support and make adjustments in response to your baby's readiness. This will help your baby use all energy for the next steps in development and growth and make your baby feel successful and strong. For instance, always first watch your baby to find out for what your baby is ready at that moment; when your baby breathes calmly, the face is pink, and your baby appears comfortable, begin to speak softly, letting your baby know that you are there; gently introduce your hands to your baby, for instance, cradle your hand softly around your baby's back and head helping your baby recognize your familiar touch to feel assured. Then open your baby's blanket slowly, use your soft voice to tell your baby what it is that you are doing, and keep your hand and voice in contact with your baby throughout any care and social interaction. With your gentle steady touch and calm voice, you help your baby wake up gradually and become ready for the next step. Your presence, soft voice, holding, and gentle touch will support your baby also to settle back into sleep after being awake for a while. Remaining calm and slowing down is a very important part of all you do with your baby. Observing your baby's behavior to see what is being communicated and to understand what may be best to offer next is always the best approach in being with your baby. This will enhance your parenting confidence to be your baby's best supporter and advocate.

6. Protect Sleep

Sleep is crucial for the development of your baby's brain. Many important processes take place while your baby sleeps, for example, the development of the sensory organs and functions, the consolidation of memory and learning, and healthy growth. Be mindful of keeping your baby's environment quiet and calm, so that sleep is steady and uninterrupted by disturbing sounds, too much activity, or bright lights. Remember that sleep is oftentimes more restful when you hold your baby skin-to-skin. Discuss with the healthcare team how to protect consistently your baby's sleep.

7. Connect and Communicate Through Touch

Touch is the earliest and most essential way of connection and communication between you and your baby. Touching your baby will help you learn about your baby's behavior and preferences. Your baby will experience comfort and safety and feel your love through your touch. Watch for how your baby responds and let that guide your interaction. Touch your baby gently, to let your baby feel the steady and calm nurturing touch of your hands; perhaps cuddle one hand around the soles of your baby's feet, and with your other hand cradle the top of your baby's head or around the baby's body while the baby's arms and legs are tucked. This will convey to your baby a sense of steadiness, safety, and trust in you that will help your baby stay calm and feel comforted. When you have questions or concerns, please speak with your baby's healthcare team in the nursery about how best to provide your baby with your touch in the gentle and comforting way that suits your baby as a unique being with particular medical conditions and circumstances.

8. Care with Skin-to-Skin Holding

Give your baby the opportunity to be really close to you. With your baby wearing only a diaper, hold your baby on your bare chest (be sure to remove your bra). This is often referred to as skin-to-skin or kangaroo care. Begin to hold your baby skin-to-skin as soon as possible after birth as your baby's medical condition allows and, when possible, for as long each day as you prefer. There is much evidence regarding the benefits to your baby, as well as to you, for skin-to-skin contact every day, especially with very small or sick babies. These benefits, among many others, include improved short- and long-term developmental and cognitive outcomes.

9. Offer Human Milk and Nursing

Human milk is by far the best nutrition for your baby, and your milk is ideal for your baby. Prior to your baby's birth, or when possible as soon as your baby is born, discuss with the healthcare team in the nursery when and how you may express milk from your breasts. The earliest part of your milk, the colostrum, is liquid gold for your baby and valuable for many reasons. Therefore, every drop of milk you express (pump) counts. Seek the support of a lactation consultant, when such a specialist is available in the nursery, or that of an experienced nurse. Make sure that you pump your breasts while looking at or touching your baby and/or holding a blanket or cloth that carries your baby's unique scent. This will help your milk flow more easily. Should for any reason there be challenges that you are not able to provide enough milk, be sure to inquire about the availability of donor human milk. Consider opportunities for your baby to rest against your bare chest to smell, lick, and nuzzle your nipples from very early on. This will help your milk flow and help your baby find your nipple gradually and suck on it. Early on your baby may receive your milk through a thin tube into the nose that goes into the stomach when smelling and nuzzling your breast. Gradually suckling will become stronger and easier for your baby. Ensure that you make all feeding a pleasurable and positive experience for your baby and yourself. Your presence and calm touch will comfort your baby during feeding; hold the milk syringe so that you can pace the milk flow according to your baby's behavior during feeding. By being part of your baby's feeding from early on, you are setting the stage for pleasurable and comfortable feeding experiences in the future. Breast feed your baby for as long as your body allows. There are many benefits to your baby, as well as to you, when you provide your milk.

10. Promote Sucking for Comfort and Security

From about 20 weeks on, while growing in the womb, babies suck on their fingers and hands. They continue to seek out their fingers to suck on when they are in the nursery. It appears to soothe and calm them. At times it may be difficult for your baby to hold a finger or thumb in the mouth long enough to suck with pleasure. This may frustrate your baby and lead to more upset and searching to suck on something. Consider gently offering a small, size-appropriate pacifier when your baby wants to suck. This likely will help your baby calm and fall asleep contently. By supporting your baby's pleasurable sucking, you are supporting your baby's competence in learning to feel soothed and calm.

Most importantly, trust your baby and trust yourself.

[Used with permission from Pearls of Wisdom Task Group, NIDCAP Federation Int'l. 2020.]

SYSTEM-WIDE NIDCAP IMPLEMENTATION: NIDCAP NURSERY SELF-ASSESSMENT AND NIDCAP NURSERY CERTIFICATION

System-integrated developmental care saves significantly on medical and educational costs, aside from assuring significantly better quality of life for infants and their families and increased staff confidence (Mohammed et al., 2014; Montirosso et al., 2012; Mosqueda et al., 2013; Solhaug et al., 2010). The comprehensive NIDCAP approach as compared with other less well-developed approaches is expected to increase these savings. Developmental care system change in the NIDCAP model requires intensive training of an interdisciplinary core team and significant up-front financial and time investment that, however, is saved in readily once care has changed nursery wide. Most important is the assurance of sustainability, which requires quality assurance of staff training and continuation of in-depth education along the main dimensions of the philosophy and implementation of care for the infant, philosophy and implementation of care for the family, for the staff, and for physical environment adaptations. These innovative transformations are highly cost-effective. Research trial–documented US care cost reductions due to NIDCAP implementation range from US $4,000 to $12,000 per NIDCAP infant. NIDCAP infants were shown to be released from intensive (level III) to lower-intensity (level II) care levels in significantly fewer days, which measurably saved on hospital cost in all healthcare systems (Petryshen et al., 1997; Stevens et al., 1996). In order to achieve the results published in the literature cited earlier, a core team consisting of interdisciplinary certified NIDCAP Professionals spanning medical, nursing, and developmental professional backgrounds guides and maintains the quality of care implementation by the other professionals and the staff in the nursery. Detailed repeated bedside observations and daily problem solving lead to environmental and care modifications geared to enhance staff competence and collaboration, and therewith enhance infants and families' unique strengths and reduce their vulnerabilities. Research has shown that, in order to effect reliable behavior change in caregivers when in action, it is critical to develop such on-site well-trained core teams who, in turn, provide one-on-one coaching, collaboration, and guidance. Under the stresses of the daily work environment, and confronted with interactive decision making, it is difficult for many adults to implement, hold on to, and grow in intended behavior change (Fixsen et al., 2007; Fixsen et al., 2005; Joyce & Showers, 2002). The NIDCAP Professionals' daily support, coupled with serially repeated up-to-date developmental care observations and recommendations, assures incremental progress in infants and families' emerging strengths. Infants and families' setbacks in the NICU often occur due to staff misinformation and miscommunication concerning the infants and families' current sensitivities and reactions. Practicing in the NIDCAP approach assures continued attunement to and awareness of each infant and family's individual trajectory in the context of the infant's hospitalization and beyond. In 2009, the NFI published on its open access website www.nidcap.org within the section of NIDCAP Nursery a detailed assessment instrument, the NIDCAP Nursery Manual (Smith et al., 2009). This manual consists of 121 scales grouped into four major categories of a nursery's characteristics and functioning, as well as of four Category Summary Scales, and one Overall Nursery Summary Scale. The individual and the summary scales address the level of individualization, family-centeredness, and developmental support that a nursery provides for the infants and families in its care, as well as for the professionals and staff involved in delivering such care. Aspects of the nursery considered are the physical environment, the care for the infants, the care for the families, and the care for the professionals and staff members in the nursery, who in turn care for the infants and families. The

individual scales are organized into the following four categories: (1) Physical Environment of the Hospital and Nursery, (2) Philosophy and Implementation of Care: Infant, (3) Philosophy and Implementation of Care: Family, and (4) Philosophy and Implementation of Care: Professionals and Staff. The five-point rating scales of the NIDCAP Nursery Manual assess a nursery's philosophy and implementation of care in reference to the NIDCAP model. Each of the five score points represents a level or degree of NIDCAP implementation as follows: (1) traditional, conventional care; (2) the beginning or a minimal degree or level of NIDCAP implementation; (3) an inconsistent, variable or moderate degree or level of NIDCAP implementation; (4) a consistent well-integrated level or degree of NIDCAP implementation; and (5) a highly attuned, distinguished level or degree of NIDCAP implementation. NA, for "not applicable," is scored when an aspect of care does not apply to a specific nursery system. Scores derived from the individual ratings within each of the four categories are utilized to describe and characterize an individual nursery to assess the nursery's level of developmental care implementation and integration and its readiness on the path to a systems-wide individualized, developmentally supportive, family-centered NIDCAP Nursery. This self-assessment process when accomplished by teams of staff and leadership formed to address the four main areas, and within them subareas as indicated, builds collaboration and the development of joint ownership of the change process. All staff members have a place in the process. The self-assessment is an excellent first step once a nursery has arrived at the joint decision to improve care delivery and implementation in the NIDCAP model. The assessment process aids a nursery in the succinct identification of the nursery's strengths already in place and of the areas requiring more in-depth discussion, planning, and strategizing of implementation of improvement. The manual is an excellent tool for repeated self-assessment on a biannual or an annual basis in order to track change and the milestones and successes achieved. Such a joint process engenders creativity, energy, and motivation in staff and leadership and leads to increased joint ownership of and engagement in a dynamic continued change process. Once scores reach a level of 3.6 or above on the summary scales, NIDCAP implementation likely is approaching a system-integrated level, and the nursery may consider application for NFI evaluation with the goal to earn the recognition of formal NIDCAP Nursery Certification. Details of the certification process itself may be found on the NFI website www.nidcap.org. The NFI site review team utilizes the same Nursery Assessment Manual in reviewing the site that the site itself utilized to guide their change process. The Nursery Assessment Manual thus is a multifaceted instrument that serves to (1) train and mentor NIDCAP Master Trainers and Trainers and NIDCAP Professionals as well as nursery staff and leadership in the integration of all aspects of developmental care within their nursery; (2) document the current standard of care within a nursery as well as track the nursery's adoption of and progress in developmental care as the comprehensive framework of care delivery; (3) examine the relationship of environment and caregiving parameters to infant, family, and staff functioning and satisfaction; (4) Provide specific developmental recommendations and suggestions for the integration of developmental care within the context of the nursery environment; the care and nurturing of the infant, family; and support the staff's professional functioning and satisfaction; (5) promote the best short- and long-term development of all infants and their families; (6) recognize a nursery system's strengths and, as indicated, seek and/or provide guidance toward growth and further development in the integration of the principles of individualized, relationship-based developmental NIDCAP care; and (7) lastly, formally evaluate, when desired, the quality of a nursery's developmental orientation and care implementation. To earn NFI certification as NIDCAP Nursery means to provide a dynamic environment for the full integration of expert medical and nursing care securely embedded within the active

pursuit of mutual respect, caring, nurturance of and collaboration with infants and families, and among all professionals and staff members.

All NICU work involves complex human interaction at many levels and the complex interface of physical and emotional vulnerability. At the core is the tiny, immature, fully dependent, highly sensitive, and rapidly developing fetal infant and this infant's hopeful, open, and vulnerable parents, who count on and trust the caregivers' attention and investment. This realization constitutes the challenge and the opportunity of NIDCAP (Als, 1992b) (Fig. 3-2).

The impact of NIDCAP is spreading to NICUs around the world. The NFI's logo states that the NFI strives to be "The Voice of the Newborn." The NFI's motto and goal is to mentor caregivers, change hospitals, and improve the future for newborns and their families in hospital settings. According to its mission, the NFI aspires for all newborns and families to receive hospital care and assessment in the relationship-based, family-integrated NIDCAP model. The

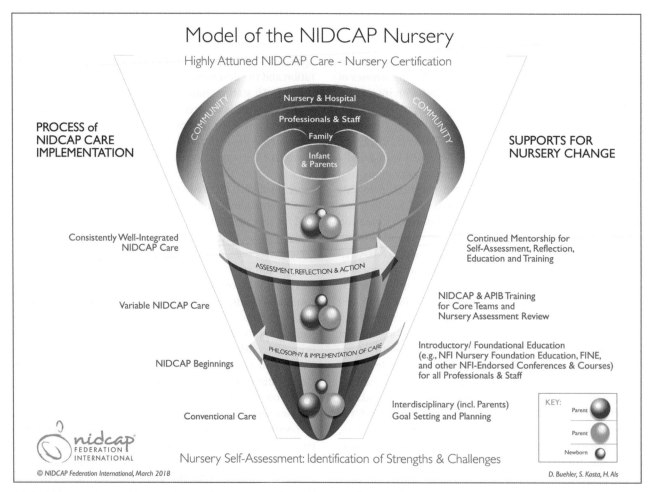

FIGURE 3-2. Depiction of the change process and the learning and education opportunities available for the staff at this point.

NFI defines its role as assurer of the quality of all NIDCAP education, training, and certification for professionals, trainers, and training centers as well as of hospital systems. Furthermore, the NFI seeks to advance the philosophy and science of such care. The NFI's quality standards of training in and implementation of the comprehensive, dynamic, and evidence- and systems-based NIDCAP approach help guard against simplified versions represented in the many generic developmental care aspects in the field, which all lack the theoretical foundation, thorough training, and scientific evidence that underlie NIDCAP. The NFI at this point oversees 24 certified NIDCAP Training Centers, 6 in the United States, 1 in Canada, 14 in Europe, 1 in South America, 1 in Israel, and 1 in Australia. Additional centers are currently in active development, e.g., in Japan, Belgium, Austria, and Sweden; several others are at the planning stages. Furthermore, since its launch in 2011 eight nursery systems have achieved NFI NIDCAP Nursery certification, three in the United States, two in France, one in Sweden, one in Denmark, and one in Israel. Additional nurseries have submitted their self-assessment documentation to the NFI and are currently engaged in preparation for the certification process. As described above, NIDCAP Nursery Certification acknowledges and declares publicly that all aspects of care in the respective NICU system meet NFI certification criteria. Successful NIDCAP Nursery Certification represents distinction in the provision of a consistently high level of NIDCAP care for infants and their families, as well as for the staff, and as such presents an inspiration for all working in this field.

Summary

In summary, the work outlined in this chapter emphasizes that trusting the preterm infant's behavior as meaningful communication moves traditional newborn intensive and other hospital care delivery into a collaborative, relationship-based, neurodevelopmental framework. The NIDCAP framework and approach leads to respect for infants and families as mutually attuned and invested in one another and as active structurers of their own developments. It sees infants, parents, and professional caregivers engaged in continuous coregulation with one another, and in turn with their social and physical environments. It highlights the mutually supportive realization of all human beings' developmentally and individually specific expectations for the increasing differentiation and modulation toward shared goals and improved outcomes, whether they are newborn infants, families, support staff or professionals, administrators, or hospital directors or presidents. Such an approach emphasizes from early on the infant's own strengths and developmental goals and institutes support for the infant's self-regulatory competence and achievement of these goals. Furthermore, the individualized, developmental approach to care as defined in the NIDCAP model improves outcome

not only medically but also behaviorally, psychologically, neurophysiologically, and in terms of brain structure. It protects the preterm brain's vulnerability and improves parent competence and staff satisfaction. It thus reduces cost in the short and long run. The NIDCAP model is based on scientific evidence. The research results indicate that increase in support to behavioral self-regulation improves developmental outcome along many dimensions. The processes involved entail prevention of inappropriate inputs during a highly sensitive period of brain development and the fostering of brain receptivity and opportunity for appropriate inputs. Furthermore, involved is the fostering of caregivers' and parents' confidence in understanding and supporting the infant as a competent individual, a fetus courageous enough to fight for survival and continuation of intrauterine development despite requiring intensive medical care. The introduction of NIDCAP into a medical system, as stated, involves considerable investment at all levels of organization. It requires substantive educational efforts; changes in the practice of care and of professionals' role and self-definition, as well as personal growth and change in each of those involved in NICU systems. Reflective process work is an essential ingredient of all such change and of the assurance of continued growth. The futures of newborns and families in hospital settings depend on the true and honest implementation of individualized, developmentally supportive, family-centered care.

Anyone who experienced the NIDCAP model of care recognizes its applicability as a comprehensive model for all care. Its expansion to all arenas of medical care is long overdue. Patients everywhere are dependent on the professionals and the systems developed in attempts to serve the patient, too often described as consumer. The vulnerability of an elderly person, a brain-impaired person, or simply an ill person, dependent on the help and care of others, prompts the many stressed and physically and/or emotionally exhausted caregivers to deny such persons their full dignity and right to be respected and recognized for the individuality and personhood that each human being possesses. Their strengths and individual identities are overlooked only too easily in the press of the day. The expansion of the NIDCAP model of care into these arenas is overdue and must be championed by those who have been afforded the training, insight, and experience. Caregivers everywhere deserve the support, training, and emotional education and nurturance to collaborate with and cherish as individuals those they care for. Care systems everywhere have the responsibility to avail themselves of the guidance and tools to build collaborative, dynamic, relationship-based nurturing care systems. The pressure for the edge in profit margins, patient days, or other business metrics misses the essence of care and diminishes and denies the dignity and humanity of caregiver and patient alike. Care that enhances the personhood of all involved in the joint process of engagement in healing interactions and relationships is the core metric upheld by NIDCAP (Table 3-1).

TABLE 3-1 NIDCAP Recommendations

Type	Recommendation	Level of Evidence	References
Preventive and/or ameliorative	NIDCAP approach toward infant care • Structuring of the infants 24-hour day • Providing restfulness • Coordinating with family presence • Introduction of self to infant at start of care • Individualized feeding method and frequency • Opportunities for skin-to-skin holding • Immersion tub bathing with containment • Supportive containment with weighing • Collaborative care with support for infant-parent involvement in care of infant • Enhancement of the physical environment -Low indirect lighting with dimmer capacity -Quiet, soothing environment for infants/parents -Free of noxious odors with parent scent present -Home-like individualized bed spaces • Direct caregiver support with developmental specialists • Multidisciplinary collaboration	VII IV II I	Als (1999); Als & Gilkerson (1997); Als & McAnulty (1998); Grunwald & Becker (1990); Lawhon (1986); Lawhon & Melzar (1991); VandenBerg (1990a); VandenBerg & Franck (1990) Als et al. (1986); Becker et al. (1991), (1993); Als & McAnulty (2011); Ferber et al. (2011); Goudarzvand et al. (2019) Duffy et al. (1990); Als et al. (1994); Buehler et al. (1995); Fleisher et al. (1995); Kleberg et al. (2000); Westrup et al. (2000); Kleberg et al. (2002); Als et al. (2004); McAnulty et al. (2009); Als et al. (2011); McAnulty et al. (2010); McAnulty et al. (2012); McAnulty et al. (2013) Ohlsson & Jacobs (2013); Symington & Pinelli (2006)

Note: Level I, evidence from a systematic review or meta-analysis of all relevant randomized controlled trials (RCTs), or evidence-based clinical practice guidelines based on systematic reviews of RCTs; level II, evidence obtained from at least one well-designed RCT; level IV, evidence from well-designed case-control and cohort studies; level VII, evidence from the opinion of authorities and/or reports of expert committees.

Potential Research Questions

Prevention

- Is the Newborn Individualized Developmental Care and Assessment Program (NIDCAP) effective for infants with cardiac surgical conditions?
- Is the Newborn Individualized Developmental Care and Assessment Program (NIDCAP) effective for healthy full-term infants?
- Is the Newborn Individualized Developmental Care and Assessment Program (NIDCAP) effective for infants exposed in the womb to drugs of abuse?
- Is the Newborn Individualized Developmental Care and Assessment Program (NIDCAP) effective for infants with intrauterine neurological and/or genetic and congenital conditions?
- Is there a critical time period for the initiation of the NIDCAP approach with infants in the NICU?

Confirmation

- Does the NIDCAP approach to care have long-term benefits for term infants who have acute medical and/or surgical issues?
- Do the effects of the NIDCAP approach to care in the newborn period last through adolescence and adulthood?

Treatment

- What effect does the NIDCAP approach have on individual staff members and the hospital system?
- Is the NIDCAP approach to care effective in a pediatric or adult intensive care unit?
- Is the NIDCAP approach to care effective in a geriatric care facility? In any care facility that serves nonverbal patients?

CONCLUSION

For the purposes of this chapter, the NIDCAP approach has been used as the exemplar to illustrate the theoretic underpinnings and comprehensive nature of developmental care.

The ultimate goal of any developmental care approach is to first adopt developmental care as the philosophic approach to care and then assure that all healthcare professionals, staff, and families work as a team to optimize infant and family outcomes (Byers, 2003).

ACKNOWLEDGMENTS

This work was in part supported by a grant from the Harris Foundation, Chicago, IL, and a grant by the Weil Foundation, Newton, MA, to H. Als.

REFERENCES

Abdulghani, N., Edvardsson, K., & Amir, L. H. (2018). Worldwide prevalence of mother-infant skin-to-skin contact after vaginal birth: A systematic review. *PLoS One, 13*(10), e0205696. https://doi.org/10.1371/journal.pone.0205696

Abidin, R. R. (1995). *Parenting stress index* (3rd ed.). Psychological Assessment Resources.

Alberts, J. R., & Cramer, C. P. (1988). Ecology and experience: Sources of means and meaning of developmental change. In Blass, E. M. (Ed.), *Handbook of behavioral neurobiology: Developmental psychobiology and behavioral ecology* (Vol. 9, pp. 1–40). Plenum Press.

Als, H. (1975). The human newborn and his mother: An ethological study of their interaction. (Doctoral dissertation, University of Pennsylvania, 1975). *Dissertation Abstract International, 36*, 5.

Als, H. (1977). The newborn communicates. *Journal of Communication, 27*, 66–73.

Als, H. (1978). Assessing an assessment: Conceptual considerations, methodological issues, and a perspective on the future of the Neonatal Behavioral Assessment Scale. *Monograph of the Society for Child Development, 43*, 14–28.

Als, H. (1979). Social interaction: Dynamic matrix for developing behavioral organization. In Uzgiris, I. C. (Ed.), *Social interaction and communication in infancy: New directions for child development* (pp. 21–41). Jossey-Bass.

Als, H. (1981 rev. 1995). *Manual for the naturalistic observation of the newborn (preterm and fullterm): Children's Hospital, Boston, Mass.* Copyright 2006. NIDCAP Federation International.

Als, H. (1982a). Toward a synactive theory of development: Promise for the assessment of infant individuality. *Infant Mental Health Journal, 3*, 229–243. https://doi.org/10.1002/1097-0355(198224)3:4<229::AID-IMHJ2280030405>3.0.CO;2-H

Als, H. (1982b). The unfolding of behavioral organization in the face of a biological violation. In Tronick, E. (Ed.), *Human communication and the joint regulation of behavior* (pp. 125–160). University Park Press.

Als, H. (1983). Infant individuality: Assessing patterns of very early development. In Call, J., Galenson, E., & Tyson, R. L. (Eds.), *Frontiers of infant psychiatry* (pp. 363–378). Basic Books.

Als, H. (1984). *Manual for the naturalistic observation of the newborn (preterm and fullterm)* (Vol. Rev). The Children's Hospital.

Als, H. (1992a). Individualized developmental care in the NICU: Estimating expectation for co-regulation. *Inflammatory Bowel Disease, 15*, 13.

Als, H. (1992b). Individualized, family-focused developmental care for the very low birthweight preterm infant in the NICU. In Friedman, S. L. & Sigman, M. D. (Eds.), *Advances in applied developmental psychology* (Vol. 6, pp. 341–388). Ablex Publishing Company.

Als, H. (1999). Reading the premature infant. In Goldson, E. (Ed.), *Developmental interventions in the neonatal intensive care nursery* (pp. 18–85). Oxford University Press.

Als, H. (2010). The preterm infant: Brain development, early experience and implications for care. In Lester, B. & Sparrow, J. (Eds.), *Nurturing children and families: Building on the legacy of T.B. Brazelton* (pp. 205–219). Blackwell Scientific, Wiley.

Als, H., & Berger, A. (1986). *Manual and scoring system for the assessment of infants' behavior: Kangaroo-Box paradigm.* Boston Children's Hospital.

Als, H., & Brazelton, T. B. (1981). A new model of assessing the behavioral organization in preterm and fullterm infants: Two case studies. *Journal American Academy Child Psychiatry, 20*, 239–263. https://doi.org/10.1016/S0002-7138(09)60987-0

Als, H., Buehler, D., Kerr, D., Feinberg, E., & Gilkerson, L. (1990, 1995. Rev. 1997). *Profile of the nursery environment and of care components. Template Manual, Part I.* Children's Hospital.

Als, H., Duffy, F. H., McAnulty, G., Butler, S., Lightbody, L., Kosta, S., Weisenfeld, N. I., Robertson, R., Parad, R. B., Ringer, S. A., Blickman, J. G., Zurakowski, D., & Warfield, S. (2012). NIDCAP improves brain function and structure in preterm infants with severe intrauterine growth restriction. *Journal of Perinatology, 32*, 797–803.

Als, H., Duffy, F. H., McAnulty, G. B., Fischer, C. B., Kosta, S., Butler, S. C., Parad, R. B., Blickman, J. G., Zurakowski, D., & Ringer, S. A. (2011). Is the Newborn Individualized Developmental Care and Assessment Program (NIDCAP) effective for preterm infants with intrauterine growth restriction? *Journal of Perinatology, 31*(2), 130–136.

Als, H., Duffy, F., McAnulty, G. B., Rivkin, M. J., Vajapeyam, S., Mulkern, R. V., Warfield, S. K., Huppi, P. S., Butler, S. C., Conneman, N., Fischer, C., Eichenwald, E. (2004). Early experience alters brain function and structure. *Pediatrics, 113*(4), 846–857.

Als, H., & Gilkerson, L. (1997). The role of relationship-based developmentally supportive newborn intensive care in strengthening outcome of preterm infants. *Seminars in Perinatology, 21*(3), 178–189. https://doi.org/10.1016/S0146-0005(97)80062-6

Als, H., Gilkerson, L., Duffy, F. H., McAnulty, G. B., Buehler, D. M., VandenBerg, K. A., Sweet, N., Sell, E., Parad, R. B., Ringer, S. A., Butler, S. C., Blickman, J. G., & Jones, K. J. (2003). A three-center randomized controlled trial of individualized developmental care for very low birth weight preterm infants: Medical, neurodevelopmental, parenting and caregiving effects. *Journal of Development Behavioral Pediatrics, 24*(6), 399–408.

Als, H., Lawhon, G., Brown, E., Gibes, R., Duffy, F. H., McAnulty, G. B., & Blickman, J. G. (1986). Individualized behavioral and environmental care for the very low birth weight preterm infant at high risk for bronchopulmonary dysplasia: Neonatal Intensive Care Unit and developmental outcome. *Pediatrics, 78*, 1123–1132.

Als, H., Lawhon, g., Duffy, F. H., McAnulty, G. B., Gibes-Grossman, R., & Blickman, J. G. (1994). Individualized developmental care for the very low birthweight preterm infant: Medical and neurofunctional effects. *Journal of American Medical Association, 272*, 853–858.

Als, H., Lester, B. M., Tronick, E. Z., & Brazelton, T. B. (1982a). Manual for the assessment of preterm infants' behavior (APIB). In Fitzgerald, H. E., Lester, B. M., & Yogman, M. W. (Eds.), *Theory and research in behavioral pediatrics* (Vol. 1, pp. 65–132). Plenum Press.

Als, H., Lester, B. M., Tronick, E. Z., & Brazelton, T. B. (1982b). Towards a research instrument for the assessment of preterm infants' behavior. In Fitzgerald, H. E., Lester, B. M. & Yogman, M. W. (Eds.), *Theory and research in behavioral pediatrics* (Vol. 1, pp. 35–63). Plenum Press.

Als, H., & McAnulty, G. (1998). *Developmental care guidelines for use in the Newborn Intensive Care Unit (NICU).* NIDCAP Federation International, Inc.

Als, H., & McAnulty, G. B. (2011). *The newborn individualized developmental care and assessment program (NIDCAP) with kangaroo mother care (KMC): Comprehensive care for preterm infants.* In On kangaroo mother care, special issue—current women's health reviews. Bentham Publishing.

Anderson, G. C., Burroughs, A. K., & Measel, C. P. (1983). Non-nutritive sucking opportunities: A safe and effective treatment for preterm neonates. In Field, T. & Sostek, A. (Eds.), *Infants born at risk* (pp. 129–147). Grune and Stratton.

Arnsten, A. (2009). Stress signalling pathways that impair prefrontal cortex structure and function. *Nature Reviews Neuroscience, 10*, 410–422. https://doi.org/10.1038/nrn2648

Avery, M. E., & First, L. R. (1994). *Pediatric medicine* (2nd ed.). Williams & Wilkins.

Babson, S. G. (1970). Growth of low birthweight infants. *Journal of Pediatrics, 77*, 11–18. https://doi.org/10.1016/S0022-3476(70)80039-7

Becker, P. T., Grunwald, P. C., Moorman, J., & Stuhr, S. (1991). Outcomes of developmentally supportive nursing care for very low birthweight infants. *Nursing Research, 40*, 150–155. https://doi.org/10.1097/00006199-199105000-00006

Becker, P. T., Grunwald, P. C., Moorman, J., & Stuhr, S. (1993). Effects of developmental care on behavioral organization in very-low-birth-weight infants. *Nursing Research, 42*, 214–220.

Beeghly, M., Perry, B. D., & Tronick, E. (2016). Self-regulatory processes in early development. In Maltzman, S. (Ed.), *Oxford library of psychology.*

The Oxford handbook of treatment processes and outcomes in psychology: A multidisciplinary, biopsychosocial approach (pp. 42–54). Oxford University Press.

Bernard, J., Seidler, R., Hassevoort, K., Benson, B., Welsh, R., Wiggins, J., Jaeggi, S. M., Buschkuehl, M., Monk, C. S., Jonides, J., & Peltier, S. (2012). Resting state cortico-cerebellar functional connectivity networks: A comparison of anatomical and self-organizing map approaches. *Frontiers in Neuroanatomy, 6*, 31. https://doi.org/10.3389/fnana.2012.00031

Bernstein, J. H., & Waber, D. P. (1996). *Developmental scoring system for the Rey-Osterrieth complex figure.* Psychological Assessment Resources.

Blickman, J. G., Brown, E. R., Als, H., Lawhon, G., & Gibes, R. (1990). Imaging procedures and developmental outcomes in the neonatal intensive care unit. *Journal of Perinatology, 10*(3), 304–306.

Boyle, E. M., Poulsen, G., Field, D. J., Kurinczuk, J. J., Wolke, D., Alfirevic, Z., & Quigley, M. A. (2012). Effects of gestational age at birth on health outcomes at 3 and 5 years of age: Population based cohort study. *British Medical Journal, 344*, e896. https://doi.org/10.1136/bmj.e896

Brazelton, T. B. (1973). *Neonatal behavioral assessment scale.* Heinemann.

Brazelton, T. B. (1984). *Neonatal behavioral assessment scale* (2nd ed.). Spastics International Medical Publications. Lippincott.

Brazelton, T. B., & Als, H. (1979). Four early stages in the development of mother-infant interaction. *The Psychoanalytic Study of the Child, 34*, 349–369.

Browne, J. V., Jaeger, C. B., & Kenner, C. (2020). Executive summary: Standards, competencies, and recommended best practices for infant- and family-centered developmental care in the intensive care unit. *Journal of Perinatology, 40*(suppl 1), 5–10. https://doi.org/10.1038/s41372-020-0767-1

Buehler, D. M., Als, H., Duffy, F. H., McAnulty, G. B., & Liederman, J. (1995). Effectiveness of individualized developmental care for low-risk preterm infants: Behavioral and electrophysiological evidence. *Pediatrics, 96*, 923–932.

Byers, J. F. (2003). Components of developmental care and the evidence for their use in the NICU. *The American Journal of Maternal/Child Nursing, 28*(3), 175–182.

Cowan, W. M. (1979). *The development of the brain the brain. A scientific American Book* (pp. 56–67). W. H. Freeman and Company.

Deng, Q., Li, Q., Wang, H., Sun, H., & Xu, X. (2018). Early father-infant skin-to-skin contact and its effect on the neurodevelopmental outcomes of moderately preterm infants in China: Study protocol for a randomized controlled trial. *Trials, 19*(1), 701. https://doi.org/10.1186/s13063-018-3060-2

Denny-Brown, D. (1962). *The basal Ganglia and their relation to disorders of movement.* Oxford University Press.

Denny-Brown, D. (1966). *The cerebral control of movement.* Charles C. Thomas.

Duffy, F. H., Als, H., & McAnulty, G. B. (1990). Behavioral and electrophysiological evidence for gestational age effects in healthy preterm and full-term infants studied 2 weeks after expected due date. *Child Development, 61*, 1271–1286.

Duffy, F. H., & Burchfiel, J. L. (1971). Somatosensory system: Organizational hierarchy from single units in monkey area 5. *Science, 172*, 273–275.

Duffy, F. H., Burchfiel, J. L., & Lombroso, C. T. (1979). Brain electrical activity mapping (BEAM): A method for extending the clinical utility of EEG and evoked potential data. *Annals of Neurology, 5*, 309–321.

Eagle, G. T. (2000). The shattering of the stimulus barrier: The case for an integrative approach in short-term treatment of psychological trauma. *Journal of Psychotherapy Integration, 310*, 301–323. https://doi.org/10.1023/A:1009453113991

Erikson, E. H. (1962). Reality and actualization. *Journal of the American Psychoanalytic Association, 10*, 451–475.

Ferber, S. G., Als, H., McAnulty, G., Peretz, H., & Zisapel, N. (2011). Melatonin and mental capacities in newborn infants. *Journal of Pediatrics, 159*(1), 99–104. https://doi.org/10.1016/j.jpeds.2010.12.032

Fischer, K. W., & Rose, S. P. (1994). Dynamic development of coordination of components in brain and behavior: A framework for theory and research. In Dawson, G. & Fischer, K. W. (Eds.), *Human behavior and the developing brain* (pp. 3–66). The Guilford Press.

Fixsen, D. L., Blase, K. A., Naoom, S. F., & Wallace, F. (2007). *Evidence-based education to benefit students and society.* University of South Florida: Louis de la Parte Florida Mental Health Institute, The National Implementation Research Network.

Fixsen, D. L., Naoom, S. F., Blase, K. A., Friedman, R. M., & Wallace, F. (2005). *Implementation research: A synthesis of the literature.* University of South Florida: Louis de la Parte Florida Mental Health Institute, The National Implementation Research Network.

Fleisher, B. F., VandenBerg, K. A., Constantinou, J., Heller, C., Benitz, W. E., Johnson, A., Rosenthal, A., & Stevenson, D. K. (1995). Individualized developmental care for very-low-birth-weight premature infants. *Clinical Pediatrics, 34*, 523–529.

Ford, M. E., & Ford, D. H., (Eds.). (1987). *Humans as self-constructing living systems: Putting the framework to work.* Lawrence Erlbaum Associates, Inc.

Franck, L. S., & Lawhon, G (2000). Environmental and behavioral strategies to prevent and manage neonatal pain. In Anand, K. J. S., Stevens, B. J. & McGrath, P. J. (Eds.), *Pain research and clinical management* (2nd Revised and Enlarged ed., Vol. 10, pp. 203–216): Elsevier Science BV.

Freud, W. E. (1991). Das "Whose baby" Syndrom. Ein Beitrag zum psychodynamischen Verständnis der Perinatologie. In Stauger, M., Conrad, F., & Haselbacher, G. (Eds.), *Psychosomatische Gynäkologie und Geburtshilfe* (pp. 123–137). Springer-Verlag.

Gilkerson, L., & Als, H. (1995). Role of reflective process in the implementation of developmentally supportive care in the newborn intensive care unit. *Infants and Young Children, 7*, 20–28.

Goudarzvand, L., Dabirian, A., Nourian, M., Jafarimanesh, H., & Ranjbaran, M. (2019). Comparison of conventional phototherapy and phototherapy along with Kangaroo mother care on cutaneous bilirubin of neonates with physiological jaundice. *Journal of Maternal-Fetal & Neonatal Medicine, 32*(8), 1280–1284.

Gouyon, J. B., Iacobelli, S., Ferdynus, C., & Bonsante, F. (2012). Neonatal problems of late and moderate preterm infants. *Seminars in Fetal and Neonatal Medicine, 17*(3), 146–152. https://doi.org/10.1016/j.siny.2012.01.015

Grossman, K. (1978). Die Wirkung des Augenoffnens von Neugeborenen auf das Verhalten ihrer Mutter. *Geburtshilfe und Frauenheilkunde, 38*, 629–635.

Grunwald, P. C., & Becker, P. T. (1990). Developmental enhancement: Implementing a program for the NICU. *Neonatal Network, 9*(6), 29–45.

Hassenstein, B. (1973). *Verhaltensbiologie des Kindes. Muenchen.* Piper Verlag.

Hepper, P. G. (2013). The developmental origins of laterality: Fetal handedness. *Development Psychobiology, 55*(6), 588–595.

Hepper, P., & Shahidullah, S. (1992). Abnormal fetal behavior in Down's Syndrome fetuses. *Quartely Journal of Clinical Psychology, 44*, 305–317.

Hepper, P., Wells, D., & Lynch, C. (2005). Prenatal thumb sucking is related to postnatal handedness. *Neuropsychologia, 43*, 313–315.

Hodel, A. S. (2018). Rapid infant prefrontal cortex development and sensitivity to early environmental experience. *Developmental Review, 48*, 113–114. https://doi.org/10.1016/j.dr.2018.02.003. PMID: 30270962; PMCID: PMC6157748.

Holmes, M., Sheldon, R., & Als, H. (1995). *Developmentally supportive and family centered care: Newborn Intensive Care Unit participation standards.* Unpublished manuscript. University of Oklahoma Health Sciences Center.

Holmes Bernstein, J., & Waber, D. P. (2007). Executive capacities from a developmental perspective. In Meltzer, L. (Ed.), *Executive function in education: From theory to practice.* Guilford Press.

Huttenlocher, P. R. (1984). Synapse elimination and plasticity in developing human cerebral cortex. *American Journal of Mental Deficiency, 88*, 488–496.

Jones, N. B. (1972). Characteristics of ethological studies of human behavior. In Jones, N. B. (Ed.), *Ethological studies of child behavior* (pp. 3–37). Cambridge University Press.

Jones, N. B. (1974). Ethology and early socialization. In Richards, M. P. M. (Ed.), *The integration of a child into a social world* (pp. 263–295). Cambridge University.

Jones, N. B. (1976). Growing points in human ethology: Another link between ethology and the social sciences. In Bateson, P. P. G. & Hinde, R. A. (Eds.), *Growing points in ethology* (pp. 427–451). Cambridge University Press.

Joyce, B., & Showers, B. (2002). *Student achievement through staff development* (3rd ed.). Association for Supervision and Curriculum Development.

Karimi, F. Z., Sadeghi, R., Maleki-Saghooni, N., & Khadivzadeh, T. (2019). The effect of mother-infant skin to skin contact on success and duration of first breastfeeding: A systematic review and meta-analysis. *Taiwanese Journal of Obstetrics Gynecology, 58*(1), 1–9. https://doi.org/10.1016/j.tjog.2018.11.002

Kasprian, G., Langs, G., Brugger, P. C., Bittner, M., Weber, M., Arantes, M., & Prayer, D. (2011). The prenatal origin of hemispheric asymmetry: An in utero neuroimaging study. *Cerebral Cortex, 21*(5), 1076–1083.

Kleberg, A., Warren, I., Norman, E., Mörelius, E., Berg, A., Mat-Ali, E., Holm, K., Fielder, A., Nelson, N., & Hellström-Westas, L. (2008). Lower stress responses after newborn individualized developmental care and assessment program care during eye screening examinations for retinopathy of prematurity: A randomized study. *Pediatrics, 121*(5), e1267–1278.

Kleberg, A., Westrup, B., & Stjernqvist, K. (2000). Developmental outcome, child behavior and mother-child interaction at 3 years of age following Newborn Individualized Developmental Care and Intervention Program (NIDCAP) intervention. *Early Human Development, 60*, 123–135.

Kleberg, A., Westrup, B., Stjernqvist, K., & Lagercrantz, H. (2002). Indications of improved cognitive development at one year of age among infants born very prematurely who received care based on the Newborn Individualized Developmental Care and Assessment Program (NIDCAP). *Early Human Development, 68*, 83–91.

Lawhon, G. (1986). Management of stress in premature infants. In Angelini, D. J., Whelan Knapp, C. M. & Gibes, R. M. (Eds.), *Perinatal neonatal nursing: A clinical handbook* (pp. 319–328). Blackwell Scientific Publications.

Lawhon, G., & Melzar, A. (1991). Developmentally supportive interventions. In Cloherty, J. P. & Stark, A. R. (Eds.), *Manual of neonatal care* (3rd ed., pp. 581–584). Little, Brown, & Co.

Lettvin, J. Y., Maturana, H., McCulloch, W., & Pitts, W. (1959). What the frog's eye tells the frog's brain. *Proceedings of the Institute of Radio Engineers, 47*, 1940–1951.

Littman, B., & Parmelee, A. H. (1974). *Manual for obstetric complications* (Infant Studies Project, Department of Pediatrics, School of Medicine, ed.). University of California.

Long, J. G., Lucey, J. F., & Philip, A. G. S. (1980). Noise and hypoxemia in the intensive care nursery. *Pedia, 65*, 143–145.

Long, J. G., Philip, A. G. S., & Lucey, J. F. (1980). Excessive handling as a cause of hypoxemia. *Pedia, 65*(2), 203–207.

Madzwamuse, S., Baumann, N., Jaekel, J., Bartmann, P., & Wolke, D. (2015). Neuro-cognitive performance of very preterm or very low birth weight adults at 26 years. *Journal of Child Psychology Psychiatry, 56*(8), 857–864.

March of Dimes. (2016). *Premature birth report card—United States.* http://www.marchofdimes.org/materials/premature-birth-report-card-united-states.pdf

March of Dimes. (2019). *2019 report card.* https://www.marchofdimes.org/materials/MOD2019_REPORT_CARD_and_POLICY_ACTIONS_BOOKLETv72.pdf

Martin, R. J., Herrell, N., Rubin, D., & Fanaroff, A. (1979). Effect of supine and prone positions on arterial oxygen tension in the preterm infant. *Pediatrics, 63*, 528–531.

Martin, R. J., Okken, A., & Rubin, D. (1979). Arterial oxygen tension during active and quiet sleep in the normal neonate. *Journal of Pediatrics, 94*, 271–274.

McAnulty, G., Duffy, F., Butler, S., Bernstein, J., Zurakowski, D., & Als, H. (2010). Effects of the newborn individualized developmental care and assessment program (NIDCAP) at age 8 years: Preliminary data. *Clinical Pediatrics, 49*(3), 258–270.

McAnulty, G., Duffy, F., Butler, S., Parad, R., Ringer, S., Zurakowski, D., & Als, H. (2009). Individualized developmental care for a large sample of very preterm infants: Health, neurobehavior and neurophysiology. *Acta Paediatrica, 98*, 1920–1926.

McAnulty, G., Duffy, F. H., Kosta, S., Weisenfeld, N. I., Warfield, S. K., Butler, S. C., & Als, H. (2013). School-age effects of the newborn individualized developmental care and assessment program for preterm infants with intrauterine growth restriction: Preliminary findings. *BioMed Central Pediatrics, 13*, 25. https://doi.org/10.1186/1471-2431-13-25

McAnulty, G., Duffy, F. H., Kosta, S., Weisenfeld, N., Warfield, S., Butler, S. C., Bernstein, J. H., Zurakowski, D., & Als, H. (2012). School age effects of the newborn individualized developmental care and assessment program for preterm medically low-risk preterm infants: Preliminary findings. *Journal of Clinical Neonatology, 1*(4), 184–194. https://doi.org/10.4103/2249-4847.105982

Ment, L. R., Vohr, B., Allan, W., Katz, K. H., Schneider, K. C., Westerveld, M., Duncan, C. C., & Makuch, R. W. (2003). Change in cognitive function over time in very low-birth-weight infants. *Journal of American Medication Association, 289*(6), 705–711.

Minde, K. K., Morton, P., Manning, D., & Hines, B. (1980). Some determinants of mother-infant interaction in the premature nursery. *Journal of the American Academy of Child Psychiatry, 19*, 1–21.

Minde, K., Whitelaw, A., Brown, J., & Fitzhardinge, P. (1983). Effect of neonatal complications in premature infants on early parent-child interactions. *Developmental Medicine and Child Neurology, 25*, 763–777.

Mohammed, S. A.-R., Bayoumi, M. H., & Mahmoud, F. S. (2014). The effect of developmentally supportive cae training program on nurses' performance and behavioral responses of newborn infants. *Journal of Education and Practice, 5*(6), 134–144.

Montirosso, R., Del Prete, A., Bellù, R., Tronick, E., Borgatti, R., & Neonatal Adequate Care for Quality of Life Study Group. (2012). Level of NICU quality of developmental care and neurobehavioral performance in very preterm infants. *Pediatrics, 129*(5), e1129–e1137. https://doi.org/10.1542/peds.2011-0813

Moore, E. R., Anderson, G. C., Bergman, N., & Dowswell, T. (2012). Early skin-to-skin contact for mothers and their healthy newborn infants. *Cochrane Database of Systematic Reviews, 5*(5), CD003519. https://doi.org/10.1002/14651858.CD003519.pub3

Mosqueda, R., Castilla, Y., Perapoch, J., de la Cruz, J., López-Maestro, M., & Pallás, C. (2013). Staff perceptions on newborn individualized developmental care and assessment program (NIDCAP) during its implementation in two Spanish neonatal units. *Early Human Development, 89*(1), 27–33. http://dx.doi.org/10.1016/j.earlhumdev.2012.07.013

Murdoch, D. R., & Darlow, B. A. (1984). Handling during neonatal intensive care. *Archives of Disease in Childhood, 29*, 957–961.

Norris, S., Campbell, L., & Brenkert, S. (1982). Nursing procedures and alterations in transcutaneous oxygen tension in premature infants. *Nursing Research, 31*, 330–336.

O'Donnell, K. J. (1986). *Assessment of maternal functioning: The mother's view of the child.* (Unpublished Manuscript). University of North Carolina, Chapel Hill.

Ohlsson, A., & Jacobs, S. E. (2013). NIDCAP: A Systematic Review and Meta-analyses of Randomized Controlled Trials. *Pediatrics, 131*(3), e881-e893. https://doi.org/10.1542/peds.2012-2121

Padilla, N., Junqué, C., Figueras, F., Sanz-Cortes, M., Bargalló, N., Arranz, A., Donaire, A., Figueras, J., & Gratacos, E. (2014). Differential vulnerability of gray matter and white matter to intrauterine growth restriction in preterm infants at 12 months corrected age. *Brain Research, 1545*, 1–11.

Patricia, P., Howard, H., Check, J., Jeffrey George, J., McKinley, P., Lewis, W., Hegwood, P., Whitfield, J. M., McLendon, D., Okuno-Jones, S., Klein, S., Moehring, J., & McConnell, C. (2003). Evaluation and development of potentially better practices for the prevention of brain hemorrhage and ischemic brain injury in very low birth weight infants. *Pediatrics, 111*(suppl E1), e489–e496.

Pearls of NIDCAP Wisdom Task Group. (2020, April 1, 2021). *Ten Pearls of NIDCAP wisdom for parents of hospitalized babies.* Retrieved April 1, 2021, from https://nidcap.org/10-pearls-of-nidcap-wisdom/

Peters, K. L., Rosychuk, R. J., Hendson, L., Cote, J. J., McPherson, C., & Tyebkhan, J. M. (2009). Improvement of short- and long-term outcomes for very low birth weight infants: The Edmonton NIDCAP trial. *Pediatrics, 124*(4), 1009–1020.

Petryshen, P., Stevens, B., Hawkins, J., & Stewart, M. (1997). Comparing nursing costs for preterm infants receiving conventional vs. developmental care. *Nursing Economics, 15*, 138–150.

Prechtl, H. (1977). *The neurological examination of the full term infant: A manual for clinical use* (2nd ed.). Lippincott.

Reppert, S. M., & Rivkees, S. A. (1989). Development of human circadian rhythms: Implications for health and disease. In Reppert, S. M. (Ed.), *Development of circadian rhythmicity and photoperiodism in mammals* (Vol. Research in Perinatal Medicine, IX, pp. 245–259). Perinatology Press.

Rey, A. (1941). L'examen psychologique dans les cas d'encephalopathie traumatique. *Archives de Psychologie, 28,* 286–340.

Robson, K. (1967). The role of eye-to-eye contact in maternal-infant attachment. *Journal of Child Psychology & Psychiatry, 8,* 13–25.

Rosenblatt, J. S. (1976). Stages in the early behavioral development of altricial young of selected species of non-primate mammals. In Bateson, P. P. G. & Hinde, R. A. (Eds.), *Growing points in ethology.* Cambridge University Press.

Sander, L. W. (1975). Infant and caretaking environment: Investigation and conceptualization of adaptive behavior in a system of increasing complexity. In Anthony, E. J. (Ed.), *Explorations in child psychiatry.* Plenum Press.

Sander, L. W. (1980). Investigation of the infant and its environment as a biological system. In Greenberg, S. I. & Pollock, G. H. (Eds.), *The course of life: Psyoanalytic contribution toward understanding personality development* (pp. 177–201). National Institute of Mental Health.

Sander, L. W., Stechler, G., Burns, P., & Lee, A. (1979). Change in infant and caregiver variables over the first two months of life: Integration of action in early development. In Thomas, E. B. (Ed.), *Origins of the infant's social responsiveness.* Lawrence Erlbaum.

Schade, J. P., & van Groenigen, D. B. (1961). Structural organization of the human cerebral cortex. I. Maturation of the middle frontal gyrus. *Acta Anatomica, 41,* 47–111.

Schneirla, T. C. (1959). An evolutionary and developmental theory of biphasic processes underlying approach and withdrawal. In Jones, M. R. (Ed.), *Nebraska symposium on motivation* (pp. 1–42). University of Nebraska Press.

Schneirla, T. C. (1965). Aspects of stimulation and organization in approach and withdrawal processes underlying vertebrate development. *Advances in Study of Behavior, 1,* 1–74.

Schneirla, T. C., & Rosenblatt, J. S. (1961). Behavioral organization and genesis of the social bond in insects and mammals. *American Journal of Orthopsychiatry, 31,* 223–253.

Schneirla, T. C., & Rosenblatt, J. S. (1963). "Critical periods" in the development of behavior. *Neuroscience, 139,* 1110–1115.

Smith, K., Buehler, D., & Als, H. (2009). *NIDCAP nursery certification criterion scales.* Copyright, NIDCAP Federation International.

Solhaug, M., Torunn Bjørk, I., & Pettersen Sandtrø, H. (2010). Staff perception one year after implementation of the the newborn individualized developmental care and assessment program (NIDCAP). *Journal of Pediatric Nursing, 25*(2), 89–97. http://dx.doi.org/10.1016/j.pedn.2009.11.004

Stevens, B., Petryshen, P., Hawkins, J., Smith, B., & Taylor, P. (1996). Developmental versus conventional care: A comparison of clinical outcomes for very low birth weight infants. *The Canadian Journal of Nursing Research, 28,* 97–113.

Svensson, K. E., Velandia, M. I., Matthiesen, A-S. T., Welles-Nyström, B. L., & Widström, A-M. E. (2013). Effects of mother-infant skin-to-skin contact on severe latch-on problems in older infants: A randomized trial. *International Breastfeeding Journal, 8*(1), 1. https://doi.org/10.1186/1746-4358-8-1

Symington, A., & Pinelli, J. (2006). Developmental care for promoting development and preventing morbidity in preterm infants. *Cochrane Database of Systematic Reviews, (2),* 1–44.

UNICEF. (2021). *The Baby Friendly Initiative: Transforming healthcare for babies, their mothers and families.*

US Department of Health and Human Services. (2019). *National vital Statistics report: Births. Final data for 2018* (Vol. 68).

VandenBerg, K. A. (1990a). Nippling management of the sick neonate in the NICU: The disorganized feeder. *Neonatal Network, 9*(1), 9–16.

VandenBerg, K. A. (1990b). Behaviorally supportive care for the extremely premature infant. In Gunderson, L. P. & Kenner, C. (Eds.), *Care of the 24–25 Week gestational age infant (small baby Protocol)* (pp. 129–157). Neonatal Network.

VandenBerg, K. A., & Franck, L. S. (1990). Behavioral issues for infants with BPD. In Lund, C. (Ed.), *BPD: Strategies for total patient care* (pp. 113–152). Neonatal Network.

Vento, T., & Feinberg, E. (1998). Developmentally supportive care. In Cloherty, J., & Stark, A., (Eds.), *Developmentally supportive care* (4th ed., pp. 151–153). Little, Brown, & Co.

Westrup, B., Böhm, B., Lagercrantz, H., & Stjernqvist, S. (2003). *Preschool outcome in children born very prematurely and cared for according to the newborn individualized development care and assessment program (NIDCAP) developmentally supportive neonatal care: A study of the newborn individualized developmental care and assessment program (NIDCAP) in Swedish settings* (pp. VI:1–21). Repro Print AB.

Westrup, B., Kleberg, A., von Eichwald, K., Stjernqvist, K., & Lagercrantz, H. (2000). A randomized controlled trial to evaluate the effects of the Newborn Individualized Developmental Care and Assessment Program in a Swedish setting. *Pediatrics, 105*(1), 66–72.

Wolke, D. (1987). Environmental and developmental neonatology. *Journal of Reproductive and Infant Psychology, 5,* 17–42.

Yakovlev, P. I., & Lecours, A. R. (1967). The myelogenic cycles of regional maturation of the brain. In Minkowsky, A. (Ed.), *Regional development of the brain in early life* (pp. 3–70). Blackwell.

CHAPTER 4

Quality Indicators for Developmental Care: A Trauma Informed Conceptual Model as an Exemplar for Change

Mary Coughlin, Tara DeWolfe, and Kristy Fuller

Developmental Care Standards for Baby, Parent, and Families in Intensive Care

Standard 2: Systems thinking

- The intensive care unit shall provide a professionally competent interprofessional collaborative practice team to support the baby, parent, and family's holistic, physical, developmental, and psychosocial needs from birth through the transition of hospital discharge to home and assure continuity to follow-up care.

INTRODUCTION

The Institute of Medicine defines quality as the degree to which health services for individuals and populations increase the likelihood of desired health outcomes and are consistent with current professional knowledge (Allen-Duck et al., 2017). Despite the existence of global healthcare standards, evidence-based best practices, accreditation requirements, countless reports, and government regulations, quality healthcare continues to elude the majority of patients and healthcare consumers. This reality begs the question "Why has quality been so difficult to achieve?" The answer may be as simple as refocusing healthcare from the conventional question of "What is wrong with you?" to "What happened to you?" From a systems thinking framework this refocusing is foundational to the concepts discussed in this chapter.

Changing this fundamental question heralds a paradigm shift to one of trauma awareness. Trauma awareness is requisite to becoming trauma informed and embracing quality indicators for trauma informed developmental care. Trauma informed care in the neonatal intensive care unit (NICU) is a biologically relevant paradigm for hospitalized babies, families, and clinicians (Coughlin, 2016, 2017, 2021; Sanders & Hall, 2018). The American Academy of Pediatrics issued a technical report and policy statement outlining the lifelong effects of early childhood adversity, toxic stress, and the role of pediatric clinicians (Shonkoff et al., 2012; Garner et al., 2012). Montirosso and Provenzi (2015), which confirms that preterm birth is an early adverse experience characterized by exposure to toxic stress and reduced buffering effects of maternal care. D'Agata et al. (2016)

introduced the Infant Medical Trauma in the NICU conceptual model (Fig. 4-1) as a vehicle to study the baby's experience in the NICU, examine associated developmental consequences, and identify effective strategies to improved care. Finally, evidence-based practice guidelines for the delivery of trauma informed care in the NICU have been endorsed by the National Association of Neonatal Nurses (Nann) for neonatal clinicians (Coughlin, 2016). This burgeoning expanse of evidence and best practice recommendations demands change across cultural, professional, practice, and personal domains.

Infants make meaning out of the world based on how the world makes them feel (Korl et al., 2019; Tronick & Beeghly, 2011). Does the baby feel safe, secure, and/or connected or do they feel unsafe, insecure, and/or isolated? These feelings create cellular memories mediated primarily by maternal caregiving experiences, which influence hypothalamic-pituitary-adrenal (HPA) axis reactivity and affect the developmental trajectory of the baby's lifelong health and well-being (Lester et al., 2018; Wright, 2018). Mitigating the iatrogenic psychological effects of medical care in the NICU and beyond is a moral and ethical imperative for quality healthcare delivery. Understanding the concepts of infant medical traumatic stress and its association with alterations in brain growth and development highlights the biologic relevance of a trauma informed developmental approach to care in the NICU and beyond (Coughlin, 2021; D'Agata et al., 2016; Montirosso et al., 2017).

The Universe of Developmental Care (UDC) Model (Fig. 4-2), introduced in 2008, was an attempt to create a visual illustration of the lived experience of the critically ill baby in the NICU and highlight opportunities to provide

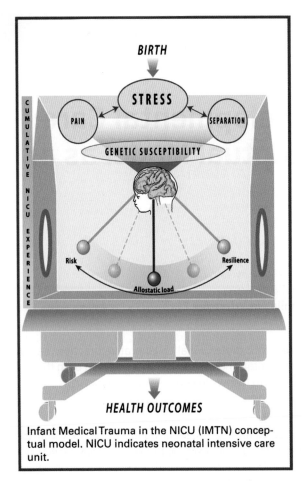

Infant Medical Trauma in the NICU (IMTN) conceptual model. NICU indicates neonatal intensive care unit.

FIGURE 4-1. Infant Medical Trauma in the NICU. [Reprinted with permission from D'Agata, A. L., Young, E. E., Cong, X., Grasso, D. J., & McGrath, J. M. [2016]. Infant medical trauma in the neonatal intensive care unit [IMTN]: A proposed concept for science and practice. *Advances in Neonatal Care, 14*[4], 289–297. https://doi.org/10.1097/ANC.0000000000000309]

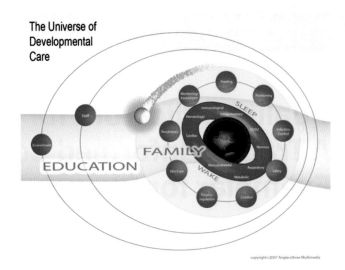

FIGURE 4-2. The Universe of Developmental Care. [Used with permission from Gibbins, A. Copyright © 2007 Anglersthree Multimedia.]

developmentally supportive care (Gibbins et al., 2008, 2010). The UDC model extended Synactive Theory beyond observable behaviors elicited by the baby reflecting central nervous system organization by emphasizing the concept of a shared surface interface. The skin and central nervous system arise from the same ectodermal germ layer and then differentiate into the surface ectoderm and the neural ectoderm sharing similar functions. The skin, representing the largest body organ, is the interface between the external and internal environments of the human body. Vital properties of the skin include the capability to locally recognize, discriminate, and integrate various signals within a heterogenous environment to launch appropriate responses (Slominski et al., 2012). Skin functions are integrated into the skin immune, pigmentary, epidermal, and adnexal systems and are in continuous communication with the systemic immune, neural, and endocrine systems (Slominski et al., 2012). The body/environment interface is where two seemingly independent surfaces with unique boundaries become intimately and seamlessly connected; each individual is affected positively or negatively by the other (Gibbins et al., 2008).

Meeting the whole person needs of the baby and family in crisis hinges on the wholeness of the clinician. One cannot give what one does not have, what one does not give to oneself. Guided by the American Psychiatric Nurses Association's position statement issued in March 2017 and revised in April 2020 entitled: "Whole Health Begins with Mental Health" the idea of a shared care interface is profoundly relevant as we understand health as a state of physical, mental, and social well-being and not merely the absence of disease (APNA Position, 2017). Consequently, during a caring encounter, embracing a whole health mindset one recognizes there are not two separate entities bumping into each other, or two separate entities with an intervening space, but a new entity formed through connection with other, one that is both individual and environment (Gibbins et al., 2008). This shared care interface emanates from healing intention and authentic presence on the part of the caregiver creating a sacred, transpersonal caring moment where patient and professional are attuned to each other's experience in deep human connection (Norman et al., 2016). Similar to a Mobius strip, when one practices authentic presence in the caring moment a shared interface emerges where the two become one. By shifting the focus from the brain, which cannot be directly viewed or touched, to the actual shared interface of care, the UDC model recognizes the dynamic, interactive, and interpersonal link between the body, mind, and spirit of the caregiver and baby/family dyad that informs the development of thoughtful, compassionate, individualized patient care plans within the complex technological environment of the NICU.

Retracing the theoretical underpinnings of nursing, from Nightingale to Newman, from Rogers to Watson and so many more, neonatal nurses are invited to embrace a whole-person unitary transformative worldview of their practice and operationalize this holistic view in everyday caring encounters. In caring for critically ill babies and their families the goal is to help these vulnerable individuals live wholly, live through their disease, through the crisis, and through the trauma, not just to survive the experience but to thrive and to flourish. This aspect of caring demands a connection with the concept of unitary caring science, an evolved worldview of one humanity, one heart, and one world (Watson, 2018). As such, the concept of the UDC and its shared care interface reflects a trauma informed approach to care. The exemplar for change begins with the clinician realigning with their purpose and mission in service to vulnerable babies and families in crisis. This is a critical and often overlooked step to ensure that the interprofessional collaborative practice team is not only competent but compassionate and aligned with their purpose, passion, and mission to support the baby, parent, and family's holistic physical, developmental, psychosocial, and spiritual needs from birth through the transition of hospital discharge to home.

WHAT IS TRAUMA INFORMED CARE?

The adverse childhood experience (ACE) study is the largest investigation to date examining the relationship between childhood abuse, neglect, and household dysfunction with adult morbidity and mortality (Felitti et al., 1998). Replicated across a multitude of demographic populations, the results stand firm. Adversity in childhood negatively impacts health and wellness across the lifespan. About 61% of Americans report at least one ACE during the first 18 years of life with 25% reporting three or more ACEs (Table 4-1) (Merrick et al., 2018, 2019). Globally, Carlson, et al. (2019) report

TABLE 4-1 Adverse Childhood Experience		
Abuse	**Household Dysfunction**	**Neglect**
• Physical • Emotional • Sexual	• Household member substance use • Household member incarceration • Household member mental illness • Parental divorce • Witnessing intimate partner violence	• Physical • Emotional

that two-thirds of youth experience adversity in childhood regardless of where they reside around the world.

Adversity in childhood is most often mediated by the child's relationship with adult caregivers and is also referred to as interpersonal trauma. Early life stress and interpersonal trauma is associated with attachment adversity and has been linked to posttraumatic stress disorder (PTSD) and developmental trauma disorder in survivors (Pervanidou et al., 2020; Spinazzola et al., 2018). Adversity in childhood is associated with significantly poorer health outcomes, risky health behaviors, and socioeconomic challenges (Fig. 4-3) (Crouch et al., 2019; Merrick et al., 2019).

Zarse et al. (2019) published a comprehensive literature review of 2 decades of research using the Adverse Childhood

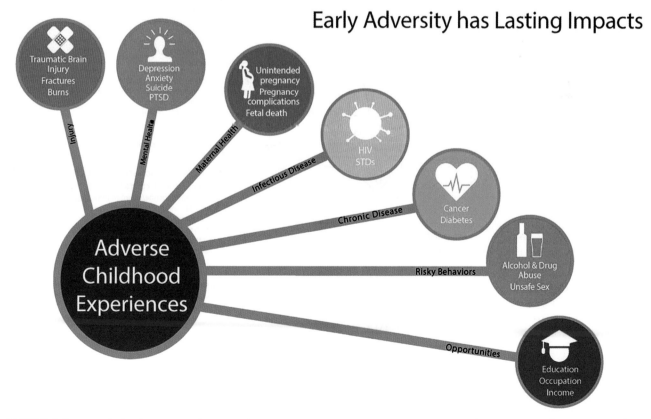

FIGURE 4-3. Association between adverse childhood experiences and negative outcomes. [Source: https://www.cdc.gov/violenceprevention/acestudy/resources.html]

Experience—Questionnaire (ACE-Q). The results highlight the dose-dependent, causal relationship between ACEs and mental illness, addictions, adult noncommunicable diseases, disrupted parenting, and insecure child rearing (Zarse et al., 2019). The perturbations in family integrity leave a transgenerational footprint of the burden of disease associated with early life adversity (Fig. 4-4) (Zarse et al., 2019).

The pervasiveness of interpersonal trauma leaves very few of us unscathed. During sensitive and critical periods of development, life experiences take on new meaning as they direct and disrupt biological processes in the wake of early life adversity. These biological processes, mediated by epigenetic mechanisms, have lifelong implications for an individual's physiologic and psychologic health and well-being (Coughlin, 2021). Individuals with a history of interpersonal trauma in childhood are highly susceptible to substance use disorders and mental and physical health challenges (Brunault et al., 2020; Lee et al., 2018; Meulewaeter et al., 2019). A preoccupation with substance use is one mechanism through which trauma and disrupted attachment are transmitted across generations (Fig. 4-5) (Chamberlain et al., 2019; Meulewaeter et al., 2019; Narayan et al., 2017).

Enlow et al. (2018) explored the relationship between maternal childhood maltreatment and child mental health in an effort to understand mechanisms and effects of intergenerational trauma. A maternal history of maltreatment during childhood was significantly associated with maltreatment of offspring, greater stress exposure, and diminished social support for the affected individuals and families (Enlow et al., 2018). In addition, when compared with children of nonmaltreated mothers, the children of maltreated mothers were more likely to present with clinically significant emotional and behavioral problems.

Less-sensitive maternal behavior has been reported in mothers who experienced adversity during childhood. Expectant mothers exposed to domestic violence (DV) during childhood demonstrate poorer prenatal attachment to their fetus and an increase in heart rate when presented with a baby-cry stimulus, and, at 6 months of age, babies of these mothers exhibited worse emotion regulation (Sancho-Rossignol et al., 2018). Toso et al. (2020) completed a systematic review examining the association between maternal prenatal exposure to violence and developmental difficulties in their children. The principal findings of this systematic review reveal an association between prenatal exposure to violence and impaired baby development (Toso et al., 2020).

Adult survivors of childhood abuse exhibit dysregulation of the HPA axis, the hypothalamic-pituitary-thyroid axis, and

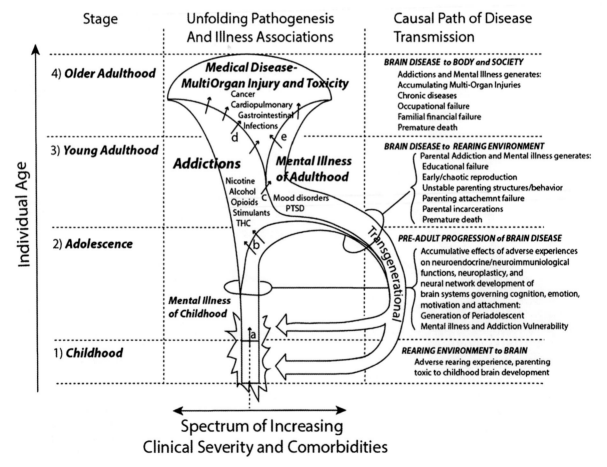

FIGURE 4-4. Neuroscience-informed causal pathway to ACEs comorbidities. [Reprinted with permission under the Creative Commons Attribution [CC-BY] 4.0 license.]

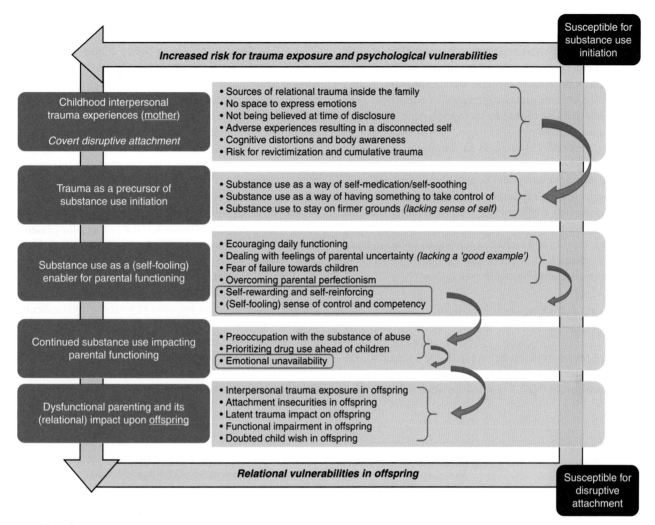

FIGURE 4-5. Mechanisms underlying the cycle of intergenerational trauma transmission in mothers with substance use disorders. [Reprinted with permission under the terms of the Creative Commons Attribution License [CC BY].]

immune function. These perturbations to maternal biology have been linked to aberrant neurodevelopmental outcomes in their offspring (Dunn et al., 2019; Roberts et al., 2018). The experience of chronic stress as a result of early life adversity and the body's biological response to the release of cortisol and a myriad of inflammatory mediators amplifies cross talk between peripheral inflammation and neural circuitry leading to chronic low-grade inflammation (Dunn et al., 2019; Nusslock & Miller, 2016). This chronic low-grade inflammation predisposes the affected individual to adiposity and insulin resistance while also acting on corticoamygdala and corticobasal ganglia threat and reward circuits that lead to self-medicating behaviors such as smoking, drug use, and the consumption of high-fat diets. The combination of inflammation/neuroinflammation and these self-medicating behaviors results in significant physical and emotional pathology, morbidity, and mortality.

Maternal separation is the most significant trauma experienced by all newborn mammals. Preterm and critically ill newborns are by all means no exception to this reality. Early maternal separation jeopardizes the physical and behavioral health of newborn humans with periods as brief as 2 hours during the first 48 hours of postnatal life negatively impacting maternal–infant bonding at 12 months of age (Csaszar-Nagy & Bokkon, 2018). Separation of mother and baby at 2 days of age for 1 hour revealed a 176% increase in autonomic activity and an 86% reduction in quiet sleep with sleep cycling almost abolished during the separation period (Morgan et al., 2011). The experience of maternal separation in the NICU becomes the foundation for cumulative toxic stress exposures to include unmanaged or undermanaged stress and pain, sleep fragmentation, susceptibility to inappropriate sensory stimuli from the physical and social environments, postural malalignment, and hazardous rituals and routines that do not honor the personhood of the baby (Weber & Harrison, 2019). All of these liabilities have a graded-dose effect on the developing baby enduring early life adversity associated with newborn intensive care (Sanders & Hall, 2018; Weber & Harrison, 2019).

The perinatal period may trigger retraumatization in individuals with a trauma history. This period presents a unique opportunity to transform the vicious cycle of trauma into a virtuous cycle of healing (Chamberlain et al., 2019a, 2019b). The opportunity begins with becoming trauma informed. To become trauma informed one must (1) realize the pervasiveness of trauma in everyday life; (2) recognize the signs and symptoms of trauma in patients, families, colleagues, and self; (3) respond to trauma by integrating knowledge and evidence-based best practices that mitigate and prevent trauma into policies, procedures, language, and annual performance appraisals; and (4) resist retraumatization by ensuring consistency in service delivery. Trauma informed care is the overarching framework for all developmental care models and strategies seeking to mitigate, manage, and ameliorate toxic stress and the negative aspects of NICU hospitalization (Fig. 4-6).

The Attributes of the Trauma Informed Professional

Healthcare transformation begins with the individual, the clinician. To provide authentic, competent, and compassionate care in the NICU it must be acknowledged that one cannot give what one does not have. One cannot give loving kindness, equanimity, respect, and dignity to other if one does not treat self with loving kindness, equanimity, and dignity (Watson, 2018). The verb "to become" has an aspirational connotation; an understanding that to become trauma informed is not a destination. Becoming trauma informed is a continuous journey of self-discovery and growth moving toward excellence in service to self and other. Each moment is an invitation to become more trauma informed, more openhearted, more knowledgeable, more courageous than the moment before. "Becoming" represents an ongoing transformation and evolution both personally and professionally. Becoming trauma informed is indeed the road less traveled, but a journey that expands the depth of service available for vulnerable babies and their families.

Eight attributes of the trauma informed professional (TIP) have been identified by an international, interdisciplinary faculty board of neonatal experts during the creation of a certification in trauma informed care (Table 4-2; Fig. 4-7). Becoming a TIP begins with unbundling one's passion, mission, and noble purpose from the myriad of tasks, rituals, and routines that often overshadow and overpower one's presence in the caring moment.

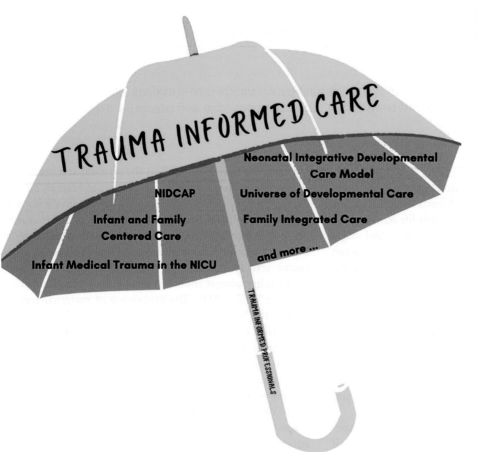

FIGURE 4-6. Trauma informed care as an overarching paradigm for all developmental care models.

TABLE 4-2 Eight Attributes of the Trauma Informed Professional	
Knowledgeable	Advocacy
Healing Intention	Role Model/Mentor
Personal Wholeness	Scholarship
Courage	Leadership for Change

TABLE 4-3 The Guiding Principles of a Trauma Informed Approach

1. Safety
2. Choice
3. Collaboration
4. Empowerment
5. Trustworthiness

An attribute is a quality or characteristic that can be learned over time. A competency is a combination of a skill and behavior that is easily identified and can be measured or validated. Each attribute represents a quality and a skill the faculty deemed critical for a leader in trauma informed developmental care. These attributes then become competencies that guide the growth and developmental trajectory of the certified TIP.

Knowledgeable

Core knowledge regarding the science and soul underpinning early life adversity and the biologic and existential sequelae associated with it is primal. Relevant research crosses all scientific realms from molecular biology to psychology, from genetics to metaphysics. Unitary caring science is a critical cornerstone of trauma informed care. Understanding the guiding principles of a trauma informed approach (Table 4-3) and the core measures for trauma informed developmental care (Table 4-4) provides the foundation to advance and expand the knowledge of the TIP.

Healing Intention

Healing means to become whole, an integrated wholeness of body, mind, and spirit. Healing is about transcendence, a movement toward wholeness and well-being over time (Zahourek, 2012). Intention is distinct and purposeful, defined as the action of directing one's mind or attention to something. Healing intention requires presence and conscious alignment with the divine essence of self to create a sense of oneness or wholeness with other during the caring moment (Sofhauser, 2016; Zahourek, 2012).

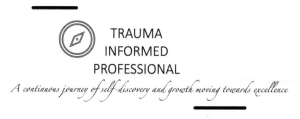

TRAUMA
INFORMED
PROFESSIONAL

A continuous journey of self-discovery and growth moving towards excellence

FIGURE 4-7. Trauma Informed Professional Certificate Program. [Reprinted with permission from Caring Essentials Collaborative, LLC.]

One may set an intention for healing at the beginning of one's shift, either as an individual or as a team. It may be a silent prayer or moment before laying hands on the patient. Practicing healing intention includes a reflection and a desire to be more present in the moment.

Personal Wholeness

Personal wholeness is a journey toward physical, psychological, social, spiritual, and existential well-being. The self-healing dimensions of personal wholeness seek to mitigate the corrosive effects of stress-reactive habits and support health-promoting activities (Loizzo et al., 2009). Upon gaining wholeness, one exudes congruence of mind, body, and spirit, experienced through relationship with self and others, resulting in a feeling of completeness and well-being. Competence comes from cultivating behaviors that realign one's acceptance and embrace of the beauty and grace that is uniquely and only self. Personal wholeness is a core attribute of the TIP that breeds resilience and compassion, for self and others, and begins when one adopts transformational practices (Table 4-5).

Courage

Courage is defined as a willful, intentional act, executed after mindful deliberation, involving objective substantial risk to the actor, primarily motivated to bring about a noble good or worthy end, despite, perhaps, the presence of the emotion of fear (Rate et al., 2007). Taking courageous action can effect change, increase self-actualization and reduce moral distress (Hawkins & Morse, 2014). To be trauma informed requires respectful courage to challenge the status quo. In further developing the attribute of courage, consider where you can step up and stand out. If you knew you could not fail, what would you do? If you knew failure would be part of it, what is worth the risk? Courage fosters clinician integrity and advocacy reducing patient suffering and ensuring the delivery of safe, compassionate, quality care (Coughlin, 2021).

Advocacy

Advocacy is any action that speaks in favor of, recommends, argues for a cause, supports or defends, or pleads on behalf of another/others. Nightingale set the precedent for advocacy in nursing as she championed safe, clean environments

TABLE 4-4 The Core Measures for Trauma Informed Developmental Care

Attributes	Examples	Level of Evidence	Sources
Healing Environment			
The physical environment is a soothing, spacious, and aesthetically pleasing healing space conducive to rest, growth, and establishing connectedness	**Infant:** Sensory input is age appropriate and aligned with best-practice recommendations: the space comfortably accommodates the 24-hour presence of the infant's family	I, II, III	Fontana et al. (2021); O'Callaghan et al. (2019); Pineda et al. (2017)
	Family: The design honors the holistic and human needs of its inhabitants integrating stress-reducing elements (nature, art, music) and ensuring personal space, privacy, and community access	I, III	Fernandez Medina et al. (2019); O'Callaghan et al. (2019); Treherne et al. (2017)
	Staff: The physical layout supports efficiency in workflow, provides protected space for staff rest and recovery, promotes collaboration and community, and ensures optimal spatial dimensions at each bedside for safe care delivery	I, III	O'Callaghan et al. (2019); Nejati et al. (2016c); Wei et al. (2018)
The human environment emanates compassion, authenticity, and healing intention while preserving the natural world and practicing environmental stewardship	**Infant:** The infant's repertoire of preverbal communication (behavioral and physiologic) is recognized, is acknowledged, and guides caring encounters	V	Weber and Harrison (2019)
	Family: Parental presence and partnerships are a system-wide priority; parents enjoy unrestricted access to their infant	I, II, III	De Bernardo et al. (2017); Hallowell et al. (2019); Sigurdson et al. (2019)
	Staff: The interprofessional team is collaborative and respectful. There is zero tolerance for behaviors that undermine safety, compromise respectful relationships, or threaten the environment (internally, interpersonally, and externally).	I	Crawford et al. (2019); Fragkos et al. (2020); Goedhart et al. (2017)
The organizational environment reflects a commitment to healing spaces and experiences that align with a trauma informed approach while fostering ecological sustainability in support for a healthy planet	**Infant:** The core measures for trauma-informed care provide the evidence-based standard for all patient encounters	I	Milette et al. (2017a); Milette et al. (2017b); Milette et al. (2019)
	Family: Families have access to physical, emotional, financial, and spiritual resources to support them through their hospital experience. Care is coordinated during the hospital stay and through the post discharge experience	I, III	Lewis et al. (2019); Sigurdson et al. (2019)
	Staff: The organization ensures staff have appropriate resources to support their holistic health and well-being while on duty to include, but not limited to, clean and restful locations to take respite, access to healthy nourishment around the clock, and dedicated staff nap areas	I, II, III	Fragkos et al. (2020); Goedhart et al. (2017); Nejati et al. (2016a), (2016b)
Protected Sleep			
Sleep integrity and circadian rhythmicity is protected for infants, families, and clinicians	**Infant:** Scheduled, nonemergent care is provided during wakeful states	I, III	Barbeau & Weiss (2017); Levy et al. (2017)
	Family: Sleep education is provided to all families; single-family rooms are equipped with sleep protection resources (cycled lighting, recommended sound levels, comfortable sleeping surfaces, etc.)	I, IV, V	Haddad et al. (2019); Georgoulas et al. (2021) Marthinsen et al. (2018)
	Staff: Shift workers are provided with sleep education for self-health and safety	I, V	Rosa et al. (2019); Wickwire et al. (2017)

TABLE 4-4 The Core Measures for Trauma Informed Developmental Care   (Continued)

Attributes	Examples	Level of Evidence	Sources
Strategies that support sleep for infants, families, and clinicians are an integral component of care and self-care	**Infant:** Skin-to-skin care is an integral component in the daily care of eligible infants	**II**	Bastani et al. (2017); Feldman et al. (2002)
	Family: Education on the importance of sleep hygiene routines for infants and families is provided	**I, II**	Bathory & Tomopoulos (2017); Martins et al. (2018)
	Staff: Supportive sleep routines are endorsed and encouraged by staff and their organization. Sleep routines are developed in partnership with family and documented to ensure consistency	**I, III**	Levy et al. (2017); van den Hoogen et al. (2017)
Safe sleep practices for infants, families, and clinicians are adopted, role modeled, and incorporated into daily routine	**Infant:** Infants are transitioned to safe sleep practices in the hospital with consistency and reliability	**I, IV, V**	AAP (2016); Naugler & DiCarlo (2018)
	Family: Parents demonstrate competency in safe sleep practices for their infant and themselves prior to discharge	**V, VI**	Naugler & DiCarlo (2018); Voos et al. (2015)
	Staff: Strategies to ensure staff safety regarding the sleep displacement/disruption associated with shift work are supported by staff, peers, and the organization at large	**I**	Joint Commission (2018); Shriane et al. (2020)
Pain & Stress			
Prevention of pain and stress is a daily expressed goal for infants, families, and clinicians	**Infants:** The prevention of pain and stress is an expressed goal of the healthcare team; each care encounter is guided by the infant's behavioral cues of readiness, stress, and pain	**I**	AAP (2020)
	Family: Families receive education and resources to effectively reduce their pain and distress during their hospital experience	**I, V**	Godoy et al. (2018); Pereira et al. (2017)
	Staff: Staff adopt proactive effective strategies aimed at managing and mitigating the pain and stress they experience as part of their daily life and their work	**I**	Stanulewicz et al. (2019); Yaribeygi et al. (2017)
Pain and/or stress is assessed, managed, and reassessed continuously for infants, families, and clinicians	**Infant:** A validated, age-appropriate, and contextually accurate tool is used to assess pain and/or stress; pain and stress behaviors guide all interventions to include the use of pharmacologic and nonpharmacologic strategies to manage and mitigate pain and/or stress	**I**	Olsson et al. (2021)
	Family: Families receive competency-based education on infant pain and stress cues and effective comfort measures for their infant; in addition, families are able to recognize and respond to their own pain and stress, adopting effective strategies to optimize their own health and wellness	**I, V**	Gates et al. (2018); McNair et al. (2020); Pereira et al. (2017); Prouhet et al. (2018)
	Staff: Staff and team members support each other in managing and mitigating the pain and/or stress experienced on duty (i.e., Code Lavender)	**IV**	Davidson et al. (2017); Graham et al. (2019)

(Continued)

TABLE 4-4 The Core Measures for Trauma Informed Developmental Care [Continued]

Attributes	Examples	Level of Evidence	Sources
Family and/or social networks are integral to the nonpharmacologic management and mitigation of pain and/or stress for their infants, families, and clinicians	**Infant:** Painful and/or stressful events and experiences are supported consistently through the presence of a dedicated person who comforts the infant during times of distress/disease	I, V	Filippa et al. [2019]; Melchior et al. [2021]; Weber & Harrison [2019]
	Family: Families, in partnership with the healthcare team, identify social and/or medical supports and resources that will assist them in managing and mitigating pain, stress, and distress over their hospital stay and beyond	I	Pados [2019]; Pados & Hess [2019]
	Staff: Strategies to ensure a healthy work environment are supported and cultivated by staff and leadership	I	Paguio & Yu [2020]; Stanulewicz et al. [2019] Wei et al. [2018]
Activities of Daily Living			
Appropriate postural alignment, mobility, and play ensure comfort, safety, and physiologic and emotional stability to support optimal neuromotor integrity	**Infant:** Skin-to-skin care in the side-lying diagonal position promotes optimal postural alignment and facilitates play with parent	III, IV	Barradas et al. [2006]; Buil et al. [2020]; Buil et al. [2016]
	Family: Accessible supportive seating for parents ensures postural alignment and comfort during attachment and play encounters	I, VI	Neu et al. [2020]; White [2020]
	Staff: Ergonomic guidelines are established to protect musculoskeletal health; organizations provide resources/benefits that promote physical activity and well-being for staff	I, IV, VI	Grimani et al. [2019]; Kotcz & Jenaszek [2020]; Lin et al. [2020]; Richardson et al. [2019]
Eating experiences are positive, pleasant, nurturing, and nourishing	**Infant:** Direct breastfeeding is encouraged and facilitated. Oral feeding encounters are guided and directed by the infant's level of readiness and engagement, supported within an age-appropriate environmental milieu	I, III, V	Fry et al. [2018]; Picaud et al. [2018]; Thomas et al. [2021]
	Family: Parents receive education on healthy nutrition for infants and families in crisis. Families have open access to healthy, nutritious meals in a quiet, clean, and relaxed setting during the hospital stay. Food security is assessed, and appropriate resources and counseling services are activated to restore food security prior to discharge	I	Health Research & Educational Trust [2017]
	Staff: Cost-conscious, nutritious food options are available 24/7; vending machines provide access to healthy snack and beverage options	I, III, V.	Grimani et al. [2019]; Nicholls et al. [2017]; Ross et al. [2019]
Appropriate hygiene and skin care routines preserve barrier function and tissue integrity while ensuring a calming and nurturing experience	**Infant:** Nonsterile glove use is reserved for encounters with blood and body fluids; continuous skin-to-skin care is facilitated to support stable, healthy microbiome	III	Crucianelli & Filippetti [2018]; Montirosso & McGlone [2020]
	Family: Swaddled bathing is provided by parents on a weekly basis	I	Fernandez and Antolin-Rodriguez [2018]
	Staff: Staff comply with hand-hygiene protocol and the appropriate use of infection control procedures; staff have easy access to alcohol-based hand sanitizers and appropriate emollients to preserve their skin integrity	I	Luangasanatip et al. [2015]

TABLE 4-4 The Core Measures for Trauma Informed Developmental Care (Continued)			
Attributes	**Examples**	**Level of Evidence**	**Sources**
Compassionate Collaborative Care			
Assessing and supporting emotional well-being is a priority	**Infant:** Parents are the infant's primary caregivers; spending quality time in physical and emotional proximity with parents is a priority	I	Scatliffe et al. (2019)
	Family: Emotional and psychological well-being of the family in crisis is assessed routinely; there is a process for appropriate referral, care, and support	III	Bry and Wigert (2019)
	Staff: Behaviors that reflect burnout and/or staff responses indicative of trauma exposure are responded to compassionately and in a timely manner	III	Ruiz-Fernandez et al. (2020); Tawfik et al. (2017)
Strategies to cultivate and maintain self-efficacy are mentored, supported, and validated	**Infant:** Infant behavioral cues and developmental capabilities are nurtured in partnership with parents and clinicians over the hospital experience	II, V	Weber & Harrison (2019); Welch et al. (2015); Welch et al. (2017)
	Family: A formal parent education program is integrated into the culture across the perinatal continuum with opportunities for return demonstration to confirm competence and confidence in skill acquisition	II, III	Gehl et al. (2020); O'Brien et al. (2018)
	Staff: Staff are mentored, coached, and supported in the adoption of new knowledge, skills, and attitudes to ensure the highest quality of care delivery	III, IV	Mansour & Mattukoyya (2019); Marcelin et al. (2019)
Communication is consistent, compassionate, and reciprocated with respectful active	**Infant:** All infant caring encounters are guided by the infant's behavioral and physiological cues for readiness	V	Sanders & Hall (2018); Weber & Harrison (2019)
	Family: Parents are valued and respected partners in care; they receive compassionate, consistent information and collaborate in shared decision making	I, III, V	Ashcraft et al. (2019); Brodsgaard et al. (2019); Ottosen et al. (2019)
	Staff: All staff receive compassionate communication training and exemplify the tenets of compassionate communication with their patients, the families, and each other	I	Patel et al. (2019); Winter et al. (2020)

and basic human rights for all (Gerber, 2018). The quality indicator of advocacy within a trauma informed approach relies on being knowledgeable and ready to take courageous action to impact others through respectful influence inspiring excellence.

Role Model and Mentor

A role model is someone others look to as an example to be emulated. A mentor is an experienced and trusted advisor. Mentoring is most effective when the mentor and mentee share similar values and interests (Burgess et al., 2018). We are called to own our role as model and mentor; guiding, engaging, and empowering our colleagues, mentees, families,

and society at large to adopt health-flourishing behaviors. Mentor–mentee rapport plays a pivotal role in a successful mentorship exchange (Pham et al., 2019). Mentorship is a bidirectional learning experience as the relationship emerges from a shared interface where one influences and effects the other. Attributes of a role model and qualities of a mentor are described in Table 4-6.

Scholarship

Pursuing scholarship invites the clinician to consider all the ways information is shared. The words we choose have power, whether we are conscious of it or not. When we are not present to the lived experience of other, our language has

TABLE 4-5 Ten Transformational Practices to support Personal Wholeness

1. Meditation	A guided practice, reflection, prayer, contemplation, pondering, quiet time, or whatever helps you slow down and gain clarity
2. Environment	Organizing or simplifying your space, lighting a candle, playing your favorite music, opening a window, buying a bouquet of flowers, or anything that brings joy to your space
3. Nutrition	Being attune to your body, optimizing hydration, and being intentional with how you fuel your body—what makes it feel good and what weighs it down
4. Movement	Moving your body regularly in a way that feels joyful: walk, run, swim, dance, yoga, cycling, etc.
5. Nature	Spending time outside everyday
6. Mind	Consider the person you want to be. A clarity word or words can help you regain focus. Use words to bring you back to who you want to be
7. Rest	Attending to ways to support your rest and rejuvenation
8. Creativity	Using journaling, drawing, painting, or brainstorming to unleash your imagination
9. Service	Celebrating acts of kindness. A smile, holding the door, a note to a friend, and all they ways you serve
10. Gratitude	Cultivating a gratitude practice such as journaling or setting daily reminders

the potential to hurt, shame, and even add to the individuals experience of trauma and isolation. The language used in our intake forms and consent forms and even the language we use in our everyday conversation must be infused with trauma awareness to become trauma informed.

In scholarship we must investigate, evaluate, and disseminate the impact of a trauma informed approach across clinical, psycho-socio-emotional, spiritual, and economic domains. Presenting at local, national, and international conferences is one example of scholarship. Collaborating and publishing research findings and/or quality improvement work is another example.

Leader for Change

The final attribute examines what it is to become a leader for change. Leaders may be formal, bearing a title in a hierarchical organization, or they may be informal, as frontline clinicians, parents, or family members. Leading change is not for the faint of heart and can feel insurmountable at times; however, when contrasted to the benefits experienced by babies, families, colleagues, and even self, it is a journey well taken. Cultivating a respectful approach to leadership as a TIP becomes transformational. In knowing one's self, one can then know other. Recognizing self in others preserves human dignity, acknowledges our shared humanity, and keeps us from reducing self and others to the moral status of object (Watson, 2018).

The Five Guiding Principles of a Trauma Informed Paradigm

Quality indicators for trauma informed developmental care are synonymous with the eight attributes/competencies of a TIP. To create change, we ourselves must embody the change

TABLE 4-6 Attributes of a Role Model and Qualities of a Mentor

Attributes of a Role Model	Qualities of a Mentor
• Approachable • Trustworthy • Empathetic • Adaptable • Knowledgeable • Good communicator • Clinically skilled • Friendly • Professional • Inspires confidence • Motivated	• Communication skills: listening, questioning, and the wise use of silence • Being a sounding board for ideas and a reality check for plans • Giving guidance without being directive • Providing feedback, suggestions, and options • Time and willingness to contribute • Confidentiality, respecting personal privacy

we wish to see in the world. We can move forward with change and transform the experience of care in the NICU for babies and families with one simple step toward trauma awareness. Trauma awareness begins with the five principles of trauma informed care to guide your human-to-human interactions (see Table 4-2).

- **SAFETY** within a trauma informed paradigm refers to the extent in which the service ensures the physical and emotional safety of the vulnerable individuals it serves. This includes not only protecting the individual(s) from immediate harm but also extends to protection from known long-term sequelae and retraumatization.

- **CHOICE** for the patient and family is crucial within the context of trauma informed care. Choice begins by informing patients and their families about treatment options and their associated pros and cons compassionately and authentically, without bias. Choice can also be seen in partnership with collaboration when baby care encounters are guided by the baby's behavioral communication of approach and avoidance.

- **COLLABORATION** is to work jointly, to cooperate with and willingly assist a group to achieve together. Collaboration without compassion produces technically correct results but misses the mark in meeting the individual's emotional, spiritual, and psychosocial needs (Lown et al., 2016). Collaborative care prioritizes respectful caring relationships, emotional support, authentic communication, and shared empowerment (Lown et al., 2016; Pfaff & Markaki, 2017).

- **EMPOWERMENT** includes sharing power with the patient and family, encouraging and facilitating patient and family partnership in decision making throughout their healthcare journey.

- **TRUSTWORTHINESS** is about transparency and creating clear expectations. Cultivating trust demands the healthcare professional be truly aligned with their purpose and their mission of service to other.

Partnering with families in crisis hinges on the emotional intelligence and well-being of the clinician. It requires the clinician to be knowledgeable; cultivate healing intention; practice personal wholeness; be a courageous advocate, role model, and mentor; be scholarly; and become a leader for change to fully give and support other. First, do no harm means that healthcare professionals and services cannot turn their back on the needs of the whole person if it is truly committed to quality and safety. The care of vulnerable babies and families cannot be framed by the scope of their diagnosis but must reflect an understanding of the continuum of need across physical, emotional, spiritual, and financial/economic domains. Availability of responsive social support networks, mental health resources, transportation options, adequate nutrition, and shelter are life saving for the family in crisis and is the responsibility of each healthcare team member to ensure.

THE CORE MEASURES OF TRAUMA INFORMED CARE

The trauma informed attributes and guiding principles translate into core competencies and performance expectations that aim to humanize the healthcare experience for vulnerable populations and the clinicians who serve them in the NICU and beyond. It is from this foundation of competence that the clinician becomes proficient at implementing supportive trauma informed developmental care practices. Coughlin (2021) has updated the original disease-independent core measures for developmentally supportive care, endorsed by Nann, to guide trauma informed developmental practices in the care of high-risk babies, families, and clinicians. These evidence-based core measures, their attributes, and examples for the baby, the family, and the clinician are described in Table 4-4. The relevance and applicability of the core measures extend from the baby, to the family to the clinician. Everyone benefits when these disease-independent domains, reflecting basic human needs, are met consistently, reliably, and compassionately.

Although the core measures are described as discrete entities, they are nevertheless intimately integrated with one another. Sleep deprivation lowers one's pain threshold and undermanaged pain impedes sleep (Krause et al., 2019; Weber & Harrison, 2019). Pleasurable and nurturing eating encounters reduce stress and promote sleep (Park et al., 2020), whereas volume-driven feeding events are distressing and painful and have lasting negative implications for the baby and the family (Wang et al., 2018; Weber & Harrison, 2019).

Consider a caregiving encounter for the baby in the NICU; it may be a vital sign assessment, diaper change, and tube feeding, or it could be a central line placement, an intubation, or really anything. Within this context the clinician is invited to consider how to evaluate the baby's experience through the lens of the five trauma informed core measures.

For the Baby

- HEALING ENVIRONMENT: Was the environment quiet, peaceful, and calm with pleasant lighting to support wakefulness and participation? Was the baby supported to be an active participant in a way that supported their self-efficacy?

- SLEEP: Did the baby demonstrate readiness for the caring encounter (i.e., opening eyes, mouthing hands, squirming/stretching)?

- PAIN AND STRESS PREVENTION and MANAGEMENT: Was the caregiver mindful of "being with" the baby rather than "doing to"? Was there meaningful connection that supported the baby during their stress? Were pain-relieving strategies required and provided?

- ACTIVITIES of DAILY LIVING (posture and play, eating and nourishment, skin care and hygiene): Did the caregiver support the baby's posture? Did the caregiver engage playfully with the baby acknowledging their developmental need to be seen? Did the encounter set a foundation for a pleasant, positive, and nurturing eating experience? If the parent was present, was every attempt made to facilitate a skin-to-skin encounter and/or a positive touch experience?

- COMPASSIONATE FAMILY COLLABORATIVE CARE: How were the parents supported to both bond and be confident in their roles? Do parents have unrestricted access to their baby to minimize parent-infant physical separation? Is skin-to-skin an integral component of the baby's and family's experience?

These moments shape the baby's and family's entire NICU stay and future relationship. In addition to recognizing the critical nature of the core measures for the baby, it is also crucial to explore the implications of these trauma informed core measures for the family and clinician. One core measure impacts the other four.

For Family and Clinicians

- HEALING ENVIRONMENT: Does the environment, physically, socially, and sensorially, support parental rest and parent–clinician connection? Does the clinician's work environment positively shape the way they show up to provide compassionate family collaborative care?

- SLEEP: Is emphasis placed on reducing parental stress to protect, support, and optimize their sleep? How is sleep valued to ensure every clinician is able to bring their best self to work?

- PAIN AND STRESS PREVENTION and MANAGEMENT: Are there strategies in place to reduce parent and clinician stress? Is the clinician mindful of the parent's postpartum pain as well as their emotional well-being?

- ACTIVITIES of DAILY LIVING
    - Posture and play: Are there opportunities to bring joy to the workplace? Are the surroundings set up to be comfortable for both the family and the clinician?
    - Eating and nourishment: Do parents and clinicians have access to nutritious meals and snacks?
    - Skin care and hygiene: Do parents and clinicians have easy access to hand sanitizers, soaps, and emollients? Do parents and clinicians understand the importance of a healthy microbiome for self and others and adopt best practices (i.e., skin-to-skin, breast feeding, nutrition, hydration)?

- COMPASSIONATE FAMILY COLLABORATIVE CARE: How is the family's and clinician's holistic physical, developmental, psychosocial, and spiritual needs supported? Is the standard of communication one that is compassionate and trauma informed?

The five core measures practice model provides clear metrics for caring actions that impact the hospital experience of baby–family dyads and healthcare professionals.

Standardized disease-independent core measures for trauma informed developmental care establish evidence-based practice expectations. These ensure that a competent interprofessional collaborative practice team is able to meet the holistic needs of the baby and family from birth through the transition of hospital discharge to home and assure continuity to follow-up care.

RECOMMENDATIONS FOR PRACTICE, EDUCATION, AND RESEARCH

Trauma informed developmental care is the framework to provide care to babies and families in crisis as well as protect and preserve the mental health and moral integrity of clinicians. Evidence-based practice guidelines for trauma informed developmental care have already been put forth, endorsed by the Nann. These guidelines can easily become another "tick box" for clinicians who are unable to unbundle themselves from their unconscious daily routines and trauma histories to discover the authentic healer that lies within. Nursing, medicine, and other healthcare professionals are invited to embrace this holistic framework. There is opportunity to integrate compassionate, authentic, and courageous caring actions and education into one's personal and professional lives. A moral duty exists to evaluate the impact of these trauma informed practices on physical, psychosocial, emotional, spiritual, clinical, and economic outcomes.

Nurse clinicians, educators, and scholars are increasingly committed to advancing the science of developmental care. The concept of a trauma informed approach to care in the NICU, presented in this chapter (Fig. 4-8), serves as a guide for professional growth and development, quality improvement initiatives, and research. This model integrates all ways of providing developmentally supportive care to ensure consistently reliable, compassionate, evidence-based care across the continuum of care and across the individual's lifespan.

Becoming trauma informed invites healthcare professionals to rediscover their individual life story, a compilation of life events and lived experiences, as a foundation for authentic and compassionate connections with the stories of others. Stories matter. Embracing our collective stories enables us to acknowledge our shared humanity and empowers clinicians to make a meaningful difference in the lives of others and self every day. Thus, individual professionals use a trauma informed framework to come together to support the baby, parent, and family's holistic physical, developmental, and psychosocial needs from birth through the transition of hospital discharge to home and assure continuity to follow-up care.

FUTURE DIRECTION

This trauma informed framework encompasses the values identified by the International Neonatal Nursing Competency Framework by the Council of International Neonatal Nurses, Inc. (COINN) (Jones, 2019). Future direction to ensure

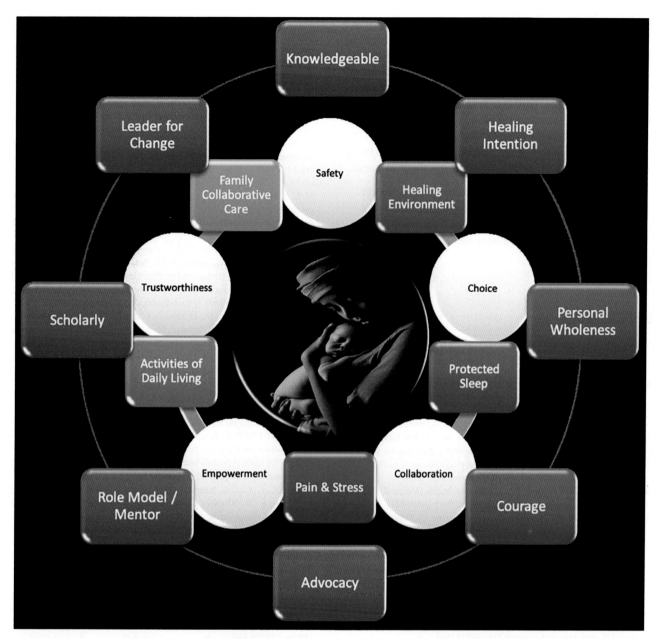

FIGURE 4-8. Trauma informed care Model and Framework. Beginning with the attributes of the trauma informed professional guided by the five principles of trauma informed care to the core measures for trauma informed developmental care. (Reprinted with permission from Caring Essentials Collaborative, LLC.)

professionally competent interprofessional collaborative practice teams would be to require trauma informed education and certification. To mitigate the risk of babies, families, and clinicians experiencing undue trauma, this education and/or certification would be a recommended prerequisite for neonatal clinicians, ancillary support professionals, leadership teams, and administrators.

CONCLUSION

The suffering alleviated through the adoption of a trauma informed approach goes beyond the physical; it is the emotional, psychological, and spiritual suffering humans experience in crisis that must be alleviated. It is the suffering of the baby and family, and also the suffering of healthcare professionals who bear witness to tragedy and trauma in the course of their service to other every day. Mental health encompasses emotional, psychological, social, and spiritual well-being. Mental health is the foundation for overall health and well-being for patients, families in crisis, healthcare professionals, and society at large (McLoughlin, 2017a, 2017b).

Awareness of the experience of trauma in the NICU for babies, families, and clinicians is a first step to transform and humanize this fragile, yet critical care environment. Developmental care has existed for centuries, dating back to Florence Nightingale, expanded upon by Drs. Brazelton and

Als, and becomes even more biologically relevant within the context of early life adversity, toxic stress, and infant medical trauma (Coughlin, 2021). The babies, families, and clinicians are each greater than the sum of their parts. The system and the service can no longer ignore the multidimensional needs of ourselves and our patients. Trauma informed developmental care is the overarching foundation encompassing all aspects of wholeness for baby, family, and self (see Fig. 4-8). This is an invitation to reignite passion and purpose to bring meaningful connection with each other and those we serve.

"I swore never to be silent whenever and wherever human beings endure suffering and humiliation. We must take sides. Neutrality helps the oppressor, never the victim. Silence encourages the tormentor, never the tormented."

—— Elie Wiesel

REFERENCES

Allen-Duck, A., Robinson, J. C., & Stewart, M. W. (2017). Healthcare quality: A concept analysis. *Nursing Forum, 52*(4), 377–386. https://dx.doi.org/10.1111%2Fnuf.12207

American Academy of Pediatrics Committee on Fetus and Newborn and Section on Anesthesiology and Pain Medicine (2016; reaffirmed 2020). Prevention and management of procedural pain in the neonate: An update. *Pediatrics, 137*(2), e20154271. https://doi.org/10.1542/peds.2015-4271

American Academy of Pediatrics Task Force on Sudden Infant Death Syndrome (2016). SIDS and other sleep-related infant deaths: Updated 2016 recommendations for a safe infant sleeping environment. *Pediatrics, 138*(5), e20162938. https://doi.org/10.1542/peds.2016-2938

APNA position: Whole health begins with mental health. (March 2017; April 2020). https://www.apna.org/i4a/pages/index.cfm?pageid=6212

Ashcraft, L. E., Asato, M., Houtrow, A. J., Kavalliertos, D., Miller, E., & Ray, K. N. (2019). Parent empowerment in pediatric healthcare settings: A systematic review of observational studies. *Patient, 12*(2), 199–212. https://doi.org/10.1007/s40271-018-0336-2

Barbeau, D. Y., & Weiss, M. D. (2017). Sleep disturbances in newborns. *Children, 4*(10), 90. https://doi.org/10.3390/children4100090

Barradas, J., Fonseca, A., Guimaraes, C. L. N., & Lima, G. M. D. S. (2006). Relationship between positioning of premature infants in kangaroo mother care and early neuromotor development. *Journal de Pediatria, 82*(6), 475–480. https://doi.org/10.2223/JPED.1565

Bastani, F., Rajai, N., Farsi, Z., & Als, H. (2017). The effects of kangaroo care on the sleep and wake states of preterm infants. *Journal of Nursing Research, 25*(3), 231–239. https://doi.org/10.1097/jnr.0000000000000194

Bathory, E., & Tomopoulos, S. (2017). Sleep regulation, physiology and development, sleep duration and patterns, and sleep hygiene in infants, toddlers, and preschool-age children. *Current Problems in Pediatric and Adolescent Health Care, 47*(2), 29–42. https://doi.org/10.1016/j.cppeds.2016.12.001

Brodsgaard, A., Pedersen, J. T., Larsen, P., & Weis, J. (2019). Parents' and nurses' experiences of partnership in neonatal intensive care units. A qualitative review and meta-synthesis. *Journal of Clinical Nursing, 28*(17–18), 3117–3139. https://doi.org/10.1111/jocn.14920

Brunault, P., Lebigre, K., Idbrik, F., Mauge, D., Adam, P., Barrault, S., Baudin, G., Courtois, R., El Ayoubi, H., Grall-Bronnec, M., Hingray, C., Ballon, N., & El-Hage, W. (2020). Childhood trauma predicts less remission from PTSD among patients with co-occurring alcohol use disorder and PTSD. *Journal of Clinical Medicine, 9*, 2054. https://doi.org/10.3390/jcm9072054

Bry, A., & Wigert, H. (2019). Psychosocial support for parents of extremely preterm infants in neonatal intensive: A qualitative interview study. *BMC Psychology, 7*, 76. https://doi.org/10.1186/s40359-019-0354-4

Buil, A., Carchon, I., Apter, G., Laborne, F. X., Granier, M., & Devouche, E. (2016). Kangaroo supported diagonal flexion positioning: New insights into skin-to-skin contact for communication between mothers and very preterm infants. *Archives of Pediatrics, 23*(9), 913–920. https://doi.org/10.1016/j.arcped.2016.04.023

Buil, A., Sankey, C., Caeymaex, L., Apter, G., Gratier, M., & Devouche, E. (2020). Fostering mother-very preterm infant communication during skin-to-skin contact through a modified positioning. *Early Human Development, 141*, 104939. https://doi.org/10.1016/j.earlhumdev.2019.104939

Burgess, A., Diggele, C., & Mellis, C. (2018). Mentorship in the health professions: A review. *The Clinical Teacher, 15*(3), 197–202. https://doi.org/10.1111/tct.12756

Carlson, J. S., Yohannan, J., Darr, C. L., Turley, M. R., Larez, N. A., & Perfect, M. M. (2019). Prevalence of adverse childhood experiences in school-aged youth: A systematic review (1990-2015). *International Journal of School & Educational Psychology, 8*, 2–23. https://doi.org/10.1080/21683603.2018.1548397

Chamberlain, C., Gee, G., Harfield, S., Campbell, S., Brennan, S., Clark, Y., Mensah, F., Arabena, K., Herrman, H., Brown, S., & Healing the Past by Nurturing the Future Group. (2019). Parenting after a history of childhood maltreatment: A scoping review and map of evidence in the perinatal period. *PLoS One, 14*(3), e0213460. https://doi.org/10.1371/journal.pone.0213460

Chamberlain, C., Ralph, N., Hokke, S., Clark, Y., Gee, G., Stansfield, C., Sutcliffe, K., Brown, S. J., Brennan, S., & Healing The Past By Nurturing The Future Group. (2019). Healing the past by nurturing the future: A qualitative systematic review and meta-synthesis of pregnancy, birth and early postpartum experiences and view of parents with a history of childhood maltreatment. *PLoS One, 14*(12), e0225441. https://doi.org/10.1371/journal.pone.0225441

Coughlin, M. (2016). *Trauma-informed care in the NICU: Evidenced-based practice guidelines for neonatal clinicians.* Springer Publishing Company.

Coughlin, M. (2017). Trauma-informed, neuroprotective care for hospitalized newborns and infants. *Infant, 13*(5), 176–179.

Coughlin, M. (2021). *Transformative nursing in the NICU: Trauma informed, age-appropriate care* (2nd ed.). Springer Publishing Company.

Crawford, C. L., Chu, F., Judson, L. H., Cuenca, E., Jadalla, A. A., Tze-Polp, L., Kawar, L. N., Runnels, C., & Garvida, R. Jr (2019). An integrative review of nurse-to-nurse incivility, hostility, and workplace violence: A GPS for nurse leaders. *Nursing Administration Quarterly, 43*(2), 138–156. https://doi.org/10.1097/naq.0000000000000338

Cricianelli, I., & Filippetti, M. I. (2018). Developmental perspectives on interpersonal affective touch. *Topoi, 39*, 575–586. https://doi.org/10.1007/s11245-018-9565-1

Crouch, E., Probst, J. C., Radcliff, E., Bennett, K. J., & Hunt McKinney, S. (2019). Prevalence of adverse childhood experiences (ACEs) among US children. *Child Abuse and Neglect, 92*, 209–218. https://doi.org/10.1016/j.chiabu.2019.04.010

Csaszar-Nagy, N., & Bokkon, I. (2018). Mother-newborn separation at birth in hospitals: A possible risk for neurodevelopmental disorders? *Neuroscience & Biobehavioral Reviews, 84*, 337–351. https://doi.org/10.1016/j.neubiorev.2017.08.013

D'Agata, A. L., Young, E. E., Cong, X., Grasso, D. J., & McGrath, J. M. (2016). Infant medical trauma in the neonatal intensive care unit (IMTN): A proposed concept for science and practice. *Advances in Neonatal Care, 16*(4), 289–297. https://doi.org/10.1097/ANC.0000000000000309

Davidson, J. E., Graham, P., Montross-Thomas, L., Norcross, W., & Zerbi, G. (2017). Code lavender: Cultivating intentional acts of kindness in response to stressful work situations. *Explore, 13*(3), 181–185. https://doi.org/10.1016/j.explore.2017.02.005

De Bernardo, G., Svelto, M., Giordano, M., Sordino, D., & Riccitelli, M. (2017). Supporting parents in taking care of their infants admitted to a neonatal intensive care unit: A prospective cohort pilot study. *Italian Journal of Pediatrics, 43*, 36. https://doi.org/10.1186/s13052-017-0352-1

Dunn, G. A., Nigg, J. T., & Sullivan, E. L. (2019). Neuroinflammation as a risk factor for attention deficit hyperactivity disorder. *Pharmacology Biochemistry and Behavior, 182*, 22–34. https://doi.org/10.1016/j.pbb.2019.05.005

Enlow, M. B., Englund, M. M., & Egeland, B. (2018). Maternal childhood maltreatment history and child mental health: Mechanisms in intergenerational effects. *Journal of Clinical Child and Adolescent Psychology, 47*(suppl 1), S47–S62. https://doi.org/10.1080/15374416.2016.1144189

Feldman, R., Weller, A., Sirota, L., & Eidelman, A. I. (2002). Skin-to-skin contact (kangaroo care) promotes self-regulation in premature infants: Sleep-wake cyclicity, arousal modulation, and sustained exploration. *Developmental Psychology, 38*(2), 194–207. https://doi.org/10.1037//0012-1649.38.2.194

Felitti, V. J., Anda, R. F., Nordenberg, D., Williamson, D. F., Spitz, A. M., Edwards, V., Koss, M. P., & Marks, J. S. (1998). Relationship of childhood abuse and household dysfunction to many of the leading causes of death in adults: The adverse childhood experiences (ACE) study. *American Journal of Preventative Medicine, 14*, 245–258. https://doi.org/10.1016/S0749-3797(98)00017-8

Fernandez Medina, I. M., Fernandez-Sola, C., Lopez-Rodriguez, M. M., Hernandez-Padilla, J. M., Jimenez Lasserrotte, M., del, M., & Granero-Molina, J. (2019). Barriers to providing mothers' own milk to extremely preterm infants in the NICU. *Advances in Neonatal Care, 19*(5), 349–360. https://doi.org/10.1097/anc.0000000000000652

Fernandez, D., & Antolin-Rodriguez, R. (2018). Bathing a premature infant in the intensive care unit: A systematic review. *Journal of Pediatric Nursing, 42*, e52–e57. https://doi.org/10.1016/j.pedn.2018.05.002

Filippa, M., Poisbeau, P., Mairesse, J., Monaci, M. G., Baud, O., Huppi, P., Grandjean, D., & Kuhn, P. (2019). Pain, parental involvement, and oxytocin in the neonatal intensive care unit. *Frontiers in Psychology, 10*, 715. https://doi.org/10.3389/fpsyg.2019.00715

Fontana, C., Marasca, F., Provitera, L., Mancinelli, S., Pesenti, N., Sinha, S., Passera, S., Abrignani, S., Mosca, F., Lodato, S., Bodega, B., & Fumagalli, M. (2021). Early maternal care restores LINE-1 methylation and enhances neurodevelopment in preterm infants. *BMC Medicine, 19*(1), 42. https://doi.org/10.1186/s12916-020-01896-0

Fragkos, K. C., Makrykosta, P., & Frangos, C. C. (2020). Structural empowerment is a strong predictor of organizational commitment in nurses: A systematic review and meta-analysis. *Journal of Advanced Nursing, 76*(4), 939–962. https://doi.org/10.1111/jan.14289

Fry, T. J., Marfurt, S., & Wengier, S. (2018). Systematic review of quality improvement initiatives related to cue-based feeding in preterm infants. *Nursing for Women's Health, 22*(5), 401–410. https://doi.org/10.1016/j.nwh.2018.07.006

Garner, A. S., Shonkoff, J. P., Committee on Psychosocial Aspects of Child and Family Health, Committee on Early Childhood, Adoption, and Dependent Care, & Section on Developmental and Behavioral Pediatrics, (2012). Early childhood adversity, toxic stress, and the role of the pediatrician: Translating developmental science into lifelong health. *Pediatrics, 129*(1), e224–e231. https://doi.org/10.1542/peds.2011-2662

Gates, A., Shave, K., Featherstone, R., Buckreus, K., Ali, S., Scott, S. D., & Hartling, L. (2018). Procedural pain: Systematic review of parent experiences and information needs. *Clinical Pediatrics, 57*(6), 672–688. https://doi.org/10.1177/0009922817733694

Gehl, M. B., Alter, C. C., Rider, N., Gunther, L. G., & Russel, R. B. (2020). Improving the efficiency and effectiveness of parent education in the neonatal intensive care unit. *Advances in Neonatal Care, 20*(1), 59–67. https://doi.org/10.1097/ANC.0000000000000644

Georgoulas, A., Jones, L., Laudiano-Dray, M. P., Meek, J., Fabrizi, L., & Whitehead, K. (2021). Sleep-wake regulation in preterm and term infants. *Sleep, 44*(1), zsaa148. https://doi.org/10.1093/sleep/zsaa148

Gerber, L. (2018). Understanding the nurse's role as a patient advocate. *Nursing, 48*(4), 55–58. https://doi.org/10.1097/01.NURSE.0000531007.02224.65

Gibbins, S., Coughlin, M., & Hoath, S. B. (2010). Quality indicators: Using the universe of developmental care model as an exemplar for change. In Kenner, C., & McGrath, J. M. (Eds.), *Developmental care of newborns & infants* (2nd ed., pp. 43–62). National Association of Neonatal Nurses.

Gibbins, S., Hoath, S. B., Coughlin, M., Gibbins, A., & Franck, L. (2008). The universe of developmental care: A new conceptual model for application in the neonatal intensive care unit. *Advances in Neonatal Care, 8*(3), 141–147. https://doi.org/10.1097/01.ANC.0000324337.01970.76

Godoy, L. D., Rossignoli, M. T., Delfino-Pereira, P., Garcia-Cairasco, N., & Henrique de Lima Umeoka, E. (2018). A comprehensive review on stress neurobiology: Basic concepts and clinical implications. *Frontiers in Behavioral Neuroscience, 12*, 127. https://dx.doi.org/10.3389%2Ffnbeh.2018.00127

Goedhart, N. S., van Oostveen, C. J., & Vermeulen, H. (2017). The effect of structural empowerment of nurses on quality outcomes in hospitals: a scoping review. *Journal of Nursing Management, 25*(3), 194–206. https://doi.org/10.1111/jonm.12455

Graham, P., Zerbi, G., Norcross, W., Montross-Thomas, L., Lobbestael, L., & Davidson, J. (2019). Testing of a caregiver support team. *Explore, 15*(1), 19–26. https://doi.org/10.1016/j.explore.2018.07.004

Grimani, A., Aboagye, E., & Kwak, L. (2019). The effectiveness of workplace nutrition and physical activity interventions in improving productivity, work performance and workability: A systematic review. *BMC Public Health, 19*(1), 1676. https://doi.org/10.1186/s12889-019-8033-1

Haddad, S., Dennis, C-L., Shah, P. S., & Stremler, R. (2019). Sleep in parents of preterm infants: A systematic review. *Midwifery, 73*, 35–48. https://doi.org/10.1016/j.midw.2019.01.009

Hallowell, S. G., Rogowski, J. A., & Lake, E. T. (2019). How nurse work environments relate to the presence of parents in neonatal intensive care. *Advances in Neonatal Care, 19*(1), 65–72. https://doi.org/10.1097/anc.0000000000000431

Hawkins, S. F., & Morse, J. (2014). The praxis of courage as a foundation for care. *Journal of Nursing Scholarship, 46*, 263–270. https://doi.org/10.1111/jnu.12077

Health Research and Educational Trust. (2017). *Social determinants of health series: Food insecurity and the role of hospitals*. Health Research & Educational Trust. https://www.aha.org/foodinsecurity

van den Hoogen, A., Teunis, C. J., Shellhaas, R. A., Pillen, S., Benders, M., & Dudink, J. (2017). How to improve sleep in a neonatal intensive care unit: A systematic review. *Early Human Development, 113*, 78–86. https://doi.org/10.1016/j.earlhumdev.2017.07.002

Joint Commission Health care worker fatigue and patient safety. (2018). https://www.jointcommission.org/-/media/tjc/documents/resources/patient-safety-topics/sentinel-event/sea_48_hcw_fatigue_final_w_2018_addendum.pdf

Jones, T. (2019). International neonatal nursing competency framework. *Journal of Neonatal Nursing, 25*, 258–264. https://doi.org/10.1016/j.jnn.2019.07.007

Kotcz, A. & Jenaszek, K. K. (2020). Assessment of pressure pain threshold at the cervical and lumbar spine region in the group of professionally active nurses: A cross-sectional study. *Journal of Occupational Health, 62*(1), e12108. https://doi.org/10.1002/1348-9585.12108

Krause, A. J., Prather, A. A., Wagner, T. D., Lindquist, M. A., & Walker, M. P. (2019). The pain of sleep loss: A brain characterization in humans. *Journal of Neuroscience, 39*(12), 2291–2300. https://doi.org/10.1523/JNEUROSCI.2408-18.2018

Krol, K. M., Moulder, R. G., Lillard, T. S., Grossmann, T., & Connelly, J. J. (2019). Epigenetic dynamics in infancy and the impact of maternal engagement. *Science Advances, 5*(10), eaay0680. https://doi.org/10.1126/sciadv.aay0680

Lee, R. S., Oswald, L. M., & Wand, G. S. (2018). Early life stress as a predictor of co-occurring alcohol use disorder and post-traumatic stress disorder. *Alcohol Research: Current Reviews, 39*(2), 147–159. PMID: 31198654.

Lester, B. M., Conradt, E., LaGasse, L. L., Tronick, E. Z., Padbury, J. F., & Marsit, C. J. (2018). Epigenetic programming by maternal behavior in the human infant. *Pediatrics, 142*(4), e20171890. https://doi.org/10.1542/peds.2017-1890

Levy, J., Hassan, F., Plegue, M. A., Sokoloff, M. D., Kushwaha, J. S., Chervin, R. D., Barks, J. D. E., & Shellhaas, R. A. (2017). Impact of hands-on care on infant sleep in the neonatal intensive care unit. *Pediatric Pulmonology, 52*(1), 84–90. https://doi.org/10.1002/ppul.23513

Lewis, T. P., Andrews, K. G., Shenberger, E., Betancourt, T. S., Fink, G., Pereira, S., & McConnell, M. (2019). Caregiving can be costly: A qualitative study of barriers and facilitators to conducting kangaroo mother care in a US tertiary hospital neonatal intensive care unit. *BMC Pregnancy and Childbirth, 19*, 227. https://doi.org/10.1186/s12884-019-2363-y

Lin, S. C., Lin, L. L., Liu, C. J., Fang, C. K., & Lin, M. L. (2020). Exploring the factors affecting musculoskeletal disorders risk among hospital nurses. *PLoS One, 15*(4), e0231319. https://doi.org/10.1371/journal.pone.0231319

Loizzo, J., Charleson, M., & Peterson, J. (2009). A program in contemplative self-healing: Stress, allostasis, and learning in the Indo-Tibetan tradition. *Annals of the New York Academy of Sciences, 1172*, 123–147. https://doi.org/10.1111/j.1749-6632.2009.04398.x

Lown, B. A., McIntosh, S., Gaines, M. E., McGuinn, K., & Hatem, D. (2016). Integrating compassionate collaborative care (the "Triple C") into health professional education to advance the triple aim of health care. *Academic Medicine, 91*(3), 310–316. https://doi.org/10.1097/ACM.0000000000001077

Luangasanatip, N., Hongsuwan, M., Limmathurotsakul, D., Lubell, Y., Lee, A. S., Harbarth, S., Day, N. P. J., Graves, N., & Cooper, B. S. (2015). Comparative efficacy of interventions to promote hand hygiene in hospital. *British Medical Journal, 351*, h3728. https://dx.doi.org/10.1136%2Fbmj.h3728

Mansour, M., & Mattukoyya, R. (2019). Development of assertive communication skills in nursing preceptorship programmes: A qualitative insight from newly qualified nurses. *Nursing Management, 26*(4), 29–35. https://doi.org/10.7748/nm.2019.e1857

Marcellin, J. R., Siraj, D. S., Victor, R., Kotadia, S., Maldonado, Y. A. (2019). The impact of unconscious bias in healthcare: How to recognize and mitigate it. *Journal of Infectious Disease, 220*(suppl 2), S62–S73. https://doi.org/10.1093/infdis/jiz214

Marthinsen, G. N., Helseth, S., & Fegran, L. (2018). Sleep and its relationship to health in parents of preterm infants: A scoping review. *BMC Pediatrics, 18*, 352. https://dx.doi.org/10.1186%2Fs12887-018-1320-7

Martins, R. M. A., Oliveira, J. R. A., Salgado, C. C. G., Marques, B. L. S., Oliveira, L. C. F., Oliveira, G. R., Rodrigues, T. S., & Ferreira, R. T. (2018). Sleep habits in infants. The role of maternal education. *Sleep Medicine, 52*, 138–144. https://doi.org/10.1016/j.sleep.2018.08.020

McLoughlin, K. A. (2017a). Five steps to engage in the concept of whole health begins with mental health. *Journal of the American Psychiatric Nurses Association, 23*(3), 230. https://doi.org/10.1177/1078390317706510

McLoughlin, K. A. (2017b). The importance of purpose in whole health and well-being. *Journal of the American Psychiatric Nurses Association, 23*(5), 375. https://doi.org/10.1177/1078390317728481

McNair, C., Chinian, N., Shah, V., McAllister, M., Franck, L. F., Stevens, B., Burry, L., & Taddio, A. (2020). Metasynthesis of factors that influence parents' participation in pain management for their infants in the NICU. *Journal of Obstetric, Gynecologic and Neonatal Nursing, 49*(3), 263–271. https://doi.org/10.1016/j.jogn.2020.02.007

Melchior, M., Kuhn, P., & Poisbeau, P. (2021). The burden of early life stress on the nociceptive system development and pain responses. *European Journal of Neuroscience.* https://doi.org/10.1111/ejn.15153

Merrick, M. T., Ford, D. C., Ports, K. A., & Guinn, A. S. (2018). Prevalence of adverse childhood experiences from 2011–2014 behavioral risk factor surveillance system in 23 states. *JAMA Pediatrics, 172*(11), 1038–1044. https://doi.org/10.1001/jamapediatrics.2018.2537

Merrick, M. T., Ford, D. C., Ports, K. A., Guinn, A. S., Chen, J., Klevens, J., Metzler, M., Jones, C. M., Simon, T. R., Daniel, V. M., Ottley, P., & Mercy, J. A. (2019). Vital signs: Estimated proportion of adult health problems attributable to adverse childhood experiences and implications for prevention—25 states, 2015—2017. *MMWR Morbidity and Mortality Weekly Report, 68*(44), 999–1005. https://doi.org/10.15585/mmwr.mm6844e1

Meulewaeter, F., De Pauw, S. S. W., & Vanderplasschen, W. (2019). Mothering, substance use disorders and intergenerational trauma transmission: An attachment-based perspective. *Frontiers in Psychiatry, 10*, 728. https://doi.org/10.3389/fpsyt.2019.00728

Milette, I., Martel, M-J., Ribeiro da Silva, M., & Coughlin McNeil, M. (2017a). Guidelines for the institutional implementation of developmental neuroprotective care in the neonatal intensive care unit. Part A: Background and the rationale. A joint position statement from the CANN, CAPWHN, Nann, and COINN. *Canadian Journal of Nursing Research, 49*(2), 46–62. https://doi.org/10.1177/0844562117706882

Milette, I., Martel, M-J., Ribeiro da Silva, M., & Coughlin McNeil, M. (2017b). Guidelines for the institutional implementation of developmental neuroprotective care in the neonatal intensive care unit. Part B: Recommendations and justification. A joint position statement from the CANN, CAPWHN, Nann, and COINN. *Canadian Journal of Nursing Research, 49*(2), 63–74. https://doi.org/10.1177/0844562117708126

Milette, I., Martel, M-J., Ribeiro da Silva, M., & Coughlin McNeil, M. (2019). Guidelines for the institutional implementation of developmental neuroprotective care in the neonatal intensive care unit. A joint position statement from the CANN, CAPWHN, Nann, and COINN. *Advances in Neonatal Care, 19*(1), 9–10. https://doi.org/10.1097/anc.0000000000000465

Montirosso, R., & McGlone, F. (2020). The body comes first. Embodied reparation and the co-creation of infant bodily-self. *Neuroscience & Biobehavioral Reviews, 113*, 77–87. https://doi.org/10.1016/j.neubiorev.2020.03.003

Montirosso, R., & Provenzi, L. (2015). Implications of epigenetics and stress regulation on research and developmental care of preterm infants. *Journal of Obstetric, Gynecologic and Neonatal Nursing, 44*(2), 174–182. https://doi.org/10.1111/1552-6909.12559

Montirosso, R., Tronick, E., & Borgatti, R. (2017). Promoting neuroprotective care in neonatal intensive care units and preterm infant development: Insights from the neonatal adequate care for quality of life study. *Child Development Perspectives, 11*(1), 9–15. https://doi.org/10.1111/cdep.12208

Morgan, B. E., Horn, A. R., & Bergman, N. J. (2011). Should neonates sleep alone? *Biological Psychiatry, 70*(9), 817–825. https://doi.org/10.1016/j.biopsych.2011.06.018

Narayan, A. J., Kalstabakken, A. W., Labella, M. H., Nerenberg, L. S., Monn, A. R., & Masten, A. S. (2017). Intergenerational continuity of adverse childhood experiences in homeless families: Unpacking exposure to maltreatment versus family dysfunction. *American Journal of Orthopsychiatry, 87*(1), 3–14. https://doi.org/10.1037/ort0000133

Naugler, M. R., & Di Carlo, K. (2018). Barriers to and interventions that increase nurses' and parents' compliance with safe sleep recommendations for preterm infants. *Nursing for Womens Health, 22*(1), 24–39. https://doi.org/10.1016/j.nwh.2017.12.009

Nejati, A., Rodiek, S., & Shepley, M. (2016b). The implications of high-quality staff break areas for nurses' health, performance, job satisfaction and retention. *Journal of Nursing Management, 24*(4), 512–523. https://doi.org/10.1111/jonm.12351

Nejati, A., Rodiek, S., & Shepley, M. (2016c). Using visual simulation to evaluate restorative qualities of access to nature in hospital staff break areas. *Landscape and Urban Planning, 148*, 132–138. https://doi.org/10.1016/j.landurbplan.2015.12.012

Nejati, A., Shepley, M., Rodiek, S., Lee, C., & Varni, J. (2016a). Restorative design features for hospital staff break areas: A multi-method study. *HERD: Health Environments Research Design Journal, 9*(2), 16–35. https://doi.org/10.1177/1937586715592632

Neu, M., Klawetter, S., Greenfield, J. C., Rotbal, K., Scott, J. L., & Hwang, S. S. (2020). Mothers' experiences in the NICU before family-centered care and in the NICUs where it is the standard of care. *Advances in Neonatal Care, 20*(1), 68–79. https://doi.org/10.1097/anc.0000000000000671

Nicholls, R., Perry, L., Duffield, C., Gallagher, R., & Pierce, H. (2017). Barriers and facilitators to healthy eating for nurses in the workplace: An integrative review. *Journal of Advanced Nursing, 73*(5), 1051–1065. https://doi.org/10.1111/jan.13185

Norman, V., Rossillo, K., & Skelton, K. (2016). Creating healing environments through the theory of caring. *AORN Journal, 104*(5), 401–409. https://doi.org/10.1016/j.aorn.2016.09.006

Nusslock, R., & Miller, G. E. (2016). Early-life adversity and physical and emotional health across the lifespan: A neuro-immune network hypothesis. *Biological Psychiatry, 80*(1), 23–32. https://doi.org/10.1016/j.biopsych.2015.05.017

O'Brien, K., Robson, K., Bracht, M., Cruz, M., Lui, K., Alvaro, R., da Silva, O., Monterosa, L., Narvey, M., Ng, E., Soraisham, A., Ye, X. Y., Mirea, L., Tarnow-Mordi, W., Lee, S. K., & the FICare Study Group and FICare Parent Advisory Board. (2018). Effectiveness of family integrated care in neonatal intensive care units on infant and parent outcomes: A multicentre, multinational, cluster-randomized controlled trial. *Lancet Child and Adolescent Health, 2*(4), 245–254. https://doi.org/10.1016/s2352-4642(18)30039-7

O'Callaghan, N., Dee, A., & Philip, R. K. (2019). Evidence-based design for neonatal units: A systematic review. *Maternal Health, Neonatology and Perinatology, 5*(6), https://doi.org/10.1186/s40748-019-0101-0

Olsson, E., Ahl, H., Bengtsson, K., Vejayaram, D. N., Norman, E., Bruschettini, M., & Eriksson, M. (2021). The use and reporting of neonatal pain scales: A systematic review of randomized trials. *Pain, 162*(2), 353–360. https://dx.doi.org/10.1097%2Fj.pain.0000000000002046

Ottosen, M. J., Engebretson, J., Etchegaray, J., Arnold, C., & Thomas, E. J. (2019). An ethnography of parents' perceptions of patient safety in the neonatal intensive care unit. *Advances in Neonatal Care, 19*(6), 500–508. https://doi.org/10.1097/anc.0000000000000657

Pados, B. F. (2019). Physiology of stress and use of skin-to-skin care as a stress-reducing intervention in the NICU. *Nursing for Women's Health, 23*(1), 59–70. https://doi.org/10.1016/j.nwh.2018.11.002

Pados, B. F. & Hess, F. (2019). Systematic review of the effects of skin-to-skin care on short-term physiologic stress outcomes in preterm infants in the neonatal intensive care unit. *Advances in Neonatal Care, 20*(1), 48–58. https://doi.org/10.1097/anc.0000000000000596

Paguio, J. T., & Yu, D. S. F. (2020). A mixed methods study to evaluate the effects of a teamwork enhancement and quality improvement initiative on nurses' work environment. *Journal of Advanced Nursing, 76*(2), 664–675. https://doi.org/10.1111/jan.14270

Park, J., Silva, S. G., Thoyre, S. M., Brandon, D. H. (2020). Sleep-wake states and feeding progression in preterm infants. *Nursing Research, 69*(1), 22–30. https://doi.org/10.1097/NNR.0000000000000395

Patel, S., Pelletier-Bui, A., Smith, S., Roberts, M. B., Kilgannon, H., Trzeciak, S., & Roberts, B. W. (2019). Curricula for empathy and compassion training in medical education: A systematic review. *PLoS One, 14*(8), e0221412. https://doi.org/10.1371/journal.pone.0221412

Pereira, T. R. C., DeSouza, F. G., & Beleza, A. C. S. (2017). Implications of pain in functional activities in the immediate postpartum period according to the mode of delivery and parity: An observational study. *Brazilian Journal of Physical Therapy, 21*(1), 37–43. https://doi.org/10.1016/j.bjpt.2016.12.003

Pervanidou, P., Makris, G., Chrousos, G., & Agorastos, A. (2020). Early life stress and pediatric posttraumatic stress disorder. *Brain Sciences, 10*(169), https://doi.org/10.3390/brainsci10030169

Pfaff, K. & Markaki, A. (2017). Compassionate collaborative care: An integrative review of quality indicators in end-of-life care. *BMC Palliative Care, 16*, 65. https://doi.org/10.1186/s12904-017-0246-4

Pham, T. T. L., Teng, C.-I., Friesner, D., Li, K., Wu, W.-E., Liao, Y.-N., Chang, Y.-T., & Chu, T.-L. (2019). The impact of mentor-mentee rapport on nurses' professional turnover intention: perspectives of social capital theory and social cognitive career theory. *Journal of Clinical Nursing, 28*(13–14), 2669–2680. https://doi.org/10.1111/jocn.14858

Picaud, J. C., Buffin, R., Gremmo-Feger, G., Rigo, J., Putet, G., Casper, C., & Working Group of the French Neonatal Society on Fresh Human Milk Use in Preterm Infants, (2018). Review concludes that specific recommendations are needed to harmonize the provision of fresh mother's milk to their preterm infants. *Acta Paediatrica, 107*(7), 1145–1155. https://doi.org/10.1111/apa.14259

Pineda, R., Guth, R., Herring, A., Reynolds, L., Oberle, S., & Smith, J. (2017). Enhancing sensory experiences for very preterm infants: An integrative review. *Journal of Perinatology, 37*(4), 323–332. https://doi.org/10.1038/jp.2016.179

Prouhet, P. M., Gregory, M. R., Russell, C. L., & Yaeger, L. H. (2018). Fathers' stress in the neonatal intensive care unit: A systematic review. *Advances in Neonatal Care, 18*(2), 105–120. https://doi.org/10.1097/anc.0000000000000472

Rate, C. R., Clarke, J. A., Lindsay, D. R., & Sternberg, R. J. (2007). Implicit theories of courage. *Journal of Positive Psychology, 2*(2), 80–98. https://doi.org/10.1080/17439760701228755

Richardson, A., Gurung, G., Derrett, S., & Harcombe, H. (2019). Perspectives on preventing musculoskeletal injuries in nurses: A qualitative study. *Nursing Open, 6*(3), 915–929. https://doi.org/10.1002/nop2.272

Roberts, A. L., Liew, Z., Lyall, K., Ascherio, A., & Weisskopf, M. G. (2018). Association of maternal exposure to childhood abuse with elevated risk for attention deficit hyperactivity disorder in offspring. *American Journal of Epidemiology, 187*(9), 1896–1906. https://doi.org/10.1093/aje/kwy098

Rolfe, A. (2017). What to look for in a mentor. *Korean Journal of Medical Education, 29*(1), 41–43. https://doi.org/10.3946/kjme.2017.52

Rosa, D., Terzoni, S., Dellafiore, F., & Destrebecq, A. (2019). Systematic review of shift work and nurses' health. *Occupational Medicine, 69*(4), 237–243. https://doi.org/10.1093/occmed/kqz063

Ross, A., Touchton-Leonard, K., Perez, A., Wehrlen, L., Kazmi, N., & Gibbons, S. (2019). Factors that influence health-promoting self-care in registered nurses: Barriers and facilitators. *Advances in Nursing Science, 42*(4), 358–373. https://doi.org/10.1097/ans.0000000000000274

Ruiz-Fernandez, M. D., Perez-Garcia, E., & Ortega-Galan, A. M. (2020). Quality of life in nursing professionals: Burnout, fatigue, and compassion satisfaction. *International Journal of Environmental Research and Public Health, 17*(4), 1253. https://doi.org/10.3390/ijerph17041253

Sancho-Rossignol, A., Schilliger, Z., Cordero, M.I., Rusconi Serpa, S., Epiney, M., Huppi, P., Ansermet, F., & Schechter, D. S. (2018). The association of maternal exposure to domestic violence during childhood with prenatal attachment, maternal-fetal heart rate and infant behavioral regulation. *Frontiers in Psychiatry, 9*, 358. https://doi.org/10.3389/fpsyt.2018.00358

Sanders, M. R., & Hall, S. L. (2018). Trauma-informed care in the newborn intensive care unit: Promoting safety, security, and connectedness. *Journal of Perinatology, 38*(1), 3–10. https://doi.org/10.1038/jp.2017.124

Scatliffe, N., Casavant, S., Vittner, D., & Cong, X. (2019). Oxytocin and early parent-infant interactions: A systematic review. *International Journal of Nursing Science, 6*(4), 445–453. https://doi.org/10.1016/j.ijnss.2019.09.009

Shonkoff, J. P., Garner, A. S., Committee on Psychosocial Aspects of Child and Family Health, Committee on Early Childhood, Adoption, and Dependent Care, & Section on Developmental and Behavioral Pediatrics, (2012). The lifelong effects of early childhood adversity and toxic stress. *Pediatrics, 129*(1), e232–e246. https://doi.org/10.1542/peds.2011-2663

Shriane, A. E., Ferguson, S. A., Jay, S. M., & Vincent, G. E. (2020). Sleep hygiene in shift workers: A systematic literature review. *Sleep Medicine Reviews, 53*, 101336. https://doi.org/10.1016/j.smrv.2020.101336

Sigurdson, K., Mitchell, B., Liu, J., Morton, C., Gould, J. B., Lee, H. C., Capdarest-Arest, N., & Profit, J. (2019). Racial/ethnic disparities in neonatal intensive care: A systematic review. *Pediatrics, 144*(2), e20183114. https://doi.org/10.1542/peds.2018-3114

Slominski, A. T., Zmijewski, M. A., Skobowiat, C., Zbytek, B., Slominski, R. M., & Steketee, J. D. (2012). Sensing the environment: Regulation of local and global homeostasis by the skin's neuroendocrine system. *Advances in Anatomy, Embryology, and Cell Biology, 212*(v,vii), 1–115. https://doi.org/10.1007/978-3-642-19683-6_1

Sofhauser, C. (2016). Intention in nursing practice. *Nursing Science Quarterly, 29*(1), 31–34. https://doi.org/10.1177/0894318413614629

Spinazzola, J., van der Kolk, B., & Ford, J. D. (2018). When nowhere is safe: Interpersonal trauma and attachment adversity as antecedents of posttraumatic stress disorder and developmental trauma disorder. *Journal of Traumatic Stress, 31*(5), 631–642. https://doi.org/10.1002/jts.22320

Stanulewicz, N., Knox, E., Narayanasamy, M., Shivji, N., Khunti, K., & Blake, H. (2019). Effectiveness of lifestyle health promotion interventions for nurses: A systematic review. *International Journal of Environmental Research and Public Health, 17*(1), 17. https://doi.org/10.3390/ijerph17010017

Tawfik, D. S., Phibbs, C. S., Sexton, J. B., Kan, P., Sharek, P. J. Nisbet, C. C., Rigdon, J., Trockel, M., & Profit, J. (2017). Factors associated with provider burnout in the NICU. *Pediatrics, 139*(5), e20164134. https://doi.org/10.1542/peds.2016-4134

Thomas, T., Kaye, R., Jacob, A., & Grabher, D. (2021). Implementation of cue-based feeding to improve preterm infant feeding outcomes and promote parent involvement. *Journal of Obstetric, Gynecologic, and Neonatal Nursing, 50*, 328–339. https://doi.org/10.1016/j.jogn.2021.02.002

Toso, K., de Cock, P., & Leavey, G. (2020). Maternal exposure to violence and offspring neurodevelopment: A systematic review. *Paediatric Perinatal Epidemiology, 34*(2), 190–203. https://doi.org/10.1111/ppe.12651

Treherne, S. C., Feeley, N., Charbonneau, L., & Axelin, A. (2017). Parents' perspectives of closeness and separation with their preterm infants in the

NICU. *Journal of Obstetric, Gynecologic, and Neonatal Nursing, 46*, 737–747. https://doi.org/10.1016/j.jogn.2017.07.005

Tronick, E., & Beeghly, M. (2011). Infants' meaning-making and the development of mental health problems. *American Psychologist, 66*(2), 107–119. https://doi.org/10.1037/a0021631

Vinales, J. J. (2015). The mentor as a role model and the importance of belongingness. *British Journal of Nursing, 24*(10), 532–535. https://doi.org/10.12968/bjon.2015.24.10.532

Voos, K. C., Terreros, A., Larimore, P., Leick-Rude, M. K., & Park, N. (2015). Implementing safe sleep practices in a neonatal intensive care unit. *Journal of Maternal-Fetal, & Neonatal Medicine, 28*(14), 1637–1640. https://doi.org/10.3109/14767058.2014.964679

Wang, Y.-W., Hung, H.-Y., Lin, C.-H., Wang, C.-J., Lin, Y.-J., & Chang, y.-J. (2018). Effect of a delayed start to oral feeding on feeding performance and physiological responses in preterm infants: A randomized clinical trial. *Journal of Nursing Research, 26*(5), 324–331. https://doi.org/10.1097/jnr.0000000000000243.

Watson, J. (2018). *Unitary caring science: The philosophy and praxis of nursing.* University Press of Colorado.

Weber, A., & Harrison, T. M. (2019). Reducing toxic stress in the NICU to improve outcomes. *Nursing Outlook, 67*(2), 169–189. https://doi.org/10.1016/j.outlook.2018.11.002

Wei, H., Sewell, K. A., Woody, G., & Rose, M. A. (2018). The state of the science of nurse work environments in the United States: A systematic review. *International Journal of Nursing Science, 5*(3), 287–300. https://doi.org/10.1016/j.ijnss.2018.04.010

Welch, M. G., Firestein, M. R., Austin, J., Hane, A. A., Stark, R. I., Hofer, M. A., Garland, M., Glickstein, S. B., Brunelli, S. A., Ludwig, R. J., & Myers, M. M. (2015). Family Nurture Intervention in the neonatal intensive care unit improves social-relatedness, attention, and neurodevelopment of preterm infants at 18 months in a randomized controlled trial. *Journal of Child Psychology and Psychiatry, 56*(11), 1202–1211. https://doi.org/10.1111/jcpp.12405

Welch, M. G., Stark, R. I., Grieve, P. G., Ludwig, R. J., Isler, J. R., Barone, J. L., & Myers, M. M. (2017). Family nurture intervention in preterm infants increases early development of cortical activity and independence of regional power trajectories. *Acta Paediatrica, 106*(12), 1952–1960. https://doi.org/10.1111/apa.14050

White, R. D. (2020). Recommended standards for newborn ICU design, 9th edition. *Journal of Perinatology, 40*, 2–4. https://doi.org/10.1038/s41372-020-0766-2

Wickwire, E. M., Geiger-Brown, J., Scharf, S. M., & Drake, C. L. (2017). Shift work and shift work sleep disorder. *Chest, 151*(5), 1156–1172. https://dx.doi.org/10.1016%2Fj.chest.2016.12.007

Winter, R., Issa, E., Roberts, N., Norman, R. I., & Howick, J. (2020). Assessing the effect of empathy-enhancing interventions in health education and training: A systematic review of randomized controlled trials. *BMJ Open, 10*(9), e036471. https://doi.org/10.1136/bmjopen-2019-036471

Wright, R. O. (2018). "Motherless children have the hardest time": Epigenetic programming and early life environment. *Pediatrics, 142*(4), e20181528. https://doi.org/10.1542/peds.2018-1528

Yaribeygi, H., Panahi, Y., Sahraei, H., Johnston, T. P., & Sahebkar, A. (2017). The impact of stress on body function: A review. *EXCLI Journal, 16*, 1057–1072. https://dx.doi.org/10.17179%2Fexcli2017-480

Zahourek, R. P. (2012). Healing through the lens of intentionality. *Holistic Nursing Practice, 26*(1), 6–21. https://doi.org/10.1097/HNP.0b013e31823bfe4c

Zarse, E. M., Neff, M. R., Yoder, R., Hulvershorn, L., Chambers, J. E., & Chambers, R. A. (2019). The adverse childhood experiences questionnaire: Two decades of research on childhood trauma as a primary cause of adult mental illness, addiction, and medical diseases. *Cogent Medicine, 6*(1), 1581447. https://doi.org/10.1080/2331205X.2019.1581447

CHAPTER 5

The Neonatal Intensive Care Unit Environment

Maryann Bozzette, Carole Kenner, Marina Boykova, Leslie B. Altimier, and Raylene M. Phillips

Standard II: Positioning and touch for the newborn.
Standard III: Sleep and arousal interventions for the newborn.
Standard IV: Skin-to-skin contact for intimate family members.
Standard V: Reducing and minimizing pain and stress in newborns and families.

INTRODUCTION

In the 1960s, the neonatal intensive care unit (NICU) was established to provide care specifically for critically ill newborn infants. Since that time, the NICU has evolved into a state-of-the-art technological center providing a myriad of healthcare services. Medical progress has been remarkable, with greater than 84% survival rate for premature infants born greater than 27 to 28 weeks' gestation at 2 years of age, and yet when only perinatal care is examined, the long-term developmental outcomes do not always differ from those infants born less premature (Morgan et al., 2020). What then can make a difference in the long-term developmental outcomes of extremely premature infants? What about the NICU environment?

The rapid progress in medical and technical innovations has been accompanied by concern for the developmental trajectories of infants receiving neonatal intensive care, particularly for extremely preterm (EPT) infants born between 23 and 27 weeks' gestation. Technology has greatly increased the cost of care both in dollars and amount of time infants are in the NICU, with little change in long-term outcomes. The earlier in gestation an infant is born, the longer time spent in the NICU and the higher the subsequent risk for developmental delay.

The normal environment for the developing fetus at 23 to 40 weeks' gestation is the maternal womb. The intrauterine environment provides protection against outside stimulation while surrounding the developing fetus in a dark, fluid setting that allows for weightless movement and intermittent filtered sounds. The uterine walls furnish boundaries that provide security for the developing human. Maternal activity and hormonal cycles provide rhythmic and cyclic stimulation. The fetus is rocked gently and moves as the mother moves. The placenta provides necessary nutrients that meet all of the metabolic needs of the growing fetus (Blackburn, 1998, 2018). The maternal–fetal system is an astonishing, self-sufficient unit for optimal development.

In contrast, the NICU's extrauterine environment exposes newly born premature infants to bright, artificial lights; frequent, loud noises; cool, dry temperatures; gravitational forces that restrict mobility, and separation from mother. For families, the NICU is far from the vision they had when they first learned they were pregnant, and NICU living arrangements are nothing like what most parents dream about for their new child. The environment can be either hostile or comforting for the infant and family, depending on the circumstances and the support healthcare professionals can provide. This caregiving environment presents the infant and family with many challenges. The infant may appear "lost" in a sea of tubes and positional supports, which is certainly not the picture most families have as the dream about their developing fetus/infant. Parents express fears about whether or not they are capable of taking care of their baby, disappointment about the birth experience, anxiety about their baby's health, and the stress of having a baby in the NICU while still having other family obligations. This chapter addresses key elements of the impact of the NICU environment on infants and their families and how Infant and Family-Centered Developmental Care (IFCDC) practices can help the family unit survive and thrive. Although this entire text is devoted to considering the macro- and micro-environment of the infant and family in the NICU, this chapter only provides highlights and examples of interventions to support the principles of IFCDC within the context of the NICU environment.

MEDICAL ADVANCES

Use of surfactant and more specialized ventilatory supports; continuous monitoring of arterial oxygen saturation, carbon dioxide levels, and cerebral blood flow; continuous amplitude integrated electroencephalography; and other physiologic supports coupled with better antenatal screening for problems and proactive intervention have significantly increased the survival rates for even the extremely premature infant (Dizenberger & Blackburn, 2020; Lodha et al., 2020). Survival for infants born at 22 weeks' gestation in 2000 to 2017 have risen from almost 0% to 7.3% of live births and 24.1% if the infant is transferred to a high-level NICU. Over the same course of time, the rate of survival without developmental impairment increased from 1.2% to 9.3% for 22 to 24 weeks' gestational age (GA) and from 40.6% to 64.2% for 25 to 27 weeks' GA (Myrhaug et al., 2019). Complex and chronic health problems of EPT infants require extended care in the NICU environment and long-term developmental intervention. Longitudinal follow-up of infants cared for in NICUs has revealed that infants who appeared normal at discharge may show signs of school performance problems, social delays, and neurologic abnormalities as they grow older (Dizenberger & Blackburn, 2020).

NICU EQUIPMENT

The first principle of all neonatal care is thermoregulation. An infant leaves the wet, warm, intrauterine environment to one that is dry and cold. The infant warmer bed is flat, borderless, and hard compared with the womb. Keeping infants warm has been among the greatest NICU challenges, particularly for very premature infants. Infants were routinely admitted on an open warmer and later transferred to an incubator. Many of the incubators used today also convert to radiant warmers so that the infant's temperature may stay steadier during procedures and requires no transfer in and out of bed. Humidification can be maintained as well. These warmers provide warmth to maintain the infant's temperature, but many other fetal regulatory mechanisms are now lost. The diurnal variation of maternal activity and sleep cycles, as well as vestibular-proprioceptive stimulation from the infant's body and movement, are no longer present (Blackburn, 2018; Dizenberger & Blackburn, 2020). Visual, auditory, and tactile stimulation suddenly dominate, and care activities occur with little change in rhythm or intensity. Intravenous lines, tapes, and ventilator tubing may restrict infant movement.

Small and sick infants experience stimuli that are unexpected, painful, frequent, and not conducive to their continued development outside of the womb. This abrupt change in environment interrupts the normal fetal experience and presents multiple challenges for growth and development. These negative effects of the NICU environment are less likely to occur if all IFCDC standards are followed.

PRIMARY AND IATROGENIC MEDICAL COMPLICATIONS

Infants who spend considerable time in the NICU can experience may negative sequelae. They are prone to respiratory infections and reactive airway disease. Extended need for artificial ventilation can lead to ventilator-associated pneumonia and potential airway complications (Zhou et al., 2020). Low-birth-weight infants requiring mechanical ventilation are at higher risk for intraventricular hemorrhage, chronic lung disease, necrotizing enterocolitis, sepsis, and retinopathy of prematurity. Some premature infants have other vision problems such as myopia and strabismus (Yadav et al., 2018). Some of the conditions are related to a preterm birth and not just postnatal treatments. Evidence-based strategies to promote neuroprotection, even in utero, have demonstrated better neurodevelopmental outcomes (Chu et al., 2020). These strategies include use of antenatal steroids magnesium sulfate, perinatal consultations, delayed cord clamping, early thermoregulation, surfactant administration, and parenteral and enteral nutrition (Chu et al., 2020). New techniques and treatments for neonatal respiratory conditions result in fewer complications. Such techniques/treatments include use of lung ultrasound to determine when to give surfactant, use of thin catheters to administer surfactant, use of nasal CPAP, and enhanced nutrition (Davis et al., 2020; Panza et al., 2020; Rodriguez-Fanjul et al., 2020). In spite of these interventions, many infants requiring an NICU stay also require some type of medical care and early intervention during the first 2 years of life, particularly for respiratory infections.

Exposure to stressors in the NICU is associated with regional alterations in brain structure and function, decreased brain size in the frontal and parietal regions, and altered brain microstructure and functional connectivity within the temporal lobes (Boggini et al., 2021; Smith et al., 2011). Many infants in the NICU do not reach the expected developmental milestones at corrected postmenstrual ages. Difficulties in attention, executive functions, cognition, language, visual–motor abilities, as well as behavior problems affect academic performance in children born very preterm and persist to adulthood (Brydges et al., 2018).

INFECTION CONTROL

Because premature infants do not have a developed immune system, their ability to respond to pathogens is limited. Handwashing remains the gold standard for protection of hospitalized neonates. Frequent use of alcohol-based hand sanitizers is recommended when hands are not soiled. Standard precautions are used with infants in the NICU with particular attention to the preterm infant's skin that is very thin and easily damaged. Absorption of products through the skin is a concern as well as disruption of skin integrity with frequent heel sticks, blood draws, and intravenous (IV) placements.

Another major concern in the NICU is central line–associated bloodstream infections (CLABSI) (Bierlaire et al., 2020; Pearlman, 2020). Strict protocols for placement by a skilled practitioner are imperative as well as daily monitoring of the catheter insertion site. Quality improvement methods such as audits and Plan-Do-Study-Act cycles regarding line and dressing changes and use of grouped evidence-based interventions or "bundles" have been shown to reduce the incidence of CLABSI (Bierlaire et al., 2020; Pearlman, 2020).

ENVIRONMENTAL CONCERNS

Sleep

In the NICU, sleep is frequently interrupted for care or treatment. One study showed that infants weighing less than 1,500 g were disturbed more than 100 times in a 24-hour period (Cong et al., 2017). In fact, infant handling seldom occurs for social and nurturing reasons and is unpredictable and often painful (Blackburn, 2018; Dizenberger & Blackburn, 2020).

There is increasing evidence to support the relationship between sleep cycles and neurosensory development. More effort is now made to allow for undisturbed periods of sleep in the NICU. The IFCDC standards address the need to promote developmentally appropriate sleep and arousal states and sleep–wake cycles (Bigsby & Salisbury, 2020). Yet, a recent study found that only 46% of the units implementing IFCDC supported positive sleep (Lopez-Maestro et al., 2019). Sleep is important for growth (Tham, Schneider, & Broekman, 2017), and interrupting sleep by touching an infant just to check their status is unnecessary. This sleep disruption is less likely to occur if IFCDC standards, including the standard for sleep and arousal, as listed in the beginning of this chapter are followed.

Pain

Painful experiences are another NICU environmental concern. Repeated painful experiences impact the infant's neurodevelopment and reaction to noxious stimuli later in life (Williams & Lascelles, 2020). Alterations in central nervous system (CNS) development can occur from frequent and noxious stimulation experienced by premature infants. Several areas of CNS development take place during the period when preterm infants are in the NICU, including neuron migration, synaptogenesis, and arborization. The patterns of dendrite connections between neurons are critical for cell-to-cell communication. This process can be particularly vulnerable to insults from the NICU environment.

Environmental experience modifies processes of cell proliferation, cell migration, or cell differentiation. The pattern of synaptic organization can be altered by chronic pain experiences. This reorganization will likely occur even if the preterm infant has a completely uncomplicated medical perinatal course, which may help explain the reason even late preterm infants can show developmental delay.

Endotracheal tube suction can be traumatic and lead to hypoxia if attention is not paid to evidence-based guidelines. Suctioning should only be done as needed according to the infant's condition and then should only be done for about 15 seconds at a time. The length of the endotracheal tube must be known/recorded and then the suction catheter size should be selected accordingly. Suctioning can be open or closed, with closed being the method of choice in neonates (Abraham & Roberston, 2020). Soothing touch and other measures to reduce pain and stress should be used during the procedure (Abraham & Roberston, 2020).

There is strong evidence to support the use of oral sucrose as a single dose to ease pain during a heel stick, blood draws, or IV insertions (Harrison et al., 2012; Lago et al., 2020; Sen & Manav, 2020). Other methods of nonpharmacologic pain reduction that demonstrated success include SSC or kangaroo mother care, use of breastmilk instead of sucrose, and sucrose combined with music (Barandouzi et al., 2020; Fitri et al., 2020; Nimbalkar et al., 2020).

Pain assessment tools have been developed and evaluated. Although pain treatment has not been adopted uniformly in all NICUs, many more pharmacological and nonpharmacological interventions are in use today, and pain and stress prevention and reduction is incorporated into the IFCDC standards (Hynan et al., 2020). The standard to reduce stress and pain incorporates the family constellation with the infant and is listed at the beginning of this chapter.

MACROENVIRONMENT

Over the last few decades evidence has mounted to support the impact of the physical environment of the NICU on the small and sick newborn. Dr. Stanley Graven led the way in the early 1990s to begin to study the various components of the physical environment such as noise, light, and space for the infant and family. This work spawned the NICU Design Standards led by Dr. Robert White and an interdisciplinary committee of experts including families. Now in its 9th edition (last published in 2019), these standards are used in over 25 countries and address Unit Configuration; Location of the NICU with the Hospital; Family Entry and Reception Entry; Signage and Art; Safety/Infant Security; Minimum Space, Clearance, and Privacy Requirements for the Infant Space; Private (Single-Family) Rooms; Couplet Care Rooms; Airborne Infection (Isolation Room(s)); Operating Rooms Intended for Use by Newborn ICU Patients; Electrical, Gas Supply, and Mechanical Needs; Ambient Temperature and Ventilation; Handwashing; General Support Space; Staff Support Space; Support Space for Ancillary Services; Administrative Space; Family Support Space; Family Transition Room(s); Ceiling Finishes; Wall and Floor Surfaces; Furnishings; Ambient Lighting in the Infant Care Areas; Illumination of Support Areas; Daylighting; Access to Nature and Other Positive Distractions; Acoustic Environment; and Usability Testing (White, 2019).

These recommendations now address far more than just light, sound, and space because all aspects of the environment and how they function to support families impact the survival of infants and how they thrive. The recommendations include neuroprotection, care that supports and protects the developing brain. This requires anticipation and knowledge of factors that impact both positively and negatively the infant's neurological development and supports the family as they adapt to their small or sick newborn.

Many units are now moving to a Single Room Design to better support the infant and family. This design takes into consideration the macro- and micro-environments. For more information please see Chapter 6.

NEONATAL INTEGRATIVE DEVELOPMENTAL CARE MODEL

The Neonatal Integrative Developmental Care Model (Philips Healthcare, Cambridge, MA), encompasses seven core measures. They are: (1) The Healing Environment, (2) Partnering with Families, (3) Positioning and Handling, (4) Safeguarding Sleep, (5) Minimizing Stress and Pain, (6) Protecting Skin, and (7) Optimizing Nutrition (Altimier & White, 2020; Altimier & Phillips, 2013, 2016).

(The next sections on the core measures are adapted with permission from Altimier, L. B., & Phillips, R. (2022). from the NICU Environment chapter in the Kenner, C., & Boykova, M. V. (Eds.), *Neonatal nursing care handbook*, 3rd ed., Copyright 2023, Springer Publishing Company, LLC. ISBN-9780826135483.)

CORE MEASURE #1: HEALING ENVIRONMENT

The healing environment encompasses the *physical environment* of space, privacy, and safety; the *people environment* of the infant and family as well as the healthcare staff; and the *sensory environment*, which influences the infant's developing sensory system. The *physical environment* involves not only the baby's space but also characteristics of the baby's NICU room or space, which affect maternal–infant attachment, parental engagement, and participation. The *people environment* highlights the infant and the family unit and equally all of the healthcare staff that help create the multidisciplinary care team for the infant and family. The *sensory system* includes the tactile (touch), vestibular (movement, proprioception, and balance), gustatory (taste), olfactory (smell), auditory (sound), and visual (light) systems.

The overarching goal is to promote healing by minimizing the negative impacts of the artificial, extrauterine NICU environment on brain development and infant behavior and its impact on the entire family.

Selected interventions include:

1. Provide a physical design that meets the neurodevelopmental needs of the infant and provides adequate private space and facilities to support a family-integrated care approach, while at the same time meeting the needs of the multidisciplinary staff that participate in that infant and family's care.
2. Provide opportunities for all staff, as well as parents, to participate in multidisciplinary rounds.
3. Promote attachment and bonding.
4. Provide respectful care.

5. Tactile: Facilitate early, frequent, and prolonged SSC to provide positive tactile experiences through gentle, safe contact with parent's bare chest. Provide gentle, yet firm gentle touch. Maintain midline, flexion, containment, and comfort when positioning. Minimize painful procedures and invasive monitoring when possible.
6. Vestibular: Change the infant's position slowly and gently using two-person/four-handed support. Use facilitative tucking and containment.
7. Olfactory: Provide mother's scent when possible. Provide nonnutritive sucking with mother's own milk (when possible) during tube feedings.
8. Gustatory: Position infant with hands near the face/mouth. Minimize adhesives around the mouth, nose, and face.
9. Auditory: Monitor noise levels in patient rooms including equipment. Set alarms at minimal effective level, and silence alarms as quickly as possible. Cover the incubator (when appropriate) and protect the incubator/bed by eliminating items placed on top of the incubator. Consider ceiling tiles with high noise reduction coefficients. Provide soft positive sounds of human voice (mother/parent whenever possible).
10. Visual: Provide adjustable light levels at the infant's bedspace through a range of at least 10 to no more than 600 lux (approximately 1 to 60 foot candles). Avoid purposeful visual stimulation prior to 38 weeks' GA Use cycle lights at 28 weeks or sooner if stable.

CORE MEASURE # 2: PARTNERING WITH FAMILIES

Families are a critical part of the healthcare team. They are to be actively involved in the care if they so desire. Parent–Professional partnerships improve neurodevelopmental outcomes and increase family satisfaction. During the time of COVID 19, families were often separated from the infants, yet the World Health Organization, European Foundation for the Care of Newborn Infants, and many others have advocated for zero separation.

The NICU design must support families, and spaces need to be family friendly. The prevalence of anxiety, posttraumatic stress disorder, and depressive symptoms in parents of preterm and full-term infants at NICU discharge is high, with 45% of parents reporting depressive symptoms and 43% reporting elevated perceived stress. Older gestational age, greater parental stress, and lower levels of social support are strong correlates of depressive symptoms (Soghier et al., 2020). Maternal anxiety and depression negatively impact maternal–infant attachment (Bonacquisti et al., 2020).

SSC promotes family integration into the care. It provides an optimal environment for the infant and promotes physiologic stability. It helps promote early breastfeeding, bonding, and attachment. It has also been useful to reduce symptoms of infants with neonatal abstinence syndrome (Kondili & Duryea, 2019).

The goal is to support families and not treat them as "visitors" but healthcare partners. Specific interventions include:

1. Promote SSC.
2. Encourage zero separation with open access to their baby in the NICU.
3. Use active listening to understand the family's feelings.
4. Encourage and support breastfeeding.
5. Encourage families to develop confidence in their caregiving.

CORE MEASURE #3: POSITIONING, HANDLING, AND CAREGIVING

Positioning and handling of the infant is aimed at minimizing positional deformities, supporting muscle tone, postural alignment, movement patterns, and ultimately positive musculoskeletal development. Careful, thoughtful positioning has been shown to preserve musculoskeletal integrity and facilitate developmental progression (Altimier & Phillips, 2020; Altimier & White, 2020). Positioning, handling, and caregiving should be performed gently and slowly with each intervention justified and intentional, rather than performing on a predetermined schedule.

The goals are to promote autonomic stability. In order to do so, caregiving tasks are performed "with" and not "to" the infant, and they are age appropriate, individualized, nurturing, and developmentally supportive.

Specific interventions include:

1. Facilitate SSC.
2. Utilize a validated and reliable positioning assessment tool.
3. Anticipate and prioritize care to minimize stress and pain.
4. Assess sleep-wake cycles before handling.
5. Provide midline, flexed, and contained positioning.
6. Educate parents about positioning, handling, and caregiving.

CORE MEASURE #4: SAFEGUARD SLEEP

Sleep is an essential part of the healing process. It also protects brain plasticity and facilitates continued brain development (Wolfe & Ralls, 2019). The release of oxytocin during SSC also makes the mother and infant relax, fall asleep, and feel safe, all of which are necessary for quality sleep (Vittner et al., 2019).

The goals are to assess the sleep–wake cycle prior to caregiving, protect uninterrupted sleep, and transition infants to back-to-sleep protocols when possible and safe to do so.

Specific interventions include:

1. Facilitate SSC to release oxytocin, supporting sleep.
2. Utilize a valid and reliable sleep scale or direct observation methods.

3. Provide nonpharmacologic developmentally supportive care.
4. Protect sleep cycles.
5. Educate parents on sleep cycles and how to promote sleep.

CORE MEASURE # 5: MINIMIZING STRESS AND PAIN

Pain and stress often occur in the NICU related to procedures, handling, multiple sources of stimulation, disease processes, and parental separation. Physiologic changes result from stress and include rising cortisol levels, increased energy expenditure, weight loss or failure to gain, and altered brain development/organization.

The goal is to promote physiologic stability and neurodevelopmental organization.

Specific interventions include:

1. Facilitation of SSC.
2. Use of a reliable and valid pain assessment tool.
3. Promotion of individualized care that minimizes stress.
4. Use of nonpharmacologic support as possible.
5. Parental education about pain and stress and how to provide comfort care.
6. Provide psychological support.

CORE MEASURE # 6: PROTECTING SKIN

Skin provides the infant with protection from environmental toxins and infectious agents. It provides thermoregulation and fluid and electrolyte balance. It is also the vehicle for sensations such as touch that can be calming or stress/pain producing. Procedures and care practices can impact skin integrity in a positive or negative way.

The goals are to promote/protect skin integrity, reduce transdermal water loss, and provide positive gentle touch and massage.

Specific interventions include:

1. Facilitate SSC to promote development of infant microbiome.
2. Use a reliable and valid skin assessment tool.
3. Provide adequate humidity.
4. Minimize use of adhesives and use caution when removing them to prevent epidermal stripping.
5. Use skin-protective products.
6. Educate parents on how to protect the infant's skin.

CORE MEASURE # 7: OPTIMIZING NUTRITION

Breastfeeding is the ideal form of infant feeding. Infants can learn to breastfeed before learning to bottle feed. When possible, breastfeeding should be supported. Feedings should be safe, effective, developmentally appropriate, and nurturing.

TABLE 5-1 Practice Recommendations

Type	Recommendation	Level of Evidence	References
Noise and noise reduction	Environmental modifications such as sound-absorbing materials and elimination of phones and pagers.	I VI	Almadhoob and Ohlsson [2020] Smith et al. [2018]
Lighting changes	Cycled lighting to promote sleep-wake states.	VI I	Marzouk et al. [2019] Morag and Ohlsson [2016]
Care routines	Kangaroo care to promote physiologic stability, bonding, and development.	IV V	Kurt et al. [2020] Mu et al. [2019]
Parent care	Promotion of collaborative partnerships with parents.	V	Lavalle et al. [2021]
Infection control	Insertion and care of PICC lines.	VI VI	Bierlaire et al. [2020] Von Dolinger deBrito et al., 2007
Unit design	Single-room designs.	VI IV	Doede & Trinkoff [2020] Feeley et al. [2020]
Pain in preterm infants	Reduction and management of pain.	I II IV I IV II II II	Boggini et al. [2021] Barandouzi et al. [2020] Cong et al. [2017] Fitri et al. [2020] Grunu et al. [2006] Lago et al. [2020] Nimbalkar et al. [2020] Sen and Manav [2020]

Note: Level I, evidence from a systematic review or meta-analysis of all relevant randomized controlled trials (RCTs), or evidence-based clinical practice guidelines based on systematic reviews of RCTs; level II, evidence obtained from at least one well-designed RCT; level III, evidence obtained from well-designed controlled trials without randomization; level IV, evidence from well-designed case–control and cohort studies; level V, evidence from systematic reviews of descriptive and qualitative studies; level VI, evidence from a single descriptive or qualitative study; level VII, evidence from the opinion of authorities and/or reports of expert committees; PICC, peripherally inserted central catheter.

The goals are to provide safe, neurosupportive feeding; optimize nutrition; prevent oral aversion; and promote breastfeeding competence before discharge.

Specific interventions include:

1. Promote SSC to facilitate breastfeeding.
2. Use a valid and reliable infant-driven feeding scale to assess feeding readiness and quality.
3. Support maternal breastfeeding.
4. Provide the taste and smell of mother's breast milk with gavage feedings.
5. Promote nonnutritive sucking at mother's breast during gavage feeds.
6. Educate parents about feeding cues and the benefits of human breastmilk.

These goals and interventions represent just some of the neuroprotective strategies that can be used to promote positive infant growth and development and to support families. The four IFCDC standards identified at the beginning of this chapter also support the core measures.

PALLIATIVE CARE

Ethical dilemmas can occur frequently in the NICU. Many infants are surviving birth at the edge of viability. There are also many infants born with serious congenital anomalies and genetic conditions such as trisomy 13. Palliative care is the provision of comfort for infants who have a life-limiting condition or a congenital defect designed to focus on quality of life and family support. A comprehensive team of healthcare providers works with the family to develop a plan of care. This team includes a physician, nurse, social worker, chaplain or other spiritual support, and sometimes a child life therapist. Others will be part of the team in cases of complex care. Collaboration and communication are key factors for success. Taking the family's values and beliefs into consideration is important to support their participation (Kenner et al., 2015).

NICUs are encouraged to develop a staff education program for health providers to learn the necessary skills to participate through honest communication and anticipatory guidance and to learn of community resources available to families. Staff should also have acceptability to debriefing sessions and counseling services. Beginning palliative care processes early helps to build trust and positive relationships with parents as they focus on making decisions and planning care for their infant and receiving support for coping with their distress (Quinn et al., 2020). Core values of palliative care include relief from suffering, approaching the infant and family with dignity and support, and the provision of compassionate care. Attention to pain assessment and comfort therapies such as skin-to-skin care and swaddling are integral parts of the plan (Marc-Aurele & English, 2017). Practice recommendations along with their level of evidence that support the NICU environment can be found in Table 5-1.

Potential Research Questions

NICU Configuration

What other environmental and care modifications may decrease stress in the NICU?

What factors promote neuroprotection in the NICU and after discharge?

Family Care

Are families benefiting from family-centered care models?

What factors promote maternal confidence in caregiving while in the NICU?

Late Preterm

Why are late preterm infants still experiencing developmental deficits?

Term Infant

Are there differences in environmental impact for term infants who are sick and require NICU care compared with preterm infants?

CONCLUSION

Neonatal intensive care units represent one of the fastest-developing areas of technology and treatment interventions in healthcare today. Numerous techniques, such as surfactant replacement, high-frequency ventilators, and percutaneously inserted central venous catheters, have greatly decreased mortality, allowing infants at early gestations to survive. With innovations such as cardiac surgical techniques and extracorporeal membrane oxygenation, critically ill newborns who would have died in the past now are surviving. All of these medical breakthroughs, however, come with the potential for health complications and developmental delays. The time has come to focus on quality of life for these infants and their early relationships.

Premature infants remain extremely vulnerable to stress. Modifying caregiving practices to reduce iatrogenic complications from the environment remains a significant challenge for all who provide care for premature infants. Continuous demands and energy depletion that affect growth and increase susceptibility to infection are a constant concern. Preventing unnecessary pain and stress is an important part of both developmental care and palliative care.

Epigenetic studies in the future may be able to uncover how much of the developmental deficits commonly seen in preterm infants are due to immature systems at birth, NICU environmental factors, or healthcare interventions. Frequent re-examination of current practices must occur to plan necessary modifications in the overall approach to neonatal care. Neuroprotective care must be a standard in all NICUs. Approaches to neonatal care that emphasize neurodevelopmental needs and disability prevention are expected to improve long-term neonatal outcomes. Implementation of the IFCDC standards and competencies will promote positive changes in the NICU environment and support infants and their families.

REFERENCES

Abraham, A., & Roberston, S. J. (2020). *Endotracheal suctioning. Neonatal intensive care unit. Guideline. Chertsey Surrey.* NHS Ashford and St. Peter's Hospitals.

Almadhoob, A., & Ohlsson, A. (2020). Sound reduction management in the neonatal intensive care unit for preterm and very low birthweight infants. *Cochrane Database of Systematic Reviews, 2020*(1), CD010333. https://doi.org/10.1002/14651858.CD010333.pub3

Altimier, L., & Phillips, R. M. (2013). The neonatal integrative developmental care model: Seven neuroprotective core measures for family-centered developmental Care. *Newborn and Infant Nursing Reviews (NAINR), 13*(1), 9–22.

Altimier, L., & Phillips, R. (2016). The neonatal integrative developmental care model: Advanced clinical applications of the seven core measures for neuroprotective family-centered developmental care. *Newborn & Infant Nursing Reviews (NAINR), 16*(4), 230–244.

Altimier, L., & Phillips, R. (2020). Neonatal diagnostic and care protocols. Neuroprotective interventions. In Kenner, C., Altimier, L., & Boykova, M. V. (Eds). *Comprehensive neonatal nursing care* (6th ed., pp. 963–977). Springer Publishing Company.

Altimier, L. B., & Phillips, R. M. (in press). The neonatal intensive care unit environment. In C. Kenner & M. Boykova, (Eds). *Neonatal nursing care handbook* (3rd ed.). Springer Publishing Company, LLC.

Altimier, L., & White, R. (2020). The NICU environment. In Kenner, C., Altimier, L. B., & Boykova, M. (Eds). *Comprehensive neonatal nursing care* (6th ed., pp. 713–726). Springer Publishing Company, LLC.

Barandouzi, Z. A., Keshavarz, M., Montazeri, A., Ashayeri, H., & Rajaei, Z. (2020). Comparison of the analgesic effect of oral sucrose and/or music in preterm neonates: A double-blind randomized clinical trial. *Complementary Therapies in Medicine, 48*, 102271. https://doi.org/10.1016/j.ctim.2019.102271

Bierlaire, S., Danhaive, O., Carkeek, K., & Piersignilli, F. (2020). How to minimize central line-associated bloodstream infections in a neonatal intensive care unit: A quality improvement intervention based on a retrospective analysis and adoption of an evidence-based bundle. *European Journal of Pediatrics, 180*, 449–460. https://doi.org/10.1007/s00431-020-03844-9

Bigsby, R., & Salisbury, A. (2020). Standard 1, Sleep and Arousal: Intensive care units (ICUs)shall promote developmentally appropriate sleep and arousal states and sleep wake cycles. In Browne, J., Jaeger, C., & on behalf of the Consensus Committee, *Developmental care standards for infants in intensive care. Report of the first consensus conference on standards, competencies, and best practices for infant and family-centered developmental care in the intensive care unit.* https://nicudesign.nd.edu/nicu-care-standards/ifcdc--recommendations-for-best-practice-to-support-sleep-and-arousal/

Blackburn, S. (1998). Environmental impact of the NICU on developmental outcomes. *Journal of Pediatric Nursing, 13*(5), 279–289.

Blackburn, S. T. (2018). *Maternal, fetal, & neonatal physiology: A clinical perspective* (5th ed.). Saunders.

Boggini, T., Pozzoli, S., Schiavolin, P., Erario, R., Mosca, F., Brambilla, P., & Fumagalli, M. (2021). Cumulative procedural pain and brain development in very preterm infants: A systematic review of clinical and preclinical studies. *Neuroscience & Biobehavioral Reviews, 123*, 320–336. https://doi.org/10.1016/j.neubiorev.2020.12.016

Bonacquisti, A., Geller, P. A., & Patterson, C. A. (2020). Maternal depression, anxiety, stress, and maternal-infant attachment in the neonatal intensive care unit. *Journal of Reproductive and Infant Psychology, 38*(3), 297–310. https://doi.org/10.1080/02646838.2019.1695041

Brydges, C. R., Landes, J. K., Reid, C. L., Campbell, C., French, N., & Anderson, M. (2018). Cognitive outcomes in children and adolescents born very preterm: A meta-analysis. *Developmental Medicine & Child Neurology, 60*(5), 452–468.

Chu, H-Y., Chu, S-M., Lin, H-Y., Tsai, M-L., Chen, Y-T., & Lin, H-C. (2020). Evidence base multi-discipline critical strategies toward better tomorrow for very preterm infants. *Pediatric & Neonatology, 61*(4), 371–377.

Cong, X., Wu, J., Vittner, D., Xu, W., Hussain, N., Galvin, S., Fitzsimons, M., McGrath, J. M., Henderson, W. A. (2017). The impact of cumulative pain/stress on neurobehavioral development of preterm infants in the NICU. *Early Human Development, 108*, 9–16.

Davis, J. M., Pursley, D. M., & on behalf of the Pediatric Policy Council. (2020). Preventing long-term respiratory morbidity in preterm neonates: Is there a path forward? *Pediatric Research, 87*, 9–10. https://doi.org/10.1038/s41390-019-0641-z

Dizenberger, G. R., & Blackburn, S. T. (2020). Neurologic system. In Kenner, C., Altimier, L. B., & Boykova, M. V. (Eds). *Comprehensive neonatal nursing care* (pp. 373–416). Springer Publishing Company.

Doede, M., & Trinkoff, A. M. (2020). Emotional work of neonatal nurses in a single-family room NICU. *Journal of Obstetric Gynecologic, & Neonatal Nursing, 49*(3), 283–292.

Feeley, N., Robins, S., Genest, C., Stremler, R., Zelkowitz, P., & Charbonneau, L. (2020). A comparative study of mothers of infants hospitalized in an open ward neonatal intensive care unit and a combined pod and single-family room design. *BMC Pediatrics, 20*, 38. https://doi.org/10.1186/s12887-020-1929-1

Fitri, S. Y. R., Lusmilasari, L., Juffrie, M., & Bellieni, C. V. (2020). Modified sensory stimulation using breastmilk for reducing pain intensity in neonates in Indonesia: A randomized controlled trial. *Journal of Pediatric Nursing, 53*, e199–e203.

Grunau, R. E., Holsti, L., & Peters, J. W. (2006). Long-term consequences of pain in human neonates. *Seminars in Fetal & Neonatal Medicine, 11*(4), 268–275. https://doi.org/10.1016/j.siny.2006.02.007. PMID: 16632415.

Harrison, D., Beggs, S., & Stevens, B. (2012). Sucrose for procedural pain management in infants. *Pediatrics, 130*(5), 918–925.

Hynan, M. T., Cicco, R., & Hatfield, B. (2020). IFCDC-recommendations for best practice reducing & managing pain & stress in newborns & families. In Browne, J., Jaeger, C., & on behalf of the Consensus Committee, (Eds). *Developmental care standards for infants in intensive care. Report of the first consensus conference on standards, competencies, and best practices for infant and family-centered developmental care in the intensive care unit.* https://nicudesign.nd.edu/nicu-care-standards/ifcdc--recommendations-for-best-practice-reducing-managing-pain-stress-in-newborns-families/

Kenner, C., Press, J., & Ryan, D. (2015). Recommendations for palliative and bereavement care in the NICU: A family-centered integrative approach. *Journal of Perinatology, 35*(1), S19–S23.

Kondili, E., & Duryea, D. G. (2019). The role of mother-infant bond in neonatal abstinence syndrome (NAS) management. *Archives of Psychiatric Nursing, 33*(3), 267–274. https://doi.org/10.1016/j.apnu.2019.02.003

Kurt, F. Y., Kucukoglu, S., Ozedmir, A. A., & Ozcan, A. (2020). The effect of kangaroo care on maternal attachment in preterm infants. *Nigerian Journal of Clinical Practice, 23*(1), 26–32.

Lago, P., Cavicchiolo, M. E., Mion, T., Cengio, V. D., Allegro, A., Daverio, M., & Frigo, A. C. (2020). Repeating a dose of sucrose for heel prick procedure in preterms is not effective in reducing pain: A randomised controlled trial. *European Journal of Pediatrics, 179*, 293–301.

Lavalle, A., Clifford-Faugere, G. D., Ballard, A., & Aita, M. (2021). Parent-infant interventions to promote parental sensitivity during NICU hospitalization: Systematic Review and Meta-Analysis. *Journal of Early Intervention,* https://doi.org/10.1177/1053815121991928

Lodha, A., Dobry, J. L., & Premji, S. S. (2020). Extremely low birth weight infant (ELBW). In Kenner, C., Altimier, L. B., & Boykova, M. V. (Eds). *Comprehensive neonatal nursing care* (pp. 631–654). Springer Publishing Company.

Lopez-Maestro, M., De Al Cruz, J., Perapoch-Lopez, J., Gimeno-Navarro, A., Vazquez-Roman, S., Alonso-Diaz, C., Munoz-Amat, B., Morales-Betancourt, C., Soriano-Ramos, M., & Pallas-Alonso, C. (2019). Eight principles for newborn care in neonatal units: Findings from a national survey. *Acta Paediatrica, 109*(7), 1361–1368.

Marc-Aurele, K. L., & English, N. K. (2017). Primary palliative care in neonatal intensive care. *Seminars in Perinatology, 41*(2), 133–139. https://doi.org/10.1053/j.semperi.2016.11.005. PMID: 28162789.

Marzouk, S. A., Hussien, A. A., & Aziz, S. M. A. (2019). Effectiveness of cycled lighting in neonatal intensive care unit on weight and cardiorespiratory function in preterm infants. *International Journal of Paediatrics and Geriatrics, 2*(1), 18–24.

Morag, I., & Ohlsson, A. (2016). Cycled light in the intensive care unit for preterm and low birth weight infants. *The Cochrane Database of Systematic Reviews, 2016*(8), CD006982. https://doi.org/10.1002/14651858.CD006982.pub4

Morgan, A. S., Khoshnood, B., Diguisto, C., l'Helias, L. F., Marchand-Martin, L., Kaminski, M., Zeitlin, J., Breart, G., Goffinet, F., & Ancel, P-Y. (2020). Intensity of perinatal care for extremely preterm babies and outcomes at a higher gestational age: Evidence from the EPIPAGE-2 cohort study. *BMC Pediatrics, 20*, 8. https://doi.org/10.1186/s12887-019-1856-1

Mu, P-F., Lee, M-Y., Chen, Y-C., Yang, H-C., & Yang, S-H. (2019). Experiences of parents providing kangaroo care to a premature infant: A qualitative systematic review. *Nursing & Health Sciences, 22*(2), 149–161.

Myrhaug, H. T., Brurberg, K. G., Hov, L., & Markestad, T. (2019). Survival and impairment of extremely premature infants: A meta-analysis. *Pediatrics, 143*(2), e20180933 https://doi.org/10.1542/peds.2018-0933

Nimbalkar, S., Shukla, V. V., Chauhan, V., Phatak, A., Patel, D., Chapla, A., & Nimbalkar, A. (2020). Blinded randomized crossover trial: Skin-to-skin care vs. sucrose for preterm neonatal pain. *Journal of Perinatology, 40*, 896–901.

Panza, R., Laforgia, N., Bellos, I., & Pandita, A. (2020). Systematic review found that using thin catheters to deliver surfactant to preterm neonates was associated with reduced bronchopulmonary dysplasia and mechanical ventilation. *Acta Paediatrica, 109*(11), 2219–2225.

Pearlman, S. A. (2020). Quality improvement to reduce neonatal CLABSI: The journey to zero. *American Journal of Perinatology, 37*(suppl 2), S14–S17.

Quinn, M., Weiss, A. B., & Crist, J. D. (2020). Early for everyone: reconceptualizing palliative care in the neonatal intensive care unit. *Advances in Neonatal Care, 20*(2), 109–117. https://doi.org/10.1097/ANC.0000000000000707. PMID: 31990696.

Rodriguez-Fanjul, J., Balaguer, J. M., Batista-Munoz, A., Ramon, M., & Bobillo-Perez, S. (2020). Early surfactant replacement guided by lung ultrasound in preterm newborns with RDS: The ULTRASURF randomized controlled trial. *European Journal of Pediatrics, 179*, 1913–1920.

Sen, E., & Manav, G. (2020). Effect of kangaroo care and oral sucrose on pain in premature infants: A randomized controlled trial. *Pain Management Nursing, 21*, 556–564. https://doi.org/10.1016/j.pmn.2020.05.003. PMID: 32768272.

Smith, G. C., Gutovich, J., Smyser, C., Pindeda, R., Newnham, C., Tjoeng, T. H., Vavasseur, C., Wallendorf, M., Neil, J., Inder, T. (2011). Neonatal intensive care unit stress is associated with brain development in preterm infants. *Annals of Neurology, 70*(4), 541–549.

Smith, S. W., Ortmann, A. J., & Clark, W. W. (2018). Noise in the neonatal intensive care unit: A new approach to examining acoustic events. *Noise Health, 20*(5), 121–130.

Soghier, L. M., Kritikos, K. I., Carty, C. L., Glass, P., Tuchman, L. K., Streisand, R., & Fratantoni, K. R. (2020). Parental depression symptoms at neonatal intensive care unit discharge and associated risk factors. *The Journal of Pediatrics, 227*, 163. https://doi.org/10.1016/j.jpeds.2020.07.040

Tham, E. K., Schneider, N., & Broekman, B. F. (2017). Infant sleep and its relation with cognition and growth: a narrative review. *Nature and Science of Sleep, 9*, 135–149. https://doi.org/10.2147/NSS.S125992. PMID: 28553151; PMCID: PMC5440010.

Vittner, D., Butler, S., Smith, K., Makris, N., Brownell, E., Samra, H., & McGrath, J. (2019). Parent engagement correlates with parent and preterm infant oxytocin release during skin-to-skin contact. *Advances in Neonatal Care, 19*(1), 73–79. https://doi.org/10.1097/ANC.0000000000000558

Von Dolinger de Brito, D., de Almeida Silva, H., Jose Oliveira, E., Arantes, A., Abdallah, V. O., Tannus Jorge, M., & Gontijo Filho, P. P. (2007). Effect of neonatal intensive care unit environment on the incidence of hospital-acquired infection in neonates. *The Journal of Hospital Infection, 65*(4), 314–318. https://doi.org/10.1016/j.jhin.2006.01.038. PMID: 17350722.

White, R., & on behalf of the Consensus Committee, . (2019). *NICU Recommended standards for newborn intensive care unit design* (9th ed.). https://nicudesign.nd.edu/nicu-standards/

Williams, M. D., & Lascelles, B. D. X. (2020). Early neonatal pain-a review of clinical and experimental implications on painful conditions later in life. *Frontiers in Pediatrics, 8*, 30. https://doi.org/10.3389/fped.2020.00030

Wolfe, K., & Ralls, F. M. (2019). Rapid eye movement sleep and neuronal development. *Current Opinion in Pulmonary Medicine, 25*(6), 555–560.

Yadav, M., Chauhan, G., Bhardwaj, A. K., & Sharma, P. D. (2018). Clinicoetiological pattern and outcome of neonates requiring ventilation: Study in a tertiary care centre. *Indian Journal of Critical Care Medicine, 22*(5), 261–363.

Zhou, Y. F., Luo, J. Y., Quan, Q. H., Li, Y. M., Jiang, H., & Fu, K. (2020). Analysis of incidence and risk factors of neonatal ventilator associated pneumonia in a hospital in Hunan Province, 216-2018). *Zhonghua Yu Fang Yi Xue Za Zhi, 54*(8), 822–827.

CHAPTER 6

Single-Family Room Design in the Neonatal Intensive Care Unit

Leslie B. Altimier and Robert D. White

IFCDC—Standard for Systems Thinking in Collaborative Practice

Standard 1: Systems Thinking

- The intensive care unit shall exhibit an infrastructure of leadership, mission, and a governance framework to guide the performance of the collaborative practice of IFCDC.

INTRODUCTION

Infants born as early as 22 weeks' gestation now have a chance of survival in part due to technologic advances. This progress comes with great costs as premature infants are in the neonatal intensive care unit (NICU) for many weeks or months, and many have impaired short- and long-term outcomes. The NICU is where an extraordinary period of growth and development will take place for premature infants. Because the infant is no longer protected in the uterus, their physiologic and neuroprotective needs have dramatically changed. Overstimulation and sensory deprivation in this population can be resilient and fragile simultaneously. The challenge is complex—not only are we unable to fully replicate the in utero environment, there are also reasons to believe that this is not always the most appropriate practice. Just as the patent ductus serves an important purpose in utero but is a medical handicap after birth, continuation of the sensory environment found in utero can be disadvantageous to neurodevelopment of the preterm infant ex utero (White, 2018).

The neonatal environment of care has a lasting impact on the patients, families, and caregivers who experience it. The NICU, unfortunately, is a replacement for the intrauterine environment during the third trimester and early fourth trimester and a home away from home for many newly expanded families (White, 2020a). Changing a "typical" NICU environment into one that is more healing encompasses the physical environment, the people in that environment, and the infant's sensory environment (Altimier, 2015b). All sensory stimuli carry social and emotional connections and characteristics. Adverse environmental sensory insults can significantly interfere with health, appropriate neurodevelopment, and neuroprocessing, resulting in lifelong alterations in brain development and function

(Aldrete-Cortez et al., 2021; Dumont et al., 2017; Lejeune et al., 2019b; Lejeune et al., 2016; Maitre et al., 2017).

Early NICUs were highly restrictive for parents, and parental viewing through a window was the norm. Most practitioners agree that moving from the old "baby barn" or open-bay room (OBR) configuration to private rooms has been initiated first and foremost to create individualized environments in which outcomes for hospitalized premature or critically ill newborns can be optimized. Some may argue that the needs of families and caregivers come secondary; however, given the disparate needs of infants, families, and caregivers, a strong case has been made for individualizing the environment in which the infant and family now live. Single-patient room and single-family room (SFR) NICUs are increasingly being adopted because they allow for this individualization and have demonstrated improved environmental and clinical outcomes in infants (Soleimani et al., 2020). This chapter discusses the implications of SFR design in the NICU by describing current knowledge about the physical NICU environment, the people in that environment, and the infant's sensory environment along with methods to optimize outcomes for infants, families, and staff.

PARTNERING WITH FAMILIES

A family partnership begins wherever and whenever a family enters the healthcare system and continues throughout the hospitalization to discharge. Families should encounter this philosophy of care before birth in antenatal care, continue it into the delivery room, and beyond into the postpartum period. Outcomes have shown that parents who are able to directly partner with the multidisciplinary NICU team develop stronger parenting skills and greater confidence and are better prepared emotionally to care for their infants when discharged home (Bracht et al., 2013; O'Brien et al., 2013).

In NICUs across the nation, true collaboration and shared decision-making with families in the care of their baby has yet to become a fully embraced standard of care. The overwhelming and often traumatic experience of being the parent of a critically ill infant can preclude such collaboration (Coughlin, 2021; D'Agata et al., 2018). Because of the high rates of developmental consequences among prematurely born children, attention is shifting to modifiable aspects of the NICU environment, including family partnerships, which can optimize developmental outcomes (Ludwig & Welch, 2019, 2020; Porges et al., 2019; Welch et al., 2020). The provision of neuroprotective, family-centered developmentally supportive care in a collaborative environment goes a step beyond the concept of family-centered care (FCC), which in its definition holds central the needs of both patients and families.

Collaborative environments are concerned not only with patients and families but also with the needs of the entire healthcare team. Staff needs include physical surroundings that, if properly designed (ergometric designs), may help reduce fatigue and stress; increase the effectiveness of care delivered; improve patient safety; and improve outcomes for infants, families, and staff. When designing a collaborative environment, the needs of staff, families, and infants are all of equal importance.

True family-centered developmental care in the NICU results in improved neonatal and neurodevelopmental outcomes, increased family satisfaction, and even enhanced employee satisfaction once the transitional cultural change is established (Als et al., 1994, 2004; Bergman, 2019a, 2019b; Bergman et al., 2019; Darcy Mahoney et al., 2020; Dittman & Hughes, 2018; Franck et al., 2020; Klawetter et al., 2019; Pineda et al., 2018; Pisoni et al., 2021). However, implementing known principles of family-centered developmental care into the NICU and creating the necessary culture changes have often been fraught with internal and external challenges (Cardin et al., 2015; Malik et al., 2015; Mörelius et al., 2020; Phillips, 2015).

When the framework of FCC is the foundation for compassionate caregiving, the family is visible, available, and supportive of their infant's needs because they are an integral aspect of every decision that affects their child, even if not present at the bedside 24 hours a day, just like any other member of the health professional team (Craig et al., 2015; Miyagishima et al., 2017). Actively fostering family involvement rather than passively accepting the mere presence of families in the NICU is a fundamental component of collaborative caregiving that supports the full integration of neuroprotective, family-centered partnerships (Altimier & Holditch-Davis, 2020; Altimier & White, 2020; Boyle & Altimier, 2019; Bruton et al., 2018; Namprom et al., 2020; Phillips, 2020). While admission to the NICU may temporarily shift some of the caregiving responsibilities, it does not negate the importance of a parent's lifelong role in their child's overall health and development (French & Altimier, 2020; French & French, 2016; Niela-Vilén et al., 2017). It is important to note that families are not replaceable

at any level in the overall development of the child (Whitehead et al., 2018).

Compassionately delivered FCC with zero separation and where skin-to-skin contact (SSC) is the norm is currently seen as the ideal model of care to encourage parental involvement, attachment, and bonding, as well as to create partnerships with the healthcare team (Altimier, 2015a, 2015b; Altimier & White, 2020; Bergman, 2015, 2019a, 2019b; Bergman et al., 2019).

A study investigated staff and parental views about SFR care following the move to an SFR-designed NICU. Results demonstrated improvements in the staffs' quality of work life and parental rankings of "family satisfaction" at each measured interval, prior to the move and two times following the move (Watson et al., 2014). Another study evaluating the perspectives of staff regarding SFR design revealed that single private rooms improved the quality of the work environment, improved the quality of the treatment environment, and increased safety for parents. They also noted a reduction in workplace stress for staff, while demonstrating an increase in family privacy (Bosch et al., 2012). Stevens et al. also demonstrated an improvement in noise and light control, as well as staff and parental satisfaction in SFRs (Stevens et al., 2015).

PHYSICAL ENVIRONMENT

The evolution from an FCC philosophy to one that supports collaborative environments for families and providers is due in part to recognition of the importance of the physical environment in which infants, families, and healthcare providers interact. The physical environment of older traditionally designed NICUs often is identified as an obstacle to the practice of FCC and developmentally supportive care for infants and is usually less than ideal in efficiency, health, and the well-being of caregivers. Creating a physical space that supports the needs of developmentally fragile infants, promotes the role of the family, and supports caregivers is the ultimate goal of creating collaborative environments. There are several key attributes of a collaborative environment that need to be considered when designing an NICU; they include the need for (1) privacy; (2) social interaction and support; (3) comfort and image; (4) functionality; and (5) core value of quality care. Each is described in more detail below.

KEY ATTRIBUTES OF A COLLABORATIVE ENVIRONMENT

Privacy

Provision of privacy is considered an essential attribute of a collaborative environment. It is important for families to bond with their newborn while learning about their condition and providing care in a private and intimate environment. By providing a sense of ownership and privacy in each infant area, families have better opportunities to participate in their infant's care. It has been shown that an increase of parental involvement in caring for their baby(s), as well as an increase in privacy, creates a positive attitude toward SFRs among parents (Gerhardsson et al., 2018). Incorporating SFR design into NICUs allows parents to "parent in private" versus "parent in public," which supports those first intimate moments of touching, stroking, singing, exploring, and experiencing emotion. An SFR design with supportive staff can encourage overnight stays by parents, which extends private time for parents and infants and increases the opportunity for parents to engage in developing their baby's plan of care. SFR design is thought to enhance opportunities for hands-on care and parents' recognition of infant cues and temperament. SFR design also increases opportunities for SSC/kangaroo care or feedings by breast or bottle. Even with the best-designed SFR NICU, simply designing SFRs does not guarantee a collaborative environment that best meets the needs of families.

Methods to further support privacy in the SFR NICU include closing doors to infant rooms and the use of privacy curtains. Dual privacy curtains can be used: one at the door to promote privacy while parents are up and moving about in the room and a second curtain between the family zone and infant care zone to allow privacy while a parent is resting or sleeping. When families are not in the room, doors may be left open, depending on the lability of the infant (Shepley et al., 2008).

The impact of early life development on later child health and development is well recognized (Santos et al., 2015). Preliminary evidence suggests that the type of NICU design may influence environmental exposures during a crucial period of brain development, which can lead to long-term health implications. A well-designed NICU has the potential to improve developmental outcomes and reduce chronic illness (Lehtonen et al., 2020; Shepley et al., 2014).

SFRs allow mothers to be present around the clock to provide SSC/kangaroo care, express milk, and breast-feed in privacy whenever they want, including during the night. Studies demonstrate that SFRs are associated with earlier initiation of expressing milk, increased milk volumes, increased breast-feeding attempts, increased breast-feeding rates among preterm infants, increased feeding of mothers' own milk, and mothers exclusively breast-feeding to a greater extent until 4 months corrected age (Grundt et al., 2020; Sharma et al., 2019; van Veenendaal et al., 2020; Vohr, 2017). Among infants who require NICU care, breast milk feeding is associated with better cognitive development; fewer rehospitalizations; greater brain volume and white matter; and lower rates of sepsis, retinopathy of prematurity, and necrotizing enterocolitis (Belfort et al., 2016; Blesa et al., 2019; Lechner & Vohr, 2017; Lefmann, 2020; Spiegler, 2016). Breast-feeding self-efficacy, or how capable a mother feels about her ability to breast-feed, is a predictor of breast-feeding duration in mothers of NICU infants (Gerhardsson et al., 2018). SFR mothers also perceived their infant's readiness for discharge to be greater than open-bay mothers (Feeley et al., 2020).

SFR NICUs have also shown benefits such as reductions in costly hospital-acquired infections (HAIs) (Domanico et al., 2011; Julian et al., 2015; Lester et al., 2014; Ortenstrand et al., 2010), shorter length of stay (LOS) (O'Callaghan et al., 2010), improved neonatal morbidity and mortality rates (Lehtonen et al., 2020; Stevens at al., 2015), and lower direct costs of care compared to OBR NICUs (Sadatsafavi et al., 2019; Stevens et al., 2014).

Social Interaction and Support

A second attribute of a collaborative environment is social interaction and support. It is important to encourage interactions and partnerships between families and caregivers to foster communication. Space must be provided for educational purposes and to promote parent-to-parent and staff-to-staff interaction.

The Recommended Standards for Newborn ICU Design (ninth edition) stress the importance of having a clearly identified entrance and reception area for families, with immediate and direct contact with staff as they arrive. Facilitating parental contact immediately with staff enhances the security for infants in the NICU (White, 2020b). The design of this area should contribute to positive first impressions for families and foster the concept that families are important members of their infant's healthcare team, not visitors (Knudson, 2017) (see Figure 6-1).

First impressions of the NICU room can be designed to be welcoming, respectful, and encouraging to families so that they experience an environment where they can develop confidence and competence in their role as parents and in caring for their infants. The critical care environment can be intimidating to families and convey subtle or not-so-subtle messages that parents do not have a significant role in the care of and decision-making for their infant and that others are in control.

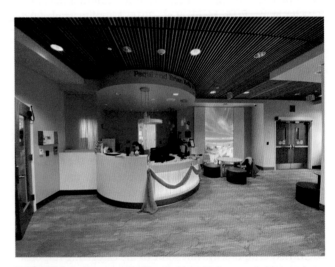

FIGURE 6-1. Beacon Children's Hospital neonatal intensive care unit entrance. (Used with permission from Beacon Children's Hospital (Memorial Hospital of South Bend), NICU.)

Family support space is also considered integral in the design of an NICU. Families of premature or critically ill newborns may experience hospitalizations that extend for weeks and months. Family support space is a space that provides for a variety of functions, including eating, toileting, showering, learning, diversional activities, access to the internet, telephones, and a locked space for valuables; all of these features facilitate parental presence and interaction (White, 2016). The physical environment in all of its aspects of space, structure, millwork, furniture, materials, flow, signage, and art has great potential to set a positive tone and invitation for families to be partners in the care of their infants (Johnson & Abraham, 2020).

Family presence and participation in bedside rounds has been lauded as a key component of family partnerships and knowledge exchange between healthcare providers and families. For most parents, the experience of participation on medical rounds helps them be less worried and anxious about their child. Nurses frequently comment that parents appear less anxious after participating in rounds (Grzyb et al., 2014). Through the development and implementation of a comprehensive multidisciplinary rounds (MDRs) quality initiative, Smith and Carver (2017) demonstrated improved parent and staff satisfaction scores in the areas of communication, teamwork, efficiency, and quality. Discharge planning during MDRs contributed to a decreased LOS (Smith & Carver, 2017).

Comfort and Image

A third attribute for a collaborative environment is attention to comfort and image, which entails providing a range of services that are appropriate for the long and stressful hours spent by both staff and families in the NICU. As single-room units are increasingly being built, they provide larger and more private spaces for families to be present and participate in their infant's care, but they also can be overwhelming and feel institutional. Many hospitals integrate themes and art that reflect the natural environment to improve wayfinding as well as create a comforting environment for families. Many SFR NICUs have incorporated "positive distraction" into unit design, notably with access to nature, to mitigate stress (Shepley et al., 2014).

Reducing light levels facilitates rest and subsequent energy conservation for the infant, as well as promotes organization and growth (Altimier, 2015b; Altimier & White, 2020; White, 2020b). Continuous bright lights in the NICU, however, can disrupt sleep–wake states, and any event, process, or drug that disrupts rapid eye movement (REM) sleep may disrupt the organization of the eye cells, structures, and connections. A Cochrane review (Morag & Ohlsson, 2013) showed that cycled lighting provided benefits compared to either continuous bright or continuous dim lighting, yet the control of light levels in many NICUs continues to be influenced more by inertia and opinion than "evidence" (White, 2020c). In the absence of compelling data, NICUs that support the continued practice of keeping babies in continuous dim lighting until the time of their discharge should change their practice, at least for infants who have passed their most critical stage of care (White, 2020c).

Preterm infants exposed to music interventions have demonstrated significantly improved white matter maturation as well as larger amygdala volumes. These results suggest a structural maturational effect of a music intervention on premature infants' auditory and emotional processing neural pathways during a key period of brain development (Sa de Almeida et al., 2020). Systematic music interactions paired with positive touch reduce hyperresponsiveness due to neurologic immaturity. This neuroprotective intervention resulted in earlier discharge of 7 to 10 days on average (Hamm et al., 2017). NICU music therapists (MTs) often provide services to parents and involve them in developmental care of their child (Dearn & Shoemark, 2014; Emery et al., 2019). An NICU MT is highly effective in reducing parental stress, enhancing parent/infant attachment, and training parents to reduce overstimulation of their infant (Detmer, 2017, 2019). A systematic review reported benefits of music therapy such as improved care, reduced time to reach discharge weight, calmer infants, more stable physiologic measures, increased oxygen saturation levels, faster weight gain, improved development, enhanced mother–infant bonding, increased nonnutritive sucking, improved feeding abilities, shortened NICU LOS, and reduced medical costs (Standley & Gutierrez, 2020).

One of the most important skills an infant must exhibit prior to discharge from the NICU is self-regulation, including a mature and stable cardiorespiratory function. In a well-designed NICU, self-regulation is more easily enhanced. For example, a music-enhanced version of the auditory, tactile, visual, and vestibular protocol, multimodal neurological enhancement (MMNE), was developed to evaluate its ability to stimulate and reinforce premature infants' acquisition of developmental behaviors in sensory, social, and motor skills. In one randomized-controlled trial, the MMNE was found to help infants achieve self-regulation (Cevasco-Trotter et al., 2019).

Functionality

A fourth attribute of a collaborative environment is functionality. Unit design should reflect a highly functional, accessible, and flexible environment. Since the first notion of applying the single-patient room concept to the neonatal care environment, caregivers for critically ill neonates have expressed concerns. In open-bay units, caregivers felt they had the ability to see and hear infants at all times and could work as a team, coming to each other's aid at a moment's notice. Concerns about isolating staff and decreasing their ability to collaborate quickly and socialize can become realities if careful attention is not given to these issues when designing an NICU.

In today's healthcare setting, the emphasis on providing high-quality care while remaining efficient and fiscally astute is paramount. There is a heightened public awareness of medical errors. The high-tech, high-stress, high-acuity, and highly emotional environment of the NICU compounds the potential for human error. A poorly designed NICU that fails to recognize the need for staff participation in unit design to ensure functionality and disregards the importance of social networking spaces, ergonomics, and workflow may later pay a price in high turnover rates, increased errors due to stress or fatigue, or serious sequelae as a result of a failure to recognize and rescue an infant in need.

Core Values of Quality Care

A fifth attribute in achieving a collaborative environment is the overall well-being of staff members. Collaborative environments feature the core values of quality care, nurse autonomy, informal and nonrigid verbal communication, innovation, bringing out the best in each individual, and striving for excellence. The nursing workforce is aging with fewer students entering nursing school. Experienced nurses often find themselves managing large patient workloads due to staffing shortages and staffing with less experienced nurses. The combination of larger workloads and working with greater inexperienced nurses leads to tension, stress, dissatisfaction, and change fatigue (Edmonson et al., 2021; McMillan & Perron, 2020). *Change fatigue* is a newer term, understood as the overwhelming feelings of stress, exhaustion, and burnout fueled by feelings of ambivalence and powerlessness associated with rapid and continuous change in the workplace. Nurses experience many of the core elements of change fatigue including exhaustion, apathy, powerlessness, and burnout (McMillan & Perron, 2020).

Healthcare staffs also, regardless of whom they are treating, have high levels of stress and may be dealing with preexisting mental health issues (Gönülal et al., 2014). Neonatal nurses caring for medically unstable infants and parents under duress have been associated with an increased risk for occupational stress and burnout. NICU nurses report greater fatigue, anxiety, and symptoms of depression than nurses on general wards, indicating that burnout in neonatal nurses remains a significant problem (Fujimaru et al., 2012; Profit et al., 2014; Tawfik et al., 2017). These are important concerns because they occur along with other challenging working conditions, including heavy workloads, time pressures, and staffing inadequacies that are associated with lower care quality, missed care, adverse events, and HAIs for patients (Lake et al., 2020; Rochefort & Clarke, 2010; Rochefort et al., 2016).

A primary nursing goal is to promote adaptive responses that positively affect health. In a collaborative environment model, the goal is the same—to create a microenvironment for the developing infant that best meets their needs and a macroenvironment that embraces family participation and to create a nursing work environment that is supportive and promotes core values such as empowerment, pride, mentoring, nurturing, respect, integrity, and teamwork.

NICU RECOMMENDED DESIGN STANDARDS

A NICU is typically in use for 10 to 30 years, over which time decisions made during its design will have human and financial impacts far beyond the initial cost (White, 2020b). Careful planning and collaboration when designing a new NICU can avoid pitfalls and bring benefit to babies, families, and caregivers alike (Soleimani et al., 2020; Thompson et al., 2020; White, 2020a, 2020b).

The information disseminated by the Consensus Committee on NICU Recommended Design Standards for Advanced Neonatal Care helps guide many decision makers who create micro- and macrocare environments for critically ill or premature newborns (https://nicudesign.nd.edu/) (White, 2020b). These standards are the result of the ongoing efforts of many people representing a multitude of professions, including healthcare professionals, architects, interior designers, state healthcare facility regulators, and parents, and are based on clinical expertise science. The NICU Recommended Design Standards, now in their ninth edition, are intended to provide entities that write standards and those that utilize them to benefit from the collective expertise of experts from all relevant fields of NICU design (White, 2020b). The full NICU Recommended Design Standards are available online at https://nicudesign.nd.edu/; however, we will discuss several standards related to single-patient rooms, SFRs, and extended family rooms (EFR) designed to provide a trending model of care—NICU couplet care (White, 2020b).

SINGLE-FAMILY ROOM

A focus on infant development and recognition of the importance of providing neuroprotective, family-centered developmentally supportive care to premature and ill newborns has characterized care delivery models in many NICUs around the world. While the term *single-patient room design* denotes one patient per room, the term *SFR design* may have subtle differences denoting not only one patient per room but also for a designated "family space" for parents to stay with their infant around the clock (see Figure 6-2). Within the neonatal intensive care environment, facilities may provide parents the opportunity to live in the NICU along with their infant(s) throughout the entire hospitalization. Designated "family space" may include a reclining chair suitable for breast-feeding or kangaroo care or a sleep surface for families. As discussed earlier, there is a paucity of research over the past decade related to benefits and outcomes of implementing SFR design in NICUs. Strong evidence demonstrating that SFRs lead to improved outcomes, reduced costs, and improved parent and staff satisfaction exists. *Standard 1* is a requirement that has been added to the ninth edition of the NICU Recommended Design Standards, which states

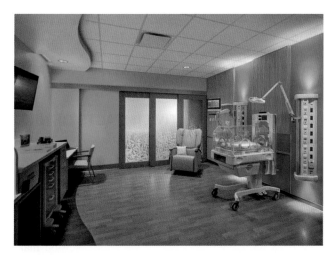

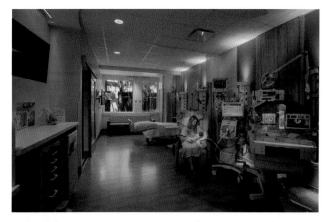

FIGURE 6-2. Single-family room at Beacon Children's Hospital, South Bend, Indiana, USA. (Used with permission from Beacon Children's Hospital (Memorial Hospital of South Bend), NICU.)

FIGURE 6-3. Extended family room (neonatal intensive care for two) at Beacon Children's Hospital, South Bend, Indiana, USA. (Used with permission from Beacon Children's Hospital (Memorial Hospital of South Bend), NICU.)

that units be designed with a sufficient number of SFRs to meet the needs of parents who wish to stay with their babies. There is also evidence that parents are the "active ingredient" to achieve improved outcomes and that placing a baby in a private room when the family is rarely present may be detrimental. These babies may be better cared for in OBRs (White, 2020b).

Expanding on the SFR model, EFRs are now trending in order to encourage zero separation between the infant and mother by coupling the care of the infant with the care of the newly delivered mother (White, 2010, 2020b). EFRs are designed with two or three bed positions intended for multiple purposes, one for multiples to stay together and another of which is couplet care (White, 2016). Couplet care begins as soon as mother is released from the labor and delivery room or recovery room and her baby is ready for transfer to the NICU from the stabilization area. Both mother and baby are admitted to an EFR so that couplet care can be established. The guiding principle of couplet care is to keep mother and baby together after delivery, even if the baby requires intensive care (White, 2016). The benefits of couplet care include early maternal attachment, skin-to-skin care, access to breast milk, and participation in care, among others. This model provides a platform for staff to consider the interdependent needs of the mother and infant(s) as a couplet in addition to each patient's individual needs. Because of the demonstrated importance of couplet care and the subsequent increase in family presence and participation, a new NICU Recommended Design *Standard (8)* recommendation was established so that design guidelines be created for couplet care rooms when they are included in the functional program (White, 2020b).

Couplet care has been practiced out of necessity for many years in resource-limited areas, but its introduction in the Western world occurred in Swedish centers in Stockholm

and Uppsala. In the United States, the first to adopt this concept was Beacon Children's Hospital in South Bend, IN, under the direction of Dr. Robert White. Rather than EFR, they coined the term *NIC2* (neonatal intensive care for two). In designing, planning, and building of the new NICU at Beacon Children's Hospital, every aspect of the environment, signage, and art was planned to encourage keeping parents and infants together (see Figure 6-3).

An atrium located in the center of the unit was built using themes of nature and access to natural light to provide respite to families and children (see Figure 6-4). Many researchers have found that views of nature and art capturing scenes of nature are positive distractions and are calming, healing, and restorative. Whichever type of private room model is chosen, there should be a focus on attention to

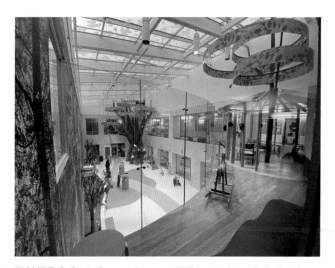

FIGURE 6-4. Atrium at Beacon Children's Hospital, South Bend, Indiana, USA. (Used with permission from Beacon Children's Hospital (Memorial Hospital of South Bend), NICU.)

privacy, social interaction and support, elements of comfort, and images that are congruent with the mission of a collaborative environment.

SPACE

NICU Design Standard 6 states that each infant space shall contain a minimum of 150 ft² (14 m²) of clear floor space, excluding handwashing stations, columns, and aisles. Within this space, there shall be sufficient furnishing to allow a parent to stay seated, reclined, or fully recumbent at the bedside. There shall be an aisle adjacent to each infant space with a minimum width of 4 ft (1.2 m) in multiple bedrooms. When single-infant rooms or fixed cubicle partitions are utilized in the NICU design, there shall be an adjacent aisle of not less than 8 ft (2.4 m) in clear and unobstructed width to permit passage of equipment and personnel (White, 2020b).

Open-bay units or areas to house multiple babies shall have a minimum of 8 ft (2.4 m) between infant beds. There shall be provision for visual privacy for each bed, and the design shall support speech privacy at a distance of 12 ft (3.6 m). The requirement for clear floor space at each infant bed has been increased to 150 ft², with the rationale that experience and space diagrams have shown that family space is compromised with the previous minimum standard of 120 ft². These numbers are minimums and often need to be increased to reflect the complexity of care rendered, bedside space needed for parenting and family involvement in care, and privacy for families (White, 2020b).

NICU Standard 7: Private (Single-Family) Rooms: The minimum size requirement for SFRs has been increased to 180 ft², and language has been added to specify that adequate space must be provided for SSC, breast-feeding, and pumping. The interpretation section has been expanded to include further guidance on the parent sleep space. The rationale for this is that experience and space diagrams have shown that family space is compromised with the previous minimum standard. Private SFRs improve the ability to provide individualized private environments for each baby and family when compared to multipatient rooms or OBRs. In order to provide adequate space at the bedside for both caregivers and families, however, these rooms need to be somewhat larger than an infant space in an open-bay, multipatient room, and they must have additional bedside storage and communication capabilities in order to avoid isolation or excessive walking by caregivers. A sleep surface for a second parent, bathroom, shower, and lockable storage for parents should be provided whenever possible (White, 2020b).

While sleep space for two parents is recommended, if that sleep space is part of the infant's room, parents may not always experience good quality sleep due to noise and staff activity. Since parents are already at risk for mental health issues related to their infant's hospitalization, protecting the quality of their sleep is important. Consider separating the infant space from the parent sleep space if possible or providing additional sleep space elsewhere on campus for parents.

The goal of providing sleep space for parents is to remove barriers to their participation and to facilitate attachment, but that should not be done at the expense of their well-being. Parents should feel invited to stay, not compelled to stay (White, 2020b).

POSITIVE AND NEGATIVE IMPACTS OF NICU ROOM TYPES

Although most studies have reported beneficial effects associated with SFR NICUs (Domanico et al., 2011; Lester et al., 2014; Stevens et al., 2011; Stevens et al., 2010), negative effects have also been reported (Pineda et al., 2012, 2014; Stevens et al., 2012).

BENEFITS OF SFR DESIGN

Lester et al. (2014) compared medical and neurobehavioral outcomes at NICU discharge between infants cared for in an open-bay and SFR NICU. Statistically significant results (all $p < .05$) showed that infants in the SFR NICU had a greater rate of weight gain, weighed more at discharge, required fewer medical procedures, had a lower gestational age at full enteral feed, had less sepsis, showed better attention, had less physiologic stress, had less hypertonicity, had less lethargy, and had less pain. The rate of weight gain, weight at discharge, and the difference in attention were mediated by increased developmental support; differences in number of medical procedures were mediated by increased maternal involvement. Differences in stress and pain were mediated by maternal involvement, and nurses reported a more positive work environment and better attitudes in the SFR NICU. This well-designed 4-year longitudinal, prospective, quasiexperimental cohort study, in short, demonstrated that SFRs are associated with improved neurobehavioral and medical outcomes and these improvements are related to increased developmental support and maternal involvement (Lester et al., 2014). In a follow-up study of infants cared for in an SFR NICU, high maternal involvement was associated with improved 18-month neurodevelopmental outcomes (Lester et al., 2016).

Another study compared emotional distress in the form of depression, anxiety, stress, and attachment scores among parents of very preterm infants cared for in a SFRs versus OBRs. Mothers in the SFRs had a significantly lower depression score from birth to 4 months corrected age compared to mothers in the open-bay unit. Both mothers and fathers in the SFRs reported significantly lower stress levels during hospitalization (Tandberg et al., 2019). Comparing the presence of parents in SFR NICUs versus OBR NICUs, it was demonstrated that parents were present 21 hours/day in SFRs versus 7 hours/day in the OBRs (Tandberg et al., 2019). Soleimani (2020) demonstrated that infants cared for in SFRs also had higher maternal involvement and had higher language and Bayley scores compared to those with lower maternal involvement. Similarly, the LOS was shorter with higher maternal involvement. The chance of infants demonstrating symptoms of autism was higher in the OBR NICU with lower maternal involvement. In general, the findings of this study demonstrated improvements in neurodevelopmental outcomes in infants benefiting from higher maternal involvement (Soleimani et al., 2020).

A variety of studies reveal substantial benefits to babies, families, and staff with SFR design such as:

- Decrease length of hospital stay (Castellucci, 2019; Mack, 2015; Ortenstrand et al., 2010; Puumala et al., 2020; Sadatsafavi et al., 2019)

- Decreased bronchopulmonary dysplasia (Ortenstrand et al., 2010)

- Decreased apnea (Domanico et al., 2011; Weisman et al., 2011)

- Decreased infections (Lester et al., 2014; Puumala et al., 2020; van Veenendaal et al., 2020)

- Increased breast-feeding or provision of human milk (Jones et al., 2016; Vohr et al., 2017)

- Improved neurodevelopmental outcomes (Lester et al., 2014; Lester et al., 2016; Puumala et al., 2020)

- Improved cognitive and language scores (Lester et al., 2016; Vohr et al., 2017b)

- Improved sleep (Levy et al., 2017; Loewy et al., 2013)

- Improved environmental controls (Almadhoob & Ohlsson, 2020; Cheong et al., 2020; Venkataraman et al., 2018)

- Increased parental presence (Abouelfettoh et al., 2011; Lester et al., 2016; Vohr, 2019; Zauche et al., 2020)

- Improved staff and parental satisfaction (Broom et al., 2019; Feeley et al., 2019; Watson et al., 2014)

- Decreased medication errors (Chaudhury et al., 2009; Montgomery et al., 2021; Tubbs-Cooley et al., 2015)

- Decreased readmissions (Shahheidari & Homer, 2012)

- Decreased costs (Ortenstrand et al., 2010; Sadatsafavi et al., 2019; Shepley et al., 2014; Soleimani et al., 2020; Stevens et al., 2014)

- Improved hand hygiene compliance (Cone et al., 2010)

NEGATIVE IMPACTS OF OPEN-BAY ENVIRONMENTS

The manipulation of early sensory experiences can demonstrate both beneficial and detrimental effects. The outcomes depend on specific conditions: when they take place, what type of sensory stimulation is provided, how is it administered, how long it lasts, and the individual reactions of the infant. The natural stimulation of a particular sensory system, at a precise time, can sustain its development. However, if the same stimulus is repeated or occurs during a different phase in the infants' development, it can have detrimental effects on the maturation processes of that system. Hyperdevelopment of certain functions can also have detrimental effects on

proximate functions that are not equally stimulated (Filippa, 2019). The sequence of this required orderly stimulation is frequently disrupted in noisy and brightly lit environments, particularly open-bay units.

NOISE

The auditory function in prematurely born children is immature and tends to be unstable, especially at a very early age. Cochlear development begins at around 10 weeks' gestation and is structurally formed by 15 weeks' gestation with auditory function commencing at around 20 weeks (Graven & Browne, 2008a). Auditory pathways to the central nervous system appear to be complete by 24 weeks' gestation. In the uterus, the fetus is exposed to lower frequency sounds and protected from higher frequency and loud external noise through absorption of sound by the maternal abdominal wall, uterus, and amniotic fluid environment (Gerhadt & Abrams, 2000). The hearing threshold (the intensity at which one perceives sound) is approximately 40 dB at 27 to 29 weeks.

Like other sensory systems, the auditory system needs stimulation to develop normally. Auditory learning is thought to start at around 28 weeks' gestation by repetitive exposure to common sounds such as voice and music during periods of wakefulness or quiet sleep, followed by a period of active or REM sleep. It is during REM sleep that the brain will create long-term synapses in the auditory cortex and brain stem that may become auditory memories (Graven & Browne, 2008a).

The environment and staff activity in the NICU can potentially alter the development of the auditory system. Environmental systems such as heating, ventilation, air conditioning, plumbing, communication systems, and foot or equipment traffic generate sounds in the NICU. High noise levels characterize older NICUs, with levels often reaching 70 to 80 dBs. The current NICU Design Standard (29) states that ambient noise levels shall be designed to mitigate a combination of continuous background sound and operational sound of at least L50 of 45 dB A-weighted, slow response and an L10 of 65 dB A-weighted, slow response, as measured three feet from any infant bed or other relevant listener position (White, 2020b). These levels are of an equivalent intensity to a quiet library and normal conversation, respectively. Average noise levels have been shown to be significantly higher in OBR NICUs compared to SFR NICUs (Ramm et al., 2017).

Studies have shown that consistent, excessive, loud noise in the NICU can increase neonates' heart rate, blood pressure, and respiratory rate; decrease systemic and cerebral oxygen saturations; and expose the infant to higher cortisol levels and increased caloric expenditure. Multiple recurring episodes of noise-induced stress reactions can result in apnea and bradycardia, which increases the risks of hypoxic episodes. Attention-deficit hyperactivity disorder and abnormal brain development have also been documented in the literature as a consequence of excessive noise levels in the NICU, as have problems with sensory development, speech, and language (Brown, 2009).

Elevated levels of speech are needed to overcome the noisy environment in the NICU, thereby increasing the negative impacts on infants, their families, and staff. It has been estimated that on average, infants are disturbed by noise 18 times a day and calculated that over a 9-week hospital stay, this could equate to 1,134 disturbances to sleep solely due to noise (Kuhn et al., 2013). Excessive and chaotic environmental noise also negatively affects staff attention and inter-staff communication (Filippa et al., 2017; Tubbs-Cooley et al., 2015). Medication errors and adverse events have been associated with increased levels of distractions, interruptions, high noise levels, and low lighting levels leading to decreased performance among staff (Chaudhury et al., 2009; Montgomery et al., 2021; Tubbs-Cooley et al., 2015).

Preterm infants exposed to prolonged excessive noise are at an increased risk for hearing loss, in addition to abnormal brain and sensory development, and speech and language problems (Brown, 2009). Additionally, preterm infants have immature auditory processing that can make it difficult for noise to be filtered out and therefore maintain self-regulation (Graven & Browne, 2008a). The inability to adjust and learn to "tune out" excessive or unwanted noise can make preterm infants increasingly vulnerable to the negative effects of noise.

The incidence of sensorineural hearing loss (SNHL) in very premature infants has been reported to be anywhere from 10 to 50 times higher than the average figure for the whole newborn population (Hof et al., 2013; Martines et al., 2013; Singh et al., 2017; Wang et al., 2017). SNHL in newborns is correlated with hospitalization in NICU. NICU infants present an increased risk for SNHL due to prematurity, hypoxia-ischemia, hyperventilation, low birth weight, and the use of ototoxic drugs (Stadio et al., 2019). More specifically, gestational age and birth weight quantify the risk of newborn hearing loss. van Dommelen et al. (2015) determined that the prevalence of newborn hearing loss consistently increases with decreasing week of gestation (1.2% to 7.5% from 31 to 24 weeks) and decreasing birth weight (1.4% to 4.8% from ≥1,500 to <750 g, all p < .002). Most vulnerable to newborn hearing loss were girls <28 weeks, boys <30 weeks, and small for gestational age neonates (van Dommelen et al., 2015). It should be noted that the risk for hearing loss is highest for very premature babies born before 32 weeks of pregnancy and having a birth weight of less than 1,500 g (Hof et al., 2013; Platt, 2014; van Dommelen et al., 2015).

Not all sound is bad; however, stimulation provided by the auditory environment plays an important role in both the auditory and emotional development of a baby. Because speech and other relevant sounds can be masked by noise, preterm infants may have difficulty making fine discriminations with respect to intonation of a voice. Research confirms that a live maternal voice makes an imprint, a memory trace in the immature cortical network during fetal life (Fellman, 2017; Filippa et al., 2019). However, enriching the NICU environment with more stimuli, for example, vocal recordings, is not always an improvement, and there are risks to increased auditory exposure on preterm infants' sensory experiences (Filippa, 2019; Lejeune, Brand, et al., 2019). The distinction between a vocal stimulus that is related, or unrelated, to the tactile task being performed by the infant needs to be connected to the infant's reactions.

Controlling noxious noise exposure for the preterm infant can protect both auditory and brain development. Average noise levels have been shown to be significantly higher in OBR NICUs compared to SFR NICUs (Ramm et al., 2017). The acoustic conditions of the NICU should favor understandable speech with normal or relaxed vocal effort for families and caregivers, as well as promote physiologic stability, uninterrupted sleep, and freedom from acoustic distractions. Neuroprotective interventions should be aimed at reducing sound levels. The implementation of "quiet times" in an NICU or utilization of single private rooms can help reduce loud sound levels. Lowering sound levels that reach the neonate can diminish stress on the cardiovascular, respiratory, neurologic, and endocrine systems, thereby promoting growth and reducing adverse neonatal outcomes. The current NICU Design Standard (29) states that ambient noise levels shall be designed to mitigate a combination of continuous background sound and operational sound of at least L50 of 45 dB A-weighted, slow response and an L10 of 65 dB A-weighted, slow response, as measured three feet from any infant bed or other relevant listener position (White, 2020b). These levels are of an equivalent intensity to a quiet library and normal conversation, respectively.

ADDITIONAL POINTS TO CONSIDER FOR NOISE ABATEMENT IN THE NICU

Methods to control noise associated with mechanical devices can be as simple as eliminating the noise from an Ambu bag flowing with oxygen or suctioning tubes, which contributes to reducing the overall noxious noise level in an environment. Attention should also be paid to how the architectural layout and the consequent choices for alarm settings and alarm distribution affect alarm pressure and by association alarm fatigue (Halpern, 2014a, 2014b, 2014c). The number of alarms and the associated noise pollution vary considerably with the open-bay NICU, generating 44% more alarms per patient per day (Joshi et al., 2018). Other simple methods to eliminate unnecessary noise include choosing chairs that can be rolled versus dragged; using parent beds that can be quickly and quietly operated for sleeping; employing rubber stoppers to prevent harsh closing of cabinets; redirecting service functions (delivering supplies and medications) via established service routes rather than passing through patient care areas; and exploring alternative product choices, such as plastic curtain pulls versus metal, use of porcelain sinks instead of metal, and use of sound-absorbing materials for ceilings and floors. When designing a neonatal care environment, attention must also be paid to methods needed to maintain environmental surfaces as well as equipment. Unit support services must remain cognizant of desired outcomes; for example, simply replacing a light bulb with one of incorrect wattage can result in a noxious buzzing, or floors that do not require more than damp mopping may inadvertently be buffed or waxed. Sound monitoring systems that indicate the noise level of patient care environments are used as another strategy to decrease noxious stimuli. Further postoccupancy data are needed not only to compare the SFR design with the OBR design but also to look at outcome data as they pertain to weight gain, intraventricular hemorrhage, sleep cycles, infections, language development, and overall LOS.

LIGHTING

The visual system is the last sense to develop functionally. Protecting the development of the visual system remains important because visual problems continue to be common among NICU graduates who were preterm births. Infants at or before 32 weeks' gestation have thin eyelids and little or no pupillary constriction. This allows little ability to limit light reaching the retina (LeVay et al., 1980). By 34 to 36 weeks' gestation, the pupillary constriction is more consistent and the eyelids are thicker, allowing some ability to limit light exposure to the retina. There is no developed pathway for an image to reach the visual cortex in utero, and the fetus in utero has minimal exposure to light or visual image. However, intrauterine light levels can exceed 50 lux, meaning that intrauterine vision is possible, because the minimum threshold for perception of light by a fetus has been estimated to be 10 lux (Banks & Shannon, 1993). The pathways from the retina to the visual cortex that transmit visual images become functional at 39 to 40 weeks' gestation. All processes involved in the development of the structure and function of the human visual system have a critical period between 20 and 40 weeks' gestation during which epigenetic events, toxic exposures, and inappropriate exogenous stimulation can produce significant alterations in the structure and function of the infant's visual system. Proper development of the visual system requires appropriate endogenous stimuli generated by the spontaneous activity of neuronal cells and the preservation of active sleep, especially REMs (Graven, 2011).

No data are available regarding the impact of visual stimulation on vision in the preterm population; however, one study compared brain growth, assessed by magnetic resonance imaging, in 47 extremely preterm infants and term newborn infants. Results showed that the preterm infants had an increased volume of gray and white matter in the cortical area, especially in the visual cortex (Padilla et al., 2015). Exposure to bright light may impair the development of the main networks of the retina because it activates photoreceptors before they have completely developed. In this circumstance, the biochemical signals from the retina are not properly transmitted to the cortex, which could lead to

disorganization of the immature visual system and possibly interfere with the development of other sensory systems, such as hearing (Lickliter, 2000). A lack of visual stimulation could also disrupt the normal development of the visual system. These results suggest that prolonged atypical visual experiences during critical periods of brain development could lead to earlier anatomic maturation of visual regions. Moreover, intense stimuli could interfere with establishing synaptic connections, either by interference with REMs or by directly suppressing neuronal activity of the visual system (Penn & Shatz, 2002). This may occur when there is a lack of focused stimuli, low exposure to moving stimuli, inappropriate environmental changes, or a total absence of light (Zores-Koenig et al., 2020).

Early postnatal exposure to constant light leads to a prolonged endogenous period of locomotor activity rhythm and affects the rhythmic gene expression in all studied brain structures later in life (Kubištová et al., 2020). Fetal circadian rhythms can be observed in utero from 30 weeks' gestation and are coupled to the maternal rhythm. The fetus receives multiple circadian cues from the mother, including transplacental hormones (e.g., melatonin and cortisol) as well as her body temperature and activity, and after birth, circadian cues come from the external environment (McKenna & Reiss, 2018; White, 2015, 2017; Whitehead et al., 2018). Preterm infants are even further deprived of these maternal factors, so they develop a sleep structure based on the NICU environment, typically sleep less, and have seriously disrupted and fragmented patterns of sleep (Fink et al., 2018; Godarzi et al., 2018; Graven & Browne, 2008b; Levy et al., 2017; Maki et al., 2017; Orsi et al., 2017; Ryan et al., 2020; White, 2015, 2018; Zores et al., 2018).

Important external cues for circadian synchronization include the light/dark cycle, the timing of feeding, and exposure to melatonin in breast milk. Disruption to these cues occur during admission to the NICU and can impair the development of circadian rhythms and influence survival and function in the neonatal period, with the potential to impact health and well-being throughout adult life.

In older NICUs, little attention was paid to lighting; overhead florescent fixtures were often used to illuminate a room, and lights did not include dimmer capabilities. As recognition grew that this practice was undesirable, lighting fixtures were often changed to house dimmable ballasts, bedside procedural lamps were introduced, and strategies to protect an infant's eyes by covering incubators/beds evolved. Most NICUs are no longer exposing infants to continuously bright ambient light; yet continuous dim lighting is not optimal, either (White, 2015). Nevertheless, studies on neuroprotective strategies lead us to believe that lighting should be individualized based on gestation and acuity, and without abrupt changes. Cycled lighting has been shown to yield improved outcomes when compared to either continuous bright or continuous dim lighting (Rivkees et al., 2004).

A primary benefit of SFR design is the ability to individualize lighting to meet the needs of developing infants while providing separately lit spaces for families and staff. *NICU Standard 24* of the NICU Design Standards states that ambient lighting levels in infant spaces shall be adjustable through a range of at least 10 to no more than 600 lux (approximately 1 to 60 foot candles), as measured on any plane at each bedside. Both natural and electric light sources shall have controls that allow immediate darkening of any bed position sufficient for transillumination when necessary (White, 2020b).

FALL PREVENTION

An increasing area for safety awareness within healthcare systems is fall prevention by patients, staff, and visitors. In the NICU, strategies include maintaining side rails in the upright position, collecting all supplies before beginning a procedure, and never turning one's back on an infant during cares. Seating choices should ensure that seats can be easily and quietly moved around the room, allow for stability during transfer of a baby from the bed to parent's arms, and ergonomically support intended functions such as kangaroo care by parents or breast-feeding by mother as well as procedures or charting by staff. Many older NICUs are overcrowded, which interferes with rapid and efficient movement of infant beds and equipment. Additional design flaws that may contribute to falls include minimal attention to cord management or ergonomics, infant swings that may extend into traffic aisles, and infant seats placed on countertops, to name a few. Carefully assessing for trip hazards should occur in any environment. SFR design provides greater opportunity to reduce falls, given the additional space provided.

STAFF

High noise levels in NICU not only affect hospitalized neonates, but harmful effects have also been reported in NICU healthcare staff. The effects include physiologic alterations such as increased blood pressure and heart rate, as well as headaches. Noisy environments also contributes to stress, burnout, and irritability of staff, all of which may produce problems in their performance, giving way to a greater number of errors and accidents (Hernández-Salazar et al., 2020). It is therefore essential to identify the intensity and factors that generate noise in the NICU to modify the environment, not only for the developing preterm or critically ill infant but also for the performance of staff.

In the NICU, stress can originate from many sources, such as a noisy environments or frequent intense interactions within families of an NICU infant. Stress, loud incessant noises, emotional exhaustion, and high demands, combined with a lack of support, may result in burned-out employees (Braithwaite, 2008; Rochefort & Clarke, 2010; Rochefort et al., 2016). A study by Profit et al. (2014) showed a high prevalence of burnout among NICU personnel, especially among nurses, nurse practitioners, and respiratory care providers. Additionally, they demonstrated a significant association between high burnout scores and poor cultures of safety (Profit et al., 2014). Provider burnout is increasing in prevalence and has been associated with adverse quality of care measures. Burnout prevalence varies across NICUs and may be associated with higher rates of healthcare-associated infections, particularly in large NICUs. In a large study associated with provider burnout, a total of 517 (26.7%) respondents reported symptoms consistent with burnout, with individual NICU burnout prevalence ranging from 7.5% to 42.9% (Tawfik et al., 2017). Interventions to reduce burnout prevalence in NICU staff is therefore of great importance.

Care should be taken when designing a new NICU because unit layout can affect the emotional work of nurses (Doede & Trinkoff, 2020). A study of 40 nurses who worked in the same NICU before and after SFR construction were found to have decreased stress after they transitioned to the new layout (Bosch et al., 2012). In a study by Feeley et al. (2019), nurses were asked to report their satisfaction with noise, light, and sightlines in SFRs compared to OBRs. Satisfaction with noise was significantly better for SFRs compared to the OBRs. Nurses were also significantly more satisfied with the lighting in SFRs (Feeley et al., 2019).

Needs of infants, families, and staff are not completely congruent; for example, staff need an area in which they can socialize away from the bedside yet be close enough to enable them to respond to their infant/family needs. A variety of lighting options must be made available for healthcare professionals working in NICUs. The degree of illumination required for accurate assessment, measurement, and effective intervention varies for each staff member and must be supported to ensure provision of safe, high-quality care. Exposure to bright light at night can help to maintain body temperature, alertness, and performance. Daylight is much less important in patient rooms than it is in areas in which adults (families or caregivers) congregate—a much different situation than in any other patient care area in a hospital. The NICU Recommended Design Standards should serve as a reference when designing new care units or addressing lighting in existing units (https://nicudesign.nd.edu/) (White, 2020b).

When creating a healthy work environment, include appropriate ergonomic seating that is adjustable for height, back, and arm support, as poor ergonomic design of patient care areas and nursing work areas can lead to back and neck stress, fatigue, and other potential injuries. Computers on wheels and workstations also should be adjustable to meet individual needs of staff. Hard flooring should be avoided whenever possible in areas in which caregivers stand for extended periods of time, especially at the bedside.

THE NICU DESIGN PROCESS

Full-scale mock-ups of patient rooms and workstations are critical when renovating or designing new patient care spaces. Framing out full-scale, multiroom mock spaces are particularly effective at enabling clinical experts to explore work as imagined in the new environment. Simulation-based deliberate practice in these mock spaces may reveal unexpected consequences of performing routine and emergent workflows in the new environment.

An essential aspect of design planning is projecting how well the NICU Recommended Design Standards 1-29 achieve functional goals, including clinical team situational awareness, communication, patient visibility, accessibility, and patient experience. Latent safety threats (LSTs) emerge when translating existing processes to the new environment. Each new NICU has unique, unexpected issues in adapting to its new space. Simulation-based operations testing help identify LSTs, improve process, and prepare staff (White, 2020b).

A new recommended *NICU Standard (30) (Usability Testing)* has been created stating that each new NICU shall perform multidisciplinary usability testing and standardization to enhance process resiliency for safety at transition. This requires simulation activities to identify latent safety hazards after design is completed but before occupancy (Adams-Chapman, 2018).

The very nature of SFR design imposes a perceived sense of isolation; healthcare providers, especially nurses, will be more physically separated from direct observation of patients. The historic "across-the-room" relationship between healthcare providers and infants is replaced with "in-another-room, down-the-hall" relationship. When choosing SFR design, there is an essential need for compensatory enhancements to stay in touch with any given patient and with one's colleagues.

The amount of change caregiving teams may experience when moving from a "baby barn" to an SFR NICU can be astronomic. Staff may be challenged both physically with a larger, less open space and philosophically as they are asked to provide developmentally supportive care and embrace families as partners in care. New, vital technology required for effective alarm management and communication in the SFR NICU is of paramount importance and can be overwhelming for those who are less technology savvy. Staffs who are educationally and emotionally prepared for change and who are involved in the decision-making and planning process will transition more smoothly to the SFR NICU.

Nursing faces a shortage that is predicted to grow in the upcoming decade. At the same time, the average age of nurses in the workforce is older than 50 years (NCSB, 2018). Attention to ergonomics; acoustic components; appropriate lighting levels; and efforts to meet the educational, spiritual, emotional, and social needs of aging nurses must be integral to the planning process. The goal of creating environments that are holistic and feature positive core values such as empowerment, pride, mentoring, nurturing, respect, and integrity is a realistic one. Institutions that can accomplish this goal will attract and retain a workforce comprising sharp, culturally diverse, and talented people. It is anticipated that collaborative practice environments that are nurturing for patients, families, and caregivers may help to ensure safety and quality care and reduce human error.

CONCLUSION

SFR NICU design can benefit patients, families, and healthcare professionals alike. Collaborative environments simply do not exist—they must be created. Attention to details of the physical space in which best collaborative practice can be demonstrated will result in best practices for developing infants, their families, and the caregivers who support them. SFRs permits the opportunities for sound and noise control, optimal lighting, infection control, and an increased opportunity to partner with families, secondary to 24/7 access. The SFR design also allows for family privacy, SSC, pumping, and intimate interactions with their baby. SFRs not only give parents an increased sense of control and belonging but they also create an optimal environment for staff to work away from the bedside, yet be within the patient care area. Research on SFR NICUs is growing and should continue to provide further evidence to support improved infant, family, and staff outcomes.

REFERENCES

Abouelfettoh, A., Ludington-Hoe, S. M., Burant, C. J., & Visscher, M. O. (2011). Effect of skin-to-skin contact on preterm infant skin barrier function and hospital-acquired infection. *Journal of Clinical Medicine Research*, 3(1), 36–46. https://doi.org/10.4021/jocmr479w

Adams-Chapman, I. (2018). Necrotizing enterocolitis and neurodevelopmental outcome. *Clinics in Perinatology*, 45(3), 453–466.

Aldrete-Cortez, V., Tafoya, S. A., Ramírez-García, L. A., & Poblano, A. (2021). Habituation alteration in infants with periventricular echogenicity as an indicator of neurocognitive impairment. *Developmental Neuropsychology*, 46, 1–11. https://doi.org/10.1080/87565641.2020.1871482

Almadhoob, A., & Ohlsson, A. (2020). Sound reduction management in the neonatal intensive care unit for preterm or very low birth weight infants. *The Cochrane Database of Systematic Reviews*, 1, CD010333. https://doi.org/10.1002/14651858.CD010333.pub3

Als, H., Duffy, F. H., McAnulty, G. B., Rivkin, M. J., Vajapeyam, S., Mulkern, R. V., Warfield, S. K., Huppi, P. S., Butler, S. C., Conneman, N., Fischer, C., & Eichenwald, E. C. (2004). Early experience alters brain function and structure. *Pediatrics*, 113(4), 846–857. https://doi.org/10.1542/peds.113.4.846

Als, H., Lawhon, G., Duffy, F. H., McAnulty, G. B., Gibes-Grossman, R., & Blickman, J. G. (1994). Individualized developmental care for the very low-birth-weight preterm infant. Medical and neurofunctional effects. *Journal of the American Medical Association*, 272(11), 853–858. http://search.ebscohost.com/login.aspx?direct=true&AuthType=ip,shib&db=cmedm&AN=8078162&site=ehost-live&scope=site&custid=s5071636

Altimier, L. B. (2015a). Compassionate family care framework: A new collaborative compassionate care model for NICU families and caregivers. *Newborn & Infant Nursing Reviews*, 15(1), 33–41. https://doi.org/10.1053/j.nainr.2015.01.005

Altimier, L. B. (2015b). Neuroprotective core measure 1: The healing NICU environment. *Newborn and Infant Nursing Reviews*, 15(3), 89–94. http://dx.doi.org/10.1053/j.nainr.2015.06.014

Altimier, L., & Holditch-Davis, D. (2020). *Neurobehavioral system*. In *Comprehensive neonatal nursing care* (6th ed., pp. 675–712). Springer Publishing Company, LLC.

Altimier, L., & White, R. (2020). The NICU environment. In Kenner, A. & Boykova, (Eds.), *Comprehensive neonatal nursing care* (6th ed., pp. 713–726). Springer Publishing Company, LLC.

Banks, M. S., & Shannon, E. (1993). *Spatial and chromatic visual efficiency in human neonates*. In *Visual perception and cognition in infancy*. Hove and London; Carl Granrud Carnegie Mellon University.

Belfort, M. B., Anderson, P. J., Nowak, V. A., Lee, K. J., Molesworth, C., Thompson, D. K., Doyle, L. W., & Inder, T. E. (2016). Breast milk feeding, brain development, and neurocognitive outcomes: A 7-year longitudinal study in infants born at less than 30 Weeks' gestation. *The Journal of Pediatrics*. 177, 133.e1–139.e1. https://doi.org/10.1016/j.jpeds.2016.06.045

Bergman, N. J. (2015). Neuroprotective core measures 1–7: Neuroprotection of skin-to-skin contact (SSC). *Newborn and Infant Nursing Reviews, 15*(3), 142–146. https://doi.org/10.1053/j.nainr.2015.06.006

Bergman, N. J. (2019a). Birth practices: Maternal-neonate separation as a source of toxic stress. *Birth Defects Research, 111*(15), 1087–1109. https://doi.org/10.1002/bdr2.1530

Bergman, N. J. (2019b). Historical background to maternal-neonate separation and neonatal care. *Birth Defects Research, 111*(15), 1081–1086. https://doi.org/10.1002/bdr2.1528

Bergman, N. J., Ludwig, R. J., Westrup, B., & Welch, M. G. (2019). Nurturescience versus neuroscience: A case for rethinking perinatal mother-infant behaviors and relationship. *Birth Defects Research, 111*(15), 1110–1127. http://search.ebscohost.com/login.aspx?direct=true&AuthType=ip,shib&db=cmedm&AN=31148386&site=ehost-live&scope=site&custid=s5071636

Blesa, M., Sullivan, G., Anblagan, D., Telford, E., Quigley, A., Sparrow, S., Serag, A., Semple, S. I., Bastin, M. E., & Boardman, J. (2019). Early breast milk exposure modifies brain connectivity in preterm infants. *NeuroImage, 184*(1), 431–439. https://doi-org.ezproxy.neu.edu/10.1016/j.neuroimage.2018.09.045

Bosch, S., Bledsoe, T., & Jenzarli, A. (2012). Staff perceptions before and after adding single-family rooms in the NICU. *Health Environments Research & Design Journal (HERD), 5*(4), 64–75. https://doi.org/10.1177/193758671200500406

Boyle, B., & Altimier, L. (2019). The role of families in providing neuroprotection for infants in the NICU. *Journal of Neonatal Nursing, 25*(4), 155–159. https://doi.org/10.1016/j.jnn.2019.05.004

Bracht, M., O'Leary, L., Lee, S. K., & O'Brien, K. (2013). Implementing family-integrated care in the NICU: A parent education and support program. *Advances in Neonatal Care, 13*(2), 115–126. https://doi.org/10.1097/ANC.0b013e318285fb5b

Braithwaite, M. (2008). Nurse burnout and stress in the NICU. *Advances in Neonatal Care, 8*(6), 343–347.

Broom, M., Kecskes, Z., Kildea, S., & Gardner, A. (2019). Exploring the impact of a dual occupancy neonatal intensive care unit on staff workflow, activity, and their perceptions. *Health Environments Research & Design Journal (HERD), 12*(2), 44–54. https://doi.org/10.1177/1937586718779360

Brown, G. (2009). NICU noise and the preterm infant. *Neonatal Network, 28*(3), 165–173. https://doi.org/10.1891/0730-0832.28.3.165

Bruton, C., Meckley, J., & Nelson, L. (2018). NICU nurses and families partnering to provide neuroprotective, family-centered, developmental care. *Neonatal Network, 37*(6), 351–357. https://doi.org/10.1891/0730-0832.37.6.351

Cardin, A., Rens, L., Stewart, S., Danner-Bowman, K., McCarley, R., & Kopsas, R. (2015). Neuroprotective core measures 1–7: A developmental care journey. Transformations in NICU design and caregiving attitudes. *Newborn and Infant Nursing Reviews, 15*(3), 132–141. http://dx.doi.org/10.1053/j.nainr.2015.06.007

Castellucci, M. (2019). Fewer tests, treatments for NICU babies reduces infections, cuts costs. *Modern Healthcare, 49*(15), 30.

Cevasco-Trotter, A. M., Hamm, E. L., Yang, X., & Parton, J. (2019). Multimodal neurological enhancement intervention for self-regulation in premature infants. *Advances in Neonatal Care, 19*(4), E3–E11. https://doi.org/10.1097/ANC.0000000000000595

Chaudhury, H., Mahmood, A., & Valente, M. (2009). The effect of environmental design on reducing nursing errors and increasing efficiency in acute care settings: A review and analysis of the literature. *Environmental Behaviors, 41*(6), 31.

Cheong, J. L. Y., Burnett, A. C., Treyvaud, K., & Spittle, A. J. (2020). Early environment and long-term outcomes of preterm infants. *Journal of Neural Transmission, 127*(1), 1–8. https://doi.org/10.1007/s00702-019-02121-w

Cone, S. K., Short, S., & Gutcher, G. (2010). From 'baby bar' to the 'single family room designed NICU': A report of staff perceptions one year post occupancy. *Newborn & Infant Nursing Reviews, 10*(2), 97–103. https://doi.org/10.1053/j.nainr.2010.03.002

Coughlin, M. (2021). *Transformative nursing in the NICU: TraumaInformed age-appropriate care* (2nd ed.). Springer Publishing.

Craig, J. W., Glick, C., Phillips, R., Hall, S. L., Smith, J., & Browne, J. (2015). Recommendations for involving the family in developmental care of the NICU baby. *Journal of Perinatology, 35*, S5–S8. https://doi.org/10.1038/jp.2015.142

D'Agata, A. L., Coughlin, M., & Sanders, M. R. (2018). Clinician perceptions of the NICU infant experience: Is the NICU hospitalization traumatic? *American Journal of Perinatology, 35*(12), 1159–1167. https://doi.org/10.1055/s-0038-1641747

Darcy Mahoney, A., White, R. D., Velasquez, A., Barrett, T. S., Clark, R. H., & Ahmad, K. A. (2020). Impact of restrictions on parental presence in neonatal intensive care units related to coronavirus disease 2019. *Journal of Perinatology, 40*, 36–46. https://doi.org/10.1038/s41372-020-0753-7

Dearn, T., & Shoemark, H. (2014). The effect of maternal presence on premature infant response to recorded music. *Journal of Obstetric, Gynecologic & Neonatal Nursing, 43*(3), 341–350. http://dx.doi.org.ezproxy.neu.edu/10.1111/1552-6909.12303

Detmer, M. R. (2017). Extending the therapeutic impact of music in the NICU through developmentally appropriate recorded music. *Imagine, 8*(1), 79–83.

Detmer, M. R. (2019). Music in the NICU: An evidence-based healthcare practice with proven benefits. *Neonatal Intensive Care, 32*(1), 20–23.

Dittman, K., & Hughes, S. (2018). Increased nursing participation in multidisciplinary rounds to enhance communication, patient safety, and parent satisfaction. *Critical Care Nursing Clinics of North America, 30*(4), 445. https://doi.org/10.1016/j.cnc.2018.07.002

Doede, M., & Trinkoff, A. M. (2020). Emotional work of neonatal nurses in a single-family room NICU. *Journal of Obstetric, Gynecologic, and Neonatal Nursing, 49*(3), 283–292. https://doi.org/10.1016/j.jogn.2020.03.001

Domanico, R., Davis, D. K., Coleman, F., & Davis, B. O. (2011). Documenting the NICU design dilemma: Comparative patient progress in open-ward and single family room units. *Journal of Perinatology, 31*(4), 281–288. https://doi.org/10.1038/jp.2010.120

van Dommelen, P., Verkerk, P. H., & van Straaten, H. L. M. (2015). Hearing loss by week of gestation and birth weight in very preterm neonates. *Journal of Pediatrics, 166*(4), 840.e841–843.e841. https://doi.org/10.1016/j.jpeds.2014.12.041

Dumont, V., Bulla, J., Bessot, N., Gonidec, J., Zabalia, M., Guillois, B., & Roche-Labarbe, N. (2017). The manual orienting response habituation to repeated tactile stimuli in preterm neonates: Discrimination of stimulus locations and interstimulus intervals. *Developmental Psychobiology, 59*(5), 590–602. https://doi.org/10.1002/dev.21526

Edmonson, C., Marshall, J., & Gogek, J. (2021). Creating a healthier workplace environment in an era of rising workforce pressures. *Nursing Administration Quarterly, 45*(1), 52–57. https://doi.org/10.1097/NAQ.0000000000000448

Emery, L., Hamm, E. L., Hague, K., Chorna, O. D., Moore-Clingenpeel, M., & Maitre, N. L. (2019). A randomised controlled trial of protocolised music therapy demonstrates developmental milestone acquisition in hospitalised infants. *Acta Paediatrica, 108*(5), 828–834. https://doi.org/10.1111/apa.14628. PMID: 30375661.

Feeley, N., Robins, S., Charbonneau, L., Genest, C., Lavigne, G., & Lavoie-Tremblay, M. (2019). NICU nurses' stress and work environment in an open ward compared to a combined pod and single-family room design. *Advances in Neonatal Care, 19*(5), 416–424. https://doi.org/10.1097/ANC.0000000000000603

Feeley, N., Robins, S., Genest, C., Stremler, R., Zelkowitz, P., & Charbonneau, L. (2020). A comparative study of mothers of infants hospitalized in an open ward neonatal intensive care unit and a combined pod and single-family room design. *BMC Pediatrics, 20*(1), 38. https://doi.org/10.1186/s12887-020-1929-1

Fellman, V. (2017). More voice, less noise in NICUs. *Acta Paediatrica, 106*(8), 1210–1211. https://doi.org/10.1111/apa.13927

Filippa, M. (2019). Auditory stimulations in the NICU: The more is it always the best? *Acta Paediatrica, 108*(3), 392–393. https://doi.org/10.1111/apa.14667

Filippa, M., Panza, C., Ferrari, F., Frassoldati, R., Kuhn, P., Balduzzi, S., & D'Amico, R. (2017). Systematic review of maternal voice interventions demonstrates increased stability in preterm infants. *Acta Paediatrica, 106*(8), 1220–1229. https://doi.org/10.1111/apa.13832

Filippa, M., Poisbeau, P., Mairesse, J., Monaci, M. G., Baud, O., Hüppi, P., Grandjean, D., & Kuhn, P. (2019). Pain, parental involvement, and oxytocin in the neonatal intensive care unit. *Frontiers in Psychology, 10*, 715. https://doi.org/10.3389/fpsyg.2019.00715

Fink, A., Bronas, U., & Calik, M. (2018). Autonomic regulation during sleep and wakefulness: A review with implications for defining the pathophysiology of neurological disorders. *Clinical Autonomic Research, 28*(6), 509–518.

Franck, L. S., Waddington, C., & O'Brien, K. (2020). Family integrated care for preterm infants. *Critical Care Nursing Clinics of North America, 32*(2), 149–165. https://doi.org/10.1016/j.cnc.2020.01.001

French, K. B., & Altimier, L. B. (2020). Through a mother's eyes. In Kenner, A., & Boykova, (Eds.), *Comprehensive neonatal nursing care* (6 ed., pp. 727–731). Springer Publishing Company, LLC.

French, K. B., & French, T. (2016). *JUNIPER, the girl who was born too soon.* Little, Brown and Company.

Fujimaru, C., Okamura, H., Kawasaki, M., Kakuma, T., Yoshii, C., & Matsuishi, T. (2012). Self-perceived work-related stress and its relation to salivary IgA, cortisol and 3-methoxy-4-hydroxyphenyl glycol levels among neonatal intensive care nurses. *Stress and Health, 28*(2), 171–174. https://doi.org/10.1002/smi.1414

Gerhardt, K. J., & Abrams, R. M. (2000). Fetal exposures to sound and vibroacoustic stimulation. *Journal of Perinatology, 20*, S21–S30.

Gerhardsson, E., Hildingsson, I., Mattsson, E., & Funkquist, E. L. (2018). Prospective questionnaire study showed that higher self-efficacy predicted longer exclusive breastfeeding by the mothers of late preterm infants. *Acta Paediatrica, 107*(5), 799–805. https://doi.org/10.1111/apa.14229

Godarzi, Z., Zarei, K., Shariat, M., Sadeghniat, K., Nikafs, N., & Sepaseh, H. (2018). Correlations of handling procedures and sleep patterns of the infants admitted to the neonatal intensive care unit. *Iranian Journal of Neonatology, 9*(3), 35–41. https://doi.org/10.22038/ijn.2018.23783.1299

Gönülal, D., Yalaz, M., Altun-Köroğlu, O., & Kültürsay, N. (2014). Both parents of neonatal intensive care unit patients are at risk of depression. *The Turkish Journal of Pediatrics, 56*(2), 171–176. http://search.ebscohost.com/login.aspx?direct=true&AuthType=ip,shib&db=cmedm&AN=24911852&site=ehost-live&scope=site&custid=s5071636

Graven, S. N. (2011). Early visual development: Implications for the neonatal intensive care unit and care. *Clinics in Perinatology, 38*(4), 671–683. https://doi.org/10.1016/j.clp.2011.08.006

Graven, S. N., & Browne, J. V. (2008a). Auditory development in the fetus and infant. *Newborn and Infant Nursing Reviews, 8*(4), 187–193. https://doi.org/10.1053/j.nainr.2008.10.010

Graven, S. N., & Browne, J. V. (2008b). Sleep and brain development: The critical role of sleep in fetal and early neonatal brain development. *Newborn & Infant Nursing Reviews, 8*(4), 173–179.

Grundt, H., Tandberg, B. S., Flacking, R., Drageset, J., & Moen, A. (2020). Associations between single-family room care and breastfeeding rates in preterm infants. *Journal of Human Lactation.* https://doi.org/10.1177/0890334420962709

Grzyb, M., Coo, H., & Dow, K. (2014). Views of parents and health-care providers regarding parental presence at bedside rounds in a neonatal intensive care unit. *Journal of Perinatology, 34*, 143–148.

Halpern, N. A. (2014a). Innovative designs for the smart ICU: Part 1. From initial thoughts to occupancy. *Chest, 145*(2), 399–403. https://doi.org/10.1378/chest.13-0003

Halpern, N. A. (2014b). Innovative designs for the smart ICU: Part 2. The ICU. *Chest, 145*(3), 646–658. https://doi.org/10.1378/chest.13-0004

Halpern, N. A. (2014c). Innovative designs for the smart ICU: Part 3. Advanced ICU informatics. *Chest, 145*(4), 903–912. https://doi.org/10.1378/chest.13-0005

Hamm, E. L., Chorna, O. D., Flanery, A., & Maitre, N. L. (2017). A parent-infant music therapy intervention to improve neurodevelopment after neonatal intensive care. *Acta Paediatrica, 106*(10), 1703–1704. https://doi.org/10.1111/apa.13952. PMID: 28631850.

Hernández-Salazar, A. D., Gallegos-Martínez, J., & Reyes-Hernández, J. (2020). Level and noise sources in the neonatal intensive care unit of a reference hospital. *Investigacion y educacion en enfermeria, 38*(3), e13. https://doi.org/10.17533/udea.iee.v38n3e13

Hof, J. R., Stokroos, R. J., Wix, E., Chenault, M., Gelders, E., & Brokx, J. (2013). Auditory maturation in premature infants: A potential pitfall for early cochlear implantation. *Laryngoscope, 123*(8), 2013–2018. https://doi.org/10.1002/lary.24054

Johnson, B. H., & Abraham, M. R. (2020). Reinforcing the essential role of families through first impressions of the physical environment. *Journal of Perinatology, 40*, 11–15. https://doi.org/10.1038/s41372-020-0747-5

Jones, L., Peters, K., Rowe, J., & Sheeran, N. (2016). The influence of neonatal nursery design on mothers' interactions in the nursery. *Journal of Pediatric Nursing, 31*(5), e301–e312. https://doi.org/10.1016/j.pedn.2016.05.005

Joshi, R., Straaten, H. V., Mortel, H. V., Long, X., Andriessen, P., & Pul, C. V. (2018). Does the architectural layout of a NICU affect alarm pressure? A comparative clinical audit of a single-family room and an open bay area NICU using a retrospective study design. *BMJ Open, 8*(6), e022813. https://doi.org/10.1136/bmjopen-2018-022813

Julian, S., Burnham, C. A. D., Sellenriek, P., Shannon, W. D., Hamvas, A., Tarr, P. I., & Warner, B. B. (2015). Impact of neonatal intensive care bed configuration on rates of late-onset bacterial sepsis and methicillin-resistant *Staphylococcus aureus* colonization. *Infection Control and Hospital Epidemiology, 36*(10), 1173–1182. https://doi.org/10.1017/ice.2015.144

Klawetter, S., Greenfield, J. C., Speer, S. R., Brown, K., & Hwang, S. S. (2019). An integrative review: Maternal engagement in the neonatal intensive care unit and health outcomes for U.S.-born preterm infants and their parents. *AIMS Public Health, 6*(2), 160–183. https://doi.org/10.3934/publichealth.2019.2.160

Knudson, J. (2017). First impression. *Healthcare Design, 17*(3), 36–40. http://search.ebscohost.com/login.aspx?direct=true&AuthType=ip,shib&db=bth&AN=122000398&site=ehost-live&scope=site&custid=s5071636

Kubištová, A., Spišská, V., Petrželková, L., Hrubcová, L., Moravcová, S., Maierová, L., & Bendová, Z. (2020). Constant light in critical postnatal days affects circadian rhythms in locomotion and gene expression in the suprachiasmatic nucleus, retina, and pineal gland later in life. *Biomedicines, 8*(12), 579. https://doi.org/10.3390/biomedicines8120579

Kuhn, P., Zores, C., Langlet, C., Escande, B., Astruc, D., & Dufour, A. (2013). Moderate acoustic changes can disrupt the sleep of very preterm infants in their incubators. *Acta Paediatrica, 102*(10), 949–954. https://doi.org/10.1111/apa.12330

Lake, E. T., Staiger, D. O., Cramer, E., Hatfield, L. A., Smith, J. G., Kalisch, B. J., & Rogowski, J. A. (2020). Association of patient acuity and missed nursing care in U.S. Neonatal intensive care units. *Medical Care Research and Review, 77*(5), 451–460. https://doi.org/10.1177/1077558718806743

Lechner, B. E., & Vohr, B. R. (2017). Neurodevelopmental outcomes of preterm infants fed human milk: A systematic review. *Clin Perinatol, 44*(1), 69–83. https://doi.org/10.1016/j.clp.2016.11.004

Lefmann, T. (2020). Breastfeeding as a best practice for mitigating the negative effects of stress. *Best Practice in Mental Health, 16*(1), 32–45.

Lehtonen, L., Lee, S. K., Kusuda, S., Lui, K., Norman, M., Bassler, D., Håkansson, S., Vento, M., Darlow, B. A., Adams, M., Puglia, M., Isayama, T., Noguchi, A., Morisaki, N., Helenius, K., Reichman, B., & Shah, P. S. (2020). Family rooms in neonatal intensive care units and neonatal outcomes: An international survey and linked cohort study. *Journal of Pediatrics, 226*, 112. https://doi.org/10.1016/j.jpeds.2020.06.009

Lejeune, F., Brand, L. A., Palama, A., Parra, J., Marcus, L., Barisnikov, K., Debillon, T., Gentaz, E., & Berne-Audéoud, F. (2019a). Preterm infant showed better object handling skills in a neonatal intensive care unit during silence than with a recorded female voice. *Acta Paediatrica, 108*(3), 460–467. https://doi.org/10.1111/apa.14552

Lejeune, F., Lordier, L., Pittet, M. P., Schoenhals, L., Grandjean, D., Hüppi, P. S., Filippa, M., & Tolsa, C. B. (2019b). Effects of an early postnatal music intervention on cognitive and emotional development in preterm children at 12 and 24 months: Preliminary findings. *Frontiers in Psychology, 10*, 494. https://doi.org/10.3389/fpsyg.2019.00494

Lejeune, F., Parra, J., Berne-Audéoud, F., Marcus, L., Barisnikov, K., Gentaz, E., & Debillon, T. (2016). Sound interferes with the early tactile manual abilities of preterm infants. *Scientific Reports, 6*, 23329. https://doi.org/10.1038/srep23329

Lester, B. M., Hawes, K., Abar, B., Sullivan, M., Miller, R., Bigsby, R., Laptook, A., Salisbury, A., Taub, M., Lagasse, L. L., & Padbury, J. F. (2014). Single-family room care and neurobehavioral and medical outcomes in preterm infants. *Pediatrics, 134*(4), 754–760.

Lester, B., Salisbury, A., Hawes, K., Dansereau, L., Bigsby, R., Laptook, A., Taub, M., Lagasse, L. L., Vohr, B. R., & Padbury, J. (2016). 18-Month follow-up of infants cared for in a single-family room neonatal intensive care unit. *The Journal of Pediatrics, 177*, 84–89.

LeVay, S., Wiesel, T. N., & Hubel, D. H. (1980). The development of ocular dominance columns in normal and visually deprived monkeys. *Journal of Complex Neurology, 191*(1), 1–51.

Levy, J., Hassan, F., Plegue, M., Sokoloff, M., Kushwaha, J., Chervin, R., Barks, J. D., & Shellhaas, R. (2017). Impact of hands-on care on infant sleep in the neonatal intensive care unit. *Pediatric Pulmonology, 52*(1), 84–90.

Lickliter, R. (2000). The role of sensory stimulation in perinatal development: Insights from comparative research for care of the high-risk infant. *Journal of Developmental and Behavioral Pediatrics, 21*(6), 437–447. https://doi.org/10.1097/00004703-200012000-00006

Loewy, J., Stewart, K., Dassler, A. M., Telsey, A., & Homel, P. (2013). The effects of music therapy on vital signs, feeding, and sleep in premature infants. *Pediatrics, 131*(5), 902–918. https://doi.org/10.1542/peds.2012-1367

Ludwig, R. J., & Welch, M. G. (2019). Darwin's other dilemmas and the theoretical roots of emotional connection. *Frontiers in Psychology, 10*, 683. https://doi.org/10.3389/fpsyg.2019.00683

Ludwig, R. J., & Welch, M. G. (2020). How babies learn: The autonomic socioemotional reflex. *Early Human Development, 151*, 105183. https://doi.org/10.1016/j.earlhumdev.2020.105183

Mack, E. (2015). Hospital cuts length of stay for babies in the NICU by four days. *Hospital Case Management, 23*(4), 49–50.

Maitre, N. L., Key, A. P., Chorna, O. D., Slaughter, J. C., Matusz, P. J., Wallace, M. T., & Murray, M. M. (2017). The dual nature of early-life experience on somatosensory processing in the human infant brain. *Current Biology, 27*(7), 1048–1054. https://doi.org/10.1016/j.cub.2017.02.036

Maki, M. T., Sbampato Calado Orsi, K. C., Tsunemi, M. H., Hallinan, M. P., Pinheiro, E. M., & Machado Avelar, A. F. (2017). The effects of handling on the sleep of preterm infants. *Acta Paulista de Enfermagem, 30*(5), 489–496. https://doi.org/10.1590/1982-0194201700071

Malik, G., McKenna, L., & Plummer, V. (2015). Perceived knowledge, skills, attitude and contextual factors affecting evidence-based practice among nurse educators, clinical coaches and nurse specialists. *International Journal of Nursing Practice, 21*, 46–57. https://doi.org/10.1111/ijn.12366

Martines, F., Martines, E., Mucia, M., Sciacca, V., & Salvago, P. (2013). Prelingual sensorineural hearing loss and infants at risk: Western Sicily report. *International Journal of Pediatric Otorhinolaryngology, 77*(4), 513–518. https://doi.org/10.1016/j.ijporl.2012.12.023

McKenna, H., & Reiss, I. (2018). The case for a chronobiological approach to neonatal care. *Early Human Development, 126*, 1–5.

McMillan, K., & Perron, A. (2020). Change fatigue in nurses: A qualitative study. *Journal of Advanced Nursing, 76*(10), 2627–2636. https://doi.org/10.1111/jan.14454

Miyagishima, S., Himuro, N., Kozuka, N., Mori, M., & Tsutsumi, H. (2017). Family-centered care for preterm infants: Parent and physical therapist perceptions. *Pediatrics International, 59*(6), 698–703. https://doi.org/10.1111/ped.13266

Montgomery, A. P., Azuero, A., Baernholdt, M., Loan, L. A., Miltner, R. S., Qu, H., Raju, D., & Patrician, P. A. (2021). Nurse burnout predicts self-reported medication administration errors in acute care hospitals. *Journal for Healthcare Quality, 43*(1), 13–23. https://doi.org/10.1097/JHQ.0000000000000274

Morag, I., & Ohlsson, A. (2013). Cycled light in the intensive care unit for preterm and low birth weight infants. *Cochrane Database of Systematic Reviews*, (8), CD006982. http://ezproxy.neu.edu/login?url=http://search.ebscohost.com/login.aspx?direct=true&db=ccm&AN=2012243491&site=ehost-live&scope=site

Mörelius, E., Olsson, E., Sahlén Helmer, C., Thernström Blomqvist, Y., & Angelhoff, C. (2020). External barriers for including parents of preterm infants in a randomised clinical trial in the neonatal intensive care unit in Sweden: A descriptive study. *BMJ Open, 10*(12), e040991. https://doi.org/10.1136/bmjopen-2020-040991

Namprom, N., Woragidpoonpol, P., Altimier, L., Jintrawet, U., Chotibang, J., & Klunklin, P. (2020). Maternal participation on preterm infants care reduces the cost of delivery of preterm neonatal healthcare services. *Journal of Neonatal Nursing, 26*(5), 291–296. https://doi.org/10.1016/j.jnn.2020.03.005

NCSB. (2018). *2017 National RN workforce survey.* https://www.ncsbn.org/workforce.htm

Niela-Vilén, H., Feeley, N., & Axelin, A. (2017). Hospital routines promote parent-infant closeness and cause separation in the birthing unit in the first 2 hours after birth: A pilot study. *Birth (Berkeley, Calif), 44*(2), 167–172. https://doi.org/10.1111/birt.12279

O'Brien, K., Bracht, M., Macdonell, K., McBride, T., Robson, K., O'Leary, L., Christie, K., Galarza, M., Dicky, T., Levin, A., & Lee, S. (2013). A pilot cohort analytic study of Family Integrated Care in a Canadian neonatal intensive care unit. *BMC Pregnancy & Childbirth, 13*(1), S12. https://doi.org/10.1186/1471-2393-13-S1-S12

O'Callaghan, F. V., Al Mamun, A., O'Callaghan, M., Clavarino, A., Williams, G. M., Bor, W., & Najman, J. M. (2010). The link between sleep problems in infancy and early childhood and attention problems at 5 and 14 years: evidence from a birth cohort study. *Early Human Development, 86*, 419–424. http://dx.doi.org/10.1016/j.earlhumdev.2010.05.020

Orsi, K. C. S. C., Avena, M. J., Lurdes de Cacia Pradella-Hallinan, M., da Luz Gonçalves Pedreira, M., Tsunemi, M. H., Machado Avelar, A. F., & Pinheiro, E. M. (2017). Effects of handling and environment on preterm newborns sleeping in incubators. *Journal of Obstetric, Gynecologic, and Neonatal Nursing, 46*(2), 238–247. https://doi.org/10.1016/j.jogn.2016.09.005

Ortenstrand, A., Westrup, B., Brostrom, E., Sarman, I., Akerström, S., Brune, T., Lindberg, L., & Waldenström, U. (2010). The Stockholm Neonatal Family Centered Care study: Effects on length of stay and infant morbidity. *Pediatrics, 125*(2), e278–e285.

Padilla, N., Alexandrou, G., Blennow, M., Lagercrantz, H., & Ådén, U. (2015). Brain growth gains and losses in extremely preterm infants at term. *Cerebral Cortex, 25*(7), 1897–1905. https://doi.org/10.1093/cercor/bht431

Penn, A. A., & Shatz, C. J. (2002). Principles of endogenous and sensory activity dependent brain development. The visual system. In Lagercrantz, H., Hanson, M., & Evrard, P. (Eds.), *The newborn brain: neuroscience and clinical applications* (pp. 204–225). Cambridge University Press.

Phillips, R. M. (2015). Seven core measures of neuroprotective family-centered developmental care: Creating an infrastructure for implementation. *Newborn & Infant Nursing Reviews, 15*, 87–90. https://doi.org/10.1053/j.nainr.2015.06.004

Phillips, R. (2020). *Guidelines for supporting skin-to-skin contact in the NICU.* In Comprehensive neonatal nursing care (6th ed., pp. 936–938). Springer Publishing.

Pineda, R., Bender, J., Hall, B., Shabosky, L., Annecca, A., & Smith, J. (2018). Parent participation in the neonatal intensive care unit: Predictors and relationships to neurobehavior and developmental outcomes. *Early Human Development, 117*, 32–38. https://doi.org/10.1016/j.earlhumdev.2017.12.008

Pineda, R. G., Neil, J., Dierker, D., Smyser, C. D., Wallendorf, M., Kidokoro, H., Reynolds, L. C., Walker, S., Rogers, C., Mathur, A. M., Van Essen, D. C., & Inder, T. (2014). Alterations in brain structure and neurodevelopmental outcome in preterm infants hospitalized in different neonatal intensive care unit environments. *Journal of Pediatrics, 164*(1), 52.e2–60.e2. https://doi.org/10.1016/j.jpeds.2013.08.047

Pineda, R. G., Stransky, K. E., Rogers, C., Duncan, M. H., Smith, G. C., Neil, J., & Inder, T. E. (2012). The single-patient room in the NICU: Maternal and family effects. *Journal of Perinatology, 32*(7), 545–551. https://doi.org/10.1038/jp.2011.144

Pisoni, C., Provenzi, L., Moncecchi, M., Caporali, C., Naboni, C., Stronati, M., Montirosso, R., Borgatti, R., & Orcesi, S. (2021). Early parenting intervention promotes 24-month psychomotor development in preterm children. *Acta Paediatrica, 110*(1), 101–108. https://doi.org/10.1111/apa.15345

Platt, M. J. (2014). Outcomes in preterm infants. *Public Health, 128*(5), 399–403. https://doi.org/10.1016/j.puhe.2014.03.010

Porges, S. W., Davila, M. I., Lewis, G. F., Kolacz, J., Okonmah-Obazee, S., Hane, A. A., Kwon, K. Y., Ludwig, R. J., Myers, M. M., & Welch, M. G. (2019). Autonomic regulation of preterm infants is enhanced by Family Nurture Intervention. *Developmental Psychobiology, 61*(6), 942–952. https://doi.org/10.1002/dev.21841

Profit, J., Sharek, P. J., Amspoker, A. B., Kowalkowski, M. A., Nisbet, C. C., Thomas, E. J., Chadwick, W. A., & Sexton, J. B. (2014). Burnout in the NICU setting and its relation to safety culture. *BMJ Quality & Safety, 23*(10), 806–813. https://doi.org/10.1136/bmjqs-2014-002831

Puumala, S. E., Rich, R. K., Roy, L., Reynolds, R., Jimenez, F. E., Opollo, J. G., & Brittin, J. (2020). Single-family room neonatal intensive care unit design: Do patient outcomes actually change? *Journal of Perinatology, 40*(6), 867–874. https://doi.org/10.1038/s41372-019-0584-6

Ramm, K., Mannix, T., Parry, Y., & Gaffney, M. P. (2017). A comparison of sound levels in open plan versus pods in a neonatal intensive care unit. *Health Environments Research & Design Journal (HERD)* (Sage Publications, Ltd.), *10*(3), 30–39. https://doi.org/10.1177/1937586716668636

Rivkees, S. A., Mayes, L., Jacobs, H., & Gross, I. (2004). Rest-activity patterns of premature infants are regulated by cycled lighting. *Pediatrics, 113*(4), 833–839. https://doi.org/10.1542/peds.113.4.833. PMID: 15060235.

Rochefort, C. M., & Clarke, S. P. (2010). Nurses' work environments, care rationing, job outcomes, and quality of care on neonatal units. *Journal of Advanced Nursing, 66*(10), 2213–2224. https://doi.org/10.1111/j.1365-2648.2010.05376.x

Rochefort, C. M., Rathwell, B. A., & Clarke, S. P. (2016). Rationing of nursing care interventions and its association with nurse-reported outcomes in the neonatal intensive care unit: A cross-sectional survey. *BMC Nursing, 15*, 1–8. https://doi.org/10.1186/s12912-016-0169-z

Ryan, M. A., Mathieson, S., Livingstone, V., O'Sullivan, M. P., Dempsey, E., & Boylan, G. B. (2020). Nocturnal sleep architecture of preterm infants in the NICU. *Infant, 16*(5), 209–214.

Sa de Almeida, J., Lordier, L., Zollinger, B., Kunz, N., Bastiani, M., Gui, L., Adam-Darque, A., Borradori-Tolsa, C., Lazeyras, F., & Hüppi, P. S. (2020). Music enhances structural maturation of emotional processing neural pathways in very preterm infants. *NeuroImage, 207*, 116391. https://doi.org/10.1016/j.neuroimage.2019.116391

Sadatsafavi, H., Niknejad, B., Shepley, M., & Sadatsafavi, M. (2019). Probabilistic return-on-investment analysis of single-family versus open-bay rooms in neonatal intensive care units-synthesis and evaluation of early evidence on nosocomial infections, length of stay, and direct cost of care. *Journal of Intensive Care Medicine, 34*(2), 115–125. https://doi.org/10.1177/0885066616689774

Santos, J., Pearce, S. E., & Stroustrup, A. (2015). Impact of hospital-based environmental exposures on neurodevelopmental outcomes of preterm infants. *Current Opinion in Pediatrics, 27*(2), 254–260. https://doi.org/10.1097/MOP.0000000000000190

Shahheidari, M., & Homer, C. (2012). Impact of the design of neonatal intensive care units on neonates, staff, and families: A systematic literature review. *Journal of Perinatal & Neonatal Nursing, 26*(3), 260–266. https://doi.org/10.1097/jpn.0b013e318261ca1d

Sharma, D., Farahbakhsh, N., Sharma, S., Sharma, P., & Sharma, A. (2019). Role of kangaroo mother care in growth and breast feeding rates in very low birth weight (VLBW) neonates: A systematic review. *Journal of Maternal-Fetal & Neonatal Medicine, 32*(1), 129–142. https://doi.org/10.1080/14767058.2017.1304535

Shepley, M. M., Harris, D. D., & White, R. (2008). Open-bay and single-family room neonatal intensive care units. *Environment & Behavior, 40*(2), 249–268. http://ezproxy.neu.edu/login?url=http://search.ebscohost.com/login.aspx?direct=true&db=aph&AN=31122664&site=ehost-live&scope=site

Shepley, M. M., Smith, J. A., Sadler, B. L., & White, R. D. (2014). The business case for building better neonatal intensive care units. *Journal of Perinatology, 34*(11), 811–815. https://doi.org/10.1038/jp.2014.174

Singh, P., Kumar, N., Kumar, D., Shrivastava, N., & Kumar, A. (2017). A prospective study for hearing screening of 4356 newborns by transient evoked oto-acoustic emissions and brainstem evoked response audiometry: A study of high risk factors for hearing loss. *International Journal of Research & Medical Science, 5*, 4. https://doi.org/10.18203/2320-6012.ijrms20171264

Smith, L., & Carver, A. (2017). Improving patient safety through daily multidisciplinary rounds. *Journal of Obstetric, Gynecologic & Neonatal Nursing, 46*, S41–S42. https://doi.org/10.1016/j.jogn.2017.04.109

Soleimani, F., Rostami, F. F., Nouri, J. M., Hatamizadeh, N., Sajedi, F., & Norouzi, M. (2020). Impacts of the design of a neonatal intensive care unit (Single-Family room care and open-ward care) on clinical and environmental outcomes. *Crescent Journal of Medical & Biological Sciences, 7*(1), 1–6. http://search.ebscohost.com/login.aspx?direct=true&AuthType=ip,shib&db=a9h&AN=141247992&site=ehost-live&scope=site&custid=s5071636

Spiegler, P., Preuß, M., Gebauer, C., Bendiks, M., Herting, E., Göpel, W., German Neonatal Network (GNN), & German Neonatal Network GNN. (2016). Does breastmilk influence the development of bronchopulmonary dysplasia? *The Journal of Pediatrics, 169*, 76.e74–80.e74.

Stadio, A. D., Molini, E., Gambacorta, V., Giommetti, G., Volpe, A. D., Ralli, M., Lapenna, R., Trabalzini, F., & Ricci, G. (2019). Sensorineural hearing loss in newborns hospitalized in neonatal intensive care unit: An observational study. *International Tinnitus Journal, 23*(1), 6. https://doi.org/10.5935/0946-5448.20190006

Standley, J. M., & Gutierrez, C. (2020). Benefits of a comprehensive evidence-based NICU-mt program: Family-centered, neurodevelopmental music therapy for premature infants. *Pediatric Nursing, 46*(1), 40–46.

Stevens, D. C., Helseth, C. C., Khan, M. A., Munson, D. P., & Reid, E. J. (2011). A comparison of parent satisfaction in an open-bay and single-family room neonatal intensive care unit. *Health Environments Research & Design Journal (HERD)* (Vendome Group LLC), *4*(3), 110–123. https://doi.org/10.1177/193758671100400309

Stevens, D., Helseth, C., Khan, M., Munson, D., & Smith, T. (2010). Neonatal intensive care nursery staff perceive enhanced workplace quality with the single-family room design. *Journal of Perinatology, 30*(5), 352–358. https://doi.org/10.1038/jp.2009.137

Stevens, D. C., Helseth, C. C., Thompson, P. A., Pottala, J. V., Khan, M. A., & Munson, D. P. (2012). A comprehensive comparison of open-bay and single-family-room neonatal intensive care units at Sanford children's hospital. *Health Environments Research & Design Journal (HERD)* (Vendome Group LLC), *5*(4), 23–39. http://search.ebscohost.com/login.aspx?direct=true&AuthType=ip,shib&db=ccm&AN=104337052&site=ehost-live&scope=site&custid=s5071636

Stevens, D. C., Thompson, P. A., Helseth, C. C., Hsu, B., Khan, M. A., & Munson, D. P. (2014). A comparison of the direct cost of care in an open-bay and single-family room NICU. *Journal of Perinatology, 34*(11), 830–835. https://doi.org/10.1038/jp.2014.178

Stevens, D., Thompson, P., Helseth, C., & Pottala, J. (2015). Mounting evidence favoring single-family room neonatal intensive car. *Journal of Neonatal-Perinatal Medicine, 8*(3), 177–188. https://doi.org/10.3233/NPM-15915035

Tandberg, B. S., Flacking, R., Markestad, T., Grundt, H., & Moen, A. (2019). Parent psychological wellbeing in a single-family room versus an open bay neonatal intensive care unit. *PLoS One, 14*(11), e0224488. https://doi.org/10.1371/journal.pone.0224488

Tawfik, D. S., Phibbs, C. S., Sexton, J. B., Kan, P., Sharek, P. J., Nisbet, C. C., Rigdon, J., Trockel, M., & Profit, J. (2017). Factors associated with provider burnout in the NICU. *Pediatrics, 139*(5), e20164134. https://doi.org/10.1542/peds.2016-4134

Thompson, T. S., White, K., Ross, J. R., Scheurer, M. A., & Smithwick, M. (2020). Human-centered design strategies in family and staff preparation for neonatal care. *Journal of Perinatology, 40*, 47–53. https://doi.org/10.1038/s41372-020-0752-8

Tubbs-Cooley, H. L., Pickler, R. H., Younger, J. B., & Mark, B. A. (2015). A descriptive study of nurse-reported missed care in neonatal intensive care units. *Journal of Advanced Nursing* (John Wiley & Sons, Inc.), 71(4), 813–824. https://doi.org/10.1111/jan.12578

van Veenendaal, N. R., van der Schoor, S., Heideman, W. H., Rijnhart, J., Heymans, M. W., Twisk, J., van Goudoever, J. B., & van Kempen, A. (2020). Family integrated care in single family rooms for preterm infants and late-onset sepsis: A retrospective study and mediation analysis. *Pediatric Research, 88*(4), 593–600. https://doi.org/10.1038/s41390-020-0875-9

Venkataraman, R., Kamaluddeen, M., Amin, H., & Lodha, A. (2018). Is less noise, light and parental/caregiver stress in the neonatal intensive care unit better for neonates? *Indian Pediatrics, 55*(1), 17–21.

Vohr, B. R. (2017). Follow-up of extremely preterm infants; the long and the short of it. *Pediatrics, 139*(6). https://doi.org/10.1542/peds.2017-0453

Vohr, B. R. (2019). The importance of parent presence and involvement in the single-family room and open-bay NICU. *Acta Paediatrica, 108*(6), 986–988. https://doi.org/10.1111/apa.14783

Vohr, B., McGowan, E., McKinley, L., Tucker, R., Keszler, L., & Alksninis, B. (2017a). Differential effects of the single-family room neonatal intensive care unit on 18- to 24-month Bayley scores of preterm infants. *The Journal of Pediatrics, 185*, 42. https://doi.org/10.1016/j.jpeds.2017.01.056

Vohr, B. R., Poggi Davis, E., Wanke, C. A., & Krebs, N. F. (2017b). Neurodevelopment: The impact of nutrition and inflammation during preconception and pregnancy in low-resource settings. *Pediatrics, 139*(Suppl. 1), S38–S49. https://doi.org/10.1542/peds.2016-2828F

Wang, C., Yang, C., Lien, R., Chu, S., Hsu, J., Fu, R., & Chiang, . (2017). Prevalence and independent risk factors for hearing impairment among very birth weight infants. *International Journal of Pediatric Otorhinolaryngology, 93*, 5. https://doi.org/10.1016/j.ijporl.2016.12.029

Watson, J., DeLand, M., Gibbins, S., MacMillan York, E., & Robson, K. (2014). Improvements in staff quality of work life and family satisfaction following the move to single-family room NICU design. *Advances in Neonatal Care, 14*(2), 8. https://doi.org/10.1097/anc.0000000000000046

Weisman, O., Magori-Cohen, R., Louzoun, Y., Eidelman, A. I., & Feldman, R. (2011). Sleep-wake transitions in premature neonates predict early development. *Pediatrics, 128*(4), 706–714. https://doi.org/10.1542/peds.2011-0047

Welch, M. G., Barone, J. L., Porges, S. W., Hane, A. A., Kwon, K. Y., Ludwig, R. J., Stark, R. I., Surman, A. L., Kolacz, J., & Myers, M. M. (2020). Family nurture intervention in the NICU increases autonomic regulation in mothers and children at 4–5 years of age: Follow-up results from a randomized controlled trial. *PLoS One, 15*(8), e0236930. https://doi.org/10.1371/journal.pone.0236930

White, R. D. (2010). Single-family room design in the neonatal intensive care unit-challenges and opportunities. *Newborn and Infant Nursing Reviews, 10*(2), 83–86. https://doi.org/10.1053/j.nainr.2010.03.011

White, R. D. (2015). Neuroprotective core measure 4: Safeguarding sleep — its value in neuroprotection of the newborn. *Newborn & Infant Nursing Reviews, 15*, 114–115. https://doi.org/10.1053/j.nainr.2015.06.012

White, R. D. (2016). The next big ideas in NICU design. *Journal of Perinatology, 36*(4), 259–262. https://doi.org/10.1038/jp.2016.6

White, R. D. (2017). Circadian variation of breast milk components and implications for care. *Breastfeeding Medicine, 12*(7), 398–400. https://doi.org/10.1089/bfm.2017.0070

White, R. D. (2018). Defining the optimal sensory environment in the NICU: An elusive task. *Acta Paediatrica, 107*(7), 1.

White, R. D. (2020a). Next steps in newborn intensive care unit design and developmental care. *Journal of Perinatology, 40*, 1. https://doi.org/10.1038/s41372-020-0748-4

White, R. D. (2020b). Recommended standards for newborn ICU design, 9th edition. *Journal of Perinatology, 40*, 2–4. https://doi.org/10.1038/s41372-020-0766-2

White, R. D. (2020c). Right lighting the NICU. *Acta Paediatrica (Oslo, Norway: 1992), 109*(7), 1288–1289. https://doi.org/10.1111/apa.15193

Whitehead, K., Laudiano-Dray, M., Meek, J., & Fabrizi, L. (2018). Emergence of mature cortical activity in wakefulness and sleep in healthy preterm and full-term infants. *Sleep, 41*(8). https://doi.org/10.1093/sleep/zsy096

Zauche, L. H., Zauche, M. S., Dunlop, A. L., & Williams, B. L. (2020). Predictors of parental presence in the neonatal intensive care unit. *Advances in Neonatal Care, 20*(3), 251–259. https://doi.org/10.1097/ANC.0000000000000687

Zores-Koenig, C., Kuhn, P., & Caeymaex, L. (2020). Recommendations on neonatal light environment from the French Neonatal Society. *Acta Paediatrica (Oslo, Norway: 1992), 109*(7), 1292–1301. https://doi.org/10.1111/apa.15173

Zores, C., Dufour, A., Pebayle, T., Dahan, I., Astruc, D., & Kuhn, P. (2018). Observational study found that even small variations in light can wake up very preterm infants in a neonatal intensive care unit. *Acta Paediatrica, 107*(7), 1191–1197. https://doi.org/10.1111/apa.14261

Infant Mental Health: Strategies for Optimal Social–Emotional Care of Infants and Families in the NICU

Jacqueline M. McGrath and Dorothy Vittner

IFCDC Standard for Systems Thinking in Collaborative Practice

Standard 1: Systems Thinking
- The intensive care unit shall exhibit an infrastructure of leadership, mission, and a governance framework to guide the performance of the collaborative practice of Infant and Family-Centered Developmental Care (IFCDC).

Standard 2: Systems Thinking
- The intensive care unit shall provide a professionally competent interprofessional collaborative practice team to support the baby, parent, and family's holistic physical, developmental, and psychosocial needs from birth through the transition of hospital discharge-to-home and assure continuity to follow-up care.

Standard 3: Systems Thinking
- The practice of IFCDC in the intensive care unit shall be based on evidence that is ethical, collaborative, safe, timely, quality driven, efficient, equitable, and cost-effective.

Standard 6: Systems Thinking
- The interprofessional collaborative team should provide IFCDC through transition to home and continuing care for the baby and family to support the optimal physiologic and psychosocial health needs of the baby and family.

Standard 2: Positioning and Touch
- Collaborative efforts among parents and ICU interprofessionals shall support optimal cranial shaping and prevent torticollis, flattening, and skull deformity.

Standard 4: Positioning and Touch
- Babies in ICU settings shall experience nurturing human touch by family and caregivers.

Standard 1: Skin-to-Skin Contact
- Parents shall be encouraged and supported in early, frequent, and prolonged skin-to-skin contact (SSC) with their babies.

Standard 2: Skin-to-Skin Contact
- Education and policies in support of SSC between parents and their baby shall be developed, implemented, monitored, and evaluated by an interprofessional collaborative team.

Standard 4: Skin-to -Skin Contact
- Parents shall be provided information about the benefits of SSC that continue for babies and parents after discharge.

Standard 1: Pain and Stress, Families
- The interprofessional team shall document increased parental/caregiver well-being and decreased emotional distress during the intensive care hospital (ICU) stay. Distress levels of baby's siblings and extended family should also be considered.

Standard 2: Pain and Stress, Babies
- The interprofessional collaborative team shall develop care practices that prioritize multiple methods to optimize baby outcomes by minimizing the impact of stressful and painful stimuli.

Standard 2: Feeding
- Every mother shall be encouraged and supported to breastfeed and/or provide human milk for her baby.

Standard 4: Feeding
- Mothers shall be supported to be the primary feeders of their baby.

Standard 11: Feeding
- Feeding management shall consider short- and long-term growth and feeding outcomes.

INTRODUCTION

This chapter uses infant mental health principles to elaborate strategies and approaches to effectively address the social and emotional needs of infants and their families in the neonatal intensive care unit (NICU). Information in this chapter is based on an extensive body of research and programmatic strategies regarding the importance of positive social relationships particularly in how these connections affect the developing infant (Barlow et al., 2015; Browne et al., 2020). Healthcare professionals can facilitate improved positive developmental outcomes using these findings as they work with infants, parents, and/or primary caregivers.

Medical fragility limits infants' capacities for interaction and, thus, impacts the developing infant–parent relationship. Typically, the medically fragile baby is more sensitive and reactive to environmental stimuli because of their immature nervous system as well as the behavioral responses that exhibit stress due to the life-saving necessary medical interventions experienced in the NICU. The baby's sensitivity and fragility mean that they will require extra human effort to facilitate self-regulation and relaxation for the infant. Sensitivity and responsiveness by the caregiver are needed so that the babies' limited physical resources are available for continued growth and healing. This sensitivity and responsiveness require encouragement from healthcare professionals for parents who may be stressed by their infant's NICU admission. Assessing the parent's responsiveness and exploring their priorities is an important first step to meet parents where they are to understand the needs of their infant during this critical or sensitive period of development.

However, in addition to recognizing the fragility of the infant, it is critical to recognize how differences in each parent's own history and current social situation may make it more difficult to address the extraordinary relational needs of the premature or medically fragile baby that requires a hospital stay. Parents come to this new relationship with their baby with personal beliefs and perspectives related to their own earlier histories, which may include loss or current or past trauma (Leahy-Warren et al., 2020). Inadequate resources, addiction, teen parenthood, mental illness, recent displacement or migration, homelessness, or other social or psychological factors complicate formation of a healthy nurturing relationship with their infant. Many of these considerations are related to the social determinants of health and are not easily modified by the individual parent or family. Preterm birth has been associated with delayed transition to parenthood (Heydarpour et al.,

2016), often owing to an inability to take on the parenting role as infants are initially cared for by NICU health professionals (Al Maghaireh et al., 2016). Parents often experience limited caregiving opportunities during NICU (Gibbs et al., 2016). Parents' active participation or level of parent engagement in infant caregiving activities has significant effects on developing infants (Vittner et al., 2019).

Past research on risk and resilience demonstrates that the number of and interaction of a multitude of risk factors is more significant than any single specific risk factor on its own. In 1998, Felitti et al., published a landmark study exploring and examining how the effects of adverse childhood exposures have long-term effects reaching into adulthood. Although this study was not particularly focused on effects of the NICU environment, there are many questions and principles to ponder and learn from their findings and those studies that followed about how the NICU environment affects long-term child development and family functioning.

Within this chapter, we intended to enable caregivers in the NICU to consider a different perspective and find ways to implement infant mental health principles as a common set of ideas and language that provide a foundation for positive strategies to work together with families and caregivers to be more effective in reducing the social–emotional and developmental risks for infants and families who must traverse the NICU. A fundamental concept in infant mental health, *parallel process,* underlies the varied strategies described in this chapter. The essential meaning of parallel process is that, when parents receive on-going support and nurturance from NICU care professionals, they are more able to provide these primary elements of healthy relationships with their infants (Lob et al., 2020). Techniques for use of an empathic stance within the parallel process will be described to operationalize infant mental health principles within the task-driven environment of the NICU.

Both developmental care and infant mental health are defined within the context of the NICU and infant care practice. Descriptions of how modalities of infant mental health services overlap and complement other services and include ways these services are different and distinct. Individualized developmental care is enriched and strengthened when concepts from the field of infant mental health are identified and routinely incorporated into care of infants and their families (Williams et al., 2018). Evidenced-based recommendations for using developmental care practices to support social and emotional development in the NICU are described in Table 7-1 and outlined in more detail through this chapter.

TABLE 7-1 Practice Recommendations That Support Social–Emotional Development in Infants and Their Parents/Primary Caregivers in the NICU

Intervention Strategy	Practice Recommendation	Level of Evidence	Citations
Facilitating parent presence	Provide welcoming environment to increase parent satisfaction	I II III	Butt et al. (2013) Craig et al. (2015) Treherne et al. (2017) See Chapter 5 for a more discussion of this evidence
	Caregivers recognize poor visitation patterns and provide concrete assistance for visiting	III	Flacking et al. (2012)
	Provide information to support parent understanding of their infants' condition	VI	Fernández Medina et al. (2018) Bry and Wigert (2019)
	Supports parents in overcoming their fear of initial physical contact through touch and holding	IV III	Phillips-Pula et al. (2013) Heydarpour et al. (2016)
	Create opportunities for parents to participate in medical rounds	III II II I	Aija et al. (2019) Rea et al. (2018) Glick et al. (2021) Tandberg et al. (2018)
Recognize maternal/paternal risk factors for postpartum depression	Caregivers recognize impact of maternal depression on the social–emotional development of the infant Screening for PPD is provided routinely to all parents with infants in the NICU	II III II	Erdei et al. (2021) Grekin and O'Hara (2014) Hynan et al. (2013) Roque et al. (2017) Heydarpour et al. (2016)
	Staff supports implementation of relationship-based developmental care through use of the reflective process	I VI	Ohlsson and Jacobs (2013) Vittner (2009)
	Recognize potential development of PTSD for parents of infants in the NICU	I II	D'Agata and McGrath (2016) Schecter et al. (2020)
Supporting parent–infant synchrony, attachment, and responsiveness	Provide support to parents to nurture parents' relationships with their infants	I II IV	Baker and McGrath (2011) Feldman (2017) Planalp et al. (2019) McFarland et al. (2020) Mathewson et al. (2017)
	"Speaking for the baby" is utilized to help parents understand the infant's nonverbal behavior	I II IV	Quinn et al. (2020) Feldman (2017) Feldman (2020) Twohig et al. (2016)
	Provide education and support parents' understanding of their infant's signals and cues	I II II	Feldman (2017) Feldman (2020) Leckey et al. (2019) Vittner (2009) Zelkowitz et al. (2011)
	Caregivers recognize maladaptive behaviors in the parent–infant relationship requiring consultation or treatment with a mental health clinician	I II III	Anderson and Cacola (2017) Hynan et al. (2013) Treyvaud et al. (2009)
Facilitating active parent participation in caregiving	Provide information and direction for provision of caregiving to increase parent confidence and competence	I I III	Zhang et al. (2021) Treyvaud et al. (2019) Vance and Brandon (2017) Vance et al. (2020) Vance et al. (2021)

(Continued)

TABLE 7-1 Practice Recommendations That Support Social–Emotional Development in Infants and Their Parents/Primary Caregivers in the NICU   (Continued)

Intervention Strategy	Practice Recommendation	Level of Evidence	Citations
	Parents are informed of the many benefits of skin-to-skin holding (SSC) and are provided support to regularly participate in SSC with their infant	II I	Ludington-Hoe et al. (2008) Kostandy and Ludington-Hoe (2019) Shorey et al. (2016) See Chapter 16 for a more discussion of this evidence
	Caregivers trained in providing infant massage modified for the medically fragile infant teach parents how to use specific strokes within a cue-based approach	II	White-Traut et al. (2013) See Chapter 17 for a more discussion of this evidence
	Caregivers collaborate with parents in using swaddled bathing to support organized infant behaviors during tub baths	I II	Ceylan and Boлşл;k, 2018 Fernández and Antolín-Rodríguez, 2018 Tasdemir and Efe (2019)
	Caregivers provide information about nutritional, medical, and developmental benefits of mother's own milk and encourage mothers to express milk and/or breastfeed whenever possible This includes supporting parents in provision of the "first" oral feeding	I I II	Zhang et al. (2021) Meier et al. (2017). Hoban et al. (2015) See Chapter 15 for more evidence
	Provide parent support groups	I III	Dahan et al. (2020) Gooding et al. (2011)
	Provide discharge planning and support to facilitate transition	II III	Pineda et al. (2020) Phillips-Pula et al. (2013)
Provide individualized developmentally supportive care strategies for infant when parents are unavailable	Provision of neuroprotective caregiving in the NICU has the potential to improve long-term developmental outcomes	I III I II II	Macho (2017) McGrath et al. (2011) Ohlsson and Jacobs (2013) Smith et al. (2011) Soleimani et al. (2020) Westrup (2007)
	Provide education and support to health professionals in provision of family center care	II III	Griffiths et al. (2019) Vittner et al. (2021)
	Provide support to improve sleep in the environment of the NICU	I	van den Hoogen et al. (2017)
	Provision of music therapy in the NICU	I	Anderson and Patel (2018) Haslbeck and Bassler (2018)
	Use of maternal voice when mother is unable to be present	I	Williamson and McGrath (2019)
	Baby clothes are available for dressing infants	VI	Bosque and Haverman (2009)
	Volunteer cuddlers trained in providing cue-based interactions are available to provide positive social support to infants whose parents or primary caregivers do not visit	II VI	Hignell et al. (2019) Insley et al. (2021)

Note: Level I, evidence from a systematic review or meta-analysis of all relevant randomized controlled trials (RCTs), or evidence-based clinical practice guidelines based on systematic reviews of RCTs; level II, evidence obtained from at least one well-designed RCT; level III, evidence obtained from well-designed controlled trials without randomization; level IV, evidence from well-designed case-control and cohort studies; level VI, evidence from a single descriptive or qualitative study.

INFANT MENTAL HEALTH SERVICES: AN OVERVIEW

Definition and Scope

Although the term "mental health" has historical associations with mental illness, the term "infant mental health" is a term that more broadly includes theory, research, and clinical practice that focuses on the emotional well-being of children from birth to 3 years within the context of the family (Anderson & Cacola, 2017; Zeanah & Zeanah, 2019). Infant mental health practice encompasses three service modalities: *promotion, prevention, and treatment. Promotion* services take place in the community and reach out to all parents. These services support wellness and positive mental health through programs that encourage parents to engage with their children. *Prevention* programs address risk factors that may be present because of the child's health or development, parental needs, or other vulnerabilities. These programs provide a variety of services designed to support relationships, expand access to needed services and resources, and reduce the identified risks (Zero to Three, 2021). *Treatment* differs from preventive intervention programs. Services are a specialized type of psychotherapy that aims to address relationship issues between parents and children. These relationship difficulties are often exacerbated by social or psychological parental risk factors. In addition, the infant's risk factors such as medical or developmental vulnerability often contribute to the kinds of interactional dysfunction targeted in infant mental health treatment (Anderson & Cacola, 2017; Zeanah & Zeanah, 2019).

Unlike the promotion and prevention service modalities, infant mental health treatment requires fully informed written parental consent that includes an agreed upon treatment plan. Licensed *mental health clinicians* may include promotion and prevention interventions within infant mental health treatment. Infant *mental health specialists* provide promotion and prevention strategies that are intended to be therapeutic (developmentally supportive) but are not psychotherapy.

Professionals working within the promotion and prevention modalities are referred to as *infant mental health specialists* and come from a range of interdisciplinary professional backgrounds: physical, occupational, and speech therapy; early childhood special education; mental health, social work, or nursing. Specialists integrate and tailor services to their particular area such as a high-risk infant follow-up program, pediatric clinic, or residential drug treatment setting. Services include support, observation, planning, and intervention; use of empathy; and promotion of age-appropriate play, developmental, and social skills (Anderson & Cacola, 2017; Zeanah & Zeanah, 2019). In the NICU, the role of the developmental specialist corresponds to the role of the infant mental health specialist providing promotion, and prevention services in the NICU is comparative to providing similar strategies in the community.

In a prevention program assessment includes observation of interactions between the baby and parents during routine activities such as feeding, diapering, and play. The parent is observed for ability to care for and respond to the baby appropriately (Interventions have typically focused on the mother–infant relationship because the mother is usually the primary caregiver; however, many practitioners and researchers have begun to find ways to more systematically involve fathers and other caregivers or partners (Arockiasamy et al., 2008; Phillips-Pula et al., 2013). Interventions include assisting parents in interpretating their baby's cues, encouraging parental skill development, and promoting mutual enjoyment and delight that fosters healthy bonding and attachment. Parent behaviors that suggest a possible developmental, psychiatric, or addiction concern are identified, and appropriate referrals for consultation and/or treatment are made (Anderson & Cacola, 2017; Zeanah & Zeanah, 2019).

When over time preventive interventions do not seem adequate to support parents and help them engage sensitively with their children*, infant mental health treatment* interventions may be needed. *Mental health clinicians* licensed as psychotherapists, clinical social workers, psychologists, or psychiatrists work with parents to understand and address concerns that can impede development of a positive relationship.

Situations often requiring mental health treatment include:

- A parent's difficulty in feeling connected to a new baby
- Distortions about baby's behavior or self as a parent
- The parents own mental health complexities such as perinatal mood disorders, which may include postpartum depression, postpartum psychosis, or other preexisting conditions such as posttraumatic stress disorder (PTSD), chronic depression, and anxiety that may intrude on parental capacities and interactions with the baby
- History of or current illicit substance use
- Persistent difficulty in responding to the infant's needs and cues, and a range of other concerns
- Familial or social difficulties such as domestic violence, lack of social support network
- Difficult adaptation to the baby or parenting role due to complications such as prematurity or developmental delays
- Perceived or actual difficulties in the baby's behavior such as fussiness and feeding and sleep issues that are overwhelming the parent's capabilities to cope and respond calmly
- Behavior issues that develop as the child grows
- History of loss is pervading and interfering with the current relationships
- Recent migration or immigration that has led to a loss of family support or a reduction in individual stability

Mayes (2003) identified three levels of involvement for infant mental health clinicians in the NICU:

1. direct involvement with the infant and parents,
2. consultation to the health care professional who are involved with the infant and family, and
3. long-term consultation to the NICU to effect changes in policy and standards of care that directly or indirectly impact parents and families. Direct involvement with the family may consist of a one-time consultation or ongoing psychotherapy.

The infant mental health clinician assesses the baby's contributions to the relationship problem; in the case of NICU infants or graduates, these include difficulties the infant has in responding, calming, and engaging. Psychotherapeutic techniques might include approaches such as exploration of the parent's own history, empathic inquiry, and reframing or other methods to help parents gain insight about their fears, feelings, and behaviors. The clinician works with the parent to understand negative meanings the parent has assigned to their inability to soothe the infant or any negative attributions the parent may have about their infant.

For treatment to be as effective as possible, the clinician collaborates with medical, developmental, nursing, and social work healthcare professionals to fully understand the needs, feelings, and behaviors of the family. The needs, feelings, and behavior of the staff are also important to understand. It is critical to note that if infant mental health treatment is required during the NICU stay, the needs for the developmental care staff to stay involved and provide emotional support and information remain constant.

Infant mental health consultation is a service that can be provided by either infant mental health specialists or licensed mental health professionals depending on the presenting problem. The infant mental health consultant assists staff to understand the complex behaviors and motivations of parents. The consultant can help healthcare professionals identify their own unarticulated feelings that may be a detriment to an empathic and supportive stance with parents. Consultation can also help healthcare professionals focus on the relationship between the parent and child, so they do not get lost in the specific needs of either parent or child. Although healthcare professionals are encouraged to understand and work closely with families, consultation can provide additional reflective support to maintain appropriate boundaries. Consultation will also be helpful to healthcare professionals as they struggle with their own feelings of anxiety, sadness, and loss with NICU experiences.

Several concepts relevant to infant mental health are outlined below. All clinicians and caregivers need to be familiar with these concepts to best care for infants and families in the NICU. D'Agata and McGrath (2016) provide a framework for understanding the complex nature of developing in the NICU where parent, nurse, and organization all must work together to support optimal outcomes for each infant.

Regulation is the baby's capacity to move from state to state smoothly. The development of regulation requires a partner who works with the infant to anticipate their needs and respond appropriately, thus the term coregulation is often used. Coregulation is a central concept in understanding and support of the parent–infant relationship in the Newborn Individualized Developmental Care and Assessment Program (NIDCAP) approach to developmental care (Als & McAnulty, 2011; Ohlsson & Jacobs, 2013; Vittner, 2009; Westrup, 2007).

Synchrony is the match between parent's and infant's activities that promotes reciprocity and mutuality in engagement. By synchronizing with the child's attentive states, parents provide structure for playful interactions, regulate infant attention, facilitate the development of verbal dialogue, and promote the infant's capacity for self-regulation (Baker & McGrath, 2011; Feldman, 2017; McFarland et al., 2020).

Attunement is the parent's ability to grasp the infant's state and needs and to respond with and provide the kind of support needed by the infant to achieve a more complex state of organization. Attunement is dependent on an individual's sensitivity to the infant's signals, especially those that indicate the need for engagement or disengagement (Feldman, 2017, 2020). Infant cues are subtle and individual, so while knowing infant cues is important, knowing *this* infant's cues is even more important in providing support for engagement (Quinn et al., 2020).

Attachment is a system in the brain that influences and organizes motivational, emotional, and memory processes with respect to significant caregivers (Feldman, 2017). The attachment system motivates the infant to seek proximity and communication with parents and other primary caregivers. The ability of the parent to provide emotionally sensitive responses to the child's signals supports the child's positive emotional states and helps to modulate negative states (Feldman, 2017; Quinn et al., 2020). Security of attachment has been shown to have long-term effects on brain development and developmental and social outcomes for children, including psychological resilience (Feldman, 2017).

STRATEGIES THAT PROMOTE DEVELOPMENT OF HEALTHY PARENT–CHILD RELATIONSHIPS IN THE NICU

All infants require positive social relationships with their parents or primary caregivers to achieve healthy developmental outcomes (D'Agata & McGrath, 2016; Pineda et al., 2017). Key concepts in infant mental healthcare that support the building of positive parent–child relationships include:

- A stance of respect and acceptance of the needs of both babies and families.
- An understanding that relationships impact relationships and that support and outreach to parents often allows parents to feel accepted in a way that will allow them to be more empathic to their children.

- An awareness of how anxiety and chronic or situational stress can derail capacity to absorb and remember information. Parents may ask the same questions repeatedly or ask the same question to multiple providers hoping to get a more optimistic answer.

- Development of the ability to consider the perspective of others and to be able to consider multiple reasons for behaviors and responses.

- The need for an awareness of self and development of the practice of examining feelings and responses and the ability to tolerate strong affect from parents.

- Development of an understanding of the developmental specialist role as being therapeutic, but not therapy, and recognizing that parents may need additional services and supports from others such as licensed mental health professionals.

- Knowledge that relationships are central to development in all areas.

- Knowledge that respectful staff interactions with parents can help them regulate their anxieties and feelings so that they are more available to their children.

- Knowledge that strong feelings and responses to parents are normal and expected but need to be discussed and reflected upon, not necessarily acted upon in the moment.

- Knowledge that relationships with parents are the medium through which information and support are most effectively delivered.

- Knowledge that the meaning a family assigns to their baby's situation is determined by their own experiences, values, and cultural beliefs.

- Recognition of family strengths and acceptance of the complexity and uniqueness of family support networks. Be aware of the absence of support and help families make appropriate connections to other families and supportive services.

- Knowledge that different cultures and family systems have different needs and respect for these differences is important.

- Recognition of the need to advance health equity and address health using the social determinants of health to successfully provide care to all who must enter the NICU environment.

Caregivers in the NICU can utilize these principles to support the developing infant–parent relationship in the following ways:

Provide Opportunities for Positive Parenting Experiences

Providing opportunities for a positive experience of parenting is key concept in infant mental health. Babies who require extended hospitalization in the NICU represent a crisis for that family and infant. The life and death atmosphere of the nursery, exposure to other families in similar situations, and the up and down nature of the child's health and future all contribute to the possibilities for parental dysregulation and distress (D'Agata & McGrath, 2016). Recognizing the primacy of the parent in the infant's life using the core principles of Family-Centered Care (Institute for Patient Family Centered Care, 2021) supports the developing of the parental role (Craig et al., 2015). These principles include provision of dignity and respect; information sharing; participation and collaboration.

The following are other interventions that support positive experiences of parenting.

Create a Warm and Welcoming Environment

Cleveland (2008) has identified the need for a welcoming environment as a priority for parents. Discenza (2009) describes interventions to help parents make a positive adjustment to NICU life and begin positive parent–caregiver partnerships.

In addition, it is important that all health professionals find ways to promote parent presence and caregiving (Behr et al., 2021). Encouraging parent closeness and while at the same time decreasing parent separation has been identified as having both short- and long-term implications for the infant's development (D'Agata & McGrath, 2016; Treherne et al., 2017). For more detailed evidence related to the NICU environment please see Chapter 5.

Provide Parent Support Groups

A parent group helps parents adjust to having a baby in the NICU by providing information and support for coping with this crisis and problem-solving communication issues with staff (Dahan et al., 2020). Other benefits may include learning developmental concepts, locating hospital and community resources, awareness of cues and ways to optimize interactions with the infant, and gaining perspective (Leckey et al., 2019; Planalp et al., 2019). The group support format may not be optimal in meeting the range of parent needs, and parents should have the choice for whether to attend or not. Feedback from parents who participate or do not participate in these programs provides opportunities to individualize care to meet parent needs as well as to improve existing programs to facilitation of family-centered care.

Provide Baby Clothes for Dressing Infants

Bosque and Haverman (2009) studied responses of mothers and nursing staff to a program of dressing infants in baby clothes as an extension of developmental care. Themes in mothers' responses included stability, mastery over the NICU environment, fewer fears, overcoming the physical appearance of the preterm, feeling better, and feeling more like a mother. Themes in nurses' responses focused on infant personhood and normalcy, contribution of dressing the infant to family-centered care and discharge teaching, and benefits versus effort. Dressing infants appears to increase mothers' sense of mastery and identity and pleasure caring for their medically fragile infant.

Invite Parents to Participate in Their Infant's Care

Parents are often treated as visitors in the NICU and not invited to participate or deliver their infant's care. Family integrated Care (FICare) is a newer model of parent-delivered caregiving that provides nursing coaching and support for the parent to assume the role of primary caregiver (Franck et al., 2020). Although this type of care is intense for parents, it does have benefits that appear to be long-lasting. For more research related to the integration of FICare please see Chapter 8. For example, infant pain is a significant source of stress for parents and participation in pain care may enhance parents' feelings of efficacy and satisfaction with the parental role in the NICU (Butt et al., 2013; Filippa et al., 2019; Franck et al., 2004). In one study, mothers of infants in the NICU who reported a greater number of memories of infant pain also experienced more symptoms associated with posttraumatic stress (Vinall et al., 2018). Explore any hesitations parents may have during care of their infant and accept their responses. Many parents want to be involved in providing comfort to their infant during or after a painful procedure, but some may not be able to tolerate the processes. Nevertheless, all parents should be invited, and nonjudgmental conversations can help parents come to a decision that works for them (Samra et al., 2015).

Encourage Mothers to Provide Milk for Their Infant

Meier et al. (2017) in the NICU at Rush University Medical Center encourage mothers who do not plan to breast feed to consider maternal breast milk as a medicine for their infant and to pump for 2 weeks, then evaluate whether they want to continue. After hearing about the benefits of breast milk, 100% of mothers in Meier's studies decided to pump, expressed milk for more than 30 days, and reported feeling rewarded by the decision to provide milk (Hoban et al., 2015). More evidence about the impact of lactation and breastfeeding on social–emotional development is described further in Chapter 15.

Promote Parent Confidence and Competence

There are several strategies for promoting parenting confidence and competence in the NICU (Vance & Brandon, 2017). In a prospective longitudinal study, Vance et al. (2020) found that parenting confidence increases over time while the infant is in the NICU and in the first few months after discharge. They also found that poorer family functioning was associated with lower degrees of parenting confidence. Supporting the family to build confidence and competence is important to optimizing outcomes for the infant (Vance

et al., 2021). There are several strategies that health professionals can use to support the development of parenting confidence and competence that are often aspects of empowerment programs that have been successful at increasing parenting abilities (Zhang et al., 2021).

- Recognize the power of the relationship you are developing with parents. Take time and allow parents to set the pace for information about the baby, caregiving, and discussion of their concerns.
- Articulate the parent's role as unique and on-going, while also acknowledging how the healthcare team and the developmental specialist are collaborating on the baby's behalf.
- Personalize the environment for each infant and the infant's parents by encouraging parents to individualize the infant's bedside with a quilt, photos, and personal clothing, when appropriate, and always use the infant's and family members' names. Take the time to ask about the extended family.
- Provide maximal privacy for parents at the infant's bedside (e.g., curtains and screens) and private consultation rooms close to the NICU where healthcare professionals can discuss the infant's care with the family in private.
- Encourage families to become familiar with and clarify the implicit and explicit expectations that healthcare professionals and the institution have of them.
- Help families to be and feel useful in the NICU. Assess families' sense of comfort with tasks like diapering, bathing, and feeding; be willing to start with small steps to support parents to be successful and competent.
- Acknowledge and diffuse feelings of anxiety that parents may have.
- Consider the development of a collaboratively developed written contract that lists roles, responsibilities, and expectations for families as well as healthcare professionals.
- Facilitate parents' participation in daily medical rounds by providing information about when rounds occur and encouraging parents to ask questions they might have.
- Welcome sibling at the bedside and assure participation in family activities at the bedside by talking with the sibling about the baby. An extra family member should be available in the event the sibling wants to leave the care area before the parent is ready.

Recognize That Mothers' and Fathers' Communication Needs May Differ

In a systematic review of the literature, Cleveland (2008) identifies six needs for parents of infants in the NICU (Table 7-2). Although this study does not distinguish between needs of mothers and fathers, other studies indicate that differences exist in parents' experiences of the NICU and preference of communication style with staff. Fernández Medina et al. (2019) found that mothers reported feeling "empty" and emotionally overwhelmed and that learning to be a mother

TABLE 7-2 Needs of Parents in the NICU

1. Accurate information and inclusion in the infant's care
2. Vigilant watching-over and protecting the infant
3. Contact with the infant
4. Being positively perceived by the nursery staff
5. Individualized care
6. A therapeutic relationship with the staff

Four nursing behaviors that assist parents in meeting these needs:
1. Emotional support
2. Parent empowerment
3. A welcoming environment with supportive unit policies
4. Parent education with an opportunity to practice new skills through guided participation

Source: Cleveland, L. M. (2008). Parenting in the neonatal intensive care unit. *Journal of Obstetric, Gynecological, and Neonatal Nursing, 37*(6), 666–691.

in the environment of the NICU was exhausting. Mothers wanted communication styles that encouraged them to participate equally in the care of their infant, whereas fathers found this style less effective in helping them meet their need to access and interpret information about their infant. Alteration in role and a sense of lack of control in the NICU may lead fathers to withhold participation and connection with the infant (Arockiasamy et al., 2008). Fathers in this study reported that communication strategies that supported information delivery and understanding the father's experience were helpful. Fathers may find communicating with male physicians and nurses about their feelings and needs especially helpful (Arockiasamy et al., 2008; Bry & Wigert, 2019). Similar parallels in the early intervention literature highlights how needs of mothers and fathers differ.

Support Parent–Infant Synchrony

The parents' ability to communicate reciprocally with their nonverbal infant supports positive development. Parent–child synchrony is the ability of the parent and child to share and match affect and behavior and is associated with higher cognitive function and greater social–emotional competence in very-low-birth-weight (VLBW) preterm infants at 2 years corrected age (Treyvaud et al., 2019). Helping parents become attuned to their infant's behavioral signals and cues and respond appropriately supports synchronicity (Zelkowitz et al., 2011). As the parent becomes successful in attunement to the infant's cues and responses, synchrony and feelings of competency increase (Baker & McGrath, 2011).

Caregivers can nurture synchronicity by "giving a voice to the infant using their behaviors and cues." Talking with parents often begins with joint observation of the infant, taking a collaborative stance and asking the parent to "Take a few minutes to watch at the beginning of your interaction, then let's talk about what behaviors we see and what the infant is trying to tell us." This kind of talking with parents about their baby's behavior allows the intervenor (in the NICU this may be the nurse or developmental specialist) to get a sense of any distortions, worries, or misperceptions the parents may have.

Parents may interpret their preterm or sick infant's unresponsiveness or signs of distress as a negative response to themselves. Bedside caregivers play a pivotal role in helping parents understand their baby's unique nonverbal messages (Twohig et al., 2016).

Additional recommendations to promote synchronicity include:

- *Support parents to continually observe and respond appropriately* to their infant's signals and cues and modify inputs to prevent overstimulation. "Let's try touching without singing first; look at your baby's face to see how they respond." Encourage parents to adjust their behavior based on the infant's response.

- *Notice and extend positive parent–infant interactions.* An example: "Look how he responded to your voice, does he look more comfortable or distressed? What do you think he is trying to tell us?"

- *Help parents observe the impact of their actions on their baby*, such as tone of voice, intensity of touch, and how parent mood affects the baby. "What did you notice right now when you whispered to him? How was that different?"

- *Lower noise levels at the bedside* so that the baby can hear the parent's voice.

- *Address vulnerabilities and stress behaviors the baby may have* (such as inability to focus, gaze aversion) and reframe these as expectable responses that are not due to dislike of the parent. Help parents notice small changes in these behaviors. "He just looked away for a second, and now look, he is trying to get your attention again."

- *Use photos* to share observations about the baby's positive responses (for example, alertness, comfort) when interacting with the parent. The caregiver might then accentuate the look of rapt attention on the baby's face. This accentuation of the parent's importance to the baby and their ability to get a baby to look with such intensity could help the parent understand their unique connection to the baby and lessen fears that the baby does not need or want them.

- *Link real-time events to the baby's progress and long-term development.* "Every minute he gets next to you is going to help him get stronger and stronger. He will remember this feeling of being held even though he won't have the words for the experience."

INTEGRATION OF RELATIONSHIP-BASED CAREGIVING

Relationship-based caregiving is an approach to service delivery that draws upon research in developmental psychology. This research and description of strategies provide evidence and details about the how relationships impact development. These approaches use the emerging relationship with the intervenor as a vehicle to support and enhance the parent–child relationship with the belief that the quality of the intervenor–parent relationship will impact the emerging parent–child relationship through a parallel relational process. Emerging evidence in the field of neuroscience validates use of relationship-based approaches and details the ways in which early relationships shape the infant and young child's brain (Smith et al., 2011; Treyvaud et al., 2019).

In a relationship-based approach to caregiving attention is given to emotional responses as well as information. Considering the relationship as the vehicle through which information, support, and needed linkages can be provided, the intervenor holds in mind the sensitivities of the parent and the child and tries to titrate interaction in a way that will help the parent feel comfortable, respected, and heard. Reflective practices that encourage observation and self-awareness in parents is considered an essential part of this approach. Although not initially framed as a mental health intervention, relationship-based developmental care can be construed as preventive infant mental health intervention aimed at helping parents develop a supportive and sensitive relationship that reduces risk to social and emotional development created by having a medically fragile infant (Griffiths et al., 2019).

Encourage Development of Supportive Relationships Between Parents and Staff

Supportive relationships between parents and staff help parents form positive relationships with their infants. Use of the parallel process to exhibit caring, concern, and acceptance for the parent as well as for the baby supports the formation of a positive parent–infant bond.

Bedside nurses are a significant source of support to parents in the NICU. Complex patient workloads often constrain nurses in the amount of time they can spend with families. The practice of primary nursing supports consistency in the infant's care and the opportunity for a nurturing bond to develop between the parents and nurse. The use of a mindful approach and reflective process in communication can increase parent's sense of their importance to their infant and the temporary nature of the NICU. Techniques such as speaking for the baby can be readily employed by nurses to enrich the parent's experience interacting with their infant. When carried out with a consistent stance of respect and welcome, even brief encounters between nurses and parent can be therapeutic support.

Developmental specialists/developmental therapists are in a unique position to provide interventions to infants that nurture optimal neurosensory and social-emotional development. These roles are less constrained by task-oriented care than bedside nurses and have more reflexibility spending time at the bedside. By listening to questions and concerns the developmental specialist/developmental therapist can reduce anxiety and fear that may interfere with the development of close feelings with the baby. Encouraging parents to talk about their feelings supports normalization of their experience and move toward acceptance and understanding of this difficult experience. Trust that builds from this connection promotes building of trust in other relationships, foremost with their baby.

The neonatal social worker can play an essential role in supporting the early parent–child relationship as a potential source of treatment, consultation, and advocacy. This role is often unrealized owing to limited resources. In some cases, neonatal social workers may not have the necessary training to fully optimize the potential of their role. Ideally, neonatal social workers will have training in infant mental health and will have appropriate amounts of time allotted in their job descriptions to meet the consultation needs of families and staff. In instances where there is risk of Child Protective Services (CPS) involvement, a team approach should be utilized to minimize identification of any particular worker as an adversary. Staff working on this team on behalf of the baby, particularly primary nurses who provide consistency of care for the baby and the family, have the responsibility to represent in great detail the needs and sensitivities of both the infant and the parents so that service planning and/or alternative placement plans can be made carefully.

Use Common Communication Frameworks

One of the challenges in the NICU for many parents is the number of people with whom they must communicate in order to spend time with their infants. These professionals include everyone from the neonatologist to the ward clerk, and we have found that communication guidelines below adapted from developmental care and infant mental health settings can be useful for staff who are seeking to create a common way of approaching parents that will lead to more feelings of cohesiveness with professional providers. Approaches to communication should be individualized and refrain from assumptions about the parent's internal experiences. For example:

- When possible, use reflective questions with parents rather than labeling their experiences or feelings (e.g., "What was it like when you held him?" versus "It must feel really good to hold him at last").
- Describe what you assume to be the child's internal response, not the parents, e.g., "When he smiles like that, I think he is telling us he is getting more relaxed being in your arms."
- Acknowledge primacy of parent in infant's life and find many ways to communicate the central role of parental relationships (e.g., "Even though she needs all this special help right now, you are the most important person in her life. As she gets better, you will be doing more and more for her and the two of you will really get to know each other").
- Find opportunities to notice and reinforce the relationship between the child and family. "I see him looking right at you, he is so curious!"
- Notice parents' efforts and support successes and efforts. Remain emotionally present with the families and try to imagine their internal responses.
- Offer information and advice as a "hypothesis testing" exercise. "I wonder what would happen right now if you just increased the pressure of your touch a little bit."
- Support family as a team/unit. Watch for any tendencies to favor or ignore either parent.

- Remain positive and supportive, but tolerate and accept parents' feelings of sadness, grief, or ambivalence.

- Do not be too perky or infer that the parent should be "grateful" or that things could be worse. Trying to cheer up parents, compare their situations with that of others, or offer overly optimistic advice is rarely effective and can be detrimental to families and babies.

- Encourage parents to ask questions about their baby's care. Parents in the NICU often receive a great deal of information, but often the real questions that they have may be difficult to formulate. With each encounter with a parent, it is a good practice to ask parents if there are other things that they would like to know, or if there are particular information of what they have just heard that were particularly meaningful.

STRATEGIES THAT PREVENT OR REDUCE DEVELOPMENTAL AND SOCIAL-EMOTIONAL RISK IN THE NICU

Developmental Care

Als formulates the goal of developmental intervention in the NICU and throughout the hospital stay is to improve child and family outcomes (Als et al., 2003). Most commonly, the term developmental care denotes interventions minimizing the stress of the NICU sensory environment by controlling excessive sensory stimuli, clustering of care activities, appropriate positioning, and provision of containment to simulate the boundaries found in the womb. A key difference between this definition and the conceptual model of developmental care proposed by Als is the inclusion of family within a framework of relationship-based caregiving (Macho, 2017).

Systematic reviews of randomly controlled studies of developmental interventions (Soleimani et al., 2020) suggest that evidence demonstrating consistent benefits of developmental care is insufficient to merit universal recommendation. Developmental care healthcare professionals dispute this finding based on years of seeing the benefits of these interventions for infants and their families. In this chapter we have incorporated evidence from the fields of developmental psychology, neuroscience, and infant mental health to support developmental care practices in the NICU.

Impact on Brain Development

Developmental interventions provided within the NIDCAP model have been shown to improve developmental outcomes (Als et al., 2003). Premature infants cared for with NIDCAP methods have enhanced brain function and structure (Als et al., 2004). In the social and emotional realms, development of secure attachment positively impacts the development of the infant's brain and its capacities to read cues, regulate emotions, and be aware of the minds and intentions of others (Feldman, 2017; Smith et al., 2011; Treyvaud et al., 2019). These data validate the use of strategies to support healthy infant–parent relationships while in the NICU (McGrath et al., 2011; Zhang et al., 2021).

Supportive Nurturing Touch, Infant Massage, and Skin-to-Skin Contact

The use of supportive nurturing human touch, infant massage, and SSC is described in more detail in other chapters in this book (please see Chapters 16 and 17). These interventions should be encouraged to support parents in overcoming their fear of initial physical contact and learn the baby's early "language" of behaviors and how to adapt touch accordingly to meet the baby's needs. Chapter 17 provides an extensive discussion of the evidence supporting the use of supportive containment and comforting touch with fragile and sensitive infants. SSC (also known as kangaroo holding or Kangaroo Care) originated in Bogota Colombia in 1979 as a technique to decrease infant mortality from cross-contamination due to infants' sharing of incubators. In SSC holding the infant is tucked against the parent's (usually mother's) bare chest inside her clothing, making it appear that she is holding her baby in a pouch on her chest. The mother and infant have much greater sensory contact with each other than in the traditionally swaddled cradle hold. The positive impact of SSC is now well documented. Benefits to infants include energy conservation, thermoregulation, improved state regulation, early breastfeeding, and decreased pain responses during procedures (Moore et al., 2016). Benefits to mothers include greater confidence and competence, better attachment, more satisfaction with the NICU experience, and increased milk volumes. Fathers also report feelings of intense connection and attachment, protectiveness, less anxiety, and more confidence (Gettler et al., 2021; Shorey et al., 2016). Studies also demonstrate long-term developmental and social–emotional benefits. See Chapter 16 for a comprehensive discussion of the evidence supporting implementation of SSC with fragile infants in the NICU.

Swaddled Bathing

In swaddled bathing the infant is wrapped in a special cloth, blanket, or towel before immersion in a tub of warm water. This technique reduces behavioral disorganization that occurs in medically fragile infants getting tub baths (Taşdemir & Efe, 2019). The infant remains calm and often becomes alert and responsive with their parents. Although long-term benefits to social–emotional development have not been studied, immediate benefits to the family experience is documented (Fernández & Antolín-Rodríguez, 2018).

Educational Materials

Written educational materials must be available to reinforce all education provided to parents in the NICU. This environment can be overwhelming to families, so much so that learning can easily be impaired. Providing education in a variety of formats may be important to reach parents at all different levels. This might include the use of written materials, pictures, text messages, videos, podcasts, webinars, and the like. It is also important to assess what the parent already knows about a topic and start the education at that point. Ask them what they want to learn and provide learning in a cooperative format will increase the likelihood that true learning will take place. Parents need to be active participants in the learning to facilitate greater uptake of the information. How the information is provided such as communication styles and tone is also important in facilitating the learning for parents and caregivers.

Parent Participation in Medical Rounds

Active participation of parents in medical rounds is becoming the standard of care in many NICUs (Aija et al., 2019). Parents are not only invited to present in rounds but they also may be asked to present on their infant or to answer questions or provide input. Parents who do participate in rounds also seem more engaged in the care of their infant and are more likely to be present more often (Rea et al., 2018; Tandberg et al., 2018). Although fears still exist from health professionals about parent presence during rounds, for the most part those fears are lessened when they experience the positive impact for families (Glick et al., 2021).

Music Therapy

The research to support the use of music during caregiving in the NICU is continuing to become more prevalent (Anderson & Patel, 2018; Haslbeck & Bassler, 2018). However, adding an additional stimulus in the NICU is not without risk and questions about how much and when must be considered. Music interventions can only be successful when the overall environment of the NICU is well controlled and the individual behavioral cues of the infant are also a part of the decision-making about what to implement and when. Although much of the research in this area seems positive, both short- and long-term costs and benefits must be considered when implementing music therapy in the NICU.

Lactation and Breastfeeding

The benefits of lactation and breastfeeding for the high-risk infant are also well documented and slowly becoming the standard of care in the NICU. Please see Chapter 15 for more details of the evidence. Research findings suggest that mothers should be encouraged to express mother's own milk or breastfeed when appropriate for their low-birth-weight infants for the developmental and health benefits to the infants and infant mental health benefits for both mothers and infants. An excellent resource for sharing information about the benefits of human milk with mothers of low-birth-weight infants is provided in an expert review by Meier et al. (2017). Numerous studies have demonstrated the positive impact of SSC on lactation in mothers of preterm infants, including longer duration of breastfeeding, higher volumes of expressed milk, higher exclusive breastfeeding rates, and higher percentage of infants breastfeeding at discharge (Elhalik & El-Atawi, 2016). Please see Chapter 14 for more details about the positive effects of SSC.

Use of Maternal Voice

The use of maternal voice as an intervention in the NICU has been found to have positive effects (Williamson & McGrath, 2019). Mothers cannot always be present in the NICU. However, their voice can be recorded and played back during caregiving and stressful procedures. The evidence to support this intervention is growing but more evidence is needed to make it standard of care. Mothers should always be supported and encouraged to be present but when they cannot be there the use of this intervention can be helpful in soothing the infant during stressful events.

Mothers at Higher Risk

Breastfeeding reduces child abuse and neglect in mothers with substantiated histories of abuse (Strathearn et al., 2009). Other studies indicate that education and support for lactation results in many-fold increases in rates of breastfeeding initiation in mothers of VLBW infants with risk factors such as low income, African-American race, single, young, and less education (Meier et al., 2017). Assistance with obtaining an electric breast pump and consistent encouragement and support, especially by a lactation counselor, are key. More evidence to support lactation and provision of human milk for high-risk mothers can be found in Chapter 15. Bedside nurses often wonder whether encouraging lactation or use of donor human milk with mothers whose initial preference is to bottle-feed will produce feelings of guilt or coercion (McGlothen-Bell et al., 2019). The ethical issues surrounding this practice are great, yet healthcare professionals need to provide the best evidence and then allow mothers to decide. This is another area where more research is needed.

WORKING WITH FAMILIES WITH PREEXISTING RISK FACTORS

Infant Factors

Medical or developmental factors, such as prematurity, birth trauma, congenital anomalies, and other chronic medical conditions, that place the child at risk for unresponsive interactions and developmental delay contribute significantly to parent stress and distress (Glenn, 2019; Roque et al., 2017). Infant factors are seldom truly modifiable, yet provision of individualized developmental care has the potential to modify and positively optimize these factors (Erdei et al., 2021). See Table 7-3.

Parent Factors

The social complexities of families at risk can present as many dilemmas as the medical care of extremely ill infants. Pre-existing factors such as substance abuse, poverty, poor family functioning, poor social support, and low level of perceived control increase difficulties in adjusting to the NICU experience (D'Agata et al., 2016). Parent factors most often related to the social determinants of health that put the infant–parent relationship at high risk are also listed in Table 7-3. Staff can anticipate that these families will need more support in engaging with their infant. The cost of the health professional not engaging with families to participate in the care of their infant increases the need for home placement with higher risks for developmental and social emotional challenges (D'Agata et al., 2016; Glenn, 2019; Roque et al., 2017). Parents with preexisting mental health problems or histories of problematic primary relationships, NICU graduates, children in foster care, and families with risk factors such as poverty, father absence, minority status, teen parent status, low parental education, substance abuse, and

TABLE 7-3 Risk Factors

Infant Risk Factors
  Birth weight
  Perinatal risk [OB history and pregnancy events]
  Gestational age
  APGAR score
  Need for ventilator
  Surgery
  Interactive capacity: responsiveness and clarity of cues
  Severity of health problems during the first year

Mother/Primary Caregiver
  History of depression, psychological disorders
  Perinatal mood disorder, postpartum depression
  Chemical dependency
  Dual diagnosis: psychological disorder and chemical
   dependency
  Father absence
  Large family size
  Low parental education
  Poverty
  Unplanned pregnancy
  Sexually transmitted disease, HIV
  Homelessness
  Lack of social supports
  Social isolation
  History of abuse [childhood, current life]
  Number of life stress events
  Chronic health problems
  Avoidant/passive coping patterns
  Teen pregnancy
  Ineffective parenting models
  Parenting history of previous CPS involvement, child
   removed from home

Source: Erdei, C., Liu, C. H., Machie, M., Church, P. T., & Heyne, R. (2021). Parent mental health and neurodevelopmental outcomes of children hospitalized in the neonatal intensive care unit. *Early Human Development*, *154*, 105278. https://doi.org/10.1016/j.earlhumdev.2020.105278

recent immigration are at higher risk for difficulties when the parents' own needs impinge on their abilities to utilize developmental support. In these cases, the developmental specialist can empathize and support the parental needs and help the parents link with additional support professionals who can help them address issues such as grief, anxiety, guilt, or relationship concerns that limit their ability to be available to respond to and support their infant.

Influence of Postpartum Depression

Postpartum depression (PPD) can have devastating effects on mothers of NICU infants and adverse effects on the infant that extend into adulthood (Erdei et al., 2021). A significant number of these preexisting high-risk parent factors overlap with predictors of PPD such as history of depression and/or anxiety, low self-esteem, inconsistent childcare, low social support, poor or no marital support, maternal sadness or blues, an infant with a difficult temperament, or an unwanted pregnancy, low socioeconomic status, and overall life stress (Heydarpour et al., 2016; Paul & Corwin, 2018; Roque et al., 2017). Given these issues, mothers of multiples, especially those who have utilized reproductive technologies, are also at heightened risk for PPD. Mothers with PPD have been found to be less affectionate, less responsive to infant cues, appeared withdrawn with a flat affect, and/or were hostile and intrusive with their infants when compared with nondepressed mothers (Erdei et al., 2021). Cultural factors related to childbirth may also impact early mental health in the NICU (Grekin & O'Hara, 2014). Many families are away from their extended families. Families also have differing perceptions and acceptance of the meaning of prematurity, developmental delay, and/or difference. The developmental specialist and bedside caregiver need to be sensitive to these differences and understand that one size does not fit all. The bedside nurse, the neonatal social worker, and developmental specialist must recognize these factors and have sufficient skill to address in a way that is acceptable to the parent. In the absence of these skills, access to consultation will help formulate appropriate questions and comments to get the parent the next level of help. In addition to screeners, it is important that all staff become aware of the risks of depression, normal mood swings associated with childbirth, and the rare but serious postpartum psychosis. Although there are many forms of treatment available for postpartum depression, recent work on maternal depression states strongly that treatment for mothers should target the mother–infant relationship in addition to the mother's depressive symptoms (Erdei et al., 2021; Hynan et al., 2013).

Influence of Mental Health Disorders

Other forms of mental health disorders are also important to assess. Intake procedures should ensure that parents have a chance to talk about their own histories including medical and mental health difficulties that they may be experiencing. Histories of addiction or current use are important to talk about as well as a complete assessment of social factors and resources. One of the difficulties in the NICU setting is that the stress of a premature birth can exacerbate or create symptoms of anxiety, depression, and paranoia. African-American mothers are more likely to have psychological distress; they have twice the risk of prematurity as white mothers and are more distressed in their response to the prematurity (Holditch-Davis et al., 2009). Mothers with a prior history of trauma will be more susceptible to the emergence of symptoms of PTSD (D'Agata et al., 2017).

Assessors must assess carefully and be cautious about categorizing someone who is adapting to an often-unexpected situation. It is essential for developmental care staff and others to maintain a positive stance toward parents with complex histories. Diagnostic terms should not be used to talk about parents, e.g., "that parent is such a typical borderline." Developmental care and nursing staff should have adequate feedback, education, and consultation so that they can monitor for any signs of danger or risk, provide support in ways that is appropriate to their role and the need of the parent, and also tailor their interventions with the parent's symptoms and sensitivities in mind. Since the developmental care staff and the nursing staff have the most contact with their parents, they are also the most likely ones to help get the parents additional services.

Factors Inhibiting Parent Presence

Parent presence in the NICU is optimal for the development of the infant. Poor visitation is considered a risk factor for parent–child relationships in the NICU (Flacking et al., 2012). Since this is a modifiable factor, the causes for poor visiting need to be evaluated on an individual basis. Transportation and childcare issues may require logistical support and concrete assistance to facilitate parent presence. Others with complex social or psychological situations or previous child protective service intervention may avoid coming to the NICU when developmental or social service staff is available. Sometimes fear, shame, or other beliefs will cause parents to stay away altogether. Parents may avoid coming to the NICU because of fear of being judged as incompetent to care for the infant (Flacking et al., 2019). Reach out to hesitant or absent parents to encourage interaction in a way that is not guilt producing, e.g., "We would love to have you see the changes that are happening with the baby. Is there anything I can do to make it easier for you to get here?" The developmental specialist and the neonatal social worker can strategize to establish relationships by texts, phone, or notes to parents left at the bedside. Take time to understand the challenges that are limiting parent presence. Sensitive outreach is needed so that parents realize their crucial importance to their child without feeling guilty for having stayed away. Avoidant parents often create negative reactions in nursing staff and developmental care personnel. Staff should be given the support and assistance as needed to examine these feelings, talk them

through, and monitor their interactions to make sure that they are not communicating in a hostile, negative, or judgmental way. It is interesting to note that the language in the literature has changed to addressing issues around parent presence rather than visiting. The same change in language in the clinical setting needs to also occur with increased support for parents to be seen as true team players that need to present rather than as visitors (Behr et al., 2021).

Volunteer Cuddlers

Infants who "grow up" in the NICU with little opportunity for reciprocal interaction from a parent or consistent caregiver are at risk for alterations in growth and development. A lack of reciprocally positive contact from a consistent, caring adult contributed to irritability and failure to thrive in hospitalized premature infants who remained in the NICU for many months. Infant cuddler programs are a way to provide the consistent positive human contact necessary for the development of normal mental health. In a recent study, Hignell et al. (2019) found that infants who were held consistently in their program went home 6 days sooner than those who did not participate in the program. Focus groups with both bedside nurses and program volunteers described a positive impact of cuddling programs on infants, families, staff, and volunteers alike. Insley et al. (2021) used preclinical medical students to provide a cuddling program in the NICU. Qualitative findings revealed these medical students felt included in patient care, empowered in their understanding of the social determinants of health, and useful in their role. For infants going into foster care, every attempt should be made to work with the foster parent to provide their care including SSC, holding, and cuddling as early as possible.

SITUATIONS REQUIRING INFANT MENTAL HEALTH TREATMENT

Infant–Parent Relationship Dysfunction

Identification of preexisting risk factors enables early assessment and intervention. Families in crisis often will need enhanced care and resources, and the developmental care staff and other intervenors are also more likely to need consultation and support to maintain an empathic stance toward both parent and child. If this stance is not nurtured parents can sense the staff's negative feelings and reactions to them and may respond by avoiding the NICU, going to multiple providers with questions, or becoming accusatory or defensive about care the baby is receiving.

Treatment of Problematic Attunement

Not uncommonly, the stress of parenting in the NICU results in maladaptive interactions such as overstimulation or other inappropriate behavior. It is sometimes difficult to know if this maladaptive behavior is caused by a response to the crisis of having a sick or preterm infant in the NICU or if the maladaptive patterns represent a general life pattern now exacerbated by the birth. Using interventions that fall within the definition of preventative infant mental health, the developmental specialist or bedside caregiver observes the infant–parent interaction and models appropriate behavior if needed (for example, providing comforting and calming touch, supporting the infant in coming to alert, demonstrating use of face and voice that does not cause desaturations). The caregiver can sensitively acknowledge the parent's efforts to connect with their child by helping them understand the infant's behavior. If the parent is able to respond in a way that supports the infant, this initially maladaptive coping behavior becomes an opportunity for relationship-based caregiving. It is impossible to know at the beginning if a parent will be able to take in and use an empathic and supportive connection with a developmental specialist. In some cases, even the most attuned efforts will not be effective, and in these instances, it is essential that the developmental specialist has opportunities for consultation with and referral to a licensed mental health clinician.

Treatment of Maladaptive Parent Coping

Maladaptive coping that threatens the well-being of the individual (parent under the influence, self-sabotaging behavior, suicidal ideation, depression), the partner (inappropriate behavior, threats, or evidence of violence), the infant (inappropriate expectations and actions that do not respond to corrective suggestions), or staff (argumentativeness, abusive language, threats) requires intervention. The neonatal social worker or developmental specialist should determine if this is a transitory difficulty or one that will require on-going support and follow-up after the NICU stay. It possible that some worrisome behaviors are culturally associated expressions of grief, anger, or anxiety that are unfamiliar to the staff. These behaviors may represent a strong risk for problematic primary relationships and always require careful assessment (Table 7-4). The parents may or may not have preexisting risk factors, and the behavior does not mean the parent is or will be a bad parent. However, observation of maladaptive behaviors always means that more time and care will be needed to sort out the nature of the difficulties and find the ways to help the parent engage with their child in a supportive way (D'Agata et al., 2016; Glenn, 2019). Ideally the developmental specialist and NICU staff would have access to a licensed infant mental health clinician for consultation and reflective support to work with families for whom respectful interaction, gentle support, and information are not enough. These families require more time-intensive interventions so that they can remain engaged with their child. When an infant mental health clinician is not available for this kind of support with families, active involvement of the NICU social worker is indicated. It is essential to assess long-term risks, strategies, and concerns in NICU interdisciplinary rounds so that appropriate infant mental health services can be put in place to protect and nurture the relationships that will shape the child's long-term developmental pathways.

THE REFLECTIVE PROCESS

Developmental care providers often develop strong emotional responses to the babies and the parents with whom they work in the NICU. Providers may experience feelings of anger or annoyance with parents who seem insensitive to their child's needs or who do not show up to even see what these needs are. Through consultation with peers, social worker, or licensed infant mental health clinicians, developmental care providers have a chance to step back from these feelings. The opportunity to consider the perspective and needs of the parents will help caregivers regain their empathy and find ways to help parents engage with their children (Gilkerson & Als, 1995). This reflective process enhances the caregiver's ability to provide relationship-based care through understanding of the self and the experience of the infant and parent (Gilkerson & Als, 1995; Vittner, 2009). The successful use of reflective process strategies to support staff in facilitating developmentally supportive care has been described by Vittner (2009) based on the work of Als. Strategies included critical incident debriefings, patient-care conferences, guided dialogues with a qualified facilitator, journaling, and guided imagery. A qualified facilitator is key to this process (Vittner, 2009). The primary goal of the use of reflective processes is increasing the ability of the staff to recognize their own internal processes, manage their reactions, and as appropriate use their feelings and responses to generate empathy and craft more effective intervention with parents.

Recognize and Acknowledge Personal Feelings

Caregivers must continually reexamine feelings to avoid becoming judgmental and moralistic. Often there are cases where the feelings generated by parents and babies are difficult to understand. Parents motives and reactions are influenced by beliefs and contextual and cultural forces that are not always apparent. Parents' behaviors or expressions of feelings may stir up feelings from the caregiver's personal experiences. In some cases, parental responses can remind the caregiver of difficult situations with former NICU families. In these instances, caregivers

TABLE 7-4 Maladaptive Parent Behaviors in the NICU

Minimal time spent with infant at bedside and missed appointments
Flat affect, or other signs of depression
Inappropriate or threatening language
Inappropriate anger or argumentativeness
Evidence of family violence/abuse
Evidence of illicit substance use/abuse

Related concerns
    Evidence of homelessness
    Incarceration of parent

should be supported to seek and use consultation from peers, and consultants such as the neonatal social worker or employee support program.

Specific Suggestions for Working With Families in Crisis

■ Deal with the here and now. Focus on current issues; do not dwell on the past. If parents are not able to focus on the present or have a need to sort out issues that are impinging on their abilities to be present with their child, the developmental specialist or bedside caregiver has a role to play in acknowledging these difficulties, clarifying the limitations of their work, and helping the parent find an appropriate source of support such as a licensed mental health clinician where intrusive concerns can be examined and worked through.

■ Be aware of the limitations of your role. Use the strength of your relationship to help parents bridge to additional services.

■ When needed, refer individual family members to treatment with licensed mental health professionals. Consult with that professional for the best practice working with this family in a collaborative manner.

CONCLUSION

The integration of strategies that promote infant mental health and reduce risk of social emotional problems into developmental care offers great promise to promote the health and well-being of NICU infants and their families during their stays in the hospital and beyond. However, for many families these interventions are not sufficient because of the number and complexity of preexisting social and psychological factors. This chapter highlights the need for licensed infant mental health clinicians to partner with hospital staff. Mobilizing the resources within hospitals to support the NICU staff in their work of providing social–emotional support to infants and their families is a critical issue. Broadening and sustaining social–emotional care for infants and families in the NICU is widely supported by research from many fields including mental health, nursing, and neuroscience. Table 7-5 contains questions that still need to be answered and should be used to direct future research in this area. However, mobilizing resources to fully integrate infant mental health principles to support families and staff will require leadership at the policy, professional, and administrative levels.

TABLE 7-5 Questions yet to Be Answered

Implementation of the infant mental health (IMH) perspective in the NICU	1. What are effective models for implementation of IMH? 2. What are the training needs for NICU professionals related to implementation and integration of IMH strategies? 3. What funding strategies will support IMH care in the NICU? 4. What is the impact of a formal IMH program in the NICU on rates of parent satisfaction, parental anxiety post discharge, and rates of out-of-home placement?
Parent/infant preexisting risk factors	1. What communication strategies support NICU staff in working with families in crisis? 2. What strategies can be put in place to decrease the stigma for mothers with preexisting risk factors for poor parenting to facilitate optimal parenting for high-risk parents?
Parent presence	1. What strategies can be used to increase parent presence in the NICU? 2. What strategies can be used to increase parent active participation in the caregiving of their infant in the NICU?
Parent–infant synchrony	1. What are parent responses to "speaking for the baby"? 2. How do we increase the use of maternal voice as an intervention when mothers are unable to be present?
Developmental care	1. What are successful strategies for overcoming barriers to individualized developmentally supportive relationship-based care?
SSC holding	1. What are barriers to consistent implementation of SSC? 2. What low-cost or no-cost methods motivate staff to promote SSC with all families? 3. How does SSC interact with the developing microbiome in relationship to the gut–brain interaction?
Infant massage	1. What strategies support staff in encouraging families to provide their infant with nurturing touch? 2. How can parent-delivered infant massage become a standard of care in the NICU?
Infant feeding	1. What strategies need to be put in place so it becomes routine that mothers provide the *"first"* oral feeding to their infant? 2. What new strategies or interventions will increase the duration of provision of human milk in the NICU? 3. How to assure opportunities for all oral feedings to create positive feeding experiences with emotional connectedness?

REFERENCES

Aija, A., Toome, L., Axelin, A., Raiskila, S., & Lehtonen, L. (2019). Parents' presence and participation in medical rounds in 11 European neonatal units. *Early Human Development, 30*, 10–16. https://doi.org/10.1016/j.earlhumdev.2019.01.003

Al Maghaireh, D. F., Abdullah, K. L., Chan, C. M., Piaw, C. Y., & Al Kawafha, M. M. (2016). Systematic review of qualitative studies exploring parental experiences in the neonatal intensive care unit. *Journal of Clinical Nursing, 25*, 2745–2756. https://doi.org/10.1111/jocn.13259

Als, H., Duffy, F. H., McAnulty, G. B., Rivkin, M. J., Vajapeyam, S., Mulkern, R. V., Warfield, S. K., Huppi, P. S., Butler, S. C., Connenman, N., Fischer, C., & Eichenwald, E. C. (2004). Early experience alters brain function and structure. *Pediatrics, 113*(4), 846–857.

Als, H., Gilkerson, L., Duffy, F. K., McAnulty, G. B., Buehler, D. M., VandenBerg, K. A., Sweet, N., Sell, E., Parad, R. B., Ringer, S. A., Butler, S. C., Blickman, J. G., & Jones, K. J. (2003). A three-center, randomized, controlled trial of individualized developmental care for very low birth weight infants: Medical, neurodevelopmental, parenting, and caregiving effects. *Journal of Developmental and Behavioral Pediatrics, 24*, 399–408.

Als, H., & McAnulty, G. B. (2011). The newborn individualized developmental care and assessment program (NIDCAP) with kangaroo mother care (KMC): Comprehensive care for preterm infants. *Current Womens' Health Review, 7*(3), 288–301. https://doi.org/10.2174/157340411796355216

Anderson, C., & Cacola, P. (2017) Implications of preterm birth for maternal mental health and infant development. *MCN: American Journal of Maternal Child Nursing, 42*(2), 108–114. https://doi.org/10.1097/NMC.0000000000000311

Anderson, D. E., & Patel, A. D. (2018). Infants born preterm, stress, and neurodevelopment in the neonatal intensive care unit: Might music have an impact? *Developmental Medicine and Child Neurology, 60*(3), 256–266. https://doi.org/10.1111/dmcn.13663

Arockiasamy, V., Holsti, L., & Albersheim, S. (2008). Fathers' experiences in the neonatal intensive care unit: A search for control. *Pediatrics, 121*(2), e215–e222. https://doi.org/10.1542/peds.2007-1005. http://www.pediatrics.org/cgi/content/full/121/2/e215

Baker, B. J, & McGrath, J. M. (2011). Maternal infant synchrony: An integrated review of the literature. *Neonatal, Paediatric and Child Health Nursing, 14*(3), 2–13.

Barlow, J., Bennett, C., Midgley, N., Larkin, S. K., & Wei, Y. (2015). Parent-infant psychotherapy for improving parental and infant mental health. *Cochrane Database of Systematic Reviews, 1*, CD010534. https://doi.org/10.1002/14651858.CD010534.pub2

Behr, J. H., Brandon, D., & McGrath, J. M. (2021) Parents are "essential" care givers. *Advances in Neonatal Care, 21*(2), 93–94. https://doi.org/10.1097/ANC.0000000000000861

Bosque, E., & Haverman, C. (2009). Making babies real: Dressing infants in the NICU. *Neonatal Network, 28*(2), 85–92.

Browne, J. E., Jaeger, C. B., Kenner, C., & Gravens Consensus Committee on Infant and Family Centered Developmental Care. (2020). Executive summary: Standards, competencies, and recommended best practices for infant- and family-centered developmental care in the intensive care unit. *Journal of Perinatology, 40*(Suppl. 1), 405–410. https://doi.org/10.1038/s41372-020-0767-1https://doi.org/10.1038/s41372-020-0767-1

Bry, A., & Wigert, H. (2019). Psychosocial support for parents of extremely preterm infants in neonatal intensive care: A qualitative interview study. *BMC Psychology, 7*(1), 76. https://doi.org/10.1186/s40359-019-0354-4

Butt, M., McGrath, J. M., & Samra, H. A. (2013). An integrative review of parent satisfaction in the NICU. *JOGNN: Journal of Obstetrical, Gynecological and Neonatal Nursing, 42*(1), 106–120.

Ceylan, S. S., & BolLŞLk, B. (2018). Effects of swaddled and sponge bathing methods on signs of stress and pain in premature newborns: Implications for evidence-based practice. *Worldviews on Evidence Based Nursing, 15*(4), 296–303. https://doi.org/10.1111/wvn.12299

Cleveland, L. M. (2008). Parenting in the neonatal intensive care unit. *Journal of Obstetrical, Gynecological, and Neonatal Nursing, 37*(6), 666–691.

Craig, J. W., Glick, C., Phillips, R., Hall, S. L., Smith, J., & Browne, J. (2015). Recommendations for involving the family in developmental care of

the NICU baby. *Journal of Perinatology, 35*(Suppl. 1), S5–S8. https://doi.org/10.1038/jp.2015.142

D'Agata, A., & McGrath, J. (2016). A framework of complex adaptive systems: Parents as partners in the NICU. *Advances in Nursing Science, 39*(3), 244–256.

D'Agata, A., Sanders, M., Grasso, D. J., Young, E., Cong, X., & McGrath, J. M. (2017). Unpacking the burden of care for infants in the NICU. *Infant Mental Health Journal, 38*(2), 306–317. https://doi.org/10.1002/imhj.21636

D'Agata, A., Young, E., Cong, X., Grasso, D. J., & McGrath, J. M. (2016). Infant medical trauma in the neonatal intensive care unit (IMTN): A proposed concept for science and practice. *Advances in Neonatal Care, 16*(4), 289–297. https://doi.org/10.1097/ANC.0000000000000309

Dahan, S., Bourque, C. J., Reichherzer, M., Prince, J., Mantha, G., Savaria, M., & Janvier, A. (2020). Peer support groups for families in neonatology: Why and how to get started? *Acta Pediatrics, 109*(12), 2525–2531. https://doi.org/10.1111/apa.15312

Discenza, D. (2009). Welcome to the NICU: Helping parents adjust to NICU life. *Neonatal Network, 28*(2), 129–130.

Elhalik, M., & El-Atawi, K. (2016). Breast feeding and kangaroo care. *Journal of Pediatric Neonatal Care, 4*(6), 160.

Erdei, C., Liu, C. H., Machie, M., Church, P. T., & Heyne, R. (2021). Parent mental health and neurodevelopmental outcomes of children hospitalized in the neonatal intensive care unit. *Early Human Development, 154*, 105278. https://doi.org/10.1016/j.earlhumdev.2020.105278

Feldman, R. (2017). The neurobiology of human attachments. *Trends in Cognitive Science, 21*(2), 80–99. https://doi.org/10.1016/j.tics.2016.11.007

Feldman, R. (2020). What is resilience: An affiliative neuroscience approach. *World Psychiatry, 19*(2), 132–150. https://doi.org/10.1002/wps.20729

Felitti, V. J., Anda, R. F., Nordenberg, D., Williamson, D. F., Spitz, A. M., Edwards, V., Koss, M. P., & Marks, J. S. (1998). Relationship of childhood abuse and household dysfunction to many of the leading causes of death in adults: The adverse childhood experiences (ACE) study. *American Journal of Preventive Medicine, 14*(4), 245–258. https://doi.org/10.1016/S0749-3797(98)00017-8

Fernández Medina, I., Fernández-Sola, C., López-Rodríguez, M., Hernández-Padilla, J., Jiménez Lasserrotte, M., & Granero-Molina, J. (2019). Barriers to providing mother's own milk to extremely preterm infants in the NICU. *Advances in Neonatal Care, 19*(5), 349–360. https://doi.org/10.1097/ANC.0000000000000652

Fernández Medina, I. M., Granero-Molina, J., Fernández-Sola, C., Hernández-Padilla, J. M., Camacho Ávila, M., & López Rodríguez, M. D. M. (2018). Bonding in neonatal intensive care units: Experiences of extremely preterm infants' mothers. *Women and Birth: Journal of the Australian College of Midwives, 31*(4), 325–330. https://doi.org/10.1016/j.wombi.2017.11.008

Fernández, D., & Antolín-Rodríguez, R. (2018). Bathing a premature infant in the intensive care unit: A systematic review. *Journal of Pediatric Nursing, 42*, e52–e57. https://doi.org/10.1016/j.pedn.2018.05.002

Filippa, M., Poisbeau, P., Mairesse, J., Monaci, M. G., Baud, O., Hüppi, P., Grandjean, D., & Kuhn, P. (2019). Pain, parental involvement, and oxytocin in the neonatal intensive care unit. *Frontiers in Psychology, 10*, 715. https://doi.org/10.3389/fpsyg.2019.00715

Flacking, R., Lehtonen, L., Thomson, G., Axelin, A., Ahlqvist, S., Moran, V. H., Ewald, U., Dykes, F., & Separation and closeness experiences in the neonatal environment (SCENE) group. (2012). Closeness and separation in neonatal intensive care. *Acta Paediatrics, 101*(10), 1032–1037. https://doi.org/10.1111/j.1651-2227.2012.02787.x

Flacking, R., Breili, C., & Eriksson, M. (2019). Facilities for presence and provision of support to parents and significant others in neonatal units. *Acta Paediatrica, 108*(12), 2186–2191. https://doi.org/10.1111/apa.14948

Franck, L. S., Cox, S., Allen, A., & Winter, I. (2004). Parental concern and distress about infant pain. *Archives of Disease in Childhood, Fetal and Neonatal Ed, 89*(1), F71–F75.

Franck, L. S., Waddington, C., & O'Brien, K. (2020). Family integrated care for preterm infants. *Critical Care Nursing Clinics of North America, 32*(2), 149–165. https://doi.org/10.1016/j.cnc.2020.01.001

Gettler, L., Kuo, P., Sarma, M., Trumble, B., Burke Lefever, J., & Braungart-Rieker, J. (2021). Father's oxytocin responses to first holding their newborns: Interactions with testosterone reactivity to predict later parenting behavior and father-infant bonds. *Developmental Psychobiology, 63*(5), 1384–1398. https://doi.org/10.1002/dev.22121

Gibbs, D. P., Boshoff, K., & Stanley, M. J. (2016). The acquisition of parenting occupations in neonatal intensive care: A preliminary perspective. *Canadian Journal of Occupational Therapy, 83*, 91–102. https://doi.org/10.1177/0008417415625421

Gilkerson, L., & Als, H. (1995). Role of reflective process in the implementation of developmentally supportive care in the newborn intensive care nursery. *Infants and Young Children, 7*(4), 20–28.

Glenn, A. L. (2019). Early life predictors of callous-unemotional and psychopathic traits. *Infant Mental Health Journal, 40*, 39–53. https://doi.org/10.1002/imhj.21757

Glick, A. F., Goonan, M., Kim, C., Sandmeyer, D., Londoño, K., & Goldvon Simson, G. (2021). Factors associated with parental participation in family-centered rounds. *Hospital Pediatrics, 11*(1), 61–70. https://doi.org/10.1542/hpeds.2020-000596

Gooding, J. S., Cooper, L. G., Blaine, A. I., Franck, L. S., Howse, J. L., & Berns, S. D. (2011). Family support and family-centered care in the neonatal intensive care unit: Origins, advances, impact. *Seminars in Perinatology, 35*(1), 20–28. https://doi.org/10.1053/j.semperi.2010.10.004

Grekin, R., & O'Hara, M. W. (2014). Prevalence and risk factors of postpartum posttraumatic stress disorder: A meta-analysis. *Clinical Psychology Review, 34*(5), 389–401.

Griffiths, N., Spence, K., Loughran-Fowlds, A., & Westrup, B. (2019). Individualized developmental care for babies and parents in the NICU: Evidence-based best practice guideline recommendations. *Early Human Development, 139*, 104840. https://doi.org/10.1016/j.earlhumdev.2019.104840

Haslbeck, F. B., & Bassler, D. (2018). Music from the very beginning- A neuroscience-based framework for music as therapy for preterm infants and their parents. *Frontiers in Behavioral Neuroscience, 5*(12), 112. https://doi.org/10.3389/fnbeh.2018.00112

Heydarpour, S., Keshavarz, Z., & Bakhtiari, M. (2016). Factors affecting adaptation to the role of motherhood in mothers of preterm infants admitted to the neonatal intensive care unit: A qualitative study. *Journal of Advanced Nursing, 73*, 138–148. https://doi.org/10.1111/jan.13099

Hignell, A., Carlyle, K., Bishop, C., Murphy, M., Valenzano, T., Turner, S., & Sgro, M. (2019). The infant cuddler study: Evaluating the effectiveness of volunteer cuddling in infants with neonatal abstinence syndrome. *Paediatric Child Health, 25*(7), 414–418. https://doi.org/10.1093/pch/pxz127

Hoban, R., Bigger, H., Patel, A. L., Rossman, B., Fogg, L. F., & Meier, P. (2015). Goals for human milk feeding in mothers of very low birth weight infants: How do goals change and are they achieved during the NICU hospitalization? *Breastfeeding Medicine, 10*(6), 305–311. https://doi.org/10.1089/bfm.2015.0047

Holditch-Davis, D., Miles, M.S., Weaver, M.A., Black, B., Beeber, L., Thoyre, S. & Engelke, S. (2009). Patterns of distress in African-American mothers of preterm infants. *Journal of Developmental & Behavioral Peidatrics, 30*(3), 193–205.

van den Hoogen, A., Teunis, C. J., Shellhaas, R. A., Pillen, S., Benders, M., & Dudink, J. (2017). How to improve sleep in a neonatal intensive care unit: A systematic review. *Early Human Development, 113*, 78–86. https://doi.org/10.1016/j.earlhumdev.2017.07.002

Hynan, M. T., Mounts, K. O., & Vanderbilt, D. L. (2013). Screening parents of high-risk infants for emotional distress: Rationale and recommendations. *Journal of Perinatology, 33*(10), 748–753. https://doi.org/10.1038/jp.2013.72

Insley, E., Tedesco, K., Litman, E. A., Mangalapally, N., Gicewicz, C., & Monaco-Brown, M. L. (2021). The NICU cuddler curriculum: A service-learning curriculum for preclinical medical students in the neonatal intensive care unit. *MedEdPORTAL: The Journal of Teaching and Learning Resources, 12*(17), 11069. https://doi.org/10.15766/mep_2374-8265.11069

Institute for Patient and Family-Centered Care. (2021). *What is family-centered care?* https://www.ipfcc.org

Kostandy, R. R., & Ludington-Hoe, S. M. (2019). The evolution of the science of kangaroo (mother) care (skin-to-skin contact). *Birth Defects Research, 111*, 1023–1043. https://doi.org/10.1002/bdr2.1565

Leahy-Warren, P., Coleman, C., Bradley, R., & Mulcahy, H. (2020). The experiences of mothers with preterm infants within the first-year post discharge from NICU: Social support, attachment and level of depressive symptoms. *BMC Pregnancy Childbirth, 20*(1), 260. https://doi.org/10.1186/s12884-020-02956-2

Leckey, Y., Hickey, G., Stokes, A., & McGilloway, S. (2019). Parent and facilitator experiences of an intensive parent and infant programme delivered in routine community settings. *Primary Health Care Research & Development, 20*, e74. https://doi.org/10.1017/S146342361900029X

Lob, E., Lacey, R., & Steptoe, A. (2020). Adverse childhood experiences and depressive symptoms in later life: Longitudinal mediation effects of inflammation. *Brain Behavior and Immunity, 90*, 97–107. https://doi.org/10.1016/j.bbi.2020.07.045

Ludington-Hoe, S. M., Morgan, K., & Abouelfettoh, A. (2008). A clinical guideline for implementation of kangaroo care with premature infants of 30 or more weeks' postmenstrual age. *Advances in Neonatal Care, 8*(5), S3–S23.

Macho, P. (2017). Individualized developmental care in the NICU: A concept analysis. *Advances in Neonatal Care, 17*(3), 162–174. https://doi.org/10.1097/ANC.0000000000000374

Mathewson, K. J., Chow, C. H., Dobson, K. G., Pope, E. I., Schmidt, L. A., & van Lieshout, R. J. (2017). Mental health of extremely low birth weight survivors: A systematic review and meta-analysis. *Psychological Bulletin, 143*(4), 347–383. https://doi.org/10.1037/bul0000091

Mayes, L. C. (2003). Child mental health consultation with families of medically compromised infants. *Child and Adolescent Psychiatric Clinics, 12*, 401–421.

McFarland, D. H., Fortin, A. J., & Polka, L. (2020). Physiological measures of mother-infant interactional synchrony. *Developmental Psychobiology, 62*(1), 50–61. https://doi.org/10.1002/dev.21913

McGlothen-Bell, K., Cleveland, L., & Pados, B. F. (2019). To consent, or not to consent, that is the question: Ethical issues of informed consent for the use of donor human milk in the NICU setting. *Advances in Neonatal Care, 19*(5), 371–375. https://doi.org/10.1097/ANC.0000000000000651

McGrath, J. M., Cone, S., & Samra, H. A. (2011). Neuroprotection in the preterm infant: Further understanding of the short- and long-term implications for brain development. *Newborn and Infant Nursing Reviews, 11*(3), 109–112. https://doi.org/10.1053/j.nainr.2011.07.00

Meier, P. P., Johnson, T. J., Patel, A. L., & Rossman, B. (2017). Evidence-based methods that promote human milk feeding of preterm infants: An expert review. *Clinics in Perinatology, 44*(1), 1–22. https://doi.org/10.1016/j.clp.2016.11.005. PMID: 28159199; PMCID: PMC5328421.

Moore, E., Bergman, N., Anderson, G., Medley, N. (2016). Early skin-to-skin contact for mothers and their healthy newborn infants. *Cochrane Database of Systematic Reviews, 11*(11), CD003519. https://doi.org/10.1002/14651858.CD003519.pub4

Ohlsson, A., & Jacobs, S. E. (2013). Nidcap: A systematic review and meta-analyses of randomized controlled trials. *Pediatrics, 131*(3), e881–e893. https://doi.org/10.1542/peds.2012-2121

Paul, S., & Corwin, E. J. (2018). Identifying clusters from multidimensional symptom trajectories in postpartum women. *Research in Nursing & Health, 42*, 119–127. https://doi.org/10.1002/nur.21935

Phillips-Pula, L., Pickler, R. H., McGrath, J. M., Brown, L. F., & Dusing, S., (2013). Caring for a preterm infant at home: A mother's perspective. *Journal of Perinatal and Neonatal Nursing, 27*(4), 335–344.

Pineda, R., Bender, J., Hall, B., Shabosky, L., Annecca, A., & Smith, J. (2017). Parent participation in the neonatal intensive care unit: Predictors and relationships to neurobehavior and developmental outcomes. *Early Human Development, 117*, 32–38. https://doi.org/10.1016/j.earlhumdev.2017.12.008

Pineda, R., Collins, R., Heiny, E., Nellis, P., Smith, J., McGrath, J. M., & Barker, A. (2020). The baby bridge program: A sustainable program that can improve therapy service delivery for preterm infants following NICU discharge. *PLoS One, 15*(5), e0233411. https://doi.org/10.1371/journal.pone.0233411

Planalp, E. M., O'Neill, M., & Braungart-Rieker, J. M. (2019). Parent mindmindedness, sensitivity, and infant affect: Implications for attachment with mothers and fathers. *Infant Behavior and Development, 57*, 101330. https://doi.org/10.1016/j.infbeh.2019.101330

Quinn, P. C., Lee, K., & Pascalis, O. (2020). Beyond perceptual development: Infant responding to social categories. *Advances in Child Developmental Behavior, 58,* 35–61. https://doi.org/10.1016/bs.acdb.2020.01.002

Rea, K. E., Rao, P., Hill, E., Saylor, K. M, & Cousino, M. K. (2018). Families' experiences with pediatric family-centered rounds: A systematic review. *Pediatrics, 141*(3), e20171883. https://doi.org/10.1542/peds.2017-1883. PMID: 29437931.

Roque, A. T. F., Lasiuk, G. C., Radünz, V., & Hegadoren, K. (2017). Scoping review of the mental health of parents of infants in the NICU. *JOGNN: Journal of Obstetrical Gynecological and Neonatal Nursing, 46*(4), 576–587. https://doi.org/10.1016/j.jogn.2017.02.005

Samra, H. A., McGrath, J. M., Fischer, S., Schumacher, B., & Hanson, J. (2015). The NICU parent risk evaluation and engagement model and instrument (PREEMI) for neonates in intensive care units. *JOGNN: Journal of Obstetrical, Gynecological and Neonatal Nursing, 44*(1), 114–126. https://doi.org/10.1111/1552-6909.12535

Schecter, R., Pham, T., Hua, A., Spinazzola, R., Sonnenklar, J., Li, D., Papaioannou, H., & Milanaik, R. (2020). Prevalence and longevity of PTSD symptoms among parents of NICU infants analyzed across gestational age categories. *Clinics in Pediatrics, 59*(2), 163–169. https://doi.org/10.1177/0009922819892046

Shorey, S., He, H. G., & Morelius, E. (2016). Skin-to-skin contact by fathers and the impact on infant and paternal outcomes: An integrative review. *Midwifery, 40,* 207–217.

Smith, G. C., Gutovich, J., Smyser, C., Pineda, R., Newnham, C., Tjoeng, T. H., Vavasseur, C., Wallendorf, M., Neil, J., & Inder, T. (2011). Neonatal intensive care unit stress is associated with brain development in preterm infants. *Annals of Neurology, 70*(4), 541–549. https://doi.org/10.1002/ana.22545

Soleimani, F., Azari, N., Ghiasvand, H., Shahrokhi, A., Rahmani, N., & Fatollahierad, S. (2020). Do NICU developmental care improve cognitive and motor outcomes for preterm infants? A systematic review and meta-analysis. *BMC Pediatrics, 20*(1), 67. https://doi.org/10.1186/s12887-020-1953-1

Strathearn, L., Mamun, A. A., Najman, J. M., & O'Callaghan, M. J. (2009). Does breastfeeding protect against substantiated child abuse and neglect? A 15-year cohort study. *Pediatrics, 123* (3), 483–493.

Tandberg, B. S., Frøslie, K. F., Flacking, R., Grundt, H., Lehtonen, L., & Moen, A. (2018). Parent-infant closeness, parents' participation, and nursing support in single-family Room and open bay NICUs. *The Journal of Perinatal Neonatal Nursing, 32*(4), E22–E32. https://doi.org/10.1097/JPN.0000000000000359

Taşdemir, H. İ., & Efe, E. (2019). The effect of tub bathing and sponge bathing on neonatal comfort and physiological parameters in late preterm infants: A randomized controlled trial. *International Journal of Nursing Studies, 99,* 103377. https://doi.org/10.1016/j.ijnurstu.2019.06.008

Treherne, S. C., Feeley, N., Charbonneau, L., & Axelin, A. (2017). Parents' perspectives of closeness and separation with their preterm infants in the NICU. *JOGNN: Journal of Obstetrical Gynecological and Neonatal Nursing, 46*(5), 737–747. https://doi.org/10.1016/j.jogn.2017.07.005

Treyvaud, K., Anderson, V. A., Howard, K., Bear, M., Hunt, R. W., Doyle, L. W., Inder, T. E., Woodward, L. & Anderson, P. J. (2009). Parenting behavior is associated with early neurobehavioral development of very preterm children. *Pediatrics, 123*(2), 555–561.

Treyvaud, K., Spittle, A., Anderson, P. J., & O'Brien, K. (2019). A multilayered approach is needed in the NICU to support parents after the preterm birth of their infant. *Early Human Development, 139,* 104838. https://doi.org/10.1016/j.earlhumdev.2019.104838

Twohig, A., Reulbach, U., Figuerdo, R., McCarthy, A., McNicholas, F., & Molloy, E. J. (2016). Supporting preterm infant attachment and socioemotional development in the neonatal intensive care unit: Staff perceptions. *Infant Mental Health Journal, 37*(2), 160–171. https://doi.org/10.1002/imhj.21556

Vance, A. J., & Brandon, D. H. (2017). Delineating among parenting confidence, parenting self-efficacy, and competence. *ANS: Advances in Nursing Science, 40*(4), E18–E37. https://doi.org/10.1097/ANS.0000000000000179

Vance, A. J., Knafl, K., & Brandon, D. H. (2021). Patterns of parenting confidence among infants with medical complexity: A mixed-methods analysis. *Advances in Neonatal Care, 21*(2), 160–168. https://doi.org/10.1097/ANC.0000000000000754

Vance, A. J., Pan, W., Malcolm, W. H., & Brandon, D. H. (2020). Development of parenting self-efficacy in mothers of high-risk infants. *Early Human Development, 141,* 104946. https://doi.org/10.1016/j.earlhumdev.2019.104946

Vinall, J., Noel, M., Disher, T., Caddell, K., & Campbell-Yeo, M. (2018). Memories of infant pain in the neonatal intensive care unit influence posttraumatic stress symptoms in mothers of infants born preterm. *The Clinical Journal of Pain, 34*(10), 936–943. https://doi.org/10.1097/AJP.0000000000000620

Vittner, D. (2009). Reflective strategies in the neonatal clinical area. *Advances in Neonatal Care, 9*(1), 43–45.

Vittner, D., Butler, S., Smith, K., Makris, N., Brownell, E., Samra, H., & McGrath, J. (2019). Parent engagement correlates with parent and preterm infant oxytocin release during skin-to-skin contact, *Advances in Neonatal Care, 19*(1), 73–79. https://doi.org/10.1097/ANC.0000000000000558

Vittner, D., Demeo, S., Jaxon, V., Parker, M. Baxter, A., & McGrath, J.M. (2021). Factors that influence NICU health care professionals' decision-making to implement family-centered care. *Advances in Neonatal Care,* (1). https://doi.org/10.1097/ANC.0000000000000846

Westrup, B. (2007). Newborn individualized developmental care and assessment program (NIDCAP) - family-centered developmentally supportive care. *Early Human Development, 83*(7), 443–449. https://doi.org/10.1016/j.earlhumdev.2007.03.006

White-Traut, R., Norr, K. F., Fabiyil, C., Rankin, K. M., Li, Z., & Liu, L. (2013). Mother-infant interactions improves with a developmental intervention for mother-preterm dyads. *Infant Behavior & Development, 36*(4), 694–706. https://doi.org/10.1016/j.infbeh.2013.07.004

Williamson, S., & McGrath, J. M. (2019). What are the effects of the maternal voice on preterm Infants in the NICU? *Advances in Neonatal Care, 19*(4), 294–310. https://doi.org/10.1097/ANC.0000000000000578

Williams, K. G., Patel, K. T., Stausmire, J. M., Bridges, C., Mathis, M. W., & Barkin, J. L. (2018). The neonatal intensive care unit: Environmental stressors and supports. *International Journal of Environmental Research and Public Health, 15*(1), 60. https://doi.org/10.3390/ijerph15010060

Zeanah, C. H., & Zeanah, P.D. (2019). Infant Mental Health: The science of early experience (Chapter 1). In Zeanah, C. H., *Handbook of infant mental health* (4th ed., pp. 5–24). Gulfund Press.

Zelkowitz, P., Feeley, N., Shrier, I., Stremler, R., Westreich, R., Dunkley, D., Steele, R., Rosberger, Z., Lefebvre, F., & Papageorgiou, A. (2011). The cues and care randomized controlled trial of a neonatal intensive care unit intervention: Effects on maternal psychological distress and mother-infant interaction. *Journal of Developmental and Behavioral Pediatrics, 32*(8), 591–599. https://doi.org/10.1097/DBP.0b013e318227b3dc

Zero to Three website. Retrieved June 34, 2021, from https://go.zerotothree.org/

Zhang, Q., Wu, J., Sheng, X., & Ni, Z. (2021). Empowerment programs for parental mental health of preterm infants: A meta-analysis. *Patient Education and Counseling, 104*(7), 1636–1643. https://doi.org/10.1016/j.pec.2021.01.021

CHAPTER 8

Partnerships in Care: Mothers, Fathers, and Health Professionals

Marina Boykova and Carole Kenner

IFCDC–Standard for Systems Thinking in Collaborative Practice

Standard 1: Systems Thinking
- The intensive care unit shall exhibit an infrastructure of leadership, mission, and a governance framework to guide the performance of the collaborative practice of IFCDC.

INTRODUCTION

The challenge for the 21st century neonatal intensive care unit (NICU) healthcare professionals does not solely lie in the mastery of neonatal physiology, pathology, and the use of technology but also in exhibiting humanness in interactions with infants, mothers, fathers, siblings, grandparents, and extended family members. Nurses' work in the NICU environment is a sacred service to infants and their families, in the period of the unique and private life events for families in which nurses participate. Family involvement into care is key component to quality care delivery and is integral to contemporary neonatal care. Individualized infant and family-centered developmental care (IFCDC) concepts, standards, and competencies provide the basis for implementation of developmental strategies that support the infant and family during this critical period. Forming a partnership with parents is the effective way to foster their parenting role development and better equip them with the skill, knowledge, and expertise needed after they leave the confines of the NICU. Such a partnership has the potential to stabilize and strengthen the family unit, support infant and family mental health, and help them to establish positive parenting behaviors that enhance infant development as well as development of the healthy family as a whole unit. In this chapter, various aspects of partnerships between families and healthcare professionals as related to developmental outcomes and family integration are presented.

PARENTING IN THE NICU

Parenting is a very complex activity. The transition into the parenting role is a major task. This transition period occurs not only after delivery but also throughout the pregnancy as parents plan for the upcoming addition to the family. During the predelivery time, parents begin to visualize their "dream" infant, discuss parenting styles, and begin to make lifestyle changes. These activities are important to initiate and carry out the parenting role.

Parenting is greatly challenged when life begins in the NICU (Loewenstein et al., 2019). The separation of mother and baby after an NICU admission affects mother–infant bonding. Bonding is described as a unique, specific, long-term emotional tie that is established at the time of first contact between mother and newborn (Klaus & Kennell, 1976). Bonding is bidirectional between mother and baby, each giving the other interactive cues and responses. Examples of infant cues to which mothers respond include crying, eye contact, and facial expressions. Closeness, proximity, skin-to-skin contact (SSC), and physical touch, as well as participation in providing care immediately after birth positively influence emotional involvement and attachment in mothers and babies (Norholt, 2020). It is important for mothers to fulfill their role and interact with the baby during this time and NICU experience that might interfere with bonding (Mäkelä et al., 2018).

An NICU admission often causes the physical separation of the mother/father and baby, which might negatively affect bonding (Treherne et al., 2017). Mothers frequently have little contact with their preterm or sick baby in the delivery room. Once the infant is stabilized, parents often are given the opportunity to quickly view the baby before they are moved to the NICU. The next encounter for the mother may be a brief visit to the NICU by cart or wheelchair. This mother–infant separation after birth and NICU environment negatively affects mother–infant attachment (Bonacquisti et al., 2020), and the first contact the mother has with her newborn in the NICU can be fraught with conflicting emotions. What should be a time of long-anticipated joy and excitement often is complicated by feelings of fear and guilt. These feelings are intensified when a mother sees her sick infant in an incubator, attached to monitors, supported by a ventilator, and requiring multiple other pieces of unfamiliar technical equipment to survive. In addition, a sick or premature infant is unable to participate as a member of the mother–infant dyad and provide adequate behavioral cues, as could a vigorous healthy term infant. All of these experiences might contribute to posttraumatic stress symptoms (aka posttraumatic stress disorder) that might last for years and decades (Schecter et al., 2020).

After the birth of sick or preterm infant, the family often "hangs" in the world of the unknown during their first stage of bonding (Haut et al., 1994). Fretful about the possibilities related to the potential birth, stabilization, or even death of their child, families may pull away at this time and be afraid to think in terms of the child yet to be born as real or as a person they can hold on to (Haut et al., 1994). The second level of bonding occurs during the long hospitalization (Haut et al., 1994). During this period, an initial look or touch by the parent advances to beginning caregiving. Although the child has been born, parents may feel more separated and distant (and this might be true) than they did during the first bonding phase. Attempts at early bonding during this stage often are complicated by the length of time a parent and child are separated, machines that surround the infant, inconsistent infant progress, and the demands of family and work lives. As hospitalization lengthens, bonding momentum is threatened by the lack of infant progression. Parents may feel they are unable to parent as they would like to, or they may not feel confident in their care compared with the care provided by NICU professionals. If their infant is very ill, they also may feel that whatever they provide is meaningless, especially when they cannot hold or comfort their infant or when they must stand by and watch their infant in pain.

Mothers and fathers respond to the birth of a sick or preterm infant and NICU environment in somewhat similar, but slightly different ways. The trauma brought by NICU experience and alteration to the parental role are equally affecting both parents and may last for a prolonged period of time (Govindaswamy et al., 2019; Kantrowitz-Gordon et al., 2016; MacKay et al., 2020; Schecter et al., 2020). Mothers usually report higher stress and higher levels of intrusive feelings than fathers (Caporali et al., 2020; Ionio et al., 2016). Maternal distress is very prominent as well as depression, anxiety, and posttraumatic symptoms (Staver et al., 2021). Mothers might concentrate more on the health status of their infant rather than their own conditions. They have many questions about the whys and hows of the early birth, with much guilt and grief associated with the event (MacKay et al., 2020). Stress is often coming from physical appearance of a sick or preterm baby, NICU environment, and inadequate parent–health provider communication (Beck & Woynar, 2017). At this critical period, mothers feel worried, depressed,

and even angry; they often need an enhanced social support (Grunberg et al., 2019; Ionio et al., 2016; Turner et al., 2015). Some mothers are also anxious to demonstrate caregiving competence to "make up" for not producing the perfect infant (Kenner, 1988, 1995). The other mothers, while relying on nursing staff, might be resentful feeling that their baby is a "child of the staff" (Turner et al., 2015). Some mothers can be struggling with claiming the maternal role and not be psychologically ready for it (Citter & Ghanouni, 2020). An inability to breast-feed increases stress levels in mothers, requiring an enhanced professionals' and partner's support (Madhoun & Dempster, 2019). The trauma of an unexpected birth giving (posttraumatic stress, symptoms, or disease) can be serious and can last for months (Brunson et al., 2021). Mothers often spend many hours alone in the NICU watching their infant, separated from the father and from their own social support network. This separation and decreased social engagement further add to the mother's stress.

Fathers also feel alteration in their parental role and high levels of stress (Prouhet et al., 2018). Although they are usually the first parent to see their baby after admission to the NICU (Saxton et al., 2020), fathers often are preoccupied by the well-being of their partner rather than on developing a relationship with their new child (Arockiasamy et al., 2008; Beck & Vo, 2020). Initially, fathers are concerned for their wife/partner rather than bonding with their baby. A recent metasynthesis of 19 qualitative studies revealed that fathers of preterm infants go through five sequential stages in their bonding process with their infants: (1) lacking emotional connection and feeling like an alien, (2) engaging in caregiving and claiming role as a father, (3) claiming the infant as their own, (4) adjusting to having an infant at home, and (5) normalizing family life (Alnuaimi & Tluczek, 2021). Many fathers need information and support in the same way mothers do. They need be close to the infant and be involved in care; they also need emotional support (Merritt, 2021).

Often, fathers feel like outsiders in the NICU, while trying to build trust with and developing a relationship with NICU staff (Logan & Dormire, 2018; Merritt, 2021). Fathers sometimes feel ignored or neglected because mothers usually spend more time in the unit (Kamphorst et al., 2018). Often the emphasis is on the maternal role or the infant's activity. In response to the lack of usual control over the situation, new fathers may simply rely on the care system or remove themselves entirely from the system (Arockiasamy et al., 2008). One study found that gestational age of the infant was negatively correlated with fathers' avoidance, depression, and even hostility; stress, anger and negative feelings are higher when hospital stay is prolonged (Ionio et al., 2016).

Fathers generally return to their homes and jobs after their baby's birth to provide means for the family at these critical times. Fathers find themselves taking on new and unexpected roles in addition to that of father. These include the role of overseer, husband, wage earner, breadwinner, and protector—in essence, taking care of everything, multiple responsibilities, which lead to increased stress (Hearn et al.,

2019; Noergaard et al., 2017, 2018). When fathers are able to visit the NICU, information about what is happening to the baby and the mother becomes very important to them as well as communication with friends and family members regarding it (Kim, 2018).

There are also some special circumstances in which parenting a baby in the NICU occurs. Extremes of parental age may affect the ability to care for a new infant due both to emotional and psychological maturity, life experiences, and knowledge. Adolescent parents often do not have the maturity to take on the magnitude of the care required (Cox et al., 2019; Ruedinger & Cox, 2012). In addition, they may lack resources, infant care knowledge, and confidence. Older parents may have additional resources but can find this huge life change very stressful as they leave the lifestyle to which they are accustomed. Time together as a couple can be helpful to defuse some of the stress. The experience of being together through other stressful events can enhance the "team" approach as parents work together for mutual support.

Another category of parents is lesbian, gay, bisexual, transgender, and queer (LGBTQ) families. Often, nonbirth and nontraditional parents are not treated as "parents" by healthcare professionals, which makes them feel more stressed and vulnerable than the couple that is viewed as traditional parents (Logan, 2020; MacLean, 2021). Often, transgender men (individuals who were assigned female sex at birth and self-identify themselves as men) experience a lack of safe care, lack of knowledge of the unique reproductive needs, and social stigma (MacLean, 2021). Misgendering (improper use of pronouns, chosen names, and gender identity descriptors) can be offensive and be a barrier for receiving adequate care. Unwanted physiologic changes before, during, and after pregnancy (chest tissue growth, weight gain, feminization) can lead to heightened mental health needs and depression (Deutsch, 2016; MacLean, 2021). Chest binding in transgender men (flattening the chest area, a coping strategy for gender dysphoria) may interfere with adequate milk supply or lead to mastitis (Garcia-Acosta et al., 2020): the issue to be addressed by the nurses in the NICU and provide nontraditional parents with needed information for informed decisions. Sometimes, there also may be some role confusion between same-sex female couples regarding breast-feeding and lactating issues (birthing vs. nonbirthing mother) that might require attention from an NICU nurse (Logan, 2020).

Nontraditional parents feel more empowered when they are treated with dignity and respect; they are committed to the parenthood just as any parents (Kerppola et al., 2020). This population tends to use midwifery services even more often than the cisgender population as they seek more individualized care and support (Richardson et al., 2019). Sometimes LGBTQ parents are not supported by their relatives, which makes their friends, a "chosen family," more important for them to provide support (Kerppola et al., 2020). This is another consideration when providing care for this particular group of parents. The unique dynamic of LGBTQ families in the NICU as well as healthcare professionals' attitudes and treatment toward these families warrants further research (Logan, 2020). Examination of unconscious bias in providing neonatal care is another area of research.

Parenting NICU infant is influenced by support systems and coping skills. Support systems may be available via a large extended family or through a close network of friends. This support system is helpful during this stressful time and provides some relief to the parents. Often, when support systems escalate for mothers of sick or preterm infants, these systems decline for fathers (Arockiasamy et al., 2008). Sometimes fathers even do not know how to ask for help (Strauss et al., 2019). One study showed that the primary social support resources for fathers of preterm infants were healthcare professionals, their partners, and peer fathers of preterm infants (Kim, 2018). Years after the initial hospitalization, fathers recalled that being in the NICU was almost a bonus during this critical parenting period: this was extra time with the infant and a place of extended learning and training of how to be a father (Hearn et al., 2019).

Relationships within the family also can influence parents' involvement in the care and the perception of the infant. Coping skills are necessary to deal with the associated stress and to survive unexpected events that might occur. Undoubtedly, parental mutual support, if possible, is an essential resource for emotional adaptation to such a distressing experience. Grandparents often are involved in infant care, but healthcare providers should disclose medical information with caution because grandparents may want more information about the infant's health than parents want them to know.

Cultural values also influence parenting in the NICU and the perceptions of the infant. Each culture can present different perspectives on parental involvement in care and the development of bonds between parents and baby. For instance, one study showed that Korean mothers perceived a strong social prejudice against infants in NICUs, which may lead to negative meaning attrition and hinder the development of parent–child relationships (Shin & White-Traut, 2007). In Russia, fathers tend to leave direct infant care to the mother and take care of other essential family issues at that time (such as financial support); this can be misinterpreted as unsupportive behavior by healthcare providers. For childbearing Orthodox Jewish couples, absence of physical support from husbands, the delay in naming a baby, laws of the Sabbath and holidays, and specifics of the postpartum period are essential for understanding the families' needs and providing culturally sensitive, supportive care (Zauderer, 2009). One Canadian study found that not all fathers want to be involved in infant care (Feeley et al., 2013). A recent study conducted in Denmark also revealed an increased stress in fathers who were involved in infant care in the NICU during infant hospitalization, suggesting this involvement is an extra stressor, an extra responsibility in addition to their work, taking care of siblings, and managing housework at home (Noergaard et al., 2018).

Parents of preterm infants deserve special attention from healthcare professionals. When the transition to parenthood is interrupted by a preterm delivery, both the infant and parents are preterm. The period needed for the psychological preparation of having a baby has been abruptly shortened. In addition, parents are thrown into a high-stress foreign environment of the NICU with many fears, unknowns, and uncertainties. They certainly did not achieve the "dream" infant, and the infant may actually look very different from the prenatal perceptions, which can make parents (especially mothers) feel inadequate and guilty, thus decreasing their parenting confidence. Due to a premature delivery/NICU hospitalization, parents often experience a number of emotions.

Upon the delivery of a preterm infant, parents might exhibit *shock*. This shock can be related to the infant's unexpected birth, appearance, or the chain of events leading up to the NICU stay. Parents may feel helpless, hopeless, out of control, and guilty that this early delivery has occurred. Anger may surface as they review their circumstances, realize they did everything they were supposed to, and still have this undesirable pregnancy outcome.

Parents might then *grieve the loss* of their "dream infant" before they can accept the current situation (MacKay et al., 2020). They can move through the *grieving process* with relative ease or become stuck within a stage. Clinical setbacks can reactivate a previously experienced stage. The pattern will differ given the individuality of each couple.

Anxiety often follows. This generally occurs a few days after the delivery as parents begin to experience the uncertainty and unpredictability of their infant's health status. Parents may begin to withdraw from the situation and fail to attach to the infant. They may spend less time with the infant. They might describe symptoms of depression, heightened anxiety, increased stress, perceived lack of social support, and disengagement with friends or families (Melnyk et al., 2006, 2007; Pinelli et al., 2008). The anxiety may interfere with the processing of information and appropriate interactions with those around them, including the infant. Friction between the two parents may be noted. Parents may not always exhibit rational behavior and they may feel stressed and out of control. Conflicts can arise as parents deny receiving information or choose to not believe the information provided. In either case, parents require additional support. A social worker, psychologist, member of the clergy, or psychiatric professional may be instrumental in assisting the family through this difficult stage.

Then parents are beginning to let go of the dream and *accept the reality*, finding some kind of an *equilibrium* when they become more comfortable with the fact of the preterm birth and infant hospitalization. Stress may decrease, enhancing interactions with their infant and care staff. Promoting positive experiences such as kangaroo mother care (KMC) (SSC) supports parents and their important role during hospitalization. Early integration of parents, as they wish, into caregiving and ongoing infant care education can alleviate some of the stress and prepare parents for successful, independent caregiving at home.

Getting back to some semblance of *normalcy* in the family's daily lives comes with discharge. Reorganization of life occurs; the family unit is stabilizing to its new set of circumstances. It may become evident as parents return to the NICU with their infant or send a photo around the first birthday or the anniversary of the discharge date.

HEALTH PROFESSIONALS AS PARTNERS

The competent neonatal nurse, or any neonatal healthcare practitioner, undergoes a lengthy evolution from a new or elsewhere-experienced professional to a professional with established competence in the NICU. This progression has been described in steps that involve learning technical skills, becoming technically competent and confident, and becoming the consummate clinician; many nurses go through the following stages: the "*technician*," the "*surrogate parent*," and the "*contracted clinician*" (Perez, 1981). Nurses often feel that their values and knowledge are the correct standard of practice, and they encounter difficulty integrating the needs and values of parents and family members into plans of care. The healthcare system is traditionally authoritarian, and parents and family members are often excluded from care provision. In the past, nurses and physicians served as highly educated experts who were not to be questioned. But today, practitioners must guard against the tendency to be overly self-assured and authoritarian in the NICU.

Nurses spend more time with family members and infants than any other caregiver. Nurses are the constant at the bedside and are positioned to advocate for patients' and parents' needs. Nursing behaviors that meet the needs of NICU parents are emotional support, parent empowerment, a welcoming respectful environment, adequate parent education, and allowing the opportunity to practice newly learned skills (Cleveland, 2008). Nurses must remain committed to the professional relationship with parents and should not cross into the area of becoming overinvolved (aka "surrogate" mothers) in the family unit. Two styles of nursing were described: facilitative and constraining (Fenwick et al., 2001a). The first style recognizes that the mother–infant bond is distinct and mutually dependent. Nurses who employ this style attempt to create meaningful ways for mothers and infants to interact while demonstrating trust, understanding, and encouragement. The second style represents inhibitive nurses who are authoritative and hierarchal and approach care as experts. Mothers describe this type of nursing practice as protecting, nurse-directed care, nurse-directed teaching, and inhibiting parent interaction. These characteristics cause mothers to feel annoyed, frustrated, angry, distressed, and bitter, which causes alienation. The ultimate result is inhibited mothering, guarded expression, and stifled communication of maternal feelings in an attempt to protect a baby who is in the care of those who provoke the negative feelings. Mothers are likely to withdraw from this type of care because they feel that contact with their child is achieved through NICU nurses. Alternatively, and much less common, some mothers in these circumstances speak out openly and risk conflict, becoming disenfranchised and earning a reputation in the NICU for "being difficult." Nurses who successfully provide neonatal care must maintain a fine balance. What is perceived as a trivial procedure in the NICU, such as changing a diaper, may start or perpetuate the process of becoming disenfranchised if it takes place at a time when the mother had planned to perform the care herself. The nurse–mother relationship can influence how a mother's role is defined and how her effectiveness is evaluated. Inhibitive nursing that dismisses the mother's responsibilities to assist in the care of her child can delay the development of normal mothering (Fenwick et al., 2001a). Most of the time, parents' perspectives of nurses providing IFCDC are positive, but it is not always the case (Reid et al., 2019). One study found that sometimes disempowerment, hierarchical relationships between parents and nurses, and peripheral role of the father are present in the NICU (Serlachius et al., 2018).

To develop an effective partnership with parents, nurses and other healthcare professionals should reevaluate their own beliefs about the role of families in the NICU. Care providers must change their focus and priorities so that families become "patients" along with their babies. This approach must include an open mind and attitude. Professionals have to be willing to reconsider their significance in the life of infants and families. They also must develop a greater understanding of an infant's need for the presence and care of parents and the parents' need to process the NICU experience. To relate to the parents' situation, it helps to explore the things that might frighten us to hear as parents. Nurses cannot wave a magic wand, but they can repeat explanations, listen to parents' fears, and affirm their role. Nurses need to understand and accept that they do not have all the answers; instead, they must work as a team of professionals and parents to individualize plans of care to support long-term outcomes for infants and families. The National Perinatal Association (NPA) provides recommendations for NICU professionals to improve family support; educational materials and tools are available not only for families but also for NICU professionals as well. For more information, visit www.Support4NICUparents.org.

Openness is the key for successful partnerships. At present, few hospitals have enacted administrative policies that support parental presence during invasive procedures. The issue of parental presence during resuscitation and medical procedures in the NICU has not been well (Stewart, 2019a, 2019b). With the advent of family-oriented birthing facilities in most hospitals and the near uniformity of family members in the delivery suite, neonatal nurses and physicians have become experienced in providing aggressive intervention in the presence of family members. Mark (2021) in her recent integrative review of pediatric research found that parent presence during invasive procedures and resuscitation reduces anxiety in parents; parents believe that this is

their right to be present because they are parents. Another narrative review of pediatric and neonatal studies revealed that parents want to be offered the opportunity to be present and they want to make their own decisions about their presence in these situations (Dainty et al., 2021). It appears that the majority of literature does not indicate any detrimental effect upon parents who were present or on the children who had such procedures performed. In fact, studies suggest there may be benefit for parents, children, and the clinician–parent relationship (Mark, 2021). However, not all families wish to be present, and their desires should be honored. Not all families react in the same way to witnessing resuscitation of their child; many parents express the comfort in seeing the process; however, it requires effective communication and support during the resuscitation procedure (Stewart, 2019a, 2019b).

Parental presence during critical procedures is not as well accepted by clinicians, but acceptance appears to be progressively increasing. Not all health professionals are comfortable with family presence during resuscitation: recent study where 395 ICU nurses where involved showed that only one-third invited family to be in the room (Powers & Reeve, 2018). A study by Brei with colleagues (2021) revealed that families were present during neonatal intubation in 10% of cases only; in this study, family presence was not associated with adverse outcomes during intubation and did not influence the success of intubation procedure (Brei et al., 2021). One study also showed that parent participation in the multidisciplinary NICU rounds did not increase/affect parental NICU-related stress (Gustafson et al., 2016). Another survey showed that overall workload in healthcare providers was actually reduced if at least one family member was present during neonatal resuscitation (Zehnder et al., 2020). One metasynthesis performed by Brazilian researchers revealed that family members, patients, and professionals have controversial perceptions regarding family presence (Barreto et al., 2019). It goes in accordance with the other recent review where a great variety of opinions were found among healthcare providers (Dainty et al., 2021). The take-home point is to let parents know that it is possible to be present during procedures, should they wish so and their choice is respected.

Inclusion of parents/family into care requires organizational changes. Nurses might be knowledgeable in family-centered care (FCC) or IFCDC, but unfortunately, there can be a discrepancy between health professionals' knowledge base for such care and its implementation due to lack of training and administrative support (Twohig et al., 2016). Neonatal staff might not feel they have adequate communication skills, needed strategies, and confidence to provide support for parents. One recent study showed that educating neonatal staff to closely collaborate with parents improved the parents' presence and increased SSC time (He et al., 2021). Another study showed that an online education course significantly improved the neonatal staffs' knowledge and attitudes toward psychosocial support to NICU parents as well as their communication techniques (Hall et al., 2019). Kasat et al. (2020) also found that personnel empathy workshops helped NICU health providers to communicate more comfortably in difficult or combative situations, discussions of the end-of-life issues, or management of parental anxiety. Following this training, healthcare professionals employed better communication skills according to families' perceptions (Kasat et al., 2020).

In addition to the need for enhanced education, hospital systems must incorporate flexibility in the planning of services and policies to allow staff time to provide emotional support to parents. FCC is hindered by poor training, staff shortages, and time constraints placed on nurses. Typical nursing staffing formulas in the NICU have been based primarily on the severity of illness of infants. Patient assignments should not focus solely on physiologic parameters and the technical skills required for the provision of care. A family-focused patient assignment should take into consideration time for parent communication, parent education, discharge planning and education, and the psychosocial demands of the family. Heavy patient assignments in a fast-paced NICU environment will result in fragmented communication with parents. It is important to recognize that fostering parent–infant interaction, teaching families specific tasks, and encouraging families to perform their infant's care take more time than if a nurse simply performs care alone. Working with parents requires time and emotional energy. The institutional philosophy should reflect care provided to parents as a practice standard, not as a bonus provided when time allows.

Staffing in the NICU is vital, and consistency of care providers and communication are key components of patient safety. Parents identify several major concerns regarding nursing staff that require them to watch their babies more closely. These concerns are inadequate staff-to-baby ratios, use of float nurses (nurses who are pulled into the NICU from other areas of the hospital), and lack of adequate support (Hurst, 2001). Due to these factors, mothers might worry about the safety of their babies. Varying messages conveyed by different nurses and physicians will impair and confuse communications with mothers (Aagaard & Hall, 2008; Fenwick et al., 2001b; Hurst, 2001). Inaccurate communications also serve to confuse the professional staff and may threaten the quality of care provided (Institute of Medicine, 2001).

The ability to successfully care for families requires support and direction from leadership of both the NICU and the larger organization. One recent study found that NICUs with positive work environments had higher parental presence, suggesting that organizational context may be a contributing factor to FCC or IFCDC and parental involvement (Hallowell et al., 2019). Each facility must support and communicate a vision of caring for families. This vision provides the guiding philosophy for making uniform choices. The formulation of the philosophy and vision statement should involve all disciplines and a family representative. Family involvement (as with a family advisory committee) is crucial for this important first step and for the entire journey. The progression from the philosophy to operational guidelines should identify critical elements and help ensure that the philosophy is in practice. Without clear guidelines, the philosophy will not be carried into practice nor will it be implemented in an effective or consistent manner. Organizational polices should be reviewed by representatives of all involved disciplines, including a family representative, to ensure they meet the needs of families. After the vision and philosophy are developed, fundamental aspects of administrative support should include communication of a clear operational definition; the provision of adequate staffing, which includes a plan for continuity of care; provision of professional education; facilitation of teamwork among disciplines; establishing family resources; and consideration of necessary environmental modifications (such as single rooms). If caring for families truly is a value in an organization, then performance improvement goals and competencies should be established and measured as they relate to caring for families. A family-centered vision and mission statement should be incorporated into the requirements for hiring new personnel. Applicants should be asked to provide their understanding of FCC and give examples of how they might incorporate FCC into their practice. This process will help to identify the applicant's knowledge as it relates to caring for families, and it will highlight the importance of FCC in the NICU.

STRATEGIES TO SUPPORT PARENTS/ DEVELOP PARTNERSHIPS IN THE NICU

It is important that healthcare providers in the NICU understand the difficult process of parenting in the NICU and maximize opportunities to facilitate parent involvement into care. There is an evidence that comprehensive family-based NICU interventions focused on partnerships with parents improve parental mental well-being and enhance positive parenting behaviors as well as children's cognitive and socioemotional development (Lean et al., 2018). There are several potential strategies for professional–parent partnership and involvement of parents and families into infant care:

- Supporting the development of parent–infant bonding
- Enhancing professional–parent communication
- Supporting of the integrity of the family unit

Supporting the Development of the Parent-Infant Bonding

The NICU presents a number of challenges to positive parenting. Separation from the infant coupled with unfamiliar sights and sounds leads to barriers to holding a baby. Sufficient contact and interaction between the mother (or father) and infant, direct involvement in care during this critical time, and sense of autonomy progressively promote attachment, bonding, and closeness between parents and their infant (Treherne et al., 2017; van den Hoogen et al., 2021). Access needs to be ensured to meet parents' need to be with their infant. This access is important for the development of attachment, which is integral to the parent–infant relationship after discharge. Encouraging gentle touching, massaging, and handling the baby decrease parental fears, providing parents with feelings of control and increased understanding of baby's behaviors (Øberg et al., 2019). During the first visit, the NICU nurse should help the parent make the transition from *visitor* in a technical environment to a *nurturing mother/father*. The nurse should observe parents' cues to encourage attachment at the level for which they is ready. At the same time, the nurse should make sure the parent is aware of normal responses for the baby's gestational age and severity of illness as they begin to interact with the baby for the first time. The nurse should provide feedback to the mother/father about the baby's responses and reassure them that the baby does know them. The first interaction should be parent driven and nurse facilitated for a collaborative parent–nurse partnership. Rather than assuming an authoritarian role of teacher and supervisor, a nurse should recognize parents' individuality and readiness to assume care and take full responsibility for a baby. It is important for parents to come away from this first visit with some sense of control. Giving NICU parents a sense of control makes them feel less like "guests" in the unit (Umberger et al., 2018). Flexible times and spaces for parents support the bonding and caring process between parents and infants. The long-term developmental and health needs of a child are contingent upon their parents' ability to care for and nurture; that parental ability is based on a strong bond of love and a sense of duty. This type of relationship must be both supported and expected in the NICU. A combination of anticipatory guidance, close communication, and asking for parental assistance with initial procedures may help to smooth the transfer of care to parents.

Parents have an acute need for learning, information, and reassurance. During infant hospitalization, parental learning needs vary depending on infant and parent characteristics (parent age, previous parenting experiences, gestational age of the baby, length of hospital stay) (Furtak et al., 2020). In the acute period, parents are concerned with their infant's medical course; later, they are eager to learn feeding, giving care, and prognosis. Information might need to be repeated or reinforced several times. It needs to be provided in a direct manner using language the parents understand rather than medical terms. Consistency in information is important, as conflicting messages will only add stress. Family meetings conducted on a regular basis, not just during times of crisis, can provide this consistency as all members of the team come together and communicate in a unified manner. Parents can hear all of the perspectives and ask questions. This gives them more control over the situation because they will have the necessary information to make decisions and plans for the coming weeks and months.

Modeling contingent caregiving is probably the most powerful tool in parent education. Parenting confidence can be enhanced and cultivated via encouragement and repeated exposure to parenting behaviors (Vance et al., 2021). When nurses demonstrate developmentally sound handling, positioning, and response to cues, parents can observe things that are difficult to "picture." Parent–infant interactions also progress more quickly and confidently to hands-on care such as diapering, positioning, and comforting infants. This positive interaction gives parents confidence, comfort, and joy in parenting. Recent randomized controlled study showed that family integration and involvement into care has certain benefits such as improved infant weight gain, exclusive breast-feeding at discharge, and decrease in parental anxiety and worry (O'Brien et al., 2018). When armed with knowledge, parents are less likely to experience anxiety and feel better prepared for discharge (Discenza, 2009). All of these activities facilitate the parenting process even in a high-risk environment. Developing a partnership with parents that incorporate them into the plan of care in a tangible, supportive, and progressive manner decreases role confusion, inconsistency, and staff and parent frustration.

Promoting bonding is of a vital importance. Parents need to hear from health professionals: you are a parent, you are not a bad parent, and you are a good parent (Haward et al., 2020). Support for the father as well as the mother is important to keep them both involved throughout hospitalization. It is critical to include fathers when information is provided for future decision-making and consistency. Initial discussions of the baby's condition often involve the father, especially if the mother is recovering from a surgical delivery. Later on, most of the communication takes place with the mother who is present in the NICU more often. Addressing issues with fathers directly if they prefer in-depth information or providing a summary of the infant's condition can help tailor the information-giving process throughout the course of an NICU hospitalization. Nurses should assess fathers' stress, situational conditions, coping strategies, and resources available (Prouhet et al., 2018). Fathers see nurses as a source of support that helps them to gain confidence and knowledge in parenting and overcome feelings of fear, uncertainty, and helplessness (Hearn et al., 2019). It is also recommended to assess fathers' cultural values and preferences to facilitate involvement to the care that they feel comfortable (Feeley et al., 2013).

Early physical contact must be encouraged to enhance bonding and attachment. The mother is much more likely to initiate early physical contact, whereas the father might be more apprehensive and reticent. A father's attachment can be delayed if he is not included in the infant's NICU care. Physical contact with the preterm infant can shift the father's perceived role from that of being a health team worker to one of being a father (Arockiasamy et al., 2008). One of the ways to increase physical contact among parent and infant is skin-to-skin care (KMC), which has been recognized as a means to secure parents' attachment/bonding to their infant, improve parental feelings, and support their babies' recovery and early development. Parents who participate in KMC identify closeness to their baby as the major benefit, a time of intimate interaction and connection. (See Chapter 16 for more information on kangaroo care or SSC.)

Consequent parental presence in the unit should be encouraged. One study revealed that mothers were present 10% of the total NICU time, while fathers were present 5% of the NICU time; fathers' and grandparents' presences were associated with a shorter hospital stay; females were present significantly more than males (Saxton et al., 2020). Mothers mostly visited younger and smaller infants more often, whereas fathers visited older infants and heavier infants; grandparents tended to visit infants of younger mothers (Saxton et al., 2020). Another study found that fathers' visitation pattern was not correlated with the gestational age of the baby, but to the socioeconomic factors (such as not living with the mother or living long distance from a hospital) (Patel et al., 2020). Children at home, neurologic comorbidities, surgical history, room type, NICU stress, and distance from home were found to be the predictors of parental presence in the unit, causing variability in parental presence (Zauche et al., 2020). The single-family room design in the NICU (see Chapter 6 for more information on the single-family room design) is perhaps the optimal model in which to provide FCC or IFCDC; however, not all NICUs have this design at present.

Socioenvironmental factors are important to consider when providing care for NICU parents in nonjudgmental and supportive way. Logistics (e.g., distance from home to a hospital) and income issues might play role for parental visitation patterns. Recent qualitative study where participants were mostly low-income and low-education parents revealed some gaps in provision of FCC within two major dimensions: lack of mutual trust and lack of power sharing (Sigurdson et al., 2020). In this study, the following challenges were described: (1) lack of knowledge/ambivalence regarding social work, (2) staff judgment or unwillingness to address barriers to bedside presence, (3) unmet need for nurse continuity of care and a meaningful relationship with nurses, and (4) inconsistent access to quality translation services (Sigurdson et al., 2020). Unfortunately, racial and ethnic disparities still exist in the NICU environment as well (Glazer et al., 2021; Sigurdson et al., 2019): Latino and African American families often perceive communication as insufficient, from parents' perspective. Strategies to support the development of parent–infant bonding must also include sensitivity to cultural values and beliefs. It must flow from a commitment to open, respectful communication between the family and the health professionals.

Enhancing Professional-Parent Communication

Open communication and sharing of information with parents are key components of parental well-being and FCC (Labrie et al., 2021). Discussions with families, especially those initiated by physicians, are best held in unhurried circumstances in a seated position at eye level with parents. Medical information must be kept confidential in accordance with Health Insurance Portability and Accountability Act, but parents should have full access and input to both written and electronic medical records (Craig et al., 2015). Family's permission should be sought before engaging in a discussion of the infant's medical status when visitors are in the room or parents are in the vicinity. Acknowledging and sincerely apologizing for the stress and difficulties the family and baby face is an often-forgotten courtesy that may greatly enhance staff–parent interactions. Common courtesies frequently are overlooked in hospitals and especially in the NICU. All members of the care team (medical and nursing staff, respiratory care, laboratory, radiology, housekeeping, secretarial, etc.) should conduct themselves in a professional manner. Upon entry into the family space, introductions including an explanation of tasks to be accomplished are appropriate.

The time after the delivery of a premature or ill infant can be a time of great frustration and confusion to new parents. Conflict can occur between the competing priorities of parental interaction and bonding and the need for medical stabilization. The NICU staff should be thorough in explaining the details of the infant's condition, the supportive care necessary, expectations, and anticipated next steps. Nurses should not overexercise their power, and role negotiation is required for successful partnership: parents need to be listened to and they should have space to learn with guidance and feel to be in control (Brødsgaard et al., 2019).

With an infant's continued hospitalization come a variety of issues regarding long-term interaction with the family. Nurses who successfully facilitate the maternal–infant interaction acknowledge the interdependent nature of this relationship and enhance opportunities for mothers to interact with their babies in meaningful ways. Conventional, constraining, authoritarian nurses who position themselves as expert caregivers or surrogate mothers tend to restrict maternal–baby interactions in a way that causes mothers to become disaffected and angry and subsequently withdraw emotionally and physically from the nursery. Neonatal nurses can assist through sensegiving communication strategies that help the families make sense of the NICU environment (Gilstrap, 2020): educating parents, personalizing information, promoting open communication, and encouraging meaningful involvement into care (Hall et al., 2016). Information giving and sharing are other key components of successful partnerships between health professionals and parents. Electronic media such as digital photographs, video streaming for the NICU, online information about the NICU facility and care team, or an NICU website may help parents understand where their baby is, the form of care provided, and who is providing the care.

A coordinated team approach to communication should be employed. Recent metasynthesis revealed four functions of adequate communication in the NICU, which are fostering parent involvement in infant care: (1) building/maintaining relationships, (2) exchanging information, (3) sharing decision-making, and (4) enabling parent self-management in care (Wreesmann et al., 2020). NICU nurses have a unique relationship with families; for physicians, the issues of communication are perhaps not quite as personal but are equally important and may be emotionally charged. Physicians or nurse practitioners are responsible for the daily management of infants. They bear responsibility for communicating the course of care and making care plans in conjunction with parents; the most communication takes place between physicians or nurse practitioners and parents during bedside rounds.

Mental health of parents is of vital importance while parenting in the NICU. Maternal/family mental health is tied to infant mental health, which is a key part of IFCDC and is aligned well with nursing practice (Gordon et al., 2020). The social and emotional aspects of building trusting relationships and developing a sense of security are the aspects of positive development and are necessary for the infant to not only survive but also thrive.

Combination of the appropriate interventions has been shown to significantly reduce maternal depressive symptoms (especially cognitive behavioral therapy), but not anxiety (Mendelson et al., 2017). This finding is understandable as parental anxiety is conceptually different from depression, and anxiety probably persists to a certain degree in any parental dyad, even when there are no infant health problems present. Supporting parents' spiritual needs, facilitating learning of parenting skills, and adapting the environment to parents' needs can help improve the NICU experience (Loewenstein et al., 2019). Years ago, Melnyk and colleagues have created a program called *COPE* (Creating Opportunities for Parent Empowerment; Melnyk & Feinstein, 2009; Melnyk et al., 2006). The premise of this program is that through educational–behavioral interventions, parents have better mental health outcomes, which in turn improve developmental and behavioral outcomes for infants. This program has been tested in a variety of settings for the last several years. Findings have supported that the COPE program decreases parental stress, improves parental mental health, and decreases length of stay and associated costs (Melnyk et al., 2006, 2007; Melnyk & Feinstein, 2009; Nieves et al., 2021). The result of such programs, well described and analyzed by Givrad with colleagues (2021), can increase both parent and staff satisfaction and lower costs—significant quality markers in healthcare today.

In addition to family-centered instruction interventions, a systematic review of hospital interventions found some evidence that complimentary or alternative medicine (acupuncture, journaling, KMC, meditation) helps to decrease trauma and distress in parents (Sabnis et al., 2019). Music therapy also was shown to provide positive effects on parent empowerment (McLean et al., 2018; Vitale et al., 2021). One pilot study (Menke et al., 2021) showed that live-improvised interactive music therapy (music aligned with infant's breathing rhythms, family's musical heritage and culture) had beneficial effects on infants and parents (decreased length of stay in infants, reduction of stress in parents).

Social services staff, chaplaincy, lactation specialists, and developmental care specialists all work to support the NICU parents. Behavioral services, counselors, or psychologists should be available to parents during hospitalization upon request, just as are drug-dependency counselors and other forms of psychological supports. The NICU social worker is an invaluable resource not only for their capability to provide guidance and emotional support during an NICU hospitalization but also for their assistance regarding emotional and financial resources during this trying time. The social worker is a valuable advocate for parents who need to complete paperwork for parental leave, insurance, and financial assistance, and they can help parents access local resources to assist with transportation, boarding, and lodging costs. The NICU social worker often can serve in the role of a lay advocate while helping parents communicate with the healthcare team and physicians.

Nationally, a variety of family support services have evolved such as support groups, one-to-one peer support, telephone support, online forums, and combinations of these methods using professional and parent volunteer staff. Parent-to-parent support programs and support groups generally have been positively perceived by parents and improved their mental health, while decreasing stress, anxiety, and depression (Bourque et al., 2018; Dahan et al., 2020; Rossman et al., 2015; Treyvaud et al., 2019; Turner et al., 2015). Parental support from veteran parents and peers was recommended as a component of FCC (Hall et al., 2015, 2019; Treyvaud et al., 2019) and should be available for both parents, mothers and fathers (Thomson-Salo et al., 2017). Peer support groups are often virtual communities that assist families to cope with a small or sick newborn/infant. These groups not only provide peer support but they also have a strong political voice to enact changes such as the inclusion of families in care, in being more involved in neonatal research, and raising awareness of structural racism in healthcare including in the NICU. Some examples of such peer support groups and information hubs for parents are PreemieWorld, https://preemieworld.com/; Preemie Crystal Ball Health, https://crystalballhealth.com/about-us/; NICU Parent Network, https://nicuparentnetwork.org/; Preemie Parent Alliance, https://www.newbornhope.org/preemie-parent-alliance/; European Foundation for the Care of Newborn Infants, https://www.efcni.org/; and Miracle Babies Foundation of Australia, https://www.miraclebabies.org.au/.

Interestingly, Fratantoni (2019) using a Patient-Centered Outcomes Research Institute grant looked at the effects of 1-year long peer support for NICU parents (in hospital and afterward). There were two groups: one group of parents treated as usual and the other group had a peer parent navigator to support parental mental health and infant development. Findings revealed that groups did not vary: stress, anxiety, and depression were not statistically significant between groups. More research needs to be done in this area. It appears that hospital-based mechanisms of support may be preferred by parents because people in their personal support network (such as family members and friends) often are unable to understand what they are going through. More research is needed in this area. Overall at present, a multilayered approach to help NICU parents is recommended: psychological and psychosocial supports, parent education programs focused on infant development, and parent–infant relationships (Treyvaud et al., 2019).

Supporting Family Unit Integrity

Having an infant in the NICU is a great stressor not only for parents but also for the entire family unit, regardless of its size or configuration. All family members might be psychologically vulnerable after the birth of a sick infant. Sibling visitation in the NICU is still contentious with some physicians and nurses causing parental dissatisfaction with care provided (Hagen et al., 2019). Much concern regarding sibling visitation is based on the possible transmission of infections to hospitalized infants, and especially the potential for the transmission of serious viral infections when they are endemic in the community. Institutional policies must be individualized on the basis of national recommendations, the literature, and, most important, the community incidence of infectious processes at the time decisions are made.

Sibling visitation should be encouraged when used in conjunction with appropriate screening procedures and institutional guidelines. Although the evidence is not strong, it appears that sibling visitation, in addition to being beneficial for the family, also is beneficial for the visiting children (Savanh et al., 2020a, 2020b). Before siblings visit the NICU, there should be a review of their medical history that includes immunization records and recent exposures to infectious diseases. Siblings should exercise appropriate hand hygiene and be supervised by a parent or responsible adult while in the NICU, especially toddlers. Staff must consider the visiting sibling's age, stage of development, and capability to understand the environment to which the sibling will be exposed. Unfortunately, siblings who participate in daycare may not be able to visit frequently because of the threat of infection. Successful expansion of sibling visitation in the NICU is dependent upon parents responsibly reporting the health status of the visiting sibling. This is another situation in which parent–professional communication and honesty are of paramount importance. Staff to assist nurses should be available; institutional support and policy are required for nursing staff to more fully implement FCC.

Another related issue is visitation by grandparents, family, and friends. With proper attention to appropriate infection control measures and hand washing, visitors should not impose added risk. At some facilities, parental permission and screening for infection are the prime factors that determine the presence of additional visitors. Parents are asked to designate a list of visitors who must undergo health screening at the door of the NICU. Digital photographs are taken at the time of the first visit for future reference if that is acceptable to the parents. Visitors are allowed at the bedside even if the parents are not present if the parents agree. Each room is equipped with a digital camera above the incubator, so images can be projected on a screen in the waiting area for viewing by visitors and siblings who cannot be at the bedside. For security, the NICU is a locked unit with access granted with an approved identification card or check-in at the receptionist's desk.

During the SARS-CoV-2 (COVID-19) pandemic, many NICUs have strictly limited family presence/NICU visitation. Support for breast-feeding, KMC, and education on caregiving strategies have also been diminished. Anecdotally, this pandemic has added the parental psychological distress of having an infant in the NICU (Bembich et al., 2021). Nursing care should be adjusted and the use of a trauma-informed approach to care (recognizing signs of psychological distress [such as anxiety, stress, grief] and responding to these and other symptoms of trauma and actively seeking to avoid triggers and retraumatization while providing care) may help decrease the stress and increase coping in NICU parents during the pandemic (Choi et al., 2020). Separation of the baby from mother and family can be devastating for parents. The Global Alliance for Newborn Care (GLANCE, 2020), a collaborative organization of parents, health professionals, and policymakers, upon the consultation with World Health Organization has advocated to promote zero separation of infants and parents in its recent campaign. However, there is a contradictory and limited evidence in regard of clinical aspects of COVID-19 infection in the neonatal population. At present time (midyear 2021), there is not enough evidence regarding intrauterine infection by vertical transmission from pregnant women to her fetus; no sound evidence is available in regard to short and long term consequences for infants born to mothers with COVID-19 (Cena et al., 2021). One research showed no viral infection in neonates born to and separated from their SARS-CoV-2–positive mothers at birth who were subsequently fed unpasteurized breast milk (Shlomai et al., 2021). For low- and middle-income countries, an international group or researchers estimated that survival of preterm infants (<2000 grams) when they were kept with mothers (KMC, no separation of infant from the mother even if she is COVID-19 positive) far overweigh the small risk of infant death due to COVID-19 (Minckas et al., 2021). However, the available evidence should be taken with caution. A large multinational study revealed that pregnant women diagnosed with COVID-19 had substantially higher risks of severe pregnancy complications (e.g., preeclampsia, eclampsia, HELLP (hemolysis, elevated liver enzymes, low platelet count), elevated liver enzymes, low platelet count syndrome); the higher neonatal morbidity and mortality risks were also estimated for newborns born to COVID-19–positive mothers (Villar et al., 2021). Hopefully, once this situation with COVID-19 is under control and more research evidence available, reasonable visitation by siblings/family members will be reinstated in many NICUs that are closed for visitation at present days.

Little is still known about the impact the separation and limited support resources have on the neurodevelopment of the infant and the resiliency/coping/mental health of families. Cena et al. (2021) also note the pandemic restrictions are taking a toll on NICU staff as they cannot support families the way they wish to do, so nor can they truly provide FCC. The lack of professional guidelines adds pressure to the overwhelmed by the pandemic staff (Rao et al., 2021). This professional stress impacts the ability to foster parent–professional partnerships.

IDENTIFICATION OF PARENTS AT RISK

Parent assessment is critical to supporting the evolving parental role. The parents' first need is to have confidence that their infant is getting the best care available. Once assured, they can respond to encouragement to care for themselves enough to actively participate in their infant's care. The professional "model" of care often seeks a "diagnosis" (i.e., something that is weak and wrong and needs treatment), while the family-centered model recognizes strengths and builds on the assets the family brings to the relationship (McGrath, 2001). Needs must be acknowledged and resources provided, but the overall partnership must build on strengths within the family unit. The scope and progression of the parental role must match the infant's developmental and medical timeline toward discharge.

It is important to identify mothers/fathers with risk factors for depression/emotional withdrawal that may inhibit bonding/attachment. It is also important to promote use of possibly needed therapeutic interventions, especially in the case of depression and mental health disorders (Loewenstein, 2018; McGowan et al., 2017; Śliwerski et al., 2020). Ongoing assessment of the NICU parents for mental health issues (feelings of guilt, shame, anxiety, posttraumatic stress) is recommended (Brunson et al., 2021; Roque et al., 2017). Structured interviews (and not self-administered questionnaires) are recommended for the diagnosis of the depressive symptoms to find out any attachment problems (Śliwerski et al., 2020). Fortunately, negative consequences of maternal depression on infant attachment can be compensated by involvement in care and appropriate interventions that are focused on maternal mental health (Barnes & Theule, 2019).

The parental visitation pattern can be a sign of bonding/attachment. Multiple factors affecting parental visitation should be considered before labeling a parent as "absent" or "difficult": distance from a hospital, inability to access the transportation problems, restricted privacy and confidentiality in the NICU with the bay design of patient rooms, maternal health after birth, and other children at home, to name a few. The specific socioenvironmental settings of every family should be considered and taken into account to prevent stigmatization of parents and create effective partnership.

PARTNERSHIPS AFTER NICU DISCHARGE: TRANSITION TO HOME

The professional–parent partnerships should be continued after discharge. For more than 30 years, researchers have found that parents' transition from hospital to home is challenging (Aydon et al., 2018; Boykova, 2016a, 2016b; Boykova & Kenner, 2012; Kenner, 1988, 1995; Lundqvist et al., 2019; Murdoch & Franck, 2012). Even when FCC is implemented in the NICU and parents were integrated into infant care, the time of discharge and transition to home with fragile infant remains one of the most stressful times for parents. This transitional period can be filled with numerous readmissions and rehospitalizations, negatively affecting infant health/well-being of the family and bringing significant financial burden to families and healthcare systems (Hannan et al., 2020). Implementation of professional–parent partnership strategies is essential for easing parental and infant transition to home, preventing infant hospital readmissions, and improving infant health outcomes and family well-being.

First of all, parents' readiness for discharge is contingent upon the completion of the bonding process and transfer of care from professionals to parents. Almost 15 years ago, Griffin and Abraham (2006) stated that nurses should strive to ensure that "no teaching is needed on the day of discharge. Parents should be able to celebrate this long-awaited milestone and go home confident that they have the experience and skills to draw upon; to care for their infant" (p. 246). Readiness for discharge and successful transition to home depends not only on nurses but on physicians as well: one study suggested that home visits should be incorporated into neonatology training to improve discharge preparation in the NICU (Hobbs et al., 2017).

Frequently, NICU staffs overestimate parents' confidence in providing an infant's care after discharge. Discharge teaching may be inadequate; some families might require more discharge education such as single mothers, families with limited resources, and at high-risk families (McGowan et al., 2019; Smith et al., 2021). Some researchers emphasize that discharge support interventions should be focused on both parents as fathers' readiness for discharge depends on maternal perceptions toward discharge and not the infant morbidities (Buck et al., 2020). Also, even at discharge, a long-waited and joyful event, about half of parents still feeling depressed, dictating depression screening, stress reduction, and mental health referrals (Soghier et al., 2020).

Often, discharge comes long after birth and follows a plateau of balancing the hospitalization and family lives. At home, parents may experience difficulty learning the tasks of caring for their infant and assuming responsibility for decisions regarding the infant's care. After discharge, parents of NICU graduates may experience difficulty developing parent–child role relationships; they may need additional information and adequate social support and interactions; and they are often stressed, isolated, and depressed (Boykova, 2016b; Kenner, 1988; Leahy-Warren et al., 2020; Stotts et al., 2019).

Just like during infant hospitalization, transition from hospital to home also can be experienced differently by mothers and fathers, with differences in the parental dyad perceptions (Garfield et al., 2014; Lundqvist et al., 2019). Often, after the discharge of a vulnerable infant, parents often feel lonely having no one who could easily understand their situation, fearing possible infections, and having ambivalent feelings filled with worry and sadness. The family dynamics can be changed as parents might have different views and feelings in regard to infant's health/growth or prematurity-related conditions. Emotional burnout and anger can be detrimental to marriage and family well-being (Baraldi et al., 2020a; Lundqvist et al., 2019). Feelings of uncertainty, isolation, and hypervigilance are often reported, especially when an infant is at risk for adverse neurodevelopmental outcome (Dorner et al., 2021; Garfield et al., 2014). At home, mothers might feel very lonely and guilty, especially with preterm infant, while fathers might be depressed and overwhelmed with partners' demands, family's difficulties, and their work responsibilities (Cyr-Alves et al., 2018; Lundqvist et al., 2019; Schuetz Haemmerli et al., 2020). One study found that after discharge, the stress level (measured as cortisol level) was higher in fathers than in mothers, suggesting that fathers might be more susceptible to stressors at this particular period (Garfield et al., 2018). Mental health services and ongoing support after discharge are recommended, especially when risk factors for child maltreatment are present (Cross, 2020).

Parents dream about being home for a long time during infant hospital stay, but after discharge they look for "normalcy," which is so desired (Murdoch & Franck, 2012; Norton & Hagstrom, 2021). They find themselves in dire straits of independent caregiving at home—stress is back! Feeding the fragile infant (one of the major parental tasks that gives parents confidence in their role) with some temporary or chronic health problems at home can be challenging, especially without adequate professional support (Madhoun & Dempster, 2019). Having a medically fragile infant causes more stress/anxiety and might lead to more intrusive/over-protecting parenting style later in life, affecting child behavioral and cognitive outcomes (Adama et al., 2016; Grunberg et al., 2019; Treyvaud et al., 2016). Social isolation and "medicalized parenting" were found in one recent study that used discourse analysis (Kantrowitz-Gordon et al., 2016).

The factors that influence parenting styles include, but are not limited to, perception of infant health, life experiences, expectations, cultural values/beliefs, social support, and psychological/emotional status of the parents. The smaller/sicker the baby, the more significant the toll on the family postdischarge: comorbidities and higher health risks might increase family burden tremendously.

After discharge, informational needs do not disappear, but probably became more prominent as the "experts from a hospital" are not around anymore. Often, relatives and grandparents are one of the major sources of support (Baraldi et al., 2020a); however, this type of support can be both positive

and negative, depending on the cultural values in the family (e.g., "prescriptive" grandparents) (Adama et al., 2018; Gulamani et al., 2013). Parents report the need for information and support after discharge and perform extensive searches in online resources regarding infant development, growth, feeding, parental self-care, and available support; unfortunately, the information available is not always of the high quality and often is considered by parents as unreliable (Alderdice et al., 2018). After discharge, families also often use peer support as a source or resilience and hope; interventions using mobile health technology were also found to be helpful to parents (Lakshmanan et al., 2019).

Quality care should be continued after discharge. Before discharge to home, primary care physicians and nurse practitioners always should be welcomed to obtain information (if the families agree) upon the NICU admission of their patients and during the infant hospitalization, so they can check on the infant and family's condition. A mechanism needs to be in place to keep referring physicians and nurse practitioners informed of an infant's progress and major changes in condition. Information sharing may be achieved via phone calls from the neonatologist that are placed on admission, discharge, or when there is a major change in the infant's condition if the parents agree. Weekly updates may be achieved by phone or written messages. After discharge, primary healthcare professionals are of crucial importance for physical and developmental screenings and health checkups as follow-up and transitional care programs are not widely available (Connors et al., 2021).

During the postdischarge period, parents benefit from having improved communication, adequate support from infant health professionals, and honest information given to them (Ballantyne et al., 2017; Boykova, 2008; Kenner, 1988). Professional checkup and reassurance by trusted healthcare professional postdischarge is vitally important for parents of healthy babies (Gilworth et al., 2020), and it is even more important for former NICU parents. Parents of technology-dependent infants often report a need for a coordinated care and transitional support (Norton & Hagstrom, 2021). Professional support is of vital importance for parents: the stress of being home, at their own, is decreased when professional support is available; coping with the situation is enhanced, promoting better parent and infant outcomes. One recent study showed that video consultations with a neonatal nurse helped to increase parental confidence in caring for their baby when home (Hägi-Pedersen et al., 2021). Another study suggested that additional postdischarge communication between parents and health professionals, even during infant's rehospitalizations, might be a reason for lower parental stress and increased parental confidence at home (Grunberg et al., 2020).

Unfortunately, there is a lack of knowledge from postdischarge healthcare professionals in regard to former NICU patients as reported by both parents and health professionals (Alderdice et al., 2018; Petty et al., 2019). The transition to home is challenging not only for parents of NICU babies but for primary and community healthcare professionals as well. The lack of knowledge of the healthcare professionals who have never cared for a small or sick newborn can also be related to the lack of resources for community-based follow-up, inconsistency of the evidence-based guidelines, and inadequate training about this vulnerable population as reported by nurses and other health professionals who take care of this population after discharge in the primary and community settings (Currie et al., 2018; Petty et al., 2019). The problems with adequate care provision can be present for a very long time: adults (aged 20 to 54 years) who were born very preterm reported physical and mental long-term sequelae of prematurity and dissatisfaction with healthcare services they received as often no individual history of the prematurity was taken into account (Perez et al., 2020). An effective interprofessional collaboration and cooperation, sometimes reorganization of services, is required postdischarge (Schuetz Haemmerli et al., 2021). Some resources are available for health professionals/families on postdischarge care and transition to home. For instance, *Transitioning Newborns from NICU to Home* toolkit is available at the Agency for Health Care Research and Quality website (AHRQ, n.d). ZERO to THREE helps those who care for infants and toddlers (https://www.zerotothree.org/), and Early Intervention Services provide support for those families whose infants/children have developmental disabilities (https://www.cdc.gov/ncbddd/actearly/parents/states.html). Another useful resource available for professionals to improve their knowledge in postdischarge care for NICU graduates with special care needs and disabilities is the Leadership Education in Neurodevelopmental Disabilities (LEND) program (Association of University Centers on Disability [AUCD], n.d.). LEND program is a network of 52 centers across 44 states, and 3 territories. Its purpose is to provide training programs for health professionals in the United States that are funded by the Maternal and Child Health Bureau of the Health Resources and Services Administration for the education of healthcare professionals in the interdisciplinary assessment and management of infants and young children with neurodevelopmental and related disabilities and their families. Faculty and graduate-level trainees are drawn from a broad range of disciplines including medicine, nursing, physical therapy, occupational therapy, nutrition, social work, psychology, school psychology, special education, communications disorders, and pediatric dentistry. Parents of infants and children with disabilities and special healthcare needs are included as paid faculty and trainees in many of these programs. In recent years, a strong national network of LEND Family Faculty was developed. LEND programs teach their trainees leadership and advocacy for the children whom they serve in a family-oriented, culturally sensitive fashion. LEND programs may serve as a regional resource for training and implementation of FCC programs upon request. LEND programs provide technical assistance and continuing education in their respective regions. A geographic listing of currently funded LEND programs may be found on the website of the Association of University Centers on Disability (AUCD, n.d.).

Participation in follow-up and transitional programs gives parents a sense of security, decreasing their stress, increasing autonomy/satisfaction with care, reducing the frequency of emergency department visits/healthcare use, and improving immunization rates and number of health checkups (Baraldi et al., 2020b; Hamline et al., 2018; Liu et al., 2018; McKelvey et al., 2021). Follow-up should occur in a medical home and be supported by the wide range of hospital and community programs available for NICU graduates (Murch & Smith, 2016). The effect of these programs is especially positive when healthcare professionals in follow-up clinics/primary settings are knowledgeable, reliable, and understanding special conditions of the baby. However, attendance in the follow-up clinics/program can be problematic, and the importance of follow-up visits should be emphasized to parents at discharge. Hintz with colleagues (2019) conducted a large study in California and found out that at least one high-risk infant follow-up (HRIF) visit was associated with older maternal age, lower birth weight, private insurance, a history of severe intracranial hemorrhage, having two parents as primary caregivers, and higher HRIF program volume. The odds of visits were lower for mothers who were African American/Black or lived farther away from a hospital. Another study (Wisconsin) also found the 62% loss to neonatal follow-up clinic visits in 2 years after discharge; the associated factors were African American race, older gestational age, and maternal cigarette smoking (Swearingen et al., 2020). In this study, protective factors were older maternal age, chronic lung disease, and longer hospital stays. Research has shown that prematurity, low birth weight, physical and neurologic impairments, continuous health problems, and family social context and health disparities can be risk factors for child maltreatment after discharge from an NICU (Cross, 2020; Owora et al., 2016). It is recommended to identify, during the infant hospitalization, any parental challenges in access to resources and possible social disparities and provide enhanced education for parents at risk about benefits of follow-up clinics and services, even when medical homes are established (Feehan et al., 2020; Hintz et al., 2019).

Unfortunately, follow-up programs and their content vary widely (from 2 weeks to 3 years, interventions might include home visits, or phone/video calls, and mobile applications) (Kang & Cho, 2021). Follow-up services also vary depending on where the infant and family lives. The Program for Infants and Toddlers with Disabilities (Part C of IDEA) is a federally funded statewide early intervention service for 0 to 2 years aged infants and toddlers with disabilities (Early Childhood Technical Assistance Center, n.d.). While this program has been in existence since 1986, many families still do not get these services for a variety of reasons. Information on this program should be part of the family's discharge preparation. Appointments for follow-up specialty services should also be clearly identified. But beyond the actual appointment and services, health professionals need to partner with the family to determine their specific individualized needs. The use of developmental timelines and activities through a professional–parent partnership supports both infant and parent needs. The positive effects of such partnerships are present even after discharge as parents undergo a transition-to-home experience and encounter new challenges. A new parent–professional partnership must develop with those outside the hospital and in the community/primary care settings. Community-based programs also can assist in building support networks especially for parents of a child with a disability. At present, there is still a lack of appropriate long-term follow-up care and inadequacies in primary care for former prematurely born children, adolescents, and young adults (Marlow et al., 2020). With the development of neonatal intensive care technologies and increasing survival of the preterm/sick infants, transitional and follow-up care (including long term) for this vulnerable population deserves more attention (Kuo et al., 2017; O'Nions et al., 2021).

PARTNERSHIP AS A MODEL OF CARE

Implementation of IFCDC means that policies and NICU systems must support the concept that families are an essential part of the healthcare team and they are partners in their infant's care. IFCDC puts the infant and families at the center of all care; recently, the standards, competencies, and recommended best practices were published (Browne et al., 2020). All FCC models must be based on mutual respect, clear and open communication, inclusion in decision-making, and recognition that each party brings unique strengths to the partnership. As with any relationship, benefits and risks are shared. Potential benefits include increased satisfaction by families and staff, improved outcomes such as decreased length of stay or in the case of death a better, more compassionate experience, and a commitment to providing high-quality care. The risks are failure to build trust or work together as a team thus potentially negatively impacting care and increasing stress for all parties. Empowerment of families and engaging them in care is crucial to enhancing the NICU experience for families (Umberger et al., 2018).

Recently, Kokorelias et al. (2019) conducted a literature review of FCC models. They found that the overarching goal for these models was to provide integrative care within the family context; they identified the key components that included family–professional collaboration, family considerations, policies and procedures that support FCC or IFCDC—a systems perspective, and education/training for all involved in such care as a necessity (Kokorelias et al., 2019). Franck and O'Brien (2019) offered an evidence-based taxonomy of parent-focused NICU interventions and parent–partnership care models that are aimed at supporting clinicians, researchers, and health systems as they change their care delivery. This taxonomy consists of three levels: interventions to support parents, parent-delivered interventions,

and models of parent-partnered neonatal care (Franck & O'Brien, 2019). Using an FCC or IFCDC approach, support for the infant, family, and health professionals is placed as a high priority. Without such support, holistic care that includes mental health support cannot be achieved. When formulating an individualized IFCDC plan, nurses should create an environment that honors the parents/family's role, facilitate collaboration and involvement into care, and establish and build a trusting relationship. Some evolving tools are available for measuring closeness in the NICU and implementation of FCC in NICU (Axelin et al., 2020).

To succeed in partnership toward a shared interest or goal, nurses may have to step outside their roles, as health professionals to more fully understand the parents' world. Professionals feel "at home" in the NICU and are familiar with its sights, sounds, and smells as they focus on the assessment, ventilation, feeding, medication administration, or procedure at hand. Parents, however, often enter a bewildering, unfamiliar environment, ill exhausted from delivery, and are emotionally drained by their current crises. When professionals step out of their scientific, technical realm and peer into the parents' social and emotional sphere, they can more effectively engage in care planning and problem-solving with the family. In 2016, Hall with colleagues presented 10 recommendations for creating comprehensive family support in the NICU, which were developed on the basis of the recommendations from the NPA (Hall & Hynan, 2015). In short, these strategies include routine mentoring of parents in the developmental care of their infants; parent participation in medical rounds and nursing shift change reports; parent-to-parent support programs; provision of psychological support with the help of trained psychologist; parental mental health services availability immediate after NICU admission; coordination of predischarge needs of families (addressing educational needs, home supplies and equipment's, scheduling appointments), follow-up, transitional care of home visiting programs, including parental screening for emotional distress; regular staff education on psychological needs of parents; and support services for staff to prevent burnout.

For a true partnership to form, families must be on an equal playing field with professionals. They must not be *visitors*. Family members should be welcomed at any time. They are not asked to leave for rounds, report, procedures, or during crisis situations. They should be encouraged to actively participate as their child's advocates in all of these events. Parents can choose who visits their child and are not included in the count if there must be a limited number of visitors at the bedside because of space. In this partnership, parents can choose when to bring in "well" siblings. They should be able to make decisions about caregiving schedules, such as when their infant will be bathed or when bottle-feedings will occur, and they can select the caregiving interventions with which they will get involved. Parents should be empowered, considered as a part of the caregiving team, and involved in decision-making discussions. They should have full disclosure and understanding of the medical record. Parents must be informed about their infant's short- and long-term problems and care needs and have confidence in their knowledge and role to believe their input will be acknowledged as equal in decision-making. All of these components are necessary for true membership in the caregiving team to exist.

Prolonged hospitalization in the NICU is a difficult setting in which to establish family–professional partnerships. However, because families are the constant in a child's environment, helping families achieve a positive outcome from their NICU experience should be a priority when providing care. Staffs' understanding of this stressful time can promote positive relationships that enhance the experience for all involved. Understanding the etiology of some of the parental behaviors can help professionals support families and cultivate much more positive relationships between families and hospital staff. Using a systems thinking approach and a framework that supports the development of a partnership in which all members are equally respected should help healthcare providers acknowledge and support family needs and expectations.

NICU staff should feel privileged to support and nurture parent–child relationships. Nurses never should underestimate the power and influence they have over families during this vulnerable segment of their lives. Nurses have this partnership for a brief time that soon ebbs from memory. Parents carry this partnership into the rest of their lives. Whether their child expires after a short stay or thrives under a long or short period of care, the ways in which nurses support and affirm parents will influence them for a long time. Parents need to be included in all aspects of care based on their ability and desire. Parents are an important part of the care team, providing parenting versus medical care. They provide comfort and calm with a soft, familiar voice and positive tactile stimulation. Full parental participation in their infant's care throughout the hospital course should now be the standard of care. Providing continuity of care and effective communication are important for the provision of safe care. Consistency in the relationship between the mother and nurse is important; it promotes communication and the sense of partnering.

CONCLUSION

This chapter has presented some aspects and strategies for partnerships in care between parents and health professionals. Professional–parent partnerships have the potential to enhance bonding/attachment to infant, improve parental role development, and make a difference in infant mental health and developmental outcomes as well as to form a solid bridge across the chasm between the NICU and home for high-risk infants and families.

Potential Research Questions

Prevention

- What are the attitudes of parents of NICU patients toward participation in rounds/presence during invasive procedures?
- What is the effect of participation in rounds/presence during invasive procedures on parents of NICU patients?
- What is the impact of COVID-19 restrictions in the NICU on growth and development of infants?
- What is the impact of COVID-19 restrictions in the NICU on parental role development and transition to home?
- What approach is more effective for reducing parental anxiety postdischarge: clinic visits, home visits, online education, or online peer support groups?
- What are the needs of healthcare professionals involved in FCC and IFCDC care?
- What are the needs of healthcare professionals involved in postdischarge and primary care of former NICU graduates?

Confirmation

- What is the reliable method for identification of parents at risk for parental role development and difficult transition to home?
- What is the reliable method for measuring discharge preparedness?
- What is the reliable method for measuring parental confidence in NICU parents?
- What is the reliable method for measuring depression and grief, specifically focusing on the NICU parents?
- What is the reliable method for measuring transition to home?

Treatment

- What FCC interventions do parents perceive as the most helpful during their infant stay in the NICU?
- What interventions do parents perceive as needed to ease the transition to home?

REFERENCES

Aagaard, H., & Hall, E. O. (2008). Mothers' experiences of having a preterm infant in the neonatal care unit: A meta-synthesis. *Journal of Pediatric Nursing, 23*(3), e26–e36.

Adama, E. A., Bayes, S., & Sundin, D. (2016). Parents' experiences of caring for preterm infants after discharge from neonatal intensive care unit: A meta-synthesis of the literature. *Journal of Neonatal Nursing, 22*(1), 27–51. https://doi.org/10.1016/j.jnn.2015.07.006

Adama, E. A., Bayes, S., & Sundin, D. (2018). Parents' experiences of caring for preterm infants after discharge with grandmothers as their main support. *Journal of Clinical Nursing, 27*(17–18), 3377–3386. https://doi.org/10.1111/jocn.13868

Agency for Health Care Research and Quality. (n.d.). *Transitioning newborns from NICU to home.* https://www.ahrq.gov/patient-safety/settings/hospital/resource/nicu/index.html

Alderdice, F., Gargan, P., McCall, E., & Franck, L. (2018). Online information for parents caring for their premature baby at home: A focus group study and systematic web search. *Health Expectations, 21,* 741–751. https://doi.org/10.1111/hex.12670

Alnuaimi, N., & Tluczek, A. (2021). Father's bonding with an infant born prematurely: A qualitative meta-synthesis. *Western Journal of Nursing Research,* 1–3. https://journals.sagepub.com/doi/10.1177/01939459211002909

Arockiasamy, V., Holsti, L., & Albersheim, S. (2008). Fathers' experiences in the neonatal intensive care unit: A search for control. *Pediatrics, 121*(2), e215–e222.

Association of University Centers on Disability. (n.d.). *About LEND.* https://www.aucd.org/template/page.cfm?id=473

Axelin, A., Raiskila, S., & Lehtonen, L. (2020). The development of data collection tools to measure parent–infant closeness and family-centered care in NICUs. *Worldviews on Evidence-Based Nursing, 17*(6), 448–456.

Aydon, L., Hauck, Y., Murdoch, J., Siu, D., & Sharp, M. (2018). Transition from hospital to home: Parents' perception of their preparation and readiness for discharge with their preterm infant. *Journal of Clinical Nursing, 27*(1–2), 269–277. https://doi.org/10.1111/jocn.13883

Ballantyne, M., Orava, T., Bernardo, S., McPherson, A. C., Church, P., & Fehlings, D. (2017). Parents' early healthcare transition experiences with preterm and acutely ill infants: A scoping review. *Child: Care, Health and Development, 43*(6), 783–796. https://doi.org/10.1111/cch.12458

Baraldi, E., Allodi, M. W., Smedler, A. C., Westrup, B., Löwing, K., & Ådén, U. (2020a). Parents' experiences of the first year at home with an infant born extremely preterm with and without post-discharge intervention: Ambivalence, loneliness, and relationship impact. *International Journal of Environmental Research and Public Health, 17*(24), 9326. https://doi.org/10.3390/ijerph17249326

Baraldi, E., Allodi, M. W., Löwing, K., Smedler, A. C., Westrup, B., & Ådén, U. (2020b). Stockholm preterm interaction-based intervention (SPIBI) - study protocol for an RCT of a 12-month parallel-group post-discharge program for extremely preterm infants and their parents. *BMC Pediatrics, 20,* 49. https://doi.org/10.1186/s12887-020-1934-4

Barnes, J., & Theule, J. (2019) Maternal depression and infant attachment security: A meta-analysis. *Infant Mental Health Journal, 40,* 817–834. https://doi.org/10.1002/imhj.21812

Barreto, M. S., Peruzzo, H. E., Garcia-Vivar, C., & Marcon, S. S. (2019). Family presence during cardiopulmonary resuscitation and invasive procedures: A meta-synthesis. *Revista da Esccol de Enfermagen da USP, 53,* e03435. http://dx.doi.org/10.1590/S1980-220X2018001303435

Beck, C. T., & Vo, T. (2020). Fathers' stress related to their infants' NICU hospitalization: A mixed research synthesis. *Archives of Psychiatric Nursing, 34*(2), 75–84. https://doi.org/10.1016/j.apnu.2020.02.001

Beck, C. T., & Woynar, J. (2017). Posttraumatic stress in mothers while their preterm infants are in the newborn intensive care unit. *Advances in Nursing Science, 40*(4), 337–355. https://doi.org/10.1097/ANS.0000000000000176

Bembich, S., Tripani, A., Mastromarino, S., Di Risio, G., Castelpietra, E., & Risso, F. M. (2021). Parents experiencing NICU visit restrictions due to COVID-19 pandemic. *Acta Paediatrica, 110,* 940–941. https://doi.org/10.1111/apa.15620

Bonacquisti, A., Geller, P. A., & Patterson, C. A. (2020). Maternal depression, anxiety, stress, and maternal-infant attachment in the neonatal intensive care unit. *Journal of Reproductive and Infant Psychology, 38*(3), 297–310. https://doi.org/10.1080/02646838.2019.1695041

Bourque, C., Dahan, S., Mantha, G., Robson, K., Reichherzer, M., & Janvier, A. (2018). Improving neonatal care with the help of veteran resource parents: An overview of current practices. *Seminars in Fetal and Neonatal Medicine, 23*(1), 44–51. https://doi.org/10.1016/j.siny.2017.10.005

Boykova, M. (2008). Follow-up care of premature babies in Russia: Evaluating parental experiences and associated services. *Infant, 4*(4), 101–105.

Boykova, M. (2016a). Transition from hospital to home in parents of preterm infants: A literature review. *Journal of Perinatal & Neonatal Nursing, 34*(4), 327–348.

Boykova, M. (2016b). Life after discharge: What parents of preterm infants say about their transition to home. *Newborn & Infant Nursing Reviews, 16*(2), 58–65.

Boykova, M., & Kenner, C. (2012). Transition from hospital to home for parents of preterm infants. *Journal of Perinatal & Neonatal Nursing, 26*(1), 81–87.

Brei, B. K., Sawyer, T., Umoren, R., Gray, M. M., Krick, J., Foglia, E. E., Ades, A., Glass, K., Kim, J. H., Singh, N., Jung, P., Johnston, L., Moussa, A., Napolitano, N., Barry, J., Zenge, J., Quek, B., DeMeo, S. D., Shults, J., … National Emergency Airway Registry for Neonates (NEAR4NEOS) Investigators, . (2021). Associations between family presence and neonatal intubation outcomes: A report from the National Emergency Airway Registry for Neonates – NEAR4NEOS. *Archives of Disease in Childhood. Fetal and Neonatal Edition, 106,* 392–397. https://doi.org/10.1136/archdischild-2020-319709

Brødsgaard, A., Pedersen, J. T., Larsen, P., & Weis, J. (2019). Parents' and nurses' experiences of partnership in neonatal intensive care units: A qualitative review and meta-synthesis. *Journal of Clinical Nursing, 28,* 3117–3139. https://doi.org/10.1111/jocn.14920

Browne, J. V., Jaeger, C. B., Kenner, C., & on behalf of the Gravens Consensus Committee on Infant and Family Centered Developmental Care. (2020). Executive summary: Standards, competencies, and recommended best practices for infant- and family-centered developmental care in the intensive care unit. *Journal of Perinatology, 40,* 5–10. https://doi.org/10.1038/s41372-020-0767-1

Brunson, E., Thierry, A., Ligier, F., Vulliez-Coady, L., Novo, A., Rolland, A. C., & Eutrope, J. (2021). Prevalences and predictive factors of maternal trauma through 18 months after premature birth: A longitudinal, observational and descriptive study. *PLoS One, 16*(2), e0246758. https://doi.org/10.1371/journal.pone.0246758

Buck, C., Richard Tucker, R., Vohr, B., & McGowan, E. (2020). Predictors of parenting readiness in fathers of high-risk infants in the neonatal intensive care unit. *The Journal of Pediatrics, 217,* 192–195. https://doi.org/10.1016/j.jpeds.2019.09.078

Caporali, C., Pisoni, C., Gasparini, L., Ballante, E., Zecca, M., Orcesi, S., & Provenzi, L. (2020). A global perspective on parental stress in the neonatal intensive care unit: A meta-analytic study. *Journal of Perinatology, 40*(12), 1739–1752. https://doi.org/10.1038/s41372-020-00798-6

Cena, L., Biban, P., Janos, J., Lavelli, M., Langfus, J., Tsai, A., Youngstrom, E. A., & Stefana, A. (2021). The collateral impact of COVID-19 emergency on neonatal intensive care units and family-centered care: Challenges and opportunities. *Frontiers in Psychology, 12,* 630594. https://www.frontiersin.org/article/10.3389/fpsyg.2021.630594

Choi, K. R., Recrods, K., Low, L. K., Alhusen, J. L., Kenner, C., Bloch, J. R., Premji, S. S., Hannan, J., Anderson, C. M., Yeo, S., & Logsdon, M. C. (2020). Promotion of maternal-infant mental health and trauma-informed care during the COVID-19 pandemic. *Journal of Obstetric, Gynecologic, & Neonatal Nursing, 49*(5), 409–415.

Citter, O., & Ghanouni, P. (2020). Becoming a mother in the neonatal intensive care unit: A narrative review. *Journal of Occupational Science.* https://doi.org/10.1080/14427591.2020.1815567

Cleveland, L. M. (2008). Parenting in the neonatal intensive care unit. *Journal of Obstetric, Gynecologic, & Neonatal Nursing, 37*(6), 666–691.

Connors, J., Havranek, T., & Campbell, D. (2021). Discharge of medically complex infants and developmental follow-up. *Pediatrics in Review, 42*(6), 316–328. https://doi.org/10.1542/pir.2020-000638

Cox, J. E., Harris, S. K., Conroy, K., Engelhart, T., Vyavaharkar, A., Federico, A., & Woods, E. R. (2019). A parenting and life skills intervention for teen mothers: A randomized controlled trial. *Pediatrics, 143*(3), e20182303. https://doi.org/10.1542/peds.2018-2303

Craig, J., Glick, C., Phillips, R., Hall, S. L., Smith, J., & Browne, J. (2015). Recommendations for involving the family in developmental care of the NICU baby. *Journal of Perinatology, 35*, S5–S8. https://doi.org/10.1038/jp.2015.142

Cross, J. (2020). Child maltreatment of NICU graduates: Focus on health disparities. *Neonatology Today, 15*(3), 26–31. https://www.neonatologytoday.net/newsletters/nt-mar20.pdf

Currie, G., Dosani, A., Premji, S. S., Reily, S., Lodha, A. K., & Young, M. (2018). Caring for late preterm infants: Public health nurses' perspective. *BMC Nursing, 17*, 16. https://doi.org/10.1186/s12912-018-0286-y

Cyr-Alves, H., Macken, L., & Hyrkas, K. (2018). Stress and symptoms of depression in fathers of infants admitted to the NICU. *Journal of Obstetric, Gynecologic & Neonatal Nursing, 47*(2), 146–157. https://doi.org/10.1016/j.jogn.2017.12.006

Dahan, S., Bourque, C. J., Reichherzer, M., Prince, J., Mantha, G., Savaria, M., & Janvier, A. (2020). Peer support groups for families in neonatology: Why and how to get started? *Acta Paediatrica, 109*(12), 2525–2531. https://doi.org/10.1111/apa.15312

Dainty, K. N., Atkins, D. L., Breckwoldt, J., Maconochie, I., Schexnayder, S. M., Skrifvars, M. B., Tijssen, J., Wyllie, J., Furuta, M., Aickin, R., Acworth, J., Atkins, D., Couto, T. B., Guerguerian, A. M., Kleinman, M., Kloeck, D., Nadkarni, V., Ng, K. C., … Yeung, J. (2021). Family presence during resuscitation in paediatric and neonatal cardiac arrest: A systematic review. *Resuscitation, 162*, 20–34. https://doi.org/10.1016/j.resuscitation.2021.01.017

Deutsch, M. B. (Ed). (2016). *Guidelines for the primary and gender-affirming care of transgender and gender nonbinary people* (2nd ed.). UCSF Transgender Care, Department of Family and Community Medicine, University of California San Francisco. https://transcare.ucsf.edu/guidelines

Discenza, D. (2009). NICU parents' top ten worries at discharge. *Neonatal Network, 28*(3), 202–203.

Dorner, R. A., Boss, R. D., Burton, V. J., Raja, K., Robinson, S., & Lemmon, M. (2021). Isolated and on guard: Preparing neonatal intensive care unit families for life with hydrocephalus. *American Journal of Perinatology.* https://doi.org/10.1055/s-0040-1722344. https://www.thieme-connect.com/products/ejournals/abstract/10.1055/s-0040-1722344

Early Childhood Technical Assistance Center. (n.d.). *Part C of IDEA.* https://ectacenter.org/partc/partc.asp

Feehan, K., Kehinde, F., Sachs, K., Mossabeb, R., Berhane, Z., Pachter, L. M., Brody, S., & Turchi, R. M. (2020). Development of a multidisciplinary medical home program for NICU graduates. *Maternal and Child Health Journal, 24*(1), 11–21. https://doi.org/10.1007/s10995-019-02818-0

Feeley, N., Sherrard, K., Waitzer, E., & Boisvert, L. (2013). The father at the bedside: Patterns of involvement in the NICU. *Journal of Perinatal & Neonatal Nursing, 27*(1), 72–80. https://doi.org/10.1097/JPN.0b013e31827fb415

Fenwick, J., Barclay, L., & Schmied, V. (2001a). Struggling to mother: A consequence of inhibitive nursing interactions in the neonatal nursery. *Journal of Neonatal Nursing, 15*(2), 49–64.

Fenwick, J., Barclay, L., & Schmied, V. (2001b). 'Chatting': An important clinical tool in facilitating mothering in neonatal nurseries. *Journal of Advanced Nursing, 33*(5), 583–593.

Franck, L. S., & O'Brien, K. (2019). The evolution of family-centered care: From supporting parent-delivered interventions to a model of family integrated care. *Birth Defects Research, 111*, 1044–1059.

Fratantoni, K. (2019). *Testing a peer-support program for parents of infants going home from the NICU.* https://www.pcori.org/sites/default/files/PCORI-Fratantoni266-English-Abstract.pdf

Furtak, S. L., Gay, C. L., Kriz, R. M., Bisgaard, R., Bolick, S. C., Lothe, B., Cormier, D. M., Joe, P., Sasinski, J. K., Kim, J. H., Lin, C. K., Sun, Y., & Franck, L. S. (2020). What parents want to know about caring for their preterm infant: A longitudinal descriptive study. *Patient Education and Counseling.* https://doi.org/10.1016/j.pec.2021.04.011

García-Acosta, J. M., San Juan-Valdivia, R. M., Fernández-Martínez, A. D., Lorenzo-Rocha, N. D., & Castro-Peraza, M. E. (2020). Trans* pregnancy and lactation: A literature review from a nursing perspective. *International Journal of Environmental Research and Public Health, 17*(1), 44. https://doi.org/10.3390/ijerph17010044

Garfield, C., Lee, Y., & Kim, H. N. (2014). Paternal and maternal concerns for their very low-birth-weight infants transitioning from the NICU to home. *Journal of Perinatal & Neonatal Nursing, 28*(4), 305–312. https://doi.org/0.1097/JPN.0000000000000021

Garfield, C. F., Simon, C. D., Rutsohn, J., & Lee, Y. S. (2018). Stress from the neonatal intensive care unit to home: Paternal and maternal cortisol rhythms in parents of premature infants. *Journal of Perinatal & Neonatal Nursing, 32*(3), 257–265. https://doi.org/10.1097/JPN.0000000000000296

Gilstrap, C. M. (2020). Organizational sensegiving in family-centered care: How NICU nurses help families make sense of the NICU experience. *Health Communication,* 1–11. https://doi.org/10.1080/10410236.2020.1785373

Gilworth, G., Milton, S., Chater, A., Nazareth, I., Roposch, A., & Green, J. (2020). Parents' expectations and experiences of the 6-week baby check: A qualitative study in primary care. *British Journal of General Practitioners, 4*(5), bjgpopen20X101110. https://doi.org/10.3399/bjgpopen20X101110

Givrad, S., Hartzell, G., & Scala, M. (2021). Promoting infant mental health in the neonatal intensive care unit (NICU): A review of nurturing factors and interventions for NICU infant-parent relationships. *Early Human Development, 154*, 105281. https://doi.org/10.1016/j.earlhumdev.2020.105281

Glazer, K. B., Sofaer, S., Balbierz, A., Wang, E., & Howell, E. A. (2021). Perinatal care experiences among racially and ethnically diverse mothers whose infants required a NICU stay. *Journal of Perinatology, 41*(3), 413–421. https://doi.org/10.1038/s41372-020-0721-2

Global Alliance for Newborn Care (GLANCE). (2020). *Joining forces in times of the pandemic-Global Alliance for Newborn Care launches its first campaign "Zero separation. Together for better care!"* https://www.glance-network.org/news/details/zero-separation-global-campaign/

Gordon, J. M., Gaffney, K., Slavvit, H. C., Williams, A., & Lauerer, J. A. (2020). Integrating infant mental health practice models in nursing. *Journal of Child and Adolescent Psychiatric Nursing, 33*(1), 7–23.

Govindaswamy, P., Laing, S., Waters, D., Walker, K., Spence, K., & Badawi, N. (2019). Needs and stressors of parents of term and near-term infants in the NICU: A systematic review with best practice guidelines. *Early Human Development, 139*, 104839. https://doi.org/10.1016/j.earlhumdev.2019.104839

Griffin, T., & Abraham, M. (2006). Transition to home from the newborn intensive care unit: Applying the principles of family-centered care to the discharge process. *Journal of Perinatal and Neonatal Nursing, 20*(3), 243–249.

Grunberg, V. A., Geller, P. A., Bonacquisti, A., & Patterson, C. (2019). A NICU infant health severity and family outcomes: a systematic review of assessments and findings in psychosocial research. *Journal of Perinatology, 39*(2), 156–172. https://doi.org/10.1038/s41372-018-0282-9. PMID: 30514968

Grunberg, V., Geller, P. A., & Patterson, C. A. (2020). Utilization of NICU infant medical indices to classify parental risk for stress and family burden. *Journal of Pediatric Health Care, 34*(1), 54–62.

Gulamani, S. S., Premji, S. S., Kanji, Z., & Azam, S. I. (2013). A review of postpartum depression, preterm birth, and culture. *Journal of Perinatal & Neonatal Nursing, 27*(1), 52–61. https://doi.org/10.1097/JPN.0b013e31827fcf24

Gustafson, K. W., LaBrecque, M. A., Graham, D. A., Tella, N. M., & Curley, M. A. Q. (2016). Effect of parent presence during multidisciplinary rounds on NICU-related parental stress. *Journal of Obstetric, Gynecologic and Neonatal Nursing, 45*(5), 661–670. https://doi.org/10.1016/j.jogn.2016.04.012

Hagen, I. H., Iversen, V. C., Nesset, E., Orner, R., & Svindseth, M. F. (2019). Parental satisfaction with neonatal intensive care units: A quantitative cross-sectional study. *BMC Health Services Research, 19*(1), 37. https://doi.org/10.1186/s12913-018-3854-7

Hägi-Pedersen, MB., Kronborg, H., & Norlyk, A. (2021). Knowledge of mothers and fathers' experiences of the early in-home care of premature infants supported by video consultations with a neonatal nurse. *BMC Nursing, 20*, 54. https://doi.org/10.1186/s12912-021-00572-9

Hall, S., & Hynan, M. (Eds.). (2015). Interdisciplinary recommendations for the psychosocial support of NICU parents. *Journal of Perinatology, 35*(Suppl. 1), S1–S4. http://www.nationalperinatal.org/resources/Documents/JP%20Psychosocial%20Support%20SupplementFinal%20(1).pdf

Hall, S. L., Famuyide, M. E., Saxton, S., Moore, T., Mosher, S., Sorrels, K., Milford, C., & Craig, J. (2019). Improving staff knowledge and attitudes toward providing psychosocial support to NICU parents through an online education course. *Advances in Neonatal Care, 19*(6), 490–499. https://doi.org/10.1097/ANC.0000000000000649

Hall, S. L., Phillips, R., & Hynan, M. (2016). Transforming NICU care to provide comprehensive family support. *Newborn and Infant Nursing Reviews, 16*(2), 69–73. https://doi.org/10.1053/j.nainr.2016.03.008

Hall, S. L., Ryan, D. L., Beatty, J., & Grubbs, L. (2015). Recommendations for peer-to-peer support for NICU parents. *Journal of Perinatology, 35*, S9–S13. https://doi.org/10.1038/jp.2015.143

Hallowell, S. G., Rogowski, J. A., & Lake, E. T. (2019). How nurse work environments relate to the presence of parents in neonatal intensive care. *Advances in Neonatal Care, 19*(1), 65–72. https://doi.org/10.1097/ANC.0000000000000431

Hamline, M. Y., Speier, R. L., Vu, P. D., Tancredi, D., Broman, A. R., Rasmussen, L. N., Tullius, B. P., Shaikh, U., & Li, S. T. (2018). Hospital-to-home interventions, use, and satisfaction: A meta-analysis. *Pediatrics, 142*(5), e20180442. https://doi.org/10.1542/peds.2018-0442

Hannan, K. E., Hwang, S. S., & Bourque, S. L. (2020). Readmissions among NICU graduates: Who, when and why? *Seminars in Perinatology, 44*(4), 151245. https://doi.org/10.1016/j.semperi.2020.151245

Haut, C., Peddicord, K., & O'Brien, E. (1994). Supporting parental bonding in the NICU: A care plan for nurses. *Neonatal Network, 13*(8), 19–25.

Haward, M. F., Lantos, J., Janvier, A., & for the POST Group. (2020). Helping parents cope in the NICU. *Pediatrics, 145*. https://doi.org/10.1542/peds.2019-3567

Hearn, G., Clarkson, G., & Day, M. (2019). The role of the NICU in father involvement, beliefs, and confidence: A follow-up qualitative study. *Advances in Neonatal Care, 20*(1), 80–89. https://doi.org/10.1097/ANC.0000000000000665

He, F. B., Axelin, A., Ahlqvist-Björkroth, S., Raiskila, S., Loyttyniemi, E., & Lehtonen, L. (2021). Effectiveness of the close collaboration with parents intervention on parent-infant closeness in NICU, *BMC Pediatrics, 21, 28*. https://doi.org/10.1186/s12887-020-02474-2

Hintz, S. R., Gould, J. B., Bennett, M. V., Lu, T., Gray, E. E., Jocson, M., Fuller, M. G., & Lee, H. C. (2019). Factors associated with successful first high-risk infant clinic visit for very low birth weight infants in California. *Journal of Pediatrics, 210*, 91–98.e1. https://doi.org/10.1016/j.jpeds.2019.03.007

Hobbs, J. E., Tschudy, M. M., Hussey-Gardner, B., Jennings, J. M., & Boss, R. D. (2017). "I don't know what I was expecting": Home visits by neonatology fellows for infants discharged from the NICU. *Birth, 44*(4), 331–336. https://doi.org/10.1111/birt.12301

van den Hoogen, A., Eijsermans, R., Ockhuijsen, H. D. L., Jenken, F., Oude Maatman, S. M., Jongmans, M. J., Verhage, L., van der Net, J., & Latour, J. M. (2021). Parents' experiences of VOICE: A novel support programme in the NICU. *Nursing in Crit Care, 26*(3), 201–208. https://doi.org/10.1111/nicc.12569

Hurst, I. (2001). Vigilant watching over: Mothers' actions to safeguard their premature babies in the newborn intensive care nursery. *Journal of Perinatal and Neonatal Nursing, 15*(3), 39–57.

Institute of Medicine (IOM). (2001). *Crossing the quality chasm: A new health system for the 21st century*. National Academies Press.

Ionio, C., Colombo, C., Brazzoduro, V., Mascheroni, E., Confalonieri, E., Castoldi, F., & Lista, G. (2016). Mothers and fathers in NICU: The impact of preterm birth on parental distress. *Europe's Journal of Psychology, 12*(4), 604–621. https://doi.org/10.5964/ejop.v12i4.1093

Kamphorst, K., Brouwer, A. J., Poslawsky, I. E., Ketelaar, M., Ockhuisen, H., & van den Hoogen, A. (2018). Parental presence and activities in a Dutchneonatal intensive care unit. *Journal of Perinatal & Neonatal Nursing, 32*(3), E3–E10.

Kang, S. R., & Cho, H. (2021). Research trends of follow-up care after neonatal intensive care unit graduation for children born preterm: A scoping review. *International Journal of Environmental Research and Public Health, 18*, 3268. https://doi.org/10.3390/ijerph18063268

Kantrowitz-Gordon, I., Altman, M. R., & Vandernause, R. (2016). Prolonged distress of parents after early preterm birth. *Journal of Obstetric, Gynecologic & Neonatal Nursing, 45*(2), 196–209. https://doi.org/10.1016/j.jogn.2015.12.004

Kasat, K., Stoffels, G., & Ellington, M. (2020). Improving parent communication: Neonatal Intensive care unit empathy workshop. *Journal of Perinatology, 40*, 1423–1432. https://doi.org/10.1038/s41372-020-0742-x

Kenner, C. A. (1988). *Parent transition from hospital to home* (Unpublished dissertation). Indiana University.

Kenner, C. (1995). Transition to parenthood. In Gunderson, L. P., & Kenner, C. (Eds.), *Care of the 24–25 week gestation age infant: A small baby protocol* (2nd ed., pp. 171–184). NICU Ink.

Kerppola, J., Halme, N., Perala, M., & Maija-Pietila, A. (2020). Empowering LGBTQ parents: How to improve maternity services and child health-care settings for this community—'She told us that we are good as a family'. *Nordic Journal of Nursing Research, 40*(1), 41–51. https://doi.org/10.1177/2057158519865844

Kim, H. N. (2018). Social support provision: Perspective of fathers with preterm infants. *Journal of Pediatric Nursing, 39*, 44–48.

Klaus, M., & Kennell, J. H. (1976). *Maternal-infant bonding*. C. V. Mosby Company.

Kokorelias, K. M., Gignac, M. A. M., Naglie, G., & Cameron, J. I. (2019). Towards a universal model of family centered care: A scoping review. *BMC Health Services Research, 19*, 564. https://doi.org/10.1186/s12913-019-4394-5

Kuo, D. Z., Lyle, R. E., Casey, P. H., & Stille, C. J. (2017). Care system redesign for preterm children after discharge from the NICU. *Pediatrics, 139*(4), e20162969. https://doi.org/10.1542/peds.2016-2969

Labrie, N. H. M., van Veenendaal, N. R., Ludolph, R. A., Ket, J. C. F., van der Schoor, S., & van Kempen, A. (2021). Effects of parent-provider communication during infant hospitalization in the NICU on parents: A systematic review with meta-synthesis and narrative synthesis. *Patient Education and Counseling, 104*(7), 1526–1552. https://doi.org/10.1016/j.pec.2021.04.023

Lakshmanan, A., Kubicek, K., Williams, R., Robles, M., Vanderbilt, D. L., Mirzaian, C. B., Friedlich, P. S., & Kipke, M. (2019). Viewpoints from families for improving transition from NICU-to-home for infants with medical complexity at a safety net hospital: A qualitative study. *BMC Pediatrics, 19*(1), 223. https://doi.org/10.1186/s12887-019-1604-6

Leahy-Warren, P., Coleman, C., Bradley, R., & Mulcahy, H. (2020). The experiences of mothers with preterm infants within the first-year post discharge from NICU: Social support, attachment and level of depressive symptoms. *BMC Pregnancy and Childbirth, 20*(1), 260. https://doi.org/10.1186/s12884-020-02956-2

Lean, R. E., Rogers, C. E., Paul, R. A. & Gerstein, E. D. (2018). NICU hospitalization: Long-term implications on parenting and child behaviors. *Current Treatment Options in Pediatrics, 4*, 49–69. https://doi.org/10.1007/s40746-018-0112-5

Liu, Y., McGowan, E., Tucker, R., Glasgow, L., Kluckman, M., & Vohr, B. (2018). Transition Home Plus Program reduces Medicaid spending and health care use for high-risk infants admitted to the neonatal intensive care unit for 5 or more days. *Journal of Pediatrics, 200*, 91–97.e3. https://doi.org/10.1016/j.jpeds.2018.04.038

Loewenstein, K. (2018). Parent psychological distress in the neonatal intensive care unit within the context of the social ecological model: A scoping review. *Journal of the American Psychiatric Nurses Association, 24*(6), 495–509. https://doi.org/10.1177/1078390318765205

Loewenstein, K., Barroso, J., & Phillips, S. (2019). The experiences of parents in the neonatal intensive care unit: An integrative review of qualitative studies within the transactional model of stress and coping. *The Journal of Perinatal & Neonatal Nursing, 33*(4), 340–349. https://doi.org/10.1097/JPN.0000000000000436

Logan, R. (2020). Gay fatherhood in the NICU: Supporting the "gayby" boom. *Advances in Neonatal Care, 20*(4), 286–293. https://doi.org/10.1097/ANC.0000000000000712. PMID: 32004185

Logan, R. M., & Dormire, S. (2018). Finding my way: A phenomenology of fathering in the NICU. *Advances in Neonatal Care, 18*(2), 154–162. https://doi.org/10.1097/ANC.0000000000000471

Lundqvist, P., Weis, J., & Sivberg, B. (2019). Parents' journey caring for a preterm infant until discharge from hospital-based neonatal home care: A challenging process to cope with. *Journal of Clinical Nursing, 28*(15–16), 2966–2978. https://doi.org/10.1111/jocn.14891

MacKay, L. J., Benzies, K., Barnard, C. B., & Bouchal, S. R. (2020). Parental experiences caring for their hospitalized medically fragile infants: A description of grief, stress and coping. *The Canadian Journal of Nursing Research.* https://doi.org/10.1177/0844562120954125

MacLean, L. R. D. (2021). Preconception, pregnancy, birthing, and lactation needs of transgender men. *Nursing for Women's Health, 25*(2), 129–138.

Madhoun, L., & Dempster, R. (2019). The psychosocial aspects of feeding in the neonatal intensive care unit and beyond. *Perspectives of the ASHA Special Interest Groups, 4*, 1507–1515..

Mäkelä, H., Axelin, A., Feeley, N., & Niela-Vilén, H. (2018). Clinging to closeness: The parental view on developing a close bond with their infants in a NICU. *Midwifery, 62*, 183–188. https://doi.org/10.1016/j.midw.2018.04.003

Mark, K. (2021). Family presence during paediatric resuscitation and invasive procedures: The parental experience—An integrative review. *Scandinavian Journal of Caring Sciences, 35*, 20–36. https://doi.org/10.1111/scs.12829. https://onlinelibrary.wiley.com/doi/epdf/10.1111/scs.12829

Marlow, N., Hoy, S., Peacock, A., & Kamphuis, J. (2020). Outcomes from the other side. *Seminars in Fetal and Neonatal Medicine, 25*(3), 101125. https://doi.org/10.1016/j.siny.2020.101125

McGowan, E. C., Abdulla, L. S., Hawes, K. K., Tucker, R., & Vohr, B. R. (2019). Maternal immigrant status and readiness to transition to home from the NICU. *Pediatrics, 143*(5), e20182657. https://doi.org/10.1542/peds.2018-2657

McGowan, E. C., Du, N., Hawes, K., Tucker, R., O'Donnell, M., & Vohr, B. (2017). Maternal mental health and neonatal intensive care unit discharge readiness in mothers of preterm infants. *The Journal of Pediatrics, 184*, 68–74. https://doi.org/10.1016/j.jpeds.2017.01.052

McGrath, J. M. (2001). Building relationships with families in the NICU: Exploring the guarded alliance. *Journal of Perinatal & Neonatal Nursing, 15*(3), 74–83.

McKelvey, L. M., Lewis, K. N., Beavers, J., Casey, P. H., Irby, C., & Goudie, A. (2021). Home visiting for NICU graduates: Impacts of following baby back home. *Pediatrics*, e2020029397. https://doi.org/10.1542/peds.2020-029397

McLean, E., Skewes, K. M., & Thompson, G. (2018). Parents' musical engagement with their baby in the neonatal unit to support emerging parental identity: A grounded theory study. *Journal of Neonatal Nursing, 25*(2), 78–85. https://doi.org/10.1016/j.jnn.2018.09.005

Melnyk, B. M., Crean, H. F., Feinstein, N. F., Fairbanks, E., & Alpert-Gillis, L. J. (2007). Testing the theoretical framework of the COPE program for mothers of critically ill children: An integrative model of young children's post-hospital adjustment behaviors. *Journal of Pediatric Psychology, 32*(4), 463–474.

Melnyk, B. M., & Feinstein, N. F. (2009). Reducing hospital expenditures with the COPE (Creating Opportunities for Parent Empowerment) program for parents and premature infants: An analysis of direct healthcare neonatal intensive care unit costs and savings. *Nursing Administration Quarterly, 33*(1), 32–37.

Melnyk, B. M., Feinstein, N. F., Alpert-Gillis, L., Fairbanks, E., Crean, H. F., Sinkin, R. A., Stone, P. W., Small, L., Tu, X., & Gross, S. J. (2006). Reducing premature infants' length of stay and improving parents' mental health outcomes with the Creating Opportunities for Parent Empowerment (COPE) neonatal intensive care unit program: A randomized, controlled trial. *Pediatrics, 118*(5), e1414–e1427.

Mendelson, T., Cluxton-Keller, F., Vullo, G. C., Tandon, D., & Noazin, S. (2017). NICU-based interventions to reduce maternal depressive and anxiety symptoms: A meta-analysis. *Pediatrics, 139*(3), 1–12. https://doi.org/10.1542/peds.2016-1870

Menke, B. M., Hass, J., Diener, C., & Pöschl, J. (2021). Family-centered music therapy—Empowering premature infants and their primary caregivers through music: Results of a pilot study. *PLoS One, 16*(5), e0250071. https://doi.org/10.1371/journal.pone.0250071

Merritt, L. (2021). An integrative review of fathers' needs in the neonatal intensive care unit. *The Journal of Perinatal & Neonatal Nursing, 35*(1), 79–91. https://doi.org/10.1097/JPN.0000000000000541

Minckas, N., Medvedev, M., Adejuyigbe, E. A., Brotherton, H., Chellani, H., Estifanos, A. S., Ezeaka, C., Gobezayehu, A. G., Irimu, G., Kawaza, K., Kumar, V., Massawe, A., Mazumder, S., Mambule, I., Medhanyie, A. A., Molyneux, E. M., Newton, S., Salim, N., Tadele, H., … on behalf of the COVID-19 Small and Sick Newborn Care Collaborative Group. (2021). Preterm care during the COVID-19 pandemic: A comparative risk analysis of neonatal deaths averted by kangaroo mother care versus mortality due to SARS-CoV-2 infection. *EClinicalMedicine (Lancet), 33*, 100733. https://doi.org/10.1016/j.eclinm.2021.100733

Murch, T. N., & Smith, V. C. (2016). Supporting families as they transition home. *Newborn and Infant Nursing Reviews, 16*(4), 298–302. https://doi.org/10.1053/j.nainr.2016.09.024

Murdoch, M. R., & Franck, L. S. (2012). Gaining confidence and perspective: A phenomenological study of mothers' lived experiences caring for infants at home after neonatal unit discharge. *Journal of Advanced Nursing, 68*(9), 2008–2020. https://doi.org/10.1111/j.1365-2648.2011.05891.x

Nieves, H., Clements-Hickman, A., & Davies, C. C. (2021). Effect of a parent empowerment program on parental stress, satisfaction, and length of stay in the neonatal intensive care unit. *The Journal of Perinatal & Neonatal Nursing, 35*(1), 92–99. https://doi.org/10.1097/JPN.0000000000000540

Noergaard, B., Ammentorp, J., Fenger-Gron, J., Kofoed, P., Johannessen, H., Thibeau, S., & Dowling, D. (2017). Fathers' needs and masculinity dilemmas in a neonatal intensive care unit in Denmark. *Advances in Neonatal Care, 17*(4), E13–E22. https://doi.org/10.1097/ANC.0000000000000395

Noergaard, B., Ammentorp, J., Garne, E., Fenger-Gron, J., & Kofoed, P. (2018). Fathers' stress in a neonatal intensive care unit. *Advances in Neonatal Care, 18*(5), 413–422.

Norholt, H. (2020). Revisiting the roots of attachment: A review of the biological and psychological effects of maternal skin-to-skin contact and carrying of full-term infants. *Infant Behavior and Development, 60*, 101441. https://doi.org/10.1016/j.infbeh.2020.101441

Norton, M., & Hagstrom, A. (2021). Finding a new normal. *Advances in Neonatal Care.* https://doi.org/10.1097/ANC.0000000000000850

O'Brien, K., Robson, K., Bracht, M., Cruz, M., Lui, K., Alvaro, R., da Silva, O., Monterrosa, L., Narvey, M., Ng, E., Soraisham, A., Ye, X. Y., Mirea, L., Tarnow-Mordi, W., Lee, S. K., & FICare Study Group and FICare Parent Advisory Board. (2018). Effectiveness of Family Integrated Care in neonatal intensive care units on infant and parent outcomes: A multicentre, multinational, cluster-randomised controlled trial. *Lancet Child & Adolescent Health, 2*(4), 245–254. https://doi.org/10.1016/S2352-4642(18)30039-7

Øberg, G. C., Ustad, T., Jørgensen, L., Kaaresen, P. I., Labori, C., & Girolami, G. L. (2019). Parents' perceptions of administering a motor intervention with their preterm infant in the NICU. *European Journal of Physiotherapy, 21*(3), 134–141. https://doi.org/10.1080/21679169.2018.1503718

O'Nions, E., Wolke, D., Johnson, S., & Kennedy, E. (2021). Preterm birth: Educational and mental health outcomes. *Clinical Child Psychology and Psychiatry, 26*(3). https://doi.org/10.1177/13591045211006754

Owora, A., Chaffin, M., Nandyal, R., Risch, E., Bonner, B., & Carabin, H. (2016). Medical surveillance and child maltreatment incidence reporting among NICU graduates. *Social Work in Public Health, 31*(7), 607–616. https://doi.org/10.1080/19371918.2016.1160348

Patel, K., Cortright, L., Tumin, D., & Kohler, J. (2020). Fathers' visitation of very low birth weight infants in the neonatal intensive care unit during the first week of life. *American Journal of Perinatology, 38*(9), 909–913. https://doi.org/10.1055/s-0039-3402750

Perez, R. H. (1981). The perinatal nurse. In Perez, R. H. (Ed.), *Protocols for perinatal nursing practice.* C. V. Mosby Company.

Perez, A., Thiede, L., Ludecke, D., Ebenebe, C. U., von dem Knesebeck, O., & Singer, D. (2020). Lost in transition: Health care experiences of adults born very preterm—A qualitative approach. *Frontiers in Public Health, 8,* 605149. https://doi.org/10.3389/fpubh.2020.605149

Petty, J., Whiting, L., Mosenthal, A., Fowler, C., Elliot, D., & Green, J. (2019). The knowledge and learning needs of health professionals in providing support for parents of premature babies at home: A mixed-methods study. *Journal of Neonatal Nursing, 25,* 277–284. https://doi.org/10.1016/j.jnn.2019.07.002

Pinelli, J., Saigal, S., Bill Wu, Y. W., Cunningham, C., Di- Censo, A., Steele, S., Austina, P., & Turnerf, S. (2008). Patterns of change in family functioning, resources, coping and parental depression in mothers and fathers of sick newborns over the first year of life. *Journal of Neonatal Nursing, 14*(5), 156–165.

Powers, K., & Reeve, C. L. (2018). Factors associated with nurses' perceptions, self-confidence, and invitations of family presence during resuscitation in the intensive care unit: A cross-sectional survey. *International Journal of Nursing Studies, 87,* 103–112. https://doi.org/10.1016/j.ijnurstu.2018.06.012

Prouhet, P. M., Gregory, M. R., Russell, C. L., & Yaeger, L. Y. (2018). Fathers' stress in the neonatal intensive care unit: A systematic review. *Advances in Neonatal Care, 18*(2), 105–120.

Rao, S. P. N., Minckas, N., Medvedev, M. M., Gathara, D., Prashantha, Y. N., Estifanos, A. S., Silitonga, A. C, Jadaun, A. S., Adejuyigbe, E. A., Brotherton, H., Arya, S., Gera, R., Ezeaka, C. V., Gai, A., Gobezayehu, A. G., Dube, Q., Kummar, A., Naburi, H., Chiume, M., … on behalf of the COVID-19 Small and Sick Newborn Care Collaborative Group. (2021). Small and sick newborn care during the COVID-19 pandemic: Global survey and thematic analysis of healthcare providers' voices and experiences. *BMJ Global Health, 6,* e004347. https://gh.bmj.com/content/6/3/e004347

Reid, S., Bredemeyer, S., & Chiarella, M. (2019). Integrative review of parents' perspectives of the nursing role in neonatal family-centered care. *Journal of Obstetric, Gynecologic, and Neonatal Nursing, 48*(4), 408–417. https://doi.org/10.1016/j.jogn.2019.05.001

Richardson, B., Price, S., & Campbell-Yeo, M. (2019). Redefining perinatal experience: A philosophical exploration of a hypothetical case of gender diversity in labour and birth. *Journal of Clinical Nursing, 28*(3–4), 703–710. https://doi.org/10.1111/jocn.14521

Roque, A. T. F., Lasiuk, G. C., Radünz, V., & Hegadoren, K. (2017). Scoping review of the mental health of parents of infants in the NICU. *Journal of Obstetric, Gynecologic & Neonatal Nursing, 46*(4), 576–587. https://doi.org/10.1016/j.jogn.2017.02.005

Rossman, B., Greene, M. M., & Meier, P. P. (2015). The role of peer support in the development of maternal identity for "NICU moms". *Journal of Obstetric, Gynecologic & Neonatal Nursing, 44*(1), 3–16. https://doi.org/10.1111/1552-6909.12527

Ruedinger, E., & Cox, J. E. (2012). Adolescent childbearing: Consequences and interventions. *Current Opinion in Pediatrics, 24*(4), 446–452. https://doi.org/10.1097/MOP.0b013e3283557b89

Sabnis, A., Fojo, S., Nayak, S. S., Lopez, E., Tarn, D. M., & Zeltzer, L. (2019). Reducing parental trauma and stress in neonatal intensive care: Systematic review and meta-analysis of hospital interventions. *Journal of Perinatology, 39,* 375–386. https://doi.org/10.1038/s41372-018-0310-9

Savanh, P., Aita, M., & Héon, M. (2020). A review of siblings' needs and interventions supporting their adaptation in the neonatal intensive care unit, *Infants & Young Children, 33*(4), 332–351. https://doi.org/10.1097/IYC.0000000000000178

Savanh, P., Aita, M., Heon, M., & Charbonneau, L. (2020). Case study of an intervention to favor siblings' adaptation during the hospitalization of a preterm infant in the neonatal intensive care unit. *Journal of Neonatal Nursing, 26*(6), 352–357.

Saxton, S. N., Walker, B., & Dykhovny, D. (2020). Parents matter: Examination of family presence in the neonatal intensive care unit. *American Journal of Perinatology.* https://doi.org/10.1055/s-0040-1701506

Schecter, R., Pham, T., Hua, A., Spinazzola, R., Sonnenklar, J., Li, D., Papaioannou, Y., & Milanaikm, R. (2020). Prevalence and longevity of PTSD symptoms among parents of NICU infants analyzed across gestational age categories. *Clinical Pediatrics, 59*(2), 163–169. https://doi.org/10.1177/0009922819892046

Schuetz Haemmerli, N., Lemola, S., Holditch-Davis, D., & Cignacco, E. (2020). Comparative evaluation of parental stress experiences up to 2 to 3 years after preterm and term birth. *Advances in Neonatal Care, 20*(4), 301–313. https://doi.org/10.1097/ANC.0000000000000714

Schuetz Haemmerli, N., von Gunten, G., Khan, J., Stoffel, L., Humpl, T., & Cignacco, E. (2021). Interprofessional collaboration in a new model of transitional care for families with preterm infants—The health care professional's perspective. *Journal of Multidisciplinary Healthcare, 14,* 897–908. https://doi.org/10.2147/jmdh.s303988

Serlachius, A., Hames, J., Juth, V., Garton, D., Rowley, S., & Petrie, K. J. (2018). Parental experiences of family-centred care from admission to discharge in the neonatal intensive care unit. *Journal of Paediatrics and Child Health, 54,* 1227–1233. https://doi.org/10.1111/jpc.14063

Shin, H., & White-Traut, R. (2007). The conceptual structure of transition to motherhood in the neonatal intensive care unit. *Journal of Advanced Nursing, 48*(1), 90–98.

Shlomai, N. O., Kasirer, Y., Strauss, T., Smolkin, T., Marom, R., Shinwell, E. C., Simmonds, A., Golan, A., Morag, I., Waisman, D., Felszer-Fisch, C., Wolf, D. G., & Eventov-Friedman, S. (2021). Neonatal SARS-CoV-2 infections in breastfeeding mothers. *Pediatrics, 147*(4), e2020010918; https://doi.org/10.1542/peds.2020-010918

Sigurdson, K., Mitchell, B., Liu, J., Morton, C., Gould, J. B., Lee, H. C., Capdarest-Arest, N., & Profit, J. (2019). Racial/ethnic disparities in neonatal intensive care: A systematic review. *Pediatrics, 144*(2), e20183114. https://doi.org/10.1542/peds.2018-3114

Sigurdson, K., Profit, J., Dhurjati, R., Morton, C., Scala, M., Vernon, L., Randolph, A., Phan, J. T., & Franck, L. S. (2020). Former NICU families describe gaps in family-centered care. *Qualitative Health Research, 309*(12), 1861–1875. https://doi.org/10.1177/1049732320932897

Śliwerski, A., Kossakowska, K., Jarecka, K., Świtalska, J., & Bielawska-Batorowicz, E. (2020). The effect of maternal depression on infant attachment: A systematic review. *International Journal of Environmental Research and Public Health, 17*(8), 2675. http://dx.doi.org/10.3390/ijerph17082675

Smith, V. C., Mao, W., & McCormick, M. C. (2021). Changes in assessment of and satisfaction with discharge preparation from the neonatal intensive care unit. *Advances in Neonatal Care.* https://doi.org/10.1097/ANC.0000000000000862

Soghier, L. M., Kritikos, K. I., Carty, C. L., Glass, P., Tuchman, L. K., Streisand, R., & Fratantoni, K. R. (2020). Parental depression symptoms at neonatal intensive care unit discharge and associated risk factors. *Journal of Pediatrics, 227,* 163. https://doi.org/10.1016/j.jpeds.2020.07.040

Staver, M. A., Moore, T. A., & Hanna, K. M. (2021). An integrative review of maternal distress during neonatal intensive care hospitalization. *Archives of Women's Mental Health, 24*(2), 217–229. https://doi.org/10.1007/s00737-020-01063-7

Stewart, S. A. (2019a). Parents' experience when present during a child's resuscitation: An integrative review. *Western Journal of Nursing Research, 41*(9), 1282–1305. https://doi.or/10.1177/0193945918822479

Stewart, S. A. (2019b). Parents' experience during a child's resuscitation: Getting through it. *Journal of Pediatric Nursing, 47,* P58–P67.

Stotts, A. L., Villarreal, Y. R., Klawans, M. R., Suchting, R., Dindo, L., Dempsey, A., Spellman, M., Green, C., & Northrup, T. F. (2019). Psychological flexibility and depression in new mothers of medically vulnerable infants: A mediational analysis. *Maternal and Child Health Journal, 23*(6), 821–829. https://doi.org/10.1007/s10995-018-02699-9

Strauss, Z., Avrech Bar, M., & Stanger, V. (2019). Fatherhood of a premature infant: "A rough roller-coaster ride." *Journal of Family Issues, 40*(8), 982–1000. https://doi.org/10.1177/0192513X19832939

Swearingen, C., Simpson, P., Cabacungan, E., & Cohen, S. (2020). Social disparities negatively impact neonatal follow-up clinic attendance of premature infants discharged from the neonatal intensive care unit. *Journal of Perinatology, 40*(5), 790–797. https://doi.org/10.1038/s41372-020-0659-4

Thomson-Salo, F., Kuschel, C. A., Kamlin, O. F., & Cuzzilla, R. (2017). A fathers' group in NICU: Recognising and responding to paternal stress, utilising peer support. *Journal of Neonatal Nursing, 23*(6), 294–298. https://doi.org/10.1016/j.jnn.2017.04.001

Treherne, S., Feeley, N., Charbonneau, L., & Axelin, A. (2017). Parents' perspectives of closeness and separation with their preterm infants in the NICU. *Journal of Obstetric, Gynecologic & Neonatal Nursing, 46*(5), 737–747. https://doi.org/10.1016/j.jogn.2017.07.005

Treyvaud, K., Doyle, L. W., Lee, K. J., Ure, A., Inder, T. E., Hunt, R. W., & Anderson, P. J. (2016). Parenting behavior at 2 years predicts school-age performance at 7 years in very preterm children. *Journal of Child Psychology and Psychiatry, and Allied Disciplines, 57*(7), 814–821. https://doi.org/10.1111/jcpp.12489

Treyvaud, K., Spittle, A., Anderson, P. J., & O'Brien, K. (2019). A multilayered approach is needed in the NICU to support parents after the preterm birth of their infant. *Early Human Development, 139*, 104838. https://doi.org/10.1016/j.earlhumdev.2019.104838

Turner, M., Chur-Hansen, A., & Winefield, H. (2015). Mothers' experiences of the NICU and a NICU support group programme. *Journal of Reproductive and Infant Psychology, 33*(2), 165–179. https://doi.org/10.1080/02646838.2014.998184

Twohig, A., Reulbach, U., Figuerdo, R., McCarthy, A., McNicholas, F., & Molloy, E. J. (2016). Supporting preterm infant attachment and socioemotional development in the neonatal intensive care unit: Staff perceptions. *Infant Mental Health Journal, 37*(2), 160–171. https://doi.org/10.1002/imhj.21556

Umberger, E., Canvasser, J., & Hall, S. L. (2018). Enhancing NICU parent engagement and empowerment. *Seminars in Pediatric Surgery, 27*(1), 19–24. https://doi.org/10.1053/j.sempedsurg.2017.11.004

Vance, A. J., Knafl, K., & Brandon, D. H. (2021). Patterns of parenting confidence among infants with medical complexity: A mixed-methods analysis. *Advances in Neonatal Care, 21*(2), 160–168. https://doi.org/10.1097/ANC.0000000000000754

Villar, J., Ariff, S., Gunier, R. B., Thiruvengadam, R., Rauch, S., Kholin, A., Roggero, P., Prefumo, F., do Vale, M. S., Cardona-Perez, J. A., Maiz, N., Cetin, I., Savasi, V., Deruelle, P., Easter, S. R., Sichitiu, J., Soto Conti, C. P., Ernawati, E., Mhatre, M., ... Papageorghiou, A. T. (2021). Maternal and neonatal morbidity and mortality among pregnant women with and without COVID-19 infection: The INTERCOVID multinational cohort study. *JAMA Pediatrics.* https://doi.org/10.1001/jamapediatrics.2021.1050

Vitale, F. M., Chirico, G., & Lentini, C. (2021). Sensory stimulation in the NICU environment: Devices, systems, and procedures to protect and stimulate Premature Babies. *Children, 8*(5), 334. https://doi.org/10.3390/children8050334

Wreesmann, W. W., Lorié, E. S., van Veenendaal, N. R., van Kempen, A., Ket, J., & Labrie, N. (2020). The functions of adequate communication in the neonatal care unit: A systematic review and meta-synthesis of qualitative research. *Patient Education and Counseling.* https://doi.org/10.1016/j.pec.2020.11.029

Zauche, L. H., Zauche, M. S. Dunlop, A. L., Williams, B. L., Dowling, D., & Schierholz, E. (2020). Predictors of parental presence in the neonatal intensive care unit. *Advances in Neonatal Care, 20*(3), 251–259. https://doi.org/10.1136/archdischild-2020-318840

Zauderer, C. (2009). Maternity care for Orthodox Jewish couples: Implications for nurses in the obstetric setting. *Nursing for Women's Health, 13*(2), 112–120.

Zehnder, E., Law, B. H. Y., & Schmolzer, G. M. (2020). Does parental presence affect workload during neonatal resuscitation? Archives of diseases in Child, *Fetal & Neonatal Edition, 105*(5), 559–561. http://dx.doi.org/10.1136/archdischild-2020-318840

CHAPTER 9

Critical Periods of Development

Carole Kenner

> **IFCDC—Standard for Systems Thinking in Collaborative Practice**
>
> **Standard 1: Systems Thinking**
> - The intensive care unit shall exhibit an infrastructure of leadership, mission, and a governance framework to guide the performance of the collaborative practice of IFCDC.

INTRODUCTION

The term *critical periods in development* refers to the concept that, as development occurs, certain events must occur at a particular time or point in the process for the next developmental steps to occur in an appropriate manner. The failure of developmental milestones to occur at a precisely defined point or within a critical period in the development of an embryo or fetus may result in malformation or death. For example, if the fusing of the neural tube does not occur in the critical period of 21 to 23 days postconception, the infant will be born with some degree of spina bifida. The purpose of this chapter is to describe the critical periods of development, including changes occurring in pregnant women, and significant points in the developmental process of an embryo or fetus. The final section of the chapter compares the developmental status of the respiratory, cardiovascular, neurologic, skin, and musculoskeletal systems of preterm infants across conceptional ages ranging from 24 to 36 weeks. Knowledge of the critical periods of development is an essential part of the philosophy of individualized, family-centered, developmental care. To minimize iatrogenic environmental hazards of extrauterine life, one must understand normal fetal development and the stage of development at which a premature infant is born.

WEEKS 1 TO 8: FERTILIZATION THROUGH THE EMBRYONIC STAGE

The first period of human development begins with fertilization and goes through the development of the zygote (weeks 0 to 2) to the embryonic stage (weeks 2 to 8). This period is characterized by fertilization and early cell division, implantation, the development of the placenta, and the beginning of organogenesis (Moore et al., 2019).

Stage 1: Fertilization Occurs (1 Day Postovulation)

Zygote size: 0.1 to 0.15 mm

Fertilization begins when one of approximately 3 million sperm penetrates an oocyte and ends with the creation of the zygote (Kenner, 2020; Moore et al., 2019). This process takes approximately 24 hours and occurs in the fallopian tube. A spermatozoon can survive for 48 hours, of which 10 hours are spent transcending the female reproductive tract to get to the oocyte. The next step is penetration of the zona pellucida, a tough membrane surrounding the oocyte. Only one spermatozoon needs to bind with the protein receptors in the zona pellucida to trigger an enzyme reaction, allowing the zona to be pierced. Penetration of the zona pellucida takes approximately 20 minutes. Within 11 hours after fertilization, the oocyte has extruded a polar body with its excess chromosomes. The fusion of the oocyte and sperm nuclei marks the creation of the zygote and the end of fertilization.

Stage 2: Cleavage; First Cell Division (1.5 to 3 Days Postovulation)

Zygote size: 0.1 to 0.2 mm

The zygote now begins to cleave, forming two cells called *blastomeres*. The zygote's first cell division begins a series of divisions, with each occurring approximately every 20 hours. Each blastomere within the zona pellucida becomes smaller and smaller with each subsequent division. When cell division has produced approximately 16 cells, the zygote becomes a morula (the shape of a mulberry). It leaves the fallopian tube and enters the uterine cavity 3 to 4 days after fertilization.

Stage 3: Early Blastocyst (4 Days Postovulation)

Zygote size: 0.1 to 0.2 mm

The morula enters the uterine cavity approximately 4 days after fertilization. Cell division continues, and a cavity known as a blastocele forms in the center of the morula (Kenner 2020; Moore et al., 2019). Cells flatten and compact on the inside of the cavity while the zona pellicuda remains the same size. With the appearance of the cavity in the center, the organism is now called a *blastocyst*. The presence of the blastocyst indicates that two cell types are forming: the embryoblast (inner cell mass inside of the blastocele) and the trophoblast (cells on the outside of the blastocele).

Stage 4: Implantation Begins (5 to 6 Days Postovulation)

Zygote size: 0.1 to 0.2 mm

The blastocyst "hatches" from the zona pellucida on approximately the sixth day after fertilization as the blastocyst cells secrete an enzyme that erodes the epithelial uterine lining and creates an implantation site for the blastocyst (Kenner, 2020; Moore et al., 2019). The ovary is induced to continue producing progesterone. The trophoblastic cells of the implanting blastocyst release human chorionic gonadotropin (hCG) in a cyclic process. Endometrial glands in the uterus enlarge in response to the blastocyst, and the implantation site becomes swollen with new capillaries. Implantation involves three distinct processes: degeneration of the zona pellucida, attachment of the blastocyst to the endometrial endothelium followed by a rapid proliferation of the trophoblast, and erosion of the endometrial epithelium with burrowing of the blastocyst beneath the surface. More research is focusing on the reciprocity of actions between the zygote (a signal from the zygote) and the receptivity of the maternal uterine surface for successful implantation. Many perinatal experts refer to this period as an all-or-nothing time, meaning that if there is a significant embryologic problem, implantation may never occur and, in some instances, a woman might have a heavier than usual menstrual flow and never know that fertilization occurred. If the "error" in the zygotic or embryonic material is not large enough, implantation may occur, but a viable fetus or long-term pregnancy may not happen. More research is needed in this vital area of perinatal/neonatal care.

Critical Points in Zygotic/Embryonic Development

Two points in this early period are of particular importance in the development of the embryo. The first critical point is that of fertilization itself and the immediately following cell divisions. It is at this initial point in human development that many chromosomal abnormalities can occur. These abnormalities may result from more than one sperm, fertilizing an egg, resulting in dispermy, or a zygote with extra chromosomes or incomplete mitotic divisions in the early zygotic period. Triploid conceptions account for approximately 20% of chromosomally abnormal abortions. Implantation problems constitute another critical point. Failure of blastocysts to implant may result from a poorly developed endometrium. Early in pregnancy, the corpus luteum increases its hormone production in preparation for implantation of the blastocyst. Degeneration of the corpus luteum is prevented by hCG. Any alterations in hCG production or corpus luteum hormone production can interfere with endometrial development and impede implantation.

DEVELOPMENT OF THE PLACENTA

Stage 5: Implantation Complete; Placental Circulation System Begins (7 to 12 Days Postovulation)

Zygote size: 0.1 to 0.2 mm

Early in the embryonic period at the point of implantation, the placenta begins to form (Kenner, 2020; Moore et al., 2019). The placenta is a temporary fetomaternal organ made of two components: a large fetal portion derived from the chorionic sac and a small maternal portion derived from the endometrium. The placenta forms the intrauterine environment in which the fetus grows and develops. The placenta, together with the umbilical cord, provides the means of transport and exchange of oxygen and nutrients from the mother to the embryo/fetus and carbon dioxide and waste from the embryo/fetus to the mother.

The functions of the placenta include:

- Fetal protection.
- Nutrition provision.
- Oxygen/carbon dioxide exchange.
- Waste removal.
- Hormone production.

DEVELOPMENT OF THE PLACENTA AND FETAL MEMBRANES

The development of the placenta begins as implantation proceeds. The invasion of the endometrium begins on the 7th day after fertilization and generally is complete by the 12th day. At this time, the trophoblast begins to differentiate into two layers: the inner cytotrophoblast and the outer syncytiotrophoblast. The cytotrophoblast is a mononucleated layer of cells that forms new trophoblast cells that migrate into the increasing mass of syncytiotrophoblast, where they fuse and lose their cell membrane. The syncytiotrophoblast is a rapidly expanding, multinuclear mass without distinct cell boundaries that invades the endometrial tissue (capillaries, glands, and connective tissue). As this occurs, the blastocyst becomes embedded in the endometrium. Proteolytic enzymes produced by the syncytiotrophoblast facilitate this process. The syncytiotrophoblast begins to produce hCG, which maintains the corpus luteum during early pregnancy and forms the basis for pregnancy tests. Eight days after conception, intercommunicating spaces, or lacunae, appear in the syncytiotrophoblast. The lacunae fill with fluid that contains maternal blood from ruptured endometrial capillaries and glandular secretions from eroded uterine glands. The nutrients in this fluid pass to the developing embryo by diffusion. The flow of maternal blood into the lacunar spaces from the maternal capillaries is the beginning of uteroplacental circulation. Both arterial and venous branches of maternal blood vessels communicate with the lacunae, and oxygenated blood enters the lacunae from the spiral arteries and deoxygenated blood is removed from the lacunae from the endometrial veins.

During implantation, endometrial tissue cells enlarge and accumulate glycogen and lipids. This cellular transformation is referred to as the "decidual reaction," and the altered endometrium is known as the decidua. Consensus is that this reaction protects the myometrium from uncontrolled invasion by the trophoblast. There are three regions of the decidua: the decidua basalis is the part that forms the maternal component of the placenta, the decidua capsularis is the superficial part of the decidua overlying the conceptus, and the decidua parietalis is the remaining part of the decidua.

By the end of the second week following fertilization, primary chorionic villi appear. Proliferation of the cytotrophoblast layer produces columns of cells or fingerlike projections that grow into the syncytiotrophoblast. A mesenchymal core grows within these projections from which blood vessels will later develop.

As the blastocyst burrows into the endometrium, small spaces appear between the inner cell mass and the cytotrophoblast. This is the early amniotic cavity that gradually enlarges to completely surround the developing fetus. Amnioblasts (amnion forming cells) from the cytotrophoblast form a thin membrane, the amnion, which encloses the amniotic cavity. The epiblast (a type of cell from the embryonic disk) forms the floor of the amniotic cavity.

Development of the Chorionic Sac

Cells from the yolk sac give rise to a layer of connective tissue, the extraembryonic mesoderm. As changes occur in the trophoblast and endometrium, spaces appear within the extraembryonic mesoderm. These spaces fuse and form a large cavity, the extraembryonic coelom. This cavity surrounds the amnion and yolk sac and splits the extraembryonic mesoderm into the extraembryonic somatic mesoderm, lining the trophoblast and covering the amnion, and the exraembryonic splanchnic mesoderm, surrounding the yolk sac. The extraembryonic somatic mesoderm together with the cytotrophoblast and the syncytiotrophoblast constitutes the chorion. The chorion forms the walls of the gestational

sac, within which the connecting stalk suspends the developing embryo and its amniotic and yolk sac. Initially, chorionic villi cover the entire chorionic sac. As the sac grows, the villi associated with the decidua capsularis are compressed and soon degenerate. This now-smooth part of the chorion is called the *chorion laeve*. The chorionic villi associated with the decidua basalis branch out profusely and enlarge, forming the fetal portion of the placenta called the *chorion frondosum* or *villus chorion*. The mature placenta is established by 4 to 10 weeks after conception but continues to grow in both size and thickness until approximately 20 weeks gestation. The fully developed placenta covers 15% to 30% of the decidua and weighs approximately one-sixth of the total fetus weight.

Placental Structure

The fetal part of the placenta (chorion frondosum) is attached to the maternal part of the placenta (decidua basalis) by anchoring villi (Kenner 2020; Moore et al., 2019). As the chorionic villi invade the decidua basalis, several wedge-shaped areas of decidua are formed, called the *placental septa*. The placental septa divide the fetal part of the placenta into irregular areas called *cotyledons*. Each cotyledon consists of two or more mainstem villi and their many branches. The space surrounding the villi contains maternal blood and secretions and is called the *intervillous space*. Maternal blood enters the intervillous space from the spiral arteries in the decidua basalis and is drained by endometrial veins. The numerous villi continuously are bathed with maternal blood that circulates throughout the intervillous space. This is the site for nutrient transfer and gas exchange. The normal growth and development of the embryo and the fetus is more dependent on the adequate bathing of the villi than on any other factor. Several layers of tissue separate maternal and fetal circulations. These tissues are called the placental membrane. A molecule of oxygen in the maternal blood surrounding the villi must diffuse through four tissue layers to reach fetal blood: the syncytiotrophoblast, the cytotrophoblast, the connective tissue of the villus, and epithelium of the fetal capillaries. This membrane has been called the placental barrier, but it is important to remember that most drugs and other substances in the maternal circulation easily pass through the placental membrane and enter the fetal circulation.

Fetal–Placental Circulation

Deoxygenated blood leaves the fetus via two umbilical arteries and passes to the placenta. The umbilical arteries, at the site of cord attachment to the placenta, branch into a number of chorionic arteries. The chorionic arteries branch further, forming an extensive arteriovenous system within each villus, bringing fetal blood extremely close to maternal blood. This system provides a large surface area for the exchange of nutrients, gases, and waste products between the maternal and fetal circulation. There is normally no intermingling of maternal and fetal blood, although, occasionally, small quantities of fetal blood may enter maternal circulation through minute defects that might develop in the placental membrane. The veins from each villus converge back into the single umbilical vein at the site of attachment of the umbilical cord. The umbilical vein then carries oxygen-rich blood to the fetus.

Although villous growth continues until term, degenerative changes also begin to occur, such as intervillous thrombi, fibrin deposits, infarcts, and calcification. These degenerative changes can alter gas and nutrient transfer and may result in fetal hypoxia and fetal growth restriction.

Placental Function

Placental metabolism, specifically, the synthesis of glycogen, cholesterol, and fatty acids, is important early in pregnancy, providing nutrition and energy for the developing embryo/fetus. The transport of substances across the placental membrane occurs as a result of simple diffusion, in which substances move from areas of higher concentration to lower concentration (e.g., oxygen, carbon dioxide, water, urea, most drugs, and drug metabolites); facilitated diffusion which requires a carrier to move a substance down a concentration gradient (e.g., glucose); active transport, which occurs when substances are transported against a concentration gradient and require energy expenditure (e.g., amino acids, water-soluble vitamins); and pinocytosis, whereby extracellular fluid containing a particular substance is engulfed by the cells of the plasma membrane (e.g., phospholipids, lipoproteins, maternal antibodies, or transferrin).

Placental Hormones

The endocrine functions of the placenta are critical to maintaining a normal, healthy pregnancy. Using precursors from both the mother and fetus, the placenta can synthesize protein and steroid hormones. The placenta (syncytiotrophoblast) begins its hormone synthesis as a blastocyst and continues this function until it is expelled from the uterus at birth. The four major hormones produced by the placenta are hCG; human placental lactogen (hPL), also called human chorionic somatomammotropin; progesterone; and estrogens.

The primary role of hCG is to maintain the corpus luteum during early pregnancy. Concentrations of hCG in maternal serum double every 1.4 to 2 days until peak values are reached by 2 to 3 months postconception. hCG is the hormone that is the basis for pregnancy testing. hPL promotes fetal growth by altering maternal protein, carbohydrate, and fat metabolism. This hormone is responsible for decreasing maternal insulin sensitivity and glucose use, which increases the amount of glucose that is available for transport to the fetus. Progesterone has many functions that are essential to maintain pregnancy. It also serves as a substrate for fetal adrenal hormone synthesis. Adequate

estrogen also is important for a normal pregnancy. During pregnancy, all three of the major estrogens—estrone, estradiol, and estriol—are markedly increased, although estriol increases the most, at approximately 1,000-fold. Placental estrogen synthesis is unique in that it requires precursors from both the fetus and the mother. Approximately 90% of the precursors for estriol are derived from the fetus, as well as 60% of the precursors for estrone and estradiol.

Critical Period of Development

The development of the placenta is a critical point in a pregnancy. Any impairment in the development of the transport system for substances passing between the mother and fetus can result in fetal growth restriction. Impairment in the endocrine function of the placenta (e.g., secretion of hCG, progesterone, or estriol) can result in loss of pregnancy because these hormones are necessary to maintain a normal pregnancy. It should be noted that at this early stage of the pregnancy, environmental factors such as exposure to cigarette smoke may result in decreased uterine blood flow, an abnormally small placenta, and intrauterine growth restriction.

Stage 6: Chorionic Villi Form; Gastrulation (13 Days Postovulation)

Embryonic size: 0.2 mm

With implantation complete and placental development in progress, this stage is the beginning of organogenesis. All major organ systems begin to develop at this point—long before many women realize they are pregnant. Chorionic villi "fingers" in the forming placenta now anchor the site to the uterus. The formation of embryo blood and blood vessels begins in this stage. The blood system appears first in the area of the "placenta" surrounding the embryo, while the yolk sac begins to produce hematopoietic or nonnucleated blood cells. By the end of the first part of this stage (6a), the embryo is attached by a connecting stalk; this eventually will become part of the umbilical cord to the developing placenta.

Stage 6b begins when a narrow line of cells appears on the surface of the embryonic disk. This primitive streak is the future axis of the embryo and marks the beginning of *gastrulation,* the process that produces the three layers of the embryo—the endoderm, mesoderm, and ectoderm.

Stage 7: Neurulation and Notochordal Process (16 Days Postovulation)

Embryonic size: 1.4 mm

Gastrulation continues with the formation of the endoderm and mesoderm, which develop from the primitive streak, changing the two-layered disk into a three-layered disk (Moore et al., 2019). The cells in the central part of the mesoderm release a chemical that causes a dramatic change in the size of the cells in the top layer (ectoderm) of the flat disk-shaped embryo. The ectoderm grows rapidly over the next few days, forming a thickened area. The three layers eventually will give rise to the:

- Endoderm: Forms the lining of the lungs, tongue, tonsils, urethra, and associated glands, bladder, and digestive tract.
- Mesoderm: Forms the muscles, bones, lymphatic tissue, spleen, blood cells, heart, lungs, and reproductive and excretory systems.
- Ectoderm: Forms the skin, nails, hair, lens of eye, lining of the internal and external ear, nose sinuses, mouth, anus, tooth enamel, pituitary gland, mammary system, and all parts of the nervous system.

Stage 8: Primitive Pit, Notochordal Canal, and Neurenteric Canals Form (17 to 19 Days Postovulation)

Embryonic size: 1.0 to 1.5 mm

The embryonic area is now shaped like a pear, and the head region is broader than the tail end. The ectoderm has thickened to form the neural plate. The edges of this plate rise and form a concave area known as the neural groove. This groove is the precursor of the embryo's nervous system and is one of the first organs to develop. The blood cells of the embryo already are developed, and they begin to form channels along the epithelial cells, which form consecutively with the blood cells.

Stage 9: Somites Appear (19 to 21 Days Postovulation)

Embryonic size: 1.5 to 2.5 mm

The top view of the embryo resembles the sole of a shoe, with the head end wider than the tail end and a slightly narrowed middle. Somites, which are condensations composed of mesoderm, appear on either side of the neural groove. The first pair of somites appear at the tail end and progress to the middle; at this time there are one to three pair of somites. Every ridge, bump, and recess now indicates cellular differentiation. A head fold rises on either side of the primitive streak. The primitive streak runs between one-fourth to one-third the length of the embryo.

Secondary blood vessels now appear in the chorion/placenta. Hematopoietic cells appear on the yolk sac simultaneously with endothelial cells that will form blood vessels for newly emerging blood cells. Endocardial (muscle) cells begin to fuse and form the two tubes that will become the embryo's heart.

Stage 10: Neural Fold Begins to Fuse; Heart Tube Fuses (21 to 23 Days Postovulation)

Embryonic size: 1.5 to 3.0 mm

Tremendous growth and change occur as the embryo becomes longer and the yolk sac expands. At this time,

on each side of the neural tube, between 4 and 12 pairs of somites can exist. The cells that become the eyes appear as thickened circles just off the neural folds. The cells of the ears also are present. Neural folds are rising and fusing at several points along the length of the neural tube concomitant with the budding somites, which appear to "zipper" the neural tube closed. Neural crest cells eventually will contribute to the embryo's skull and face.

The two endocardial tubes fuse to form one single tube derived from the roof of the neural tube; it becomes S-shaped and makes the primitive heart asymmetric. As the S shape forms, the cardiac muscle begins to contract.

Stage 11: 13 to 20 Somite Pairs Have Formed; Rostral Neuropore Closes; Optic Vesicle, Two Pharyngeal Arches Appear (23 to 25 Days Postovulation)

Embryonic size: 2.5 to 3.0 mm

Thirteen to 20 pairs of somites are present and shaped in a modified S curve. The embryo has a bulblike tail and a connecting stalk to the developing placenta. A primitive S-shaped tubal heart is beating, resulting in the rhythmic flow of fluids being propelled throughout the body. However, this is not true circulation because blood vessel development still is incomplete.

At this stage, the neural tube determines the form of the embryo. Although the primary blood vessels along the central nervous system (CNS) are connecting, the CNS appears to be the most developed system. When 20 somites are present in the embryo, the forebrain is completely closed.

Stage 12: 21 to 29 Somite Pairs Are Present; Caudal Neuropore Closes; 3 to 4 Pharyngeal Arches Appear; Upper Limb Buds Appear (25 to 27 Days Postovulation)

Embryonic size: 3.0 to 5.0 mm

At this time, the embryo has a distinctive C shape. The arches that form the face and neck now are becoming evident under the enlarging forebrain. By the time the neural tube is closed, both the eyes and ears will have begun to form. At this stage, the brain and spinal cord together are the largest and most compact tissue of the embryo.

The blood system continues to develop. Blood cells follow the surface of the yolk sac, where they originate, move along the CNS, and move in the chorionic villi and the maternal blood system. Valves and the septa might appear. The digestive epithelium layer begins to differentiate into the future locations of the liver, lungs, stomach, and pancreas. Liver formation begins, with a few cells appearing before the remaining portions of the digestive system develop.

Stage 13: Four Limb Buds, Lens Disc and Optic Vesicle, 30 to 40 Somite Pairs Can Be Found (Approximately 27 to 29 Days Postovulation)

Embryonic size: 4.0 to 6.0 mm

The brain differentiates into three main parts: the forebrain, midbrain, and hindbrain. The forebrain consists of lobes that translate input from the senses and will be responsible for memory formation, thinking, reasoning, and problem solving. The midbrain will serve as a relay station, coordinating messages to their final destination. The hindbrain will be responsible for regulating the heart, breathing, and muscle movements. The thyroid continues to develop, and the lymphatic system, which filters out bacteria, starts to form.

The optic placode invaginates and forms the optic vesicles, which will develop into the structures needed for hearing and maintenance of equilibrium. Retinal discs press outward and touch the surface ectoderm. In response, the ectoderm proliferates, forming the lens disc. Specific parts of the eye such as the retina, the future pigment of the retina, and the optic stalk are identifiable. The primitive mouth with a tongue is recognizable.

Heart chambers now are filled with plasma and blood cells, making the heart seem distended and prominent. The heart and liver combined are equal in volume to the head at this stage. Blood circulation is well-established, although true valves are not yet present. The villous network is in place to accommodate the exchange of blood between the woman and the embryo. Aortic arches 4 and 6 develop and 5 might appear. Lung buds continue to form.

The gallbladder, stomach, intestines, and pancreas continue to form, and the metamorphic bud appears in the chest cavity. The stomach is in the shape of a spindle, and the pancreas can be detected in the intestinal tube. The developing liver receives blood from the placenta via the umbilical cord. The amnion encloses the connecting stalk, helping to fuse it with the longer and slenderer umbilical vesicle (the remnant of the yolk sac).

Upper-limb buds now are visible as ridges and the lower limb buds begin to develop. Folding is complete, and the embryo now is three-dimensional and is completely enclosed in the amniotic sac. The somites will be involved in building bones and muscles. The first, thin surface layer of skin appears, covering the embryo.

Stage 14: Lens Pit and Optic Cup Appear; Endolymphatic Appendages Are Distinct (4 to 8 Weeks Postfertilization)

Embryonic size: 5.0 to 7.0 mm

Head and Neck

The brain and head grow rapidly during these periods. The mandibular and hyoid arches are noticeable and form the beginning of the neck and jawbones. Ridges appear that demarcate the three future sections of the brain. The spinal cord wall at this stage contains three zones: the ventricular, the mantle, and the marginal. The ventricular zone will form neurons, glial cells, and ependymal cells; the intermediate mantle will form neuron clusters; and the marginal zone will contain processes of neurons. The adenohypophyseal pouch, which will develop into the anterior pituitary, is defined. The lens vesicles open to the surface and are nestled within the optic cup. The optic vesicle increases its size by approximately one-fourth, and its endolymphatic appendage is more defined. Nasal plates can be detected by thickened ectoderm.

Thorax

The esophagus now forms from a groove of tissue that separates from the trachea, which also is visible. Semilunar valves begin to form in the heart. Four major subdivisions of the heart (the trabeculated left and right ventricles, the conus cords, and the truncus arteriosus) clearly are defined during this time. Two sprouts, a ventral sprout from the aortic sac and a dorsal sprout from the aorta, form the pulmonary arch. Right and left lung sacs lie on either side of the esophagus.

Abdominal and Pelvic Regions

Ureteric buds appear. Metanephroi, which eventually will form the permanent kidney, now are developing.

Limbs: Upper

Upper limbs elongate into cylindrically shaped buds, tapering at the tip to eventually form the hand plate. Nerve distribution and innervation begins in the upper limbs.

Stage 15: Lens Vesicles, Nasal Pit, and Hand Plate Develop; Trunk Widens; Future Cerebral Hemispheres are Distinct (6 to 8 Weeks Postfertilization)

Embryonic size: 7.0 to 9.0 mm

Head and Neck

The brain has increased in size by 33%; it still is larger than the trunk. The rostral neuropore is closed and four pairs of pharyngeal arches now are visible, although the fourth still is quite small. The maxillary and mandibular prominences of the first arch are clearly delineated. The stomodeum, the depression in the ectoderm, which will develop into the mouth and oral cavity, appears between the prominent forebrain and the fused mandibular prominence. Swellings of the external ear begin to appear on both sides of the head, formed by the mandibular arch. The lens pit has closed, retinal pigment may appear in the external layer of the optic cup, and lens fibers form the lens body. Two symmetrical and separate nasal pits may appear as depressions in the nasal disc.

Thorax

The esophagus continues to lengthen. Blood flow through the atrioventricular canal is divided into left and right streams, which continue through the outflow tract and aortic sac. The left ventricle is larger than the right and has a thicker wall. Lobar buds appear in the bronchial tree.

Abdominal and Pelvic Regions

The intestine lengthens. Ureteric buds lengthen and the tip expands, beginning the formation of the final and permanent set of kidneys.

Limbs: Upper and Lower

Distinct regions of the hand plate, forearm, and arm now can be discerned in the upper limb bud. The lower limb bud begins to round at the top, and the tip of its tapering end eventually will form the foot. Innervation, the distribution of nerves, begins in the lower limb buds.

Spine

The relative width of the trunk increases from the growth of the spinal ganglia, the muscular plate, and the corresponding mesenchymal tissues.

Stage 16: Growth Spurt (6 to 8 Weeks Postfertilization)

Embryonic size: 9.0 to 11.0 mm

Head and Neck

The brain is well marked by its cerebral hemispheres. The hindbrain, which is responsible for heart regulation, breathing, and muscle movements, begins to develop. The future lower jaw, the first part of the face to be established, now is visible, while the future upper jaw is present but not demarcated. Mesenchymal cells originating in the primitive streak, neural crest, and prechordal plate continue to form the skull and face. External retina pigment is visible and the lens pit has grown into a D shape. Nasal pits still are two separate plates, but they rotate to face ventrally as the head widens.

Thorax

Primary cardiac tubes separate into aortic and pulmonary channels, and the ventricular pouches deepen and enlarge, forming a common wall with their myocardial shells. Mammary gland tissue begins to mature.

Abdominal and Pelvic Regions

The mesentery—which attaches the intestines to the rear abdominal wall; holds them in position; and supplies them with blood, nerves, and lymphatics— now is clearly defined. The ureter, the tube that will convey urine from the kidney to the bladder, continues to lengthen. Proliferation of the coelomic epithelium indicates the gonadal primordium.

Limbs: Upper and Lower

Hand regions of upper limb buds differentiate further to form a central carpal part and a digital plate. The thigh, leg, and foot areas can be distinguished in the lower limb buds.

Stage 17: A Four-Chamber Heart and a Sense of Smell (Approximately 41 Days Postovulation)

Embryonic size: 10 to 13 mm

Head and Neck

Jaw and facial muscles now are developing. The nasofrontal groove becomes distinct, and an olfactory bulb forms in the brain. Auricular hillocks become recognizable. The dental laminae or teeth buds begin to form. The pituitary, which is the master gland responsible for growth of hormones that regulate other glands such as the thyroid, adrenal, and gonads, begins to form. The trachea, the larynx, and the bronchi begin to form.

Thorax

The heart begins to separate into four chambers. The diaphragm, the tissue that separates the chest cavity from the abdomen, forms.

Abdominal and Pelvic Regions

Intestines begin to develop within the umbilical cord and later will migrate into the abdomen when the embryo's body is large enough to accommodate them. In the area of the future pelvis, primitive germ cells arrive at the genital area and will respond to genetic instructions to develop into either female or male genitalia.

Limbs: Upper and Lower

Digital rays begin to appear in the footplates, and finger rays are more distinct.

Spine

The trunk becomes straighter.

Stage 18: Ossification of the Skeleton Begins (42 to 46 Days Postovulation)

Embryonic size: 11 to 14 mm

Head and Neck

Nerve plexuses begin to develop in the region of the scalp. Eyes are pigmented and eyelids begin to develop and may fold.

Thorax

Within the heart, the trunk of the pulmonary artery separates from the trunk of the aorta. Nipples appear on the chest. The body appears more like a cube.

Abdominal and Pelvic Regions

Kidneys begin to produce urine for the first time. The genital tubercle, urogenital membrane, and anal membrane appear.

Limbs: Upper and Lower

The critical period of arm development ends, and the arms are at their proper location, roughly proportional to the embryo. The hand plates are not finished, but develop further in the next 2 days. The wrists are clearly visible, and the hands have ridges or notches indicating the future separation of the fingers and the thumbs.

Spine and Skeleton

Ossification of the skeleton begins.

Stage 19: Brain Waves and Muscles (Approximately 47 to 48 Days Postovulation)

Embryonic size: 13 to 18 mm

Head and Neck

The brain has the first detectable brain waves. The head is more erect, and semicircular canals start to form in the inner ear, which will enable a sense of balance and body position.

Thorax

The septum primum fuses with the septum intermedium in the heart.

Abdominal and Pelvic Regions

The gonads form. In approximately 1 week, the gender of the embryo will be recognizable in the form of testes or ovaries.

Limbs: Upper and Lower

Knee and ankle locations are indicated by indentations. Legs are now at their proper location, proportional to the embryo. The critical period for the lower limbs is about to end. Toes are almost completely notched, and toenails begin to appear. Joints grow more distinct.

Spine, Skeleton, and Muscles

The trunk elongates and straightens, and the bone cartilage begins to form a more solid structure. Muscles develop and get stronger.

Stage 20: Spontaneous Involuntary Movement (49 to 51 Days Postovulation)

Embryonic size: 19 to 20 mm

Head and Neck

The brain now is connected to tiny muscles and nerves, enabling the embryo to make spontaneous movements. The scalp plexus now is present. Nasal openings and the tip of the nose are fully formed.

Limbs: Upper and Lower

The upper limbs become longer and continue to bend at the elbows and extend forward. Skin on the footplate folds down between the future toes, each distinguishable from the other.

Stage 21: Intestines Begin to Recede Into Body Cavity (Approximately 52 Days Postovulation)

Embryonic size: 17 to 21 mm

Head and Neck

Eyes are well-developed but still are located on the side of the head. As head development continues, they will migrate forward. External ears are set low on the embryo's head but will move up as the head enlarges. During the next few days, tongue development is completed.

Abdominal and Pelvic Regions

Intestines begin migration within the umbilical cord toward the embryo. The liver causes a ventral prominence of the abdomen.

Limbs: Upper and Lower

Fingers lengthen while distinct grooves form between the fingers, which also lengthen as the hands approach each other across the abdomen. Feet approach each other but still are fan-shaped, and toe digits still are webbed.

Stage 22: Heart Development Ends (53 to 55 Days Postovulation)

Embryonic size: 19 to 24 mm

Head and Neck

The head is beginning to develop fissures that make it more characteristic of what we recognize as "humanness." Eyelids and external ears are more developed, and the upper lip is fully formed.

Thorax

The critical period of heart development is completed. The major structures are in place, and the conducting system of the heart has developed.

Abdominal and Pelvic Regions

In female embryos, the clitoris is beginning to form. The penis will develop from the same tissue.

Limbs: Upper and Lower

Primary ossification centers appear in the long bones, directing the replacement of cartilage by bone. This process usually begins in the upper limbs. Fingers overlap those of the opposite hand, and the digits of the fingers fully separate. Feet lengthen and become more defined.

Abdominal and Pelvic Regions

The anal membrane is perforated. Urogenital membranes differentiate in the male and female embryos. Testes or ovaries are distinguishable.

Stage 23: Essential External and Internal Structures Are Complete (Approximately 56 to 57 Days Postovulation)

Embryonic size: 23 to 26 mm

Head and Neck

The head is erect and rounded. The external ear is completely developed. The eyes are closed, but the retina is fully pigmented. The eyelids begin to unite and are only half-closed. Taste buds begin to form on the surface of the tongue. The primary teeth are at cap stage. Bones of the palate begin to fuse. The scalp plexus reaches head vertex.

Abdominal and Pelvic Regions

Intestines begin to migrate from the umbilical cord into the body cavity. The external genitals still are difficult to recognize.

Limbs: Upper and Lower

Upper and lower limbs are well-formed. Fingers get longer, and toes are no longer webbed; all digits are separated and distinct.

Spine, Skeleton, Muscles, and Skin

A layer of rather flattened cells, the precursor of the surface layer of the skin, replaces the thin ectoderm of the embryo. The tail has disappeared.

At this point, at the end of the eighth week of gestation, the embryonic phase of development is complete as is the period of rapid organogenesis. Although each organ system will continue to develop and mature, the basic structures of each system are in place. It is during this early period that the developing embryo is most vulnerable to the effects of exposure to external substances such as cigarette smoke, alcohol, and teratogenic drugs that will adversely affect the course of development.

WEEKS 9 TO 40: FETAL DEVELOPMENT

Fetal development begins in week 9 and continues through the end of the pregnancy. During this period, organogenesis is complete, the fetus undergoes a period of rapid growth, and critical developmental milestones are reached that allow for the survival of the infant in the extrauterine environment. In this section, we review the sequencing of fetal development and discuss the critical periods in the development of the neurosensory and respiratory systems that affect preterm infant survival.

Weeks 9 to 11

Head and Neck

The basic brain structure is complete, and brain mass increases rapidly through this period. Sockets for all 20 teeth are formed in gums. The face now has a human appearance. Separate folds of the mouth fuse to form the palate, and early facial hair follicles begin to develop.

Thorax

Vocal cords form in the larynx, and the fetus can make sounds.

Abdominal and Pelvic Regions

The intestines have migrated into the abdomen from the umbilical cord. Digestive tract muscles are functional and practice contracting. Nutrient-extracting villi line the now-folded intestines. The liver and gallbladder are formed, and the liver starts to secrete bile that is stored in the gallbladder. Development of the thyroid, pancreas, and gallbladder is complete, and the pancreas starts to produce insulin. Genitalia continue to develop more differentiated female characteristics (labium minus, and labium majora) and male characteristics (glans, penis, urethral groove, scrotum). Neither male nor female genitalia are fully formed.

Limbs: Upper and Lower

Fingernails begin to grow from nail beds.

Skin and Muscles

Fetus develops primitive reflexes, and the skin is very sensitive.

Weeks 12 to 15

The fetus is more flexible, with the ability to move the head, mouth, lips, arms, wrists, hands, legs, feet, and toes, although the mother likely cannot feel these movements yet.

The somatesthetic system is the first in the fetal sensory developmental systems to become functional during this period (Fig. 9-1). This system includes the sense of touch, pressure, and, probably, pain. Its focus is on the sensory nerve ending of the palms of hands, soles of feet, and perioral and perinasal areas of the face.

Head and Neck

The head is approximately 50% of the crown-to-rump length and rests on the well-defined neck instead of shoulders. The developing sucking muscles of the mouth fill out cheeks, tooth buds continue to develop, and salivary glands begin to function. The scalp hair pattern is discernible.

The head and neck are straighter and almost erect as muscles strengthen and additional bone texture forms in the

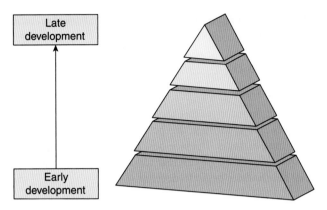

FIGURE 9-1. Progression of fetal sensory development by system. Top to bottom: visual, auditory, chemosensory, vestibular, and somatesthetic.

back. Eyes are now oriented in a forward manner, and the ears are close to their final position.

Thorax

The heartbeat can be detected with external instruments. Lungs develop further as the fetus inhales and exhales amniotic fluid, which is essential for air sacs within the lungs to function properly. The fetal heart pumps approximately 25 quarts of blood per day and increases to 300 quarts per day by the time of delivery.

Abdominal and Pelvic Regions

The fully functional spleen will assume functions supervised by the liver such as removal of old red blood cells and production of antibodies. The fetus' gender can be detected on ultrasound as genitalia become clearly visible.

Limbs: Upper and Lower

Arms have almost reached final proportion and length, although legs still are quite short relative to the fetus' body.

Hands, particularly the thumbs, become functional. Toenails begin to grow from the nail beds.

Skin, Muscles, and Glands

Muscles function more smoothly. The fetus is more flexible and has advanced movements of the head, mouth and lips, arms, wrists, hands, legs, feet, and toes. Fetal positioning, even at this early time, begins to influence later musculoskeletal development (see Table 9-1 for practice recommendations). Muscles and the nervous system continue to advance. The sweat glands appear, and body hair begins to grow.

Placenta

By approximately the fourth month (10 to 12 weeks after fertilization), the placenta has achieved its full thickness, with no further development of new cotyledons. Circumferential placental growth continues, with further branching of the villi and growth of the placental capillaries. As a result, the surface area for placental exchange continues to expand until late in gestation, increasing its functional efficiency.

Weeks 16 to 20

No new structures form after this point, but each system continues to develop in complexity and the fetus enters a period of rapid growth.

Behavior

During this period, the vestibular system is becoming functional. The fetus can now experience changes in position and orientation, has phases of sleep and waking, and may prefer a favorite sleep position. Also, at this point, ultrasound can show the fetus beginning to suck on a thumb or toe. When

TABLE 9-1 **Practice Recommendations**			
Type	Recommendation	Level of Evidence	References
Prevention	Increased knowledge among health professionals regarding fetal alcohol spectrum disorders (FASDs) and recognition of screening barriers for perinatal alcohol use may decrease the occurrence of FASD. What is the relationship between prenatal opioid exposure (POE) and brain and later child development?	IV IV VII IV	Chiodo et al., 2019 Ordean et al., 2020 Larson et al., 2019 Boggess & Risher, 2020
Intervention	Provision of adequate iron in premature or low-birth-weight infants should be considered within the context of central nervous system development. Prenatal *Cannabis* use should be considered within the context of long-term psychopathology during middle childhood. Use of kangaroo mother care (KMC) should be considered within the context of neonatal growth and development, especially of the very-low-birth-weight infant.	V IV IV	Moreno-Fernandez et al., 2019 Paul et al., 2020 Sharma et al., 2017

Note: Level I = evidence from a systematic review or meta-analysis of all relevant randomized controlled trials (RCTs), or evidence-based clinical practice guidelines based on systematic reviews of RCTs; level II = evidence obtained from at least one well-designed RCT; level III = evidence obtained from well-designed controlled trials without randomization; level IV = evidence from well-designed case–control and cohort studies; level V = evidence from systematic reviews of descriptive and qualitative studies; level VI = evidence from a single descriptive or qualitative study; level VII = evidence from the opinion of authorities and/or reports of expert committees.

a family views these pictures, the fetus becomes more "real" to them. With the help of today's technology, it is becoming easier to incorporate the fetus into family life.

Head and Neck

Eyes are in their final position, facing forward, and primitive reflexes such as blinking develop. Ears move to their final position and stand out from head. Eyebrows begin to form.

Abdominal and Pelvic Regions

Meconium begins to form and accumulate in the bowels. Meconium is the product of cell loss, digestive secretion, and swallowed amniotic fluid. Ovaries of female fetuses contain primitive egg cells—all of the eggs a woman will have for her entire life. The uterus of the female fetus is fully formed.

Limbs: Upper and Lower

Fingertips and toes develop the unique swirls and creases of fingerprints and toe prints.

Nervous System

The nerve pathways continue to mature and are undergoing myelinization.

Blood

Fetal circulation is completely functional. The umbilical cord system continues to grow and thicken as blood travels with considerable force through the body to nurture the fetus.

Skin

Brown fat (colored by capillary growth) coats the neck, chest, and crotch areas around the lymphatic system. The vernix (consisting of dead skin, lanugo cells, and oil from glands) now is clearly formed and visible covering the skin.

Placenta

The placenta is fully formed and grows in diameter, but not in thickness. The fetus' viability now is dependent on the production of progesterone via the placenta as the corpus luteum is no longer functional. Progesterone is responsible for continued enrichment of the uterine lining and rich vascular support of the pregnancy.

Weeks 20 to 24

In this period, the infant begins to approach the age of extrauterine viability. The cardiovascular system is functional, and by 24 weeks the respiratory system is sufficiently developed to support rudimentary gas exchange. The next sections focus on describing the characteristics of the normally developing fetus that will influence the functioning and care of the preterm infant.

Behavior

The next fetal sensory system to become functional is the chemosensory system (the senses of smell and taste). This sensory system is not well defined until 24 weeks gestation. However,

the fetus is practicing sucking, swallowing, and breathing, and there are indications from research that the smell and taste of amniotic fluid is similar to that of the mother's breast milk to help with orientation to suckling and breastfeeding. Exposure to flavors through amniotic fluid and later breast milk potentially lays down lifelong eating patterns and preferences (Forestal, 2017). If mothers can be encouraged to pursue healthy eating habits during pregnancy and they then they breastfeed, research findings suggest the infant/child will be influenced (Forestal, 2017). Bottle-fed babies do not have the same advantages. Maternal healthy eating may lead to less childhood obesity—an area in need of further research.

Head and Neck

At this point, extremely rapid brain growth begins, which lasts until 5 years after birth. Eyebrows and scalp hair become more visible, and the fetus blinks more often. Lanugo covers the body completely, although it is concentrated around the head, neck, and face. The bones of the ear—the hammer, anvil, and stirrup—harden at this point, making sound conduction possible. At this time, the fetus might be aware of maternal sounds such as breathing, heartbeat, digestion, and, possibly, voice. During this period, the fetus also begins to respond to sound originating outside the uterus, resulting in changes in physiologic perimeters. The fetus also is capable of reacting to light. Permanent teeth buds appear high in the gums. The nostrils begin to open.

Respiratory System

The maturation of the lungs has evolved to the canalicular stage. In this stage, the lung tissue is becoming highly vascularized, and the bronchioles are dividing into two or more respiratory bronchioles that will further divide into three to six alveolar ducts. By 24 weeks conceptional age, extrauterine respiration becomes possible because some of the primitive alveoli have developed in areas that are sufficiently vascularized to allow an exchange of gas. Surfactant production begins at approximately 20 weeks conceptional age, but in very small amounts. Surfactant production will not reach adequate levels until approximately 28 weeks conceptional age.

Abdominal and Pelvic Regions

Testes of male fetuses begin descending from the pelvis into the scrotum.

Limbs: Upper and Lower

Legs approach the final length and proportion relative to the body. Arms and legs move with more force as muscles strengthen. The skeleton hardens. Hand strength improves.

Blood vessels, bones, and organs are visible beneath a thin layer of wrinkled, translucent, pink skin. The fetus is thin, with little subcutaneous fat.

Weeks 24 to 28

Head and Neck

The forebrain enlarges to cover all other developed brain structures while maintaining its hemisphere divisions. Eyes are partially open and eyelashes are present. Sucking and swallowing improves. Brain-wave patterns resemble those of a full-term baby at birth.

Respiratory System

Lung development now enters the terminal sac period (24 weeks to birth). This stage is characterized by the proliferation of terminal sacs that are the site of gas exchange in the lungs. As the terminal sacs develop, the epithelium becomes thin and capillaries begin to bulge into the sac to form the intersection for gas exchange. At 24 weeks conceptional age, the sacs are lined primarily with type I alveolar cells, also known as squamous epithelial cells. By 28 weeks, the type II alveolar cells will largely replace type I cells. The type II cells secrete pulmonary surfactant. It should be noted that the rate of maturation of type II cells and the level of surfactant production varies widely among individuals. Full surfactant production usually is present by 38 to 40 weeks conceptional age.

Nervous System

The brain continues a period of rapid development. As the brain develops, it increases in complexity and in the degree of convolutions. If born, the infant is at the mercy of the environment and is unable to habituate or adapt responses to stimuli. The infant cannot shut out noises and is easily overstimulated; stressors are exacerbated by the infant's poor muscle tone and control of responses. Interventions during this time should be directed at protecting the infant from environmental stimulation and can include nesting, positioning with flexion, nonnutritive sucking, and kangaroo mother care; however, each intervention must be individually evaluated. Paternal holding is suggested; even when the benefits to the infant are limited, careful consideration of both risks and benefits is recommended.

Skin and Muscles

During this period of rapid weight gain, the fetus has 2% to 3% body fat. Production of red blood cells is taken over entirely by the bone marrow. Physiologic flexion is beginning to develop as the infant continues to grow into the limited space of the womb.

Abdominal and Pelvic Regions

Testes of male fetuses are completely descended.

Weeks 28 to 32

During this period of development, the auditory system matures, resulting from the maturation of hair cells and their connection through the appropriate ganglion to the auditory cortex. Before this period, the response to auditory stimulation is at the brain-stem level, affecting physiologic parameters. Subsequent recall or recognition

of auditory stimulation can be perceived, and an apparent memory pattern can be established at the cortical level at 32 weeks' gestation. Eyes open during alert times and close during sleep. The fetal brain creates endogenous visual stimuli to the visual cortex during rapid eye movement (REM) sleep; this visual development during REM sleep is essential for normal development of the cortex. The visual sensory system is the last of the primary sensory systems to mature. Also, during this period, the fetus begins to develop its own immune system. If born, the infant can be alert for short periods of time; however, periods of deep sleep, when most growth hormone is secreted, may be limited by environmental stimulation. The infant can suck on a pacifier and be put to the breast for sucking experiences; nutritive sucking abilities are very immature and not recommended. Interventions such as nesting, positioning with flexion, nonnutritive sucking, kangaroo mother care, and/or cycled lighting might be beneficial during this time.

Head and Neck

Rapid brain growth continues, and head size pushes the skull outward, creating more surface convolutions. This quick growth increases the number of interconnections between individual nerve cells. The iris is colored, and the pupil reflexes respond to light.

Limbs: Upper and Lower

Toenails are fully formed. Because of the lack of space in the uterus, the legs are drawn up in what is known as the fetal position.

Weeks 32 to 36

*Late preterm infants are those born 34 to 36 weeks

The placenta now is one-sixth of fetal weight. The surface area for placental exchange has continued to expand through the late gestational period, increasing its functional efficiency and continuing to provide adequate support for the growing fetus. This rate of growth decreases after 34 to 36 weeks; however, cellular hypertrophy continues until term. At term, the average placenta weighs between 500 and 600 g, is 15 to 20 cm in diameter, and is 2- to 3-cm thick. Although villous growth continues until term, degenerative changes such as intervillous thrombi, fibrin deposits, infarcts, and calcification begin to occur in the last few weeks of pregnancy. These degenerative changes may alter gas and nutrient transfer and can result in fetal hypoxia and fetal growth restriction.

Gastrointestinal System

The gastrointestinal system is very immature and will stay that way until 3 or 4 years after birth. The fetus stores approximately 15% of its weight in fat to keep the body warm. The fetus receives and eliminates nutrition through the umbilical cord. If born, the ability to coordinate nutritive sucking (sucking, swallowing, and breathing) matures between 34 to 36 weeks postconception; the breast or bottle can be offered after this point.

Respiratory System

The respiratory system continues to develop, increasing the number of terminal sacs, continuing to increase vascularization of the area, and increasing the percentage of type II alveolar cells and surfactant production.

Abdominal and Pelvic Regions

Increased fat stores improve the ability of the fetus to maintain temperature stability.

Limbs

Upper and lower space limitations continue to restrict fetal movement. Limbs are bent and drawn close to the body.

Weeks 36 to Term

The final weeks of gestational development are devoted to continue the overall fetal growth and maturation. The laying down of adipose tissue assists in eventual thermoregulation and insulation of the body. Beyond 36 weeks' gestation, the fetus, if born, is considered term even though a human pregnancy is noted to last 40 weeks. Lung development at 36 weeks and beyond will support life with minimal problems. From a developmental standpoint, a fetus that reaches this point and is born without major illness or congenital anomalies generally will survive and prosper. The infant's positive development in extrauterine life is dependent upon an appreciation of what has gone before.

Critical Periods of Development and External Influences

There are many known teratogens or factors that may influence fetal development. For the most part, the impact is related to the timing of the exposure, the duration and volume of the exposure, and the maternal–fetal genotype. This chapter has reviewed the critical periods of development; now these must be put into the context of a family history (of diabetes, for example), congenital anomalies, and the mother's preconceptual and prenatal health practices. Some examples to consider are maternal drug use (including alcohol, cigarette, opioids, street, and prescription drug use), exposure to toxins at work (chemical, stress, radiation), and changes in altitude. Maternal diet is important, as is the context of chronic illnesses or previous treatment for conditions such as cancer.

Another area of research is the use of kangaroo mother care or skin-to-skin immediately following birth. What is the KMC's relationship to self-regulation and is infant behavior during KMC reflective of "learned fetal behavior"? (Widstrom et al., 2020; Widstrom et al., 2019).

CONCLUSION

This chapter briefly reviews the critical periods of normal and (to some extent) abnormal embryonic and fetal development. An understanding of in-utero development is crucial if caregivers are to provide neonatal care that supports positive extrauterine growth and development. Developmental care incorporates the principles of development during both fetal and postnatal life.

Potential Research Questions

Prevention

- What is the relationship between maternal eating patterns during pregnancy and when breast-feeding to an infant's flavor or food preferences?
- Is the potential for increased neonatal infection only a threat to those exposed to maternal prenatal alcohol and smoking, or can this risk be related to maternal health and nutrition, too?
- What is the relationship between alcohol prenatal use and brain activity, including sleep patterns?
- What is the relationship to prenatal opioid use and long-term neurocognitive outcomes?

Intervention

- What is the relationship between postnatal nutrition and brain development in the extremely low-birth-weight infant?
- What is the relationship between the postnatal environment and developmental brain plasticity?
- What is the relationship between maternal supplements during pregnancy and fetal and neonatal growth patterns?
- What is the relationship between breast-feeding and long-term growth and development of the small or sick newborn?
- What is the impact of kangaroo mother care (KMC) on neonatal growth and development?

REFERENCES

Boggess, T., & Risher, W. C. (2020). Clinical and basic research investigations into the long-term effects of prenatal opioid exposure on brain development. *Journal of Neuroscience Research.* https://doi.org/10.1002/jnr.24642. PMID: 32459039.

Chiodo, L. M., Cosmian, C., Pereira, K., Kent, N., Sokol, R. J., & Hannigan, J. H. (2019). Prenatal alcohol screening during pregnancy by midwives and nurses. *Alcoholism, Clinical and Experimental Research, 43*(8), 1747–1758. https://doi.org/10.1111/acer.14114. PMID: 31184777; PMCID: PMC6772020.

Forestal, C. A. (2017). Flavor perception and preference development in human infants. *Annuals of Nutrition and Metabolism, 70*(Suppl. 3), 17–25. https://doi.org/10.1159/000478759. PMID: 28903110.

Kenner, C. (2020). Fetal development: Environmental influences and critical periods. In Kenner, C., Altimier, L.B., & Boykova, M. (Eds.), *Comprehensive neonatal nursing care* (6th ed., pp. 1–20). Elsevier.

Larson, J. J., Graham, D. L., Singer, L. T., Beckwith, A. M., Terplan, M., Davis, J. M., Martinez, J., & Bada, H. S. (2019). Cognitive and behavioral impact on children exposed to opioids during pregnancy. *Pediatrics, 144*(2), e20190514. https://doi.org/10.1542/peds.2019-0514

Moore, K. L., Persaud, T. V. N., & Torchia, M. G. (2019). *The developing human. Clinically oriented embryology* (11th ed.). Saunders.

Moreno-Fernandez, J., Ochoa, J. J., Latunde-Dada, G. O., & Diaz-Castro, J. (2019). Iron deficiency and iron homeostasis in low birth weight preterm infants: A systematic review. *Nutrients, 11*(5), 1090.

Ordean, A., Foret, M., Selby, P., & Grennell, E. (2020). Screening, brief intervention, and referral to treatment for prenatal alcohol use and cigarette smoking: A survey of academic and community health care providers. *Journal of Addiction Medicine, 14*(4), e76–e82.

Paul, S. E., Hatoum, A. S., Fine, J. D., Johnson, E. C., Hansen, I., Karcher, N. R., Moreau, A. L., Bondy, E., Qu, Y., Carter, E. B., Rogers, C. E., Agrawal, A., Barch, D., & Bogdan, R. (2020). Associations between prenatal cannabis exposure and childhood outcomes: Results from the ABCD study. *JAMA Psychiatry, 78*(1), 64–76. https://doi.org/10.1001/jamapsychiatry.2020.2902

Sharma, D., Farahbakhsh, N., Sharma, S., Sharma, P., & Sharma, A. (2017). Role of kangaroo mother care in growth and breastfeeding rates in very low birth weight (VLBW) neonates: A systematic review. *The Journal of Maternal-Fetal & Neonatal Medicine, 32*(1), 129–142. https://doi.org/10.1080/14767058.2017.1304535

Widstrom, A.-M., Brimdyr, K., Svensson, K., Cadwell, K., & Nissen, E. (2019). Skin-to-skin contact the first hour after birth, underlying implications and clinical practice. *Acta Paediatrics, 108*, 1192–1204.

Widstrom, A.-M., Brimdyr, K., Svensson, K., Cadwell, K., & Nissen, E. (2020). A plausible pathway of imprinted behaviors: Skin-to-skin actions of the newborn immediately after birth follow the order of fetal development and intrauterine training of movements. *Medical Hypothese, 134*, 109432. https://doi.org/10.1016/j.mehy.2019.109432

CHAPTER 10

Factors Influencing Development

Susan Tucker Blackburn

IFCDC Standards in Collaborative Practice

Standard 1: Systems Thinking

- The intensive care unit shall exhibit an infrastructure of leadership, mission, and a governance framework to guide the performance of the collaborative practice of IFCDC.

Standard 2: Pain and Stress, Families

- The interprofessional team shall document increased parental/caregiver well-being and decreased emotional distress during the intensive care hospital stay. Distress of baby's siblings and extended family should also be considered.

INTRODUCTION

Numerous factors influence growth and development during the prenatal, perinatal, and postnatal periods. These factors also affect neurobehavioral development and outcomes of the fetus and newborn. The normal growth and development of a fetus is influenced by a complex interaction of genes and environment. An infant's genetic endowment reflects traits that are inherited from their parents and previous generations, as well as new chromosomal alterations or gene mutations. The intrauterine environment in which a fetus develops is influenced by biological, physical, and social factors. Maternal, fetal, and placental risk factors and disorders can alter this environment and an infant's developmental trajectory. This chapter provides an overview of these factors and their potential influence on infants.

This chapter is organized around factors that characterize the prenatal, perinatal, and postnatal periods. Within each period, examples of developmental influences are described. Many of the factors from the prenatal period extend through the perinatal period. Individual maternal and fetal differences influence development during the prenatal, perinatal, and postnatal periods. Individuality is developed at an early stage of intrauterine existence and continues throughout the lifespan. From an individualized, family-centered, developmental care philosophy, these influences and differences can affect how a newborn and family respond to the extrauterine environment and to each other. The content in this chapter provides background that addresses the Developmental Care Specialist's practice.

PRENATAL FACTORS INFLUENCING DEVELOPMENT

The prenatal period is a critical period during which the many factors influence development and implementation of individualized, family-centered, developmental care. Factors present in all pregnancies include maternal age, race, height–weight ratio at conception, height, and parity. Other factors that may influence fetal development include a woman's health history, environmental and fetal factors (i.e., multiple births, fetal infections), medical and obstetric complications during pregnancy, maternal lifestyle (e.g., no or minimal prenatal care, cigarette smoking, substance abuse), drug exposures, genetic/family history, and history of previous pregnancies. For example, if a mother had a previous infant with fetal growth restriction (FGR, also referred to as intrauterine growth restriction or IUGR) or low birth weight (LBW; birth weight less than 2,500 g) or a preterm or stillborn delivery, the current infant may be at increased risk for these and other complications (American College of Obstetrics and Gynecologists (ACOG) and Society for Maternal Fetal Medicine, 2019).

Maternal Socioeconomic and Demographic Factors

Adolescent mothers (especially those younger than 16 years) or mothers of advanced maternal age (those older than 35 years) are at greater risk for fetal and neonatal complications. An adolescent mother might have an altered nutritional status related to her own growth and development or an eating disorder and is at greater risk for a growth-restricted fetus and preterm birth, whereas advanced maternal age has been associated with an increased risk of chromosomal abnormalities such as Down syndrome (Blackburn, 2018). The older a woman is at conception, the higher the risk of chromosomal abnormalities. In addition, older women are more likely to have chronic disorders such as preexisting diabetes or hypertension, which can affect pregnancy outcomes, and are at greater risk for pregnancy-related problems such as preeclampsia and gestational diabetes. Women who weigh less than 100 lb or more than 200 lb at conception also are at risk for altered fetal nutrition and pregnancy complications. Mothers who were LBW babies themselves are at increased risk to give birth to LBW infants. A primigravida has no previous history of pregnancy or delivery to indicate potential pregnancy-related problems. A multigravida who has had more than four previous deliveries has a uterus that has been stretched several times and organs that have been reshaped and may be approaching advanced maternal age. All of these factors can increase the risk of complications. In addition, a short interval between pregnancies and births does not allow a woman's body the time to rebuild essential nutrients, muscle tissue and tone, and hormonal balance to support another developing fetus (Blackburn, 2018).

Race and ethnicity are other risk factors that affect preterm and LBW birth rates. Racial and ethnic disparities are reported, with differences in maternal and infant outcomes varying with the ethnicity and race of the mother and infant including differences in maternal and infant outcomes (Centers for Disease Control (CDC) and Prevention, 2019a, 2019b). For example, non-Hispanic black infants have a higher mortality compared with other racial and ethnic groups (CDC, 2019a). Preterm birth rates are highest for black infants (14%), followed by American Indian/Alaska Natives (11.7%), Hispanic (9.8%), white (9.2%), and Asian/Pacific Islander (8.8%) infants (National Center for Health Statistics, 2021). The LBW rate also is highest for infants who are black (13.9%), followed by Asian/Pacific Islander (8.5%), American Indian/Alaskan Native (7.5%), Hispanic (7.5%), and white infants (7.0%) (National Center for Health Statistics, 2021). On average, black infants are two times as likely as white infants to be born low birth weight (National Center for Health Statistics, 2021). Simpson notes that "instead of race as a factor, racism and racial inequality in how healthcare is available, accessed and provided are more likely causative" (Simpson, 2021, p. 8). Understanding, respecting, and supporting cultural diversity and individual sociocultural and spiritual aspects is essential during the perinatal period (Callister, 2021).

Maternal Nutrition and Lifestyle

Maternal lifestyle is an important factor. Being a single mother and/or an adolescent, having lower socioeconomic status (SES), or a lower educational level are risk factors. A combination of low SES and low maternal educational level is linked with an increased incidence of FGR and LBW. These women might live in inadequate housing and lack access to adequate nutrition and consistent prenatal care. Inadequate prenatal care coupled with these or other risk factors can lead to adverse maternal and neonatal outcomes (Adams, 2021; Callister, 2021). The nutritional status of these women might be substandard, affecting fetal growth and development and placing them at risk for FGR, LBW, and adverse neonatal outcomes.

The nutrition of the mother is one of the major determinants of fetal growth and the weight and health of an infant at birth. A mother's poor diet places an infant at risk for fetal malnutrition, FGR, LBW, and preterm birth and may alter brain growth (Blackburn, 2018; Callister, 2021). Most LBW infants have small placentas because placental growth precedes fetal growth. Placental size has been linked with decreased maternal carbohydrate intake early in pregnancy and decreased fetal size at birth with decreased protein intake later in the pregnancy (Blackburn, 2018).

Certain nutrient supplements may promote better fetal outcomes. For example, periconceptional folic acid supplementation had been documented to reduce the risk for neural tube defects and other anomalies (American Academy of Pediatrics, 1999, reaffirmed 2012; Kancherla et al., 2021). Periconceptional folic acid supplementation also has been reported to increase fetal growth with higher placental and birth weights and reduce the risk of LBW and small-for-gestational-age (SGA) infants (American Academy of Pediatrics Committee, 1999, reaffirmed 2012; Kancherla et al., 2021). Vitamin D deficiency during pregnancy has been associated with a risk of preeclampsia (Palacios et al., 2019).

Fetal growth is a complex process influenced by genetic, environmental, placental, maternal, and fetal factors. Fetal growth occurs in two main phases. Deprivation of essential nutrients in either phase can lead to altered fetal growth and development. For example, during the first trimester growth phase (hyperplasia) when cells rapidly divide and multiply, folic acid and vitamin B12, which play a role in the synthesis of nucleic acids, are required. The second fetal growth phase, hypertrophy, occurs during the second and third trimesters of pregnancy when cells increase in size and require amino acids and vitamin B12 for protein synthesis (Blackburn, 2018). Alterations in placental function can lead to failure of the fetus to reach their intrauterine growth potential and development of FGR (Nardozza et al., 2017). FGR is seen in approximately 5% to 10% of all pregnancies (Nardozza et al., 2017). Prenatal influences on growth and development can have lifelong implications including later development of metabolic diseases such as type 2 diabetes, hypertension, and obesity (Monteiro et al., 2016). Maternal nutrition during pregnancy is thought to have a role in "programming" of fetal tissues so that altered nutrition has long-term consequences for later neurobehavioral development and health (Blackburn, 2018; Cao-Leia et al., 2020; Monteiro et al., 2016; Van den Bergh et al., 2020).

Maternal Disorders

Maternal disease can adversely influence fetal development. Maternal complications may arise due to preexisting maternal conditions such as diabetes, hypertension, or thyroid disorders. Other complications such as preeclampsia may arise as a consequence of pregnancy. In addition, more women with chronic genetic conditions and congenital defects are giving birth. These conditions include sickle cell anemia, cystic fibrosis, phenylketonuria, and congenital heart disease (CHD). Until recently, women with these conditions either did not live until childbearing age or were counseled to not conceive or were often unable to carry a pregnancy to term.

Diabetes

Diabetes (type 1, type 2, gestational) in pregnancy has long been recognized as a serious maternal, fetal, and neonatal problem. Alterations in metabolic processes in a woman with diabetes increase the risk of fetal and neonatal problems and may alter metabolic programming increasing the risk of long-term disorders. The effects of diabetes on the fetus are related to the degree of glucose control before and during conception and the presence of maternal cardiovascular complications. The development of fetal and neonatal problems also is linked to the severity of the mother's diabetes and how well her disorder is controlled before and during pregnancy (Blackburn, 2018; Moore et al., 2018; Pearson et al., 2007; Roth, 2021). Women with severe diabetes with vascular compromise may experience placental insufficiency that can lead to varying degrees of nutritional or hypoxic damage to the fetus resulting in FGR and oligohydramnios.

Congenital defects are more likely to occur and are seen in 5% to 6% of women with pregestational diabetes and 10% to 12% of women on insulin therapy (Kallema et al., 2020; Moore et al., 2018). Congenital anomalies are related to diabetic control in the 3-month period before conception and the first 2 months of pregnancy, a time at which mothers might not be preparing for pregnancy or know they are pregnant. Women with excellent glycemic control during this time have a significantly lower risk of having an infant with an anomaly (Kallema et al., 2020; Moore et al., 2018; Pearson et al., 2007). Common fetal anomalies seen in infants of diabetic mothers include neural tube defects, cardiac defects, gastrointestinal malformations, and renal anomalies. Two-thirds of these defects involve the cardiovascular and central nervous system (Kallema et al., 2020; Moore et al., 2018). The risk of congenital anomalies is not increased in women who develop gestational diabetes after the first trimester (Kallema et al., 2020).

Macrosomia (greater than the 90th percentile of weight for gestational age or a birthweight of greater than 4,000 g) also is a common problem that occurs in response to elevated maternal glucose, with subsequent increased transfer of glucose and other fuels across the placenta. As a result, fetal insulin production is elevated with increased growth and fat deposition in the infant. These infants are at increased risk for birth trauma, particularly shoulder dystocia (increased 2- to 4-fold), brachial plexus injuries, facial nerve injuries, clavicle or humeral fractions, and asphyxia. Infants of diabetic mothers with altered renal function or hypertension may have poor growth and be SGA (Kallema et al., 2020; Roth, 2021). Neonatal hypoglycemia is common and related to a sudden decrease in glucose in the blood stream after birth at a time when the infant's insulin production still is elevated (Kallema et al., 2020). Infants of mothers with diabetes also are at risk for hypocalcemia, hypomagnesemia, polycythemia, hyperbilirubinemia, and respiratory distress due to delayed lung maturity and alterations in production of pulmonary surfactant. Much has been learned about the effects of diabetes on pregnancy, and, with good control before conception, and during pregnancy, negative outcomes can be reduced (Moore et al., 2018; Roth, 2021). Preconception education and prenatal care are essential in this population. Infants of women with diabetes are at increased risk for obesity in childhood and adolescence and for later development of diabetes (Monteiro, 2016; Moore et al., 2018; Tam et al., 2017). Infants of diabetic mothers are at increased risk for later development of type 1 and type 2 diabetes (Blackburn, 2018; Moore et al., 2018).

Cardiovascular Problems

The incidence of cardiac disease in the pregnant population is between 1% and 4% and is a leading cause of maternal morbidity and mortality (ACOG, 2019; Ghandi & Martin, 2015; Ramlakhan et al., 2020). CHD plays a more prominent role today than in years past because with better early management of CHD, children now are growing to adulthood and becoming parents (Ramlakhan et al., 2020). If either parent has a congenital heart defect, the fetus has an increased risk for having a congenital cardiac defect. If the mother is the affected parent, she adds an environmental risk in the form of altered hemodynamics during pregnancy. When maternal systemic circulation is compromised, uterine blood flow can be severely diminished, leading to decreased fetal oxygenation, altered fetal growth and development, and an increased risk that the infant will be LBW or delivered prematurely. Decreases in fetal oxygenation increase the risk of hypoxia; fetal distress; and cardiorespiratory, neurologic, and other problems (Blackburn, 2018). More emphasis is being placed on prenatal screening for cardiac disease and CHD that might otherwise go undetected and on early detection of fetal cardiac problems. Preconception counseling evaluates potential risks, treatment options, and preventative strategies to reduce risk and promote optimal pregnancy outcomes for mother and fetus (ACOG, 2019).

Maternal anemia also has fetal and neonatal implications related to decreased oxygen-carrying capacity and inadequate nutrient availability, leading to decreased growth and increased mortality due to lack of an adequate oxygen supply. Maternal anemia in the first trimester is related to increased risk of preterm birth (Blackburn, 2018; Georgieff, 2020; Rahmati et al., 2020). The most common cause of maternal anemia is iron deficiency anemia. Fetal and neonatal risks in pregnant women with iron deficiency anemia include growth restriction, preterm birth, infection, and altered metabolic programming (ACOG, 2019; Breymann, 2015). Low maternal iron intake during the third trimester may alter fetal brain development and influence neurodevelopmental sequelae (Blackburn, 2018; Georgieff, 2020).

Hypertensive States in Pregnancy

Hypertension is one of the more common complications of pregnancy and a leading cause of maternal and neonatal mortality and morbidity (Battarbee et al., 2020; Umesawa & Kobashi, 2017). Maternal hypertension may be chronic, develop during pregnancy (gestational hypertension or pre-eclampsia), or both. Preeclampsia occurs in 5% to 8% of all pregnancies (Burgess, 2021; Umesawa & Kobashi, 2017). Preeclampsia is a multisystem disorder characterized by placental dysfunction triggered by not yet completely understood immunologic, genetic, and environmental factors that lead to maternal systemic endothelial cell dysfunction with increased systemic vascular resistance, enhanced platelet aggregation, and activation of the coagulation system. Genetic and immunologic components also may influence preeclampsia (ACOG, 2013; Blackburn, 2018; Umesawa & Kobashi, 2017). Risk factors for preeclampsia include multiple gestations, chronic hypertension, diabetes mellitus, or renal disorders. Higher rates of gestational and chronic hypertension are reported in non-Hispanic black women and in women over 30 years of age across all ethnic groups (Batterbee et al., 2020). Preeclampsia can alter placental blood flow and increase the risk of placental abruption and other problems for the fetus and neonate. Owing to alterations in maternal renal, pulmonary, and hepatic systems with this disorder, fetal complications include LBW, FGR, and hypoxia; altered cardiovascular and neurodevelopmental outcomes are also reported (ACOG, 2013). Fetal and neonatal effects may be increased if hemolysis, elevated liver enzymes, and low platelets syndrome (HELLP) occurs. These women are at high risk for acute renal failure (ACOG, 2013). Guidelines are available regarding the classification, diagnosis, and management of hypertension during pregnancy (ACOG, 2013).

Renal Disease

Maternal renal disease can be attributed to a maternal anomaly such as polycystic kidney or other genetic disorders or may be secondary to another condition such as diabetes, HELLP syndrome, preeclampsia, systemic lupus erythematosus, or perinatal infections (Thadhani & Young, 2018). Fetal fluid and electrolyte balance depends on maternal renal and fluid and electrolyte homeostasis; infants of mothers with renal problems are at increased risk for FGR and prematurity (Blackburn, 2018; Thadhani & Young, 2018).

Thyroid Disorders

Maternal thyroid disorders also are associated with fetal and neonatal problems (ACOG, 2020; Lee et al., 2020). Maternal T4 is essential during the first trimester for early development of the brain and other systems since the fetal thyroid gland is not functional during this time (Blackburn, 2018). Women with hyperthyroidism are at higher risk for placental abruption, preterm labor, and FGR, and their infants may develop transient hyperthyroidism (from transplacental-passage maternal antibodies) or hypothyroidism due to maternal antithyroid drugs (ACOG, 2020; Blackburn, 2018; Lee et al., 2020). Hypothyroidism increases the risk of prematurity, LBW, placenta abruption, and impaired neurological outcome in infants (ACOG, 2020; Lee et al., 2020).

Exposure to Drugs and Other Potential Teratogens

Teratogens are substances, organisms, physical agents, or deficiency states to which a fetus is exposed during gestation that have the potential to alter normal structural or functional development (biochemical and behavioral) (Blackburn, 2018). The dose of the agent, timing of exposure, agent synergism, rate of metabolism, host susceptibility of both mother and fetus, and maternal chronic disorders play a role in fetal outcome. The degree to which exposure adversely affects fetal development in part depends on the interplay between the genotypes of the mother and fetus, along with environmental effects. Drugs, both prescription and over the counter, can have a variety of effects on a fetus. Polydrug use (which may involve use of prescription drugs, street drugs, or herbal agents in various combinations) further complicates the problem. Issues related to drug use are not just limited to the mother but can have an adverse effect on future offspring. In addition, environmental exposures or drugs taken by a male might damage spermatozoa, leading to abnormal spermatozoa and risk of congenital malformations. Many agents in addition to drugs have teratogenic potential. For example, the fetus is susceptible to adverse effects from maternal infections, nutritional deficiencies, maternal chronic disorders, ionizing radiation, and environmental agents.

Principles of teratogenesis, originally outlined by Wilson (1977), include:

- Susceptibility to a teratogenic agent is dependent on the genotype of the embryo and the manner in which the agent interacts with environmental factors.
- Susceptibility to teratogenic agents is dependent on the timing of the exposure and the developmental stage of the embryo.
- Teratogenic agents act in specific ways on cells or tissues to cause pathogenesis.
- The final manifestations of abnormal development are death, malformation, growth alterations, and functional disorders.
- Access to the embryo by environmental teratogens depends on the nature of the agent.
- As the dosage increases, manifestations of deviant development increase (Blackburn, 2018; Chambers & Freidman, 2018).

The mechanisms leading to teratogenic alterations are: (1) gene mutation; (2) chromosome breaks and nondisjunction;

(3) mitotic interference and cell death; (4) altered nucleic acid integrity or function; (5) lack of or excess of precursors, substrates, or coenzymes needed for biosynthesis; (6) altered energy sources; (7) enzyme and growth factor inhibitions; (8) osmolar imbalance; (9) altered membrane characteristics; and (10) altered cell and neuronal migration or central nervous system (CNS) organization (Blackburn, 2018).

The effects of any pharmacologic or other teratogenic agents will depend on the critical period of development or stage of fetal development at the time of the exposure. The rapidly developing neurologic system is always a concern, even in the last trimester of gestation, because this system is still undergoing critical changes well into the postbirth period.

Several examples of the effects of prescribed drugs on the fetus and neonate are described in this section. Anticoagulants such as warfarin (Coumadin) can lead to growth and developmental restriction, deafness, and scoliosis when exposure is in the first trimester. When exposure takes place in the second and third trimesters, effects include eye anomalies, hydrocephaly, and other CNS defects and/or neonatal hemorrhage. Risks of FGR and preterm birth also are increased in these infants (Blackburn, 2018; Kiernan & Jones, 2019). Potential adverse fetal effects, including congenital anomalies, growth restriction, seizure-related hypoxia, and altered cognitive abilities, have been described for infants of mothers with epilepsy treated with antiepileptic drugs such as phenytoin (Dilantin), valproate, carbamazepine, and topiramate (Harden & Lu, 2019; Ornoy et al., 2017). The risk of congenital anomalies is higher in infants exposed to antiepileptic drug polytherapy than monotherapy.

Some antianxiety agents or mood stabilizers have been associated with an increased risk of congenital malformations when taken in the first trimester (Sutter-Dallay et al., 2015). Use of selective serotonin uptake inhibitors (SSRIs) during pregnancy, particularly in the first trimester, has been associated with an increased risk of congenital defects in some studies, although data are inconsistent (Bałkowiec-Iskra et al., 2017; Reefhuis et al., 2015). Other findings include a possible increased risk of persistent pulmonary hypertension with use in late pregnancy and a transient neonatal withdrawal pattern during the first few weeks after birth (Bailey & Diaz-Barbosa, 2018; Bałkowiec-Iskra et al., 2017; Reefhus et al., 2015). In addition, use of SSRIs and antidepressants throughout pregnancy has been associated with an increased risk of preterm birth (Sutter-Dallay et al., 2015). Exposure to first- and second-generation antipsychotic agents is associated with LBW, preterm birth, altered perinatal adaptation, jaundice, and extrapyramidal symptoms (Sutter-Dallay et al., 2015). Exposure of the fetus to psychotropic drugs usually produces mild responses, but it can be more serious including altered neonatal adaptation, neonatal withdrawal symptoms, and residual pharmacological effects after birth (Convertino et al., 2016).

The use of herbal preparations by pregnant women also is growing. Little research outside of animal studies has been completed for many herbal agents to determine the effects on the developing fetus and the neonate. Women often have questions about the safety of such products. There are often no definitive answers, but the use of herbs, both ingested and topical, must be discussed in the maternal history review. Ginger has been reported to be an effective therapy for nausea and vomiting during pregnancy (Kennedy et al., 2016). Kennedy et al. (2016) review herbs used to prevent and treat pregnancy-related issues.

Maternal Substance Abuse

Maternal substance abuse and the number of abused drugs has increased in the past decade, including use of prescribed drugs, with a concomitant increase in numbers of infants with neonatal abstinence syndrome (NAS) or neonatal opioid withdrawal syndrome (Cook et al., 2017; Jansson & Patrick, 2019). Abused drugs include marijuana, heroin, cocaine, methylenedioxymethamphetamine (MDMA, or "ecstasy"), and alcohol, as well as prescribed opiates and other pain relievers, such as fentanyl, methadone, and buprenorphine (Cook et al., 2017; Jansson & Patrick, 2019; Smid et al., 2019) Abuse of these agents can lead to prematurity, FGR, developmental delays, tremulousness, exaggerated startle reflex, and alterations in visual processing. The quality of alertness in infants can be affected, and frontal lobe dysfunction also can become apparent later in development. Developmental outcomes continue to be a major focus, with studies examining the effects of drugs, maternal lifestyle, and interaction patterns with infants and children (Jansson & Patrick, 2019; Smid et al., 2019).

A maternal history must include all substances to anticipate potential developmental problems. Polydrug use has become common. This may or may not include legal as well as illegal substances. It may be difficult to distinguish between specific drug exposures, polydrug use, and maternal comorbidities (Bailey & Diaz-Barbosa, 2018; Cook et al., 2017; Smid et al., 2019). In addition to affecting the medical well-being of mother and fetus, substance abuse may also influence whether or when a mother will seek prenatal care, comply with suggested prenatal care, obtain proper nutrition, acquire sexually transmitted infections, or reside in adequate housing. Obstetric complications associated with substance abuse that affect maternal and fetal well-being include maternal hypertension, urinary tract infections, preeclampsia, premature rupture of membranes, preterm labor and delivery, LBW, and FGR and its associated complications (Prasad & Jones, 2018). Effects of maternal substance abuse on neonates of women who engage in substance abuse may include altered bonding; exaggerated startle response; generalized growth restriction; increased risk for FGR, LBW, and other neonatal complications; neurobehavioral abnormalities; altered sleep patterns; irritability; jitteriness; tremors; depressed sucking; and smaller head circumference (Bailey & Diaz-Barbosa, 2018; Cook et al., 2017; Smid et al., 2019). Studies of maternal substances extend beyond the effects on fetal development to specific neurodevelopment outcomes that include the postnatal environment as a variable.

The fetal effects of cocaine may include small head circumference and adverse neurologic outcomes (hypertonia, tremors, and extensor leg posturing). Cocaine use may increase the risk of placental abruption and preterm birth. Other consequences include LBW, SGA, FGR, developmental delays, and altered neurobehavioral development (Cook et al., 2017; Jansson & Patrick, 2019; Smid et al., 2019; Sutter-Dallay et al., 2015).

Opioid abuse during pregnancy is associated with increased risk of microcephaly, NAS, LBW, sudden infant death syndrome, prematurity, and long-term neurobehavioral and neurocognitive issues (Bailey & Diaz-Barbosa, 2018; Cook et al., 2017; Jansson & Patrick, 2019). Another aspect of substance abuse is the risk for human immunodeficiency virus (HIV). Perinatal transmission to the fetus has decreased as a result of medication protocols given to mothers to reduce fetal transmission. However, HIV infection secondary to substance abuse remains a global problem (Wedi et al., 2016).

Cannabis use has increased in the United States with state deregulation. Regular high-dose use during pregnancy may lead to LBW and a risk of long-term neurocognitive effects. Cannabis use does not cause significant withdrawal but may lead to subtle newborn alterations (Bailey & Diaz-Barbosa, 2018; Cook et al., 2017). Amphetamines and methamphetamines can result in FGR, prematurity, LBW, and neonatal withdrawal, which usually does not require pharmacologic therapy (Cook et al., 2017; Smid et al., 2019; Smith & Santos, 2016).

Nicotine

Although cigarette smoking has decreased in the United States, nicotine is the most abused substance during pregnancy (Bailey & Diaz-Barbosa, 2018). Many women still smoke during pregnancy, and women may not fully comprehend the dangers of smoking nor of exposure to second-hand or third-hand smoke on a developing infant (Bailey & Diaz-Barbosa, 2018). Nicotine and cotinine readily cross the placenta; levels in fetal blood may be higher than in maternal blood (Gould et al., 2020). Nicotine and cotinine may lead to vasoconstriction of the placental vessels (leading to less oxygen for mother and fetus) and possible hypoxic episodes, as well as disruptions in cell replication (Bailey & Diaz-Barbosa, 2018; Gould et al., 2020). Fetal tachycardia decreased oxygen saturations, and polycythemia can occur. Maternal smoking during pregnancy increases the risk of obstetrical complications, spontaneous abortion, ectopic pregnancy, placental abruption and previa, preterm labor, SGA, and later respiratory problems in offspring (Gould et al., 2020). The maternal and fetal genotypes influence the degree of fetal and neonatal effects (Blackburn, 2018).

There is a dose-related impact of smoking on risk of LBW and preterm birth. Owing to the effect of reduction in uteroplacental blood flow, there is an increased risk for a fetus to be exposed to lower oxygen and available nutrients. As a result, the infant is at increased risk for LBW, FGR, prematurity, and neurobehavioral abnormalities (Bailey & Diaz-Barbosa, 2018; Blackburn, 2018). Smoking cessation programs during pregnancy reduce the number of women who continue to smoke, improve fetal growth, and reduce the risk of LBW and preterm birth (Gould et al., 2020).

Alcohol

Ethanol is another drug that is commonly abused during pregnancy. Alcohol teratogenicity can occur any time during pregnancy with effects varying depending on tissues and structures undergoing critical development at the time of exposure (Cook et al., 2017). No level of drinking has been proven safe because alcohol consumption at any stage of pregnancy can affect the brain and other areas of development (Blackburn, 2018).

Infants exposed to alcohol in utero are at increased risk for a range of alcohol-related damage. Fetal alcohol spectrum disorder (FASD) is characterized by the triad of prenatal or postnatal growth restriction, CNS involvement, and specific craniofacial features. Other features may include increased irritability, microcephaly, mild to moderate mental retardation, poor sucking, FGR, short palpebral fissures, strabismus, ptosis, and myopia. Other forms of fetal-alcohol-related damage (e.g., fetal alcohol effects) might be part of the continuum of FASD. Affected children may have physical defects (such as congenital heart defects) without the characteristic facial features of FASD or may have mental and behavioral abnormalities without congenital defects or FASD facial features. These deficits often are not detected until preschool or school age (Blackburn, 2018; Cook et al., 2017).

Maternal/Fetal Infections

Maternal infections are known potential teratogens that can adversely affect fetal development. In addition, researchers are examining the link between perinatal infections and cerebral palsy (Korzeniewski et al., 2019). Intrauterine infections and inflammation are frequently associated with asphyxia, and the combination of these events can lead to brain injury, especially in immature infants. Chorioamnionitis is one of the most common maternal infections and often is related to premature or prolonged rupture of membranes with subsequent premature labor and delivery. These mothers and infants should be monitored closely. Organism-specific antibiotic therapy is recommended for the maternal–fetal dyad and the newborn.

Cytomegalovirus infection is most likely to occur with maternal primary infection. Ninety percent of infected infants are free of symptoms at birth, but 5% to 15% of these infants might have long-term sequelae. Fewer than 5% of these infants will have severe involvement at birth, including FGR, microcephaly, periventricular calcifications, encephalopathy, deafness, blindness, chorioretinitis, cerebellar hypoplasia, brain developmental disorders, and hepatosplenomegaly (Kwak et al., 2018). Another maternal infection of concern to the fetus is herpes simplex virus (HSV). The mortality rate may be high, especially if the neonate is exposed to an active primary HSV infection. Many of these children exhibit neurologic or ophthalmic sequelae. Disseminated infection occurs in 70% of cases with jaundice, respiratory distress syndrome, and CNS involvement. Since herpes can be transmitted even when the mother's herpes appears inactive, careful assessment is needed (James & Kimberlin, 2015). Maternal rubella also can pose danger for a fetus. The most severe sequelae occur with first-trimester infections and may include deafness, eye defects including cataracts and glaucoma, CNS anomalies, CHD, microcephaly, and psychomotor retardation (Blackburn, 2018). Toxoplasmosis also can have fetal effects. Severity varies with gestation (earlier infection results in more severe effects). Fetal effects can include IUGR, hydrocephalus, microcephaly, chorioretinitis (with risk of subsequent vision loss if untreated), seizures, and psychomotor retardation. These neurologic, ophthalmologic, and other sequelae are variable and most prominent in untreated infants (Rudd, 2021). Human immunodeficiency is also of concern for the fetus. The chance of perinatal transmission continues to drop with new medication combinations. Maternal treatment with antiretroviral drugs markedly reduces the risk of HIV transmission to the fetus from the mother and the risk of fetal infection (Rudd, 2021; Wedi et al., 2016). New tests allow for the detection of the virus early in an infant's life, but prevention through treatment during pregnancy shows the most promise. Untreated women are at increased risk for preterm birth (Wedi et al., 2016). Gonorrhea and syphilis infections also have fetal effects including sepsis or meningitis, stillbirth, IUGR, nonimmune hydrops, or premature labor. Varicella zoster affects 30% to 49% of fetuses born to mothers with active disease. Congenital varicella syndrome includes IUGR, cataracts, microphthalmos, chorioretinitis, and microcephaly (Blackburn, 2018; Rudd, 2021).

Infection with SARS-CoV-2 (Covid-19) is a recent issue, and effects on the pregnant woman, fetus, and newborn are still being investigated. The risk of severe disease during pregnancy appears to be higher than in the general population (Wastnedge et al., 2021). An increased incidence of preterm birth, LBW, and neonatal intensive care unit (NICU) admission has been reported (Allotey et al., 2020; Dubey et al., 2020; Shalish et al., 2020; Smith et al., 2020). In general, neonatal infection is not common and generally is acquired postnatally with favorable respiratory outcomes.

Maternal Trauma

A growing trend in our society is violence against pregnant women. Trauma is the most common nonobstetric cause of maternal mortality (Mauricio La Rosa et al., 2020). The prevalence of violence during pregnancy is up to 8%, with 3

to 4 per 1,000 requiring hospitalization (Mauricio La Rosa et al., 2020). Traumatic injury occurs in every trimester; the frequency increases as pregnancy progresses (Kilpatrick, 2017; Mauricio La Rosa et al., 2020). The postpartum period also may be a period of increased risk. The most frequent cause of trauma in the pregnant woman is domestic violence, followed by motor vehicle accidents, falls, and penetrating trauma. When trauma occurs, the effects to both the mother and the fetus must be considered. The fetus is vulnerable to the effects of maternal trauma, especially blunt or penetrating trauma to the abdomen. Effects on the fetus include preterm rupture of membranes, premature labor and delivery, fetal demise, placental abruption with fetomaternal bleed, fetal skull injuries (especially when the head is engaged and there is a maternal pelvic fracture), uterine rupture, hypoxic compromise secondary to maternal respiratory embarrassment, shock, disseminated intravascular coagulopathy, and maternal cardiac arrest (Mauricio La Rosa et al., 2020; Kilpatrick, 2017; Sakamoto et al., 2019).

Perinatal Stress and Fetal Programming

Exposure of the fetus to stress during the perinatal period can increase the risk of preterm birth and alter physiologic programming (Cao-Leia et al., 2020; Van den Bergh et al., 2020). "Programming refers to changes in physiologic systems in the fetus suggesting that behavioral and health outcomes in offspring may result from long lasting alterations in the structure and function of fetal organs" (Cao-Leia et al., 2020, p. 198). In utero stress exposure may lead to long-term adverse effects on offspring. One way this may occur is through epigenetic mechanisms such as changes in DNA methylation and other factors (Cao-Leia et al., 2020; Van den Bergh et al., 2020). Stress in the intrauterine environment may include depression, anxiety, psychosocial distress, and altered metabolic processes. Perinatal stress can increase maternal cortisol levels and alter programming of the fetal hypothalamic-pituitary-adrenal (HPA) axis (Cao-Leia et al., 2020; Van den Bergh et al., 2020). Thus, the fetal environment can have long-term influences on the individual mediated by changes in the programming and development of systems such as the CNS, autonomic system, HPA axis, cardiovascular system, and immune system. This may alter prenatal and postnatal growth and increase susceptibility to later development of adult-onset cardiovascular, metabolic, neurodevelopmental, and psychologic disorders in offspring (Blackburn, 2018; Cao-Leia et al., 2020; Ramlakhan et al., 2020; Van den Bergh et al., 2020).

Fetal Complications

Other complications that occur during pregnancy are related to the fetus and intrinsic factors. One example of such complications is hydrops fetalis. Hydrops fetalis is generalized subcutaneous edema in a fetus or neonate, usually accompanied by ascites and pleural and/or pericardial effusions. In immune hydrops, maternal antibodies cross the placenta and destroy fetal erythrocytes, similar to what occurs with ABO and Rh incompatibility between fetal and maternal blood types. Nonimmune hydrops occurs for several reasons: cardiovascular (the most frequent cause); hematologic, such as alpha-thalassemia; glucose-6-phosphate dehydrogenase deficiency; chronic fetal–maternal or twin-to-twin transfusion; renal; infectious disease such as parvovirus b19, syphilis, rubella, cytomegalovirus; pulmonary; gastrointestinal such as in utero volvulus and meconium peritonitis; and chromosomal, such as achondroplasia, Turner syndrome, trisomies (13, 18, and 21), triploidy, and aneuploidy (Blackburn, 2018).

Genes and Genetic History

Research continues on the role of genes in mediating prenatal exposures, including exposures to maternal diseases, medications, and environmental agents. With growing knowledge of the human genome, and newer technologies such as exome and genetic sequencing, many genes and gene sequences that are involved in genetic disorders and congenital anomalies have been identified. In addition, genetic variations may help in the understanding of gene–environment interactions in the etiology and risk of complex disorders such as preterm birth and susceptibility to teratogens (Blackburn, 2018; Jorde et al., 2019).

Genetic polymorphisms (variations in genome sequence) may alter the expression of a protein, which may increase the risk of disease; this risk may be modified by exposure to specific drugs or environmental agents. Polymorphic genes and environmental influences may increase susceptibility to preterm labor and may increase susceptibility to preeclampsia and birth defects (Gregg & Kuller, 2018; Jorde et al., 2019). Genetic differences in folate metabolism may increase the risk for neural tube defects and miscarriage; other genetic variations may increase the risk of preterm birth or oral facial clefts with exposure to cigarette smoke or alter alcohol metabolism, increasing the risk of fetal alcohol spectrum disorders (Blackburn, 2018). These risks may be modified by exposure to specific pharmacologic or environmental agents.

Genetic disorders can be passed from one generation to the next via characteristic patterns of inheritance. With autosomal-dominant disorders, males and females are affected equally, and either parent can pass the gene to sons or daughters. An affected infant has an affected parent unless there is a new mutation, and if an individual has the affected gene, they will have the disorder unless there is altered penetrance. Unaffected offspring of an affected parent will have normal offspring if their mate is an unaffected person. If one parent is affected, and assuming that parent has only one of the affected genes, there is a 50% risk with each pregnancy that their child also will be affected; if both parents carry one of the altered genes, the risk of having an affected child is 75% with each pregnancy. Family history often indicates a vertical route of transmission through successive generations on one side of the family. Examples of autosomal dominant disorders include myotonic dystrophy, Huntington disease, neurofibromatosis, and coronary artery disease.

Autosomal recessive disorders also affect males and females equally. Parents of affected offspring rarely are affected and usually are heterozygous carriers, meaning they each carry one of the affected genes. To develop an autosomal recessive disorder, a person must carry two of the affected genes. With carrier parents, there is a 25% chance with each pregnancy of having an affected offspring, and a 50% chance the offspring will be a carrier. Examples of autosomal recessive disorders include cystic fibrosis, sickle cell anemia, Tay–Sachs disease, beta thalassemia, congenital adrenal hyperplasia, and many other inherited metabolic disorders.

Another pattern of inheritance is X-linked recessive, in which usually only male offspring are affected with a disorder. Carrier women transmit the disorder from mother to son. All sons of affected men are normal. All daughters of affected men are carriers. A daughter may develop an X-linked recessive disorder if she has an affected father and carrier mother. Examples of X-linked recessive disorders include Duchene muscular dystrophy, hemophilia, color blindness, and glucose-6-phosphate dehydrogenase deficiency.

Multifactorial inheritance is attributable to the interaction of genetic and environmental factors. A person has a genetic predisposition to develop a specific disorder, but that disorder will not be expressed without interaction with certain environmental factors. Multifactorial disorders include birth defects (e.g., congenital heart defects, cleft lip and palate, neural tube defects, congenital dislocated hips) and many adult-onset disorders (some forms of cancer, coronary artery disease, bipolar affective disorders, and diabetes mellitus). Birth defects also arise from purely environmental causes (e.g., teratogens), although in some cases, as noted above, there may be a genetic predisposition that increases the likelihood a teratogen will cause damage. Nontraditional patterns of inheritance (that do not follow traditional Mendelian patterns) are less common. An example of this pattern is genomic imprinting, which is seen in Prader–Willi syndrome (PWS) and Angelman syndrome (AS). In this complex pattern of inheritance, genes on part of the long arm of chromosome 13 are deleted. If this deletion is on the chromosome 13 that the infant received from the mother, the child has AS; if the deletion is on the paternal chromosome, the child has PWS.

Prenatal Detection of Congenital Anomalies

Technology to screen and assess fetal development has become highly sophisticated, and the ability to detect many anomalies before birth is becoming precise using techniques such as prenatal ultrasonography, fetal magnetic resonance imaging, and Doppler flow studies. With three-dimensional ultrasound imaging, the picture quality is well defined, allowing clinicians to view, anticipate, and prepare for an infant with detectable anomalies (Wojcik et al., 2020).

Diagnostic procedures include chorionic villous sampling, amniocentesis, and percutaneous umbilical blood sampling. Other techniques include maternal screening for genetic disorders during the first and, less frequently in recent years, second trimesters, family history, preimplantation testing of embryos with assisted reproductive technologies, and cell-free DNA (cfDNA) testing (Sabbagh & Van den Veyver, 2020; Wojcik et al., 2020). cfDNA testing is a more recent technique involving analysis of fetal cell-free DNA in maternal serum. cfDNA is primarily produced in the placenta and can be found in maternal serum from about 4 weeks' gestation (Zhang et al., 2019). Fetal genome sequencing studies are currently in progress (Sabbagh & Van den Veyver, 2020).

Techniques for diagnosis of fetal anomalies have been accompanied by development of fetal surgery techniques for disorders such as congenital diaphragmatic hernia, open spina bifida, twin–twin transfusion syndrome, thoracic malformations, airway obstruction, lower urinary tract obstruction, sacrococcygeal teratoma, and aortic valve stenosis (Vaughn et al., 2020). Strategies to assess fetal status and placental function in the third trimester include fetal movement analysis, antenatal fetal heart rate surveillance, nonstress and contraction stress testing, biochemical monitoring, umbilical artery Doppler velocimetry, fetal blood gas monitoring, and the biophysical profile (Blackburn, 2018). Biomarker algorithms have been evaluated to predict later development of preeclampsia in the mother (Wojcik et al., 2020; Zhang et al., 2019).

PERINATAL FACTORS INFLUENCING DEVELOPMENT

Perinatal factors that influence development include maternal, placental, and fetal issues. Maternal and fetal perinatal history during this time is also a critical component of care. Factors that may affect fetal/neonatal/infant outcomes during this period include all of those covered in the previous section on prenatal influences, as well as alterations in placental structure and function, premature rupture of membranes, preterm labor, abnormal presentation, and fetal stress and distress during labor and delivery.

Preterm Labor and Birth

In the United States in 2019, 1 in 10 infants (10.2% of live births) was born premature; 1.6% of live births were very preterm, and 8.6% were moderately preterm (National Center for Health Statistics, 2021). Preterm birth is a major contributor to perinatal mortality and morbidity. Maternal history and current pregnancy are evaluated for risks for preterm labor and delivery. A history of having a previous spontaneous preterm birth increases the risk of a subsequent preterm delivery, with the recurrence rate inversely related to the gestational age of the previous preterm birth (Blackburn, 2018). The rate of preterm birth increases with multiple

gestation and as the number of multiples increases. Twin birth rates have been increasing in recent years (da Fonsecs et al., 2020).

The four major mechanisms proposed for preterm labor are (1) infection or inflammation, (2) decidual hemorrhage or placental abruption; (3) maternal and fetal stress with activation of the maternal or fetal HPA axis; and (4) uterine overdistension or physical stress (Buhimschi et al., 2018). Infections (bacterial vaginosis, chorioamnionitis, chlamydia, gonorrhea, syphilis, asymptomatic bacterial infection, urinary tract infection, and pyelonephritis) are found in approximately one-fourth of preterm births (Buhimschi et al., 2018). Other risks include multiple pregnancy (with the risk of preterm birth increasing as number of multiples increase), cervical incompetence, uterine abnormalities, placenta previa or abruption, reduced maternal body mass index, drug/alcohol use, and obstetric complications such as hypertension, and a short cervical length at 18 to 20 weeks' gestation (Blackburn, 2018; da Fonsecs et al., 2020).

Socioeconomic, ethnic/racial, and familial genetic risk factors also are seen. In addition, economically disadvantaged women have a higher rate of preterm birth, as do adolescents or women with advanced maternal age, maternal stress or depression, or absence of prenatal care. However, many women who give birth prematurely have no specific identifiable risk factors for preterm labor.

Premature labor is defined as contractions that start the delivery process before 37 weeks' gestation. Prematurity/LBW is the second leading cause of infant mortality in the United States, and respiratory distress syndrome (RDS) is the fourth leading cause of death (National Center for Health Statistics, 2021).

The use of antenatal corticosteroids (ACS) has increased the survival rate for babies delivered because of preterm labor. A single course of ACS given to women in preterm labor decreases RDS, germinal matrix/intraventricular hemorrhage (GMH/IVH), neonatal death, need for respiratory support, systemic infection in the first 48 hours, and necrotizing enterocolitis (Roberts et al., 2017). Use of prophylactic antibiotics in women during the intrapartum period who meet specific criteria can reduce the risk of perinatal group B streptococcal infection in their offspring (ACOG, 2019; Verani et al., 2010).

Short cervical length may be used for screening at-risk women, with the risk of preterm birth inversely related to cervical length (da Fonsecs et al., 2020; Norman, 2020). Progesterone has been used prophylactically in women with a singleton pregnancy and a history of a previous preterm infants to prevent recurrent preterm delivery (Boelig et al., 2019; Dodd et al., 2013; Jardie et al., 2019; Medley et al., 2018; Norman, 2020).

Strategies demonstrated to be effective in preventing or reducing preterm birth in specific populations of pregnant women include midwife-led continuity models of care; screening for lower genital tract infections for pregnant women less than 37 weeks' gestation and without signs of labor, bleeding, or infection; zinc supplementation for pregnant women without systemic illness; and cervical cerclage for women with singleton pregnancy and high-risk preterm birth (Medley et al., 2018). Administration of magnesium sulfate to women at imminent risk of preterm delivery has a neuroprotective effect and reduces the risk of cerebral palsy in offspring (Shepherd et al., 2017; Wolf et al., 2020).

Placental Dysfunction and Abnormalities

Placental dysfunction can be related either to a maternal condition altering blood flow or to changes in the growth or structure of the placenta itself. Because the placenta is responsible for nourishing the fetus and regulating the oxygen supply and removal of toxins, anything that changes the placental growth, surface, or circulation potentially can affect fetal growth and development. Placental anomalies are associated with poor fetal/neonatal outcomes including LBW and prematurity and may be markers for risks (Blackburn, 2018).

The most common placental abnormality is abruptio placentae or abruption. Perinatal mortality for affected infants is increased. Abruption can be caused by uteroplacental insufficiency from separation or decreased perfusion from maternal hypovolemia, uterine hypertonus, or fetal hemorrhage. Abruption increases the risk of fetal hypoxia and anoxia, preterm birth, and SGA infants. Even if the bleeding stops and the pregnancy continues, the decreased placental surface area might not be adequate to meet the nutritional needs of the fetus. As a result, these infants are at higher risk for neurobehavioral alterations. Placenta previa is also associated with an increased risk for preterm birth. These infants may be SGA if placental exchange of nutrients is chronically compromised. The risk of CNS, cardiovascular, respiratory, or gastrointestinal tract abnormalities and anemia also increases with placenta previa.

Premature Rupture of Membranes

Premature rupture of the membranes (PROM), or rupture before onset of uterine contractions, may be due to mechanical stress (polyhydramnios, multiple gestation), alterations in membranous collagen, or chorioamnionitis (Blackburn, 2018). The neonatal outcome is dependent on the gestational age of the fetus at the time of the rupture and delivery and the underlying cause. Risks are similar to that of preterm delivery.

POSTNATAL INFLUENCES ON DEVELOPMENT

Prenatal influences often result in variations in birth weight and gestational age. Infants must be assessed for neonatal variations. LBW is defined as less than 2,500 g. Very low birth weight (VLBW) is weight less than 1,500 g; extremely low birth weight (ELBW) are infants born at less than 1,000 g.

An infant can be average, small, or large for gestational age (AGA, SGA, or LGA, respectively) depending on comparisons with normal growth curves for gestational age groups. All of these infants can be term, preterm, or post term. A SGA infant is one whose weight at birth falls below the 10th percentile for gestation or more than 2 standard deviations (SDs) below the mean. The reason these infants are SGA may be due to pathologic processes or to factors such as parity or body mass index/parental. Infants whose weight falls beneath the 3rd percentile are severely undergrown. LGA infants are those whose weight is more than the 90th percentile or 2 SDs above the mean (Tappero & Honeyfield, 2019). These data help assess the risk of problems for neonates or infants.

Infants are classified at birth by birth weight and gestational age. FGR infants, also referred to as IUGR, are infants who have not grown at the expected in utero rate for weight, length, or head circumference owing to pathologic processes in utero. These infants often are SGA but may not be if their weight is not below the 10th percentile for gestation. Symmetric FGR occurs when the weight, length, and head circumference all fall below the 10th percentile. This is more common in fetuses with congenital infections and anomalies. Asymmetric FGR occurs when head circumference and length are within the normal range for their gestational age, with weight below the 10th percentile. This finding often is related to impaired placental functioning or poor nutrition, with sparing of brain growth. Neonatal outcome for these children is variable and often is related to the underlying cause of the growth restriction as well as gestational age at delivery. In the absence of major anomalies, viral infections, or chromosomal abnormalities, growth-restricted newborns may have few complications. Through antenatal testing, absent or reversed-end diastolic flow on Doppler flow studies has been related to a high incidence of FGR and an increased incidence of abnormal neurologic signs in newborns. Head circumference below the 10th percentile at birth and abnormal results from a newborn neurologic examination are associated with poor growth, later microcephaly, and neurologic deficits.

Assessment of gestational age and severity of illness can have many implications for the developing infant. Gestational age may be determined prior to birth using fetal ultrasound examinations. Methods of assessing gestational age after birth include the Dubowitz and Ballard assessments of gestational age. The New Ballard Score is used most often in clinical settings. This score was modified from the Dubowitz assessment, with later expansion to include characteristics of extremely preterm infants (Tappero & Honeyfield, 2019). There are multiple severity-of-illness and mortality-risk scoring systems. Examples of these include: (1) Score for Neonatal Acute Physiology (SNAP-II), which correlates chronic physiologic instability and neurodevelopment morbidity; (2) Score for Neonatal Acute Physiology—Perinatal Extension (SNAP + PE-II), in which the SNAP was extended for use as a mortality risk predictor by inclusion of points for birthweight, SGA, and low Apgar scores; and (3) Clinical

Risk Index for Babies (CRIB, CRIB-II), which includes birth weight, gestational age, congenital anomalies, and physiologic measures that are weighted according to their risk of mortality (Garg et al., 2018).

Complications Experienced by Newborns

The complications that are experienced by a newborn and infant can often be anticipated when prenatal and intrapartum exposures are known. The more common medical complications of newborns that affect development generally, and neurobehavioral development in particular, are associated with disturbances in the endocrine, respiratory, and neurologic systems. Theoretically, any system can be affected, but in terms of neurobehavioral development, these are the most common. These areas should be considered, and questions should be asked as the maternal/neonatal history is reviewed and an infant is assessed. Complications that will be briefly reviewed in this section include hypoglycemia and hyperglycemia, RDS, bronchopulmonary dysplasia (BPD), necrotizing enterocolitis (NEC), hyperbilirubinemia, and retinopathy of prematurity (ROP), neonatal seizures, meningitis, hypoxic–ischemic encephalopathy (HIE), intercranial hemorrhage, white matter injury (WMI)/periventricular leukomalacia (PVL), and cerebellar injury.

Hypoglycemia/Hyperglycemia

Hypoglycemia occurs because of decreased substrate availability, altered endocrine regulation, or increased glucose use. This disorder is most often found in infants who are LBW, SGA, preterm, or born to a diabetic mother; it also can occur after perinatal asphyxia. Clinical signs of hypoglycemia include tremors, jitteriness, irregular respiration, hypotonia, apnea, cyanosis, poor feeding, high-pitched cry, lethargy, irritability, hypothermia, and seizures (Blackburn, 2018). Hyperglycemia is common in small infants who are receiving concentrated glucose solutions and often is an iatrogenic complication of neonatal therapy. Adverse effects include dehydration (especially in extremely LBW infants), hyperosmolarity, osmotic diuresis, risk of bacterial and fungal infection, and an increased risk of intercranial hemorrhage.

Cardiorespiratory Disorders

RDS occurs due to a developmental deficiency of pulmonary surfactant along with lung immaturity, hypoperfusion, and oxidative stress. RDS is the most common respiratory problem seen in preterm infants, although survival has increased with the use of exogenous surfactant and other therapies. RDS may interfere with oxygen availability to the rapidly developing brain, which increases the risk of neurologic impairment. The incidence of RDS inversely is related to gestational age. Multisystem complications may occur in infants with RDS, including pulmonary (bronchopulmonary dysplasia, air leak), cardiovascular (patent ductus arteriosus, hypotension, and shock), renal (oliguria), metabolic (acidosis, fluid and electrolyte alterations), hematologic (anemia, hyperbilirubinemia), neurologic disorders (seizures, GMH/IVH), retinopathy of prematurity, and secondary nosocomial infections (Frasier, 2021). The lower the gestational age and the higher the number of associated complications, the greater the risk for adverse neurodevelopment outcomes.

BPD is a chronic lung disease involving perinatal and postnatal mechanisms that injure the developing lung, alter lung function, and result in pathologic changes. Risk factors for BPD include extremely low birth weight, LBW, hyperoxia (overcoming protective antioxidant systems), mechanical ventilation, sepsis, and extrauterine growth restriction (Bonadies et al., 2020). The current pattern of BPD, seen primarily in infants weighing less than 1,000 g or those who are older than 30 weeks gestation at birth, is characterized by oxygen requirements at 36 weeks postmenstrual age (Bonadies et al., 2020; Higgins et al., 2018). From a developmental standpoint, BPD adversely affects NICU graduates. BPD is the most common respiratory illness seen in infants who were born prematurely and is reported in 15% to 35% of infants born at less than 32 weeks (Bonadies et al., 2020). Complications include intermittent bronchospasm, recurrent infections (especially ear infections, pneumonia, and upper respiratory infection), congestive heart failure, gastroesophageal reflux disease, developmental delays, neurologic and developmental sequelae including cerebral palsy, and sensorineural hearing loss.

Neurologic Complications

Seizures occur in 1.8% to 5% per 1,000 term births and 30 to 130 per 1,000 live preterm births and are the most common neonatal neurologic sign and indicator of any underlying problem (Ditzenberger & Blackburn, 2020). Prognosis is influenced by time of onset, cause, response to treatment, electroencephalogram findings, type of seizure, frequency, and duration of the seizure. Cerebral dysgenesis and hypoxic–ischemic injury with early-onset seizures have been associated with poorer outcomes. Causative factors in the etiology of seizures include HIE (the most common cause); metabolic alterations (hyponatremia or hypernatremia, hypocalcemia, hypomagnesemia, inherited metabolic problems, pyridoxine dependency, and hyperammonemia); intercranial hemorrhage, structural anomalies such as cerebral cortical dysgenesis, CNS infections (meningitis) due to either bacteria (group B streptococcus, *Escherichia coli*, or *Listeria monocytogenes*) or other organisms such as TORCH (toxoplasmosis, rubella, cytomegalovirus, and herpes simplex) organisms; withdrawal from maternal drugs (e.g., narcotic-analgesics, sedative-hypnotics, and alcohol); and familial seizures with a genetic basis with onset during the first 3 days of life (Abend et al., 2018; Ditzenberger & Blackburn, 2020).

Meningitis occurs as both an early-onset (from vaginal flora) and late-onset (from environmental pathogens) infection. Common causative agents are group B streptococci and *E. coli*. The outcome depends on rapidity of detection and initiation of adequate drug therapy. Survivors of bacterial meningitis may have neurologic sequelae including motor and mental disabilities, convulsions, hydrocephalus, and hearing loss (Ditzenberger & Blackburn, 2020).

HIE is an injury to the brain that results from a combination of a systemic hypoxemia and decreased cerebral perfusion leading to ischemia. The site of injury varies with gestational age. Full-term infants are at increased risk for gray matter injury, whereas preterm infants are at greater risk for white matter injury (Ditzenberger & Blackburn, 2020). Most of these insults occur in the antepartum and intrapartum periods, with few occurring after birth. Outcomes vary with the site, extent, and severity of the injury. Infants with mild HIE generally do well, as do infants with moderate HIE (duration less than 5 days). Infants with moderate (lasting more than 5 days) or severe HIE have a higher mortality and a higher incidence of cognitive and motor deficits including cerebral palsy. Other outcomes include cortical blindness, deafness, epilepsy, and microcephaly (Ditzenberger & Blackburn, 2020; Gunn & Thoresen, 2019). Risk factors for HIE include maternal preeclampsia, abruption, prolonged labor, FGR, sepsis, and fetal distress. Therapies include use of head or total body cooling in term infants to reduce cerebral edema and injury (Jacobs et al., 2013; Natarajan et al., 2018).

Intracranial hemorrhages also can affect outcomes. The major types seen in neonates are subdural, subarachnoid, intracerebellar, and GMH/IVH. Subdural hemorrhage usually occurs in term infants with collection of blood in the subdural space due to lacerations of superficial cerebral veins over cerebral hemispheres, and the prognosis generally is good. Bleeding over the posterior fossa or tentorial lacerations has a poorer prognosis. Hydrocephalus occasionally develops. Risk factors for subdural hemorrhage include primipara, rapid or difficult delivery, and LGA infants. Subarachnoid hemorrhage involves bleeding of venous origin in the subarachnoid space. The hemorrhage most likely is precipitated by trauma in term infants and hypoxia in preterm infants. Unless the hemorrhage is massive, outcome is good (Ditzenberger & Blackburn, 2020). Intracerebellar hemorrhages are associated with RDS, hypoxic events, prematurity, and traumatic delivery. Outcome is poor with severe intracerebellar hemorrhage (Tam, 2018).

Brain Injury in Preterm Infants

Preterm infants are vulnerable to alterations in brain maturation and brain injury from pathophysiologic events before they are born as well as after birth when they are cared for in the NICU "at a time of peak brain growth, synaptogenesis, developmental regulation of specific receptor populations, and central nervous system organization and differentiation" (Symes, 2016, p. 1157). Significant neurobehavioral sequelae have been described in 5% to 15% of ELBW infants. Milder cognitive defects, learning disabilities, and behavioral sequelae are seen in up to 25% to 50% of these infants (Gotardo et al., 2019; Schneider & Miller, 2019). The major pathophysiologic events leading to brain injury in preterm infants are hypoxemia–ischemia and inflammation–infection (Back & Miller, 2018; Back & Volpe, 2018). The most common brain lesions are the result of GMH-IVH, including periventricular hemorrhagic infarction (PVHI); white matter injury (WMI; periventricular leukomalacia [PVL]); and cerebellar injury. These disorders are the leading causes of neurologic disability in preterm infants with motor, cognitive, learning, and neurobehavioral sequelae (Back & Miller, 2018; Back & Volpe, 2018; Ditzenberger & Blackburn, 2020; Neil & Volpe, 2018).

GMH/IVH most often is seen in infants born before 34 weeks' gestation. The incidence increases with decreasing gestational age at birth. Perinatal risk factors for GMH/IVH include preterm labor, fetal or neonatal hypoxic–ischemic events, maternal infection, prolonged labor, chorioamnionitis, prolonged PROM, and ominous fetal heart rate tracings. Postnatal factors associated with GMH/IVH include prematurity, LBW, acidosis, hypo- or hypertension, low hematocrit, respiratory distress requiring mechanical ventilation, rapid administration of sodium bicarbonate or volume expansion, infusion of hyperosmolar solutions, altered hemostasis, and pneumothorax (Inder et al., 2018). The overall incidence of GMH/IVH has decreased in recent years. GMH/IVH is categorized on a small-to-severe or grades I–IV scale depending on the location and extent of the hemorrhage. The most severe form (PVHI) involves both intraventricular and brain parenchymal hemorrhage with acute ventricular dilation; these infants have the greatest risk of neurologic sequelae (Leijser & de Vries, 2019). The incidence of major neurologic sequelae ranges from 15% to 20% for infants with moderate hemorrhage up to 50% to 75% with infants with severe hemorrhage, especially PVHI (Gotardo et al., 2019; Inder et al., 2018).

Since GMH/IVH usually occurs in the first 72 hours after birth, prevention bundles have been implemented during this time to minimize activities that increase intracranial pressure or lead to alterations in venous and arterial pressure or hypoxemia and promote neutral head positioning (Bissinger et al., 2019; Chiriboga et al., 2018; de Bijl-Marcus et al., 2020). Data from randomized controlled trials of the effects of neutral head positioning on the incidence of GMH/IVH are inconclusive (Romantsik et al., 2020).

WMI/PVL are often seen along with associated neuronal and axonal alterations. This has been referred to as the encephalopathy of prematurity and is the most common severe neurological insult and the major form of brain injury in preterm infants. Three forms of WMI are seen: (1) focal cystic necrotic lesions (seen in less than 5% of infants born less than 32 weeks' gestation); (2) noncystic lesions; and (3) diffuse lesions. Noncystic and diffuse lesions are seen in 25% to 50% of VLBW infants and associated with alterations in myelination leading to PVL (Back & Miller, 2018; Neil & Volpe, 2018; Schneider & Miller, 2019). PVL involves lesions deep in white matter with loss of all cellular elements and diffuse injury in central cerebral white matter with damage to premyelinating oligodendrocytes with astrogliosis and microglial infiltration (Back & Miller, 2018; Ditzenberger & Blackburn, 2020; Neil & Volpe, 2018; Schneider & Miller, 2019). The time of onset is variable. Major risk factors for WMI are cerebral ischemia (due to asphyxia, hypoxia, GMH/IVH, hypercarbia, or hypotension) and inflammation/infection (toxins alter cerebral blood flow with the highest risks seen in infants younger than 23 to 32 weeks postmenstrual age and weighing less than 1,000 g [Ditzenberger & Blackburn, 2020]). The major risk factors are asphyxia/ischemia and inflammation/infection. WMI is a leading cause of neurological disability in infants born preterm with motor, cognitive, learning, and behavioral sequelae (Back & Volpe, 2018; Gotardo et al., 2019; Neil & Volpe, 2018; Schneider & Miller, 2019). The most common sequelae are spastic diplegia with or without hydrocephalus and vision impairment. Infants with diffuse WMI are more likely to develop visual, cognitive, and neurobehavioral impairments such as autism spectrum disorder (Gotardo et al., 2019; Neil & Volpe, 2018; Schneider & Miller, 2019).

Two forms of cerebellar injury are seen in preterm infants: primary (usually due to cerebellar hemorrhage or infarction) and secondary (cerebral hypoplasia with alterations in cerebellar growth and development (Gano & Barkovich, 2019; Limperopoulos et al., 2018; Tam, 2018). The cerebellum is one of the later brain structures to mature and undergo critical developmental events (including neuronal proliferation, migration, and arborization) in the late second and early third trimesters, when preterm infants are in the NICU (Gano & Barkovich, 2019; Tam, 2018). Risk factors are similar to those for GMH-IVH and WMI. Mortality is high for infants with severe cerebellar hemorrhage, at risk of microcephaly, hypotonia, and developmental delay in survivors; infants with smaller hemorrhages are at increased risk of mild to moderate motor impairments (Tam, 2018). Infants with cerebellar hypoplasia are at risk for altered cognitive and motor outcomes.

Other Complications

NEC is a multifactorial gastrointestinal disorder seen in preterm infants, including 5% to 10% of VLBW infants, with a mortality of up to 25% (Xiong et al., 2020). Up to half of these infants may require surgical intervention. The risk of NEC is reported to be reduced by probiotics, use of maternal antenatal corticosteroids, prebiotics, and breast milk (Blackburn, 2018; Xiong et al., 2020).

Hyperbilirubinemia is another risk factor for later neurodevelopment problems with development of bilirubin encephalopathy and kernicterus. Bilirubin encephalopathy refers to early, acute clinical symptoms of bilirubin toxicity, whereas kernicterus is chronic, permanent change to the brain with yellow staining due to deposition of bilirubin in basal ganglia and other areas of the brain and neuronal injury and necrosis (Blackburn, 2018). The goal of treatment for hyperbilirubinemia is to prevent bilirubin toxic effects. Hyperbilirubinemia management in LBW infants is determined by clinical status, age, weight, and history.

ROP is a neovascularizing disorder seen primarily in preterm infants whose retinal vasculature still is developing. Damage occurs in two phases: initial injury and ischemia, followed by abnormal proliferation. The normal vasculogenesis process is arrested and followed by rapid, excessive, irregular vascular growth and shunt formation. ROP is a complex multifactorial disorder whose incidence and severity are inversely proportional to gestational age and birthweight. ROP is classified by location (zone) and severity (stage) and the presence of "plus" disease (signs of rapidly progressing disease); the outcome depends on stage. Up to 90% of cases resolve spontaneously; others may require surgical or pharmacological intervention (Tailoi et al., 2018). Close monitoring of oximetry settings and use of oxygen saturation targets with prevention of repeated episodes of hypoxia/hyperoxia may help reduce the incidence of ROP (Higgins, 2019).

CONCLUSION

This chapter reviews factors that influence fetal and neonatal development, with an emphasis on neurodevelopmental outcomes. Long-term developmental outcomes for these infants are part of individualized family-centered plans. These outcomes are affected by the prenatal, perinatal, and postnatal influences described in this chapter. The philosophy of developmental care requires that assessment and plans be holistic, individualized, family centered, and developmentally supportive. Part of understanding individual differences is recognizing the biological risks for each that influence developmental outcomes. All caregivers of infants should advocate for strategies before and during pregnancy that may prevent preterm birth and other problems and improve outcomes, including ensuring healthcare is available and accessible to all women. Table 10-1 provides recommendations for the periconceptional period to improve perinatal outcomes.

TABLE 10-1 Examples of Recommendations for the Periconceptional and Prenatal Period to Improve Perinatal Outcomes

Type	Recommendation	Level of Evidence	References
Prevention	Folic acid supplementation to women of childbearing age to decrease the risk of neural tube and other anomalies	I VII	Goh et al. (2006) American Academy of Pediatrics Committee on Genetics. (1999, reaffirmed 2012)
Intervention	Provide periconceptional and prenatal care and counseling to women with diabetes mellitus to reduce fetal and neonatal morbidity	I	Pearson et al. (2007)
	Use smoking cessation programs in pregnancy to reduce the proportion of women who continue to smoke and the risk of low birth weight and preterm birth	I I	Gould et al. (2020) Chamberlain et al. (2017)
	Use prophylactic antibiotics in women who meet criteria to prevent perinatal group B streptococcal infection	VII VII	Verani et al. (2010) American College of Obstetricians and Gynecologists (2019)
	Use antiretroviral regimens to reduce risk of HIV transmission to fetus from mothers and fetal infection in HIV-positive women	I	Wedi et al. (2016)
	Use prophylactic progesterone supplementation in women with a history of previous preterm infants who meet selection criteria	I I	Jardie et al. (2019) Dodd et al. (2013)
	Use a single course of antenatal corticosteroids to decrease respiratory distress syndrome, intraventricular hemorrhage, neonatal death, and other complications in preterm infants Administer magnesium sulfate to women at imminent risk of preterm delivery	I I I	Roberts et al. (2017) Wolf et al. (2020) Shepherd et al. (2017)

Note: Level I, evidence from a systematic review or meta-analysis of all relevant randomized controlled trials (RCTs), or evidence-based clinical practice guidelines based on systematic reviews of RCTs; level VII, evidence from the opinion of authorities and/or reports of expert committees.

Potential Research Questions

- What effects does a maternal history of eating disorders before pregnancy have on fetal development and infant growth?
- What are the effects of abused drugs, including illegal, legal, and prescribed drugs, during pregnancy and breastfeeding on fetal and neonatal development?
- How does the use of maternal nutritional supplements and herbal agents affect fetal and neonatal development?
- What effects does a maternal pure vegan diet have on long-term development?
- What are the effects of strategies to reduce perinatal stress in the mother and fetus on long-term development?
- If there is a history of intimate-partner violence in the pregnancy, what will the long-term effect be on infant/mother bonding and family stability?
- What care strategies can practitioners use to reduce the risk of brain injury in preterm infants?

REFERENCES

Abend, N. S., Jensen, F. E., Inder, T. E., & Volpe, J. J. (2018). Neonatal seizures. In Volpe, J. J., Inder, T. E., Darras, B. T., de Vries, L. S., du Plessis, A. J., Neil, J., & Perlman, J. M. (Eds.), *Volpe's Neurology of the newborn* (6th ed., pp. 275–372). Elsevier.

Adams, E. D. (2021). Antenatal care. In Simpson, K. R., Creehand, P. A., O'Brien-Abel, N., Roth, C. K., & Rohan, A. J. (Eds.), *Perinatal nursing* (5th ed., pp. 66–98). Wolters Kluwer.

Allotey, J., Stallings, E., Bonet, M., Yap, M., Chatterjee, S., Kew, T., Debenham, L., Llavall, A.C., Dixit, A., Zhou, D. R., Balaji, R., Lee, S. I., Qui, X., Yuan, M., Coomar, D., van Wely, M., van Leeuwen, E., Kostova, E., Kunst, H., … Thangaratinam, S. (2020). Clinical manifestations, risk factors, and maternal and perinatal outcomes of coronavirus disease 2019 in pregnancy: Systematic review and meta-analysis. *British Medical Journal, 370*, m3320. https://doi.org/10.1136/bmj.m3320

American Academy of Pediatrics Committee on Genetics. (1999, reaffirmed 2012). Folic acid for the prevention of neural tube defects. *Pediatrics, 100*(2), 143–152.

American College of Obstetricians and Gynecologists. (2013). *Hypertension in pregnancy*. ACOG.

American College of Obstetricians and Gynecologists, 2019 American College of Obstetricians and Gynecologists. (2019). *Prevention of perinatal group B streptococcal disease.* (Committee Opinion No. 782). ACOG.

American College of Obstetricians and Gynecologists, 2019 American College of Obstetricians and Gynecologists. (2019). *Pregnancy and heart disease* (Practice Bulletin No, 212). ACOG.

American College of Obstetricians and Gynecologists and Society for Maternal Fetal Medicine. (2019). *Fetal growth restriction* (Practice Bulletin No, 204). ACOG.

American College of Obstetricians and Gynecology. (2020). Thyroid disease in pregnancy: ACOG practice bulletin, number 223. *Obstetrics and Gynecology, 135*, e261–e274.

Back, S. A., & Miller, S. P. (2018). Brain injury in the preterm infant. In Gleason, C. A. & Juul, S. E. (Eds.), *Avery's diseases of the newborn* (10th ed., pp. 879–896). Elsevier.

Back, S. A., & Volpe, J. J. (2018). Encephalopathy of prematurity: Pathophysiology. In Volpe, J. J., Inder, T. E., Darras, B. T., deVries, L. S., du Plessis, A. J.. Perlman, J. M. (Eds.), *Volpe's neurology of the newborn* (6th ed., pp. 405–424). Elsevier.

Bailey, N. A., & Diaz-Barbosa, M. (2018). Effect of maternal substance abuse on the fetus, neonate, and child. *Pediatric Reviews, 39*, 550–559.

Battarbee, A. N., Sinkey, R. G., Harper, L. M., Oparil, S., & Tita, A. T. N. (2020). Chronic hypertension in pregnancy. *American Journal of Obstetrics and Gynecology, 222*, 532–541.

Bałkowiec-Iskra, E., Mirowska-Guzel, D. M., & Wielgos, M. (2017). Effect of antidepressants use in pregnancy on foetus development and adverse effects in newborns. *Ginekologia Polska, 88*, 36–42.

de Bijl-Marcus, K., Brouwer, A. J., de Vries, L. S., Groenendaal, F., & van Wezel-Meijler, G. (2020). Neonatal care bundles are associated with a reduction in the incidence of intraventricular haemorrhage in preterm infants: A multicentre cohort study. *Archives of Disease in Childhood Fetal and Neonatal Edition, 5*, F419–F424.

Bissinger, R. L., Annibale, D. J., & Fanning, B. (2019). *Golden hours: Care of the very low birth weight infant* (2nd ed.). The National Certification Corporation (NCC).

Blackburn, S. T. (2018). *Maternal, fetal, and neonatal physiology: A clinical perspective* (5th ed.). Elsevier.

Boelig, R. C., Della Corte, L., Ashoush, S., McKenna, D., Saccone, G., Rajaram, S., & Berghella, V. (2019). Oral progesterone for the prevention of recurrent preterm birth: Systematic review and metaanalysis. *American Journal of Obstetrics and Gynecology MFM, 1*, 50–62.

Bonadies, L., Zaramella, P., Porzionato, A., Perilongo, G., Muraca, M., & Baraldi, E. (2020). Present and future of bronchopulmonary dysplasia. *Journal of Clinical Medicine, 9*(5), 1539. https://doi.org/10.3390/jcm9051539

Breymann, C. (2015). Iron deficiency anemia in pregnancy. *Seminars in Hematology, 52*, 339–437.

Buhimschi, C. S., Mesiano, S., & Muglia, L. J. (2018). Pathogenesis of spontaneous preterm birth. In Resnik, R., Lockwood, C. J., Moore, T. R., Greene, M. F., Copal, J. A., & Silver, R. M. (Eds.), *Creasy & resnik's maternal-fetal medicine: Principles and practice* (8th ed., pp. 96–126). Elsevier.

Burgess, A. (2021). Hypertensive disorders of pregnancy. In Simpson, K. R., Creehand, P. A., O'Brien-Abel, N., Roth, C. K., & Rohan, A. J. (Eds.), *Perinatal nursing* (5th ed., pp. 99–121). Wolters Kluwer.

Callister, L. C. (2021). Integrating cultural beliefs and practices when caring for childbearing women and families. In Simpson, K. R., Creehand, P. A., O'Brien-Abel, N., Roth, C. K., & Rohan, A. J. (Eds.), *Perinatal nursing* (5th ed., pp. 18–43). Wolters Kluwar.

Cao-Leia, L., de Rooijb, S. R., Kinga, S., Matthews, S. G., Metzd, G. A. S., Roseboome, T. J., & Szyf, M. (2020). Prenatal stress and epigenetics. *Neuroscience & Biobehavioral Reviews, 117*, 198–210.

Centers for Disease Control (CDC) and Prevention. (2019a). *Infant mortality*. CDC.

Centers for Disease Control CDC and Prevention. (2019b). *Pregnancy mortality surveillance system*. CDC.

Chamberlain, C., O'Mara-Eves, A., Porter, J., Coleman, T., Perlen, S. M., Thomas, J., & McKenzie, J. E. (2017). Psychosocial interventions for supporting women to stop smoking in pregnancy. *Cochrane Database of Systematic Reviews, 2*(2), CD001055. https://doi.org/10.1002/14651858.CD001055.pub5

Chambers, C., & Freidman, J. M. (2018). Teratogenesis and environmental exposures. In Resnik, R., Lockwood, C. J., Moore, T. R., Greene, M. F., Copal, J. A., & Silver, R. M. (Eds.), *Creasy & resnik's maternal-fetal medicine: Principles and practice* (8th ed., pp. 539–548). Elsevier.

Chiriboga, N., Cortez, J., Pena-Ariet, A., Makker, K., Smotherman, C., Gautam, S., Trikardos, A. B., Knight, H., Yeoman, M., Burnett, E., Beier, A., Cohen, I., & Hudak, M. L. (2018). Successful implementation of an intracranial hemorrhage (ICH) bundle in reducing severe ICH: A quality improvement project. *Journal of Perinatology, 39*, 143–151.

Convertino, I., Sansone, A. C., Marino, A., Galiulo, M. T., Mantarro, S. Antoni, L., Fornai, M., Blandizzi, C., & Tuccori, M. (2016). Neonatal adaptation issues after maternal exposure to prescription drugs: Withdrawal syndromes and residual pharmacological effects. *Drug Safety, 39*, 903–924.

Cook, J. L., Green, C. R., de la Ronde, S., Dell, C. A., Graves, L., Ordean, A. Ruiter, J., Steeves, M., & Wong, S. (2017). Epidemiology and effects of substance use in pregnancy. *Journal of Obstetrics and Gynaecology Canada, 39*, 906–915.

Ditzenberger, G. R., & Blackburn, S. T. (2020). Neurologic system. In Kenner, C., Altimer, L. B., & Boykova, M. V. (Eds.), *Comprehensive neonatal nursing care* (6th ed., pp. 373–416). Springer.

Dodd, J. M., Jones, L., Flenady, V., Cincotta, R., & Crowther, C. A. (2013). Prenatal administration of progesterone for preventing preterm birth in women considered to be at risk of preterm birth. *Cochrane Database of Systematic Reviews*, (7), CD004947.

Dubey, P., Reddy, S.Y., Manuel, S., & Dwivedi, A.K. (2020). Maternal and neonatal characteristics and outcomes among COVID-19 infected women: An updated systematic review and meta-analysis. *European Journal of Obstetrics, Gynecology, and Reproductive Biology, 252*, 490–501.

da Fonseca, E. B., Damiao, R., & Moreira, D. A. (2020). Preterm birth prevention. *Best Practice & Research Clinical Obstetrics & Gynaecology, 69*, 40–49.

Frasier, D. (2021). Respiratory distress. In Verklan, M. T., Walden, M., & Forest, S. (Eds.), *Core curriculum for neonatal intensive care* (6th ed., pp. 396–399). Elsevier.

Gano, D., & Barkovich, J. (2019). Cerebellar hypoplasia of prematurity: Causes and consequences. In de Vries, L. S. & Glass, H. C. (Eds.), *Handbook of clinical neurology* (Vol. 162, pp. 201–206). Elsevier.

Garg, B., Sharma, D., & Farahbakhsh, N. (2018). Assessment of sickness severity of illness in neonates: Review of various neonatal illness scoring systems. *Journal of Maternal-Fetal & Neonatal Medicine, 31*, 1373–1380.

Georgieff, M. K. (2020). Iron deficiency in pregnancy. *American Journal of Obstetrics and Gynecology, 223*, 516–524.

Ghandi, M. M., & Martin, S. R. (2015). Cardiac disease in pregnancy. *Obstetrics and Gynecology Clinics, 42*, 315–433.

Goh, Y. I., Bollano, E., Einarson, T. R., & Koren, G. (2006). Prenatal multivitamin supplementation and rates of congenital anomalies: A meta-analysis. *Journal of Obstetrics and Gynaecology Canada, 28*, 680–689.

Gotardo, J. W., Volkmer, N. V., Stangler, G. P., Dornelles, A. D., Bohrer, B. B., & Carvalho, C. G. (2019). Impact of peri-intraventricular haemorrhage and periventricular leukomalacia in the neurodevelopment of preterms: A systematic review and meta-analysis. *PLoS One, 14*(10), e02234275.

Gould, G. S., Havard, A., Lim, L. L., & Kumar, R. (2020). Exposure to tobacco, environmental tobacco smoke and nicotine in pregnancy: A pragmatic overview of reviews of maternal and child outcomes, effectiveness of interventions and barriers and facilitators to quitting. *International Journal of Environmental Research in Public Health, 17*, 2034. https://doi.org/10.3390/ijerph17062034

Gregg, A. R., & Kuller, J. A. (2018). Human genetics and patterns of inheritance. In Resnik, R., Lockwood, C. J., Moore, T. R., Greene, M. F., Copal, J. A., & Silver, R. M. (Eds.), *Creasy & resnik's maternal-fetal medicine: Principles and practice* (8th ed., pp. 3–14). Elsevier.

Gunn, A. J., & Thoresen, M. (2019). Neonatal encephalopathy and hypoxic-ischemic encephalopathy. *Handbook of Clinical Neurology, 162*, 217–237.

Harden, C., & Lu, C. (2019). Management of epilepsy in pregnancy. *Neurologic Clinics, 37*, 53–62.

Higgins, R. D. (2019). Oxygen saturation and retinopathy of prematurity, *Clinics in Perinatology, 46*, 593–599.

Higgins, R. D., Jobe, A. H., Koso-Thomas, M., Bancalari, E., Viscardi, R. M., Hartert, T. V., Ryan, R. M., Kallapur, S. G., Steinhorn, R. H., Konduri, G. G., Davis, S. D., Thebaud, B., Clyman, R. I., Collaco, J. M., Martin, C. R., Woods, J. C., Finer, N. N., & Raju, T. N. K. (2018). Bronchopulmonary dysplasia: Executive summary of a workshop. *Journal of Pediatrics, 197*, 300–308.

Inder, T. E., Perlman, J. M., & Volpe, J. J. (2018). Preterm intraventricular hemorrhage/posthemorrhagic hydrocephalus. In Volpe, J. J., Inder, T. E., Darras, B. T., deVries, L. S., du Plessis, A. J., & Perlman, J. M. (Eds.), *Volpe's neurology of the newborn* (6th ed., pp. 637–698). Elsevier.

Jacobs, S. E., Berg, M., Hunt, R., Tarnow-Mordi, W. O., Inder, T. E., & Davis, P. G. (2013). Cooling for newborns with hypoxic ischaemic encephalopathy (review). *Cochrane Database of Systematic Reviews, 2013*(1), CD003311.

James, S. H., & Kimberlin, D. W. (2015). Neonatal herpes simplex virus infection. *Infectious Disease Clinics of North America, 29*, 391–400.

Jansson, L. M., & Patrick, S. W. (2019). Neonatal abstinence syndrome. *Pediatric Clinics of North America, 66*, 353–367.

Jardie, A., Lutsiv, O., Beyene, J., & McDonals, S. D. (2019). Vaginal progesterone, oral progesterone, 17-OHPC, cerclage, and pessary for preventing preterm birth in at-risk singleton pregnancies: An updated systematic review and network metaanalysis. *BJOG: An International Journal of Obstetrics and Gynaecology, 126*, 556–567.

Jorde, L. B., Carey, J. C., & Bamshad, M. (2019). *Medical genetics* (6th ed.). Elsevier.

Kallema, V. R., Panditab, A., & Pillaic, A. (2020). Infant of diabetic mother: What one needs to know. *Journal of Maternal-Fetal & Neonatal Medicine, 33*, 482–492.

Kancherla, V., & Black, R. E. (2018). Historical perspective on folic acid and challenges in estimating global prevalence of neural tube defects. *Annals of the New York Academy of Sciences, 1414*, 20–30.

Kancherla, V., Wagh, K., Pachón, H., & Oakley, G. P., Jr. (2021). A 2019 global update on folic acid-preventable spina bifida and anencephaly. *Birth Defects Research, 113*, 77–89.

Kennedy, D. A., Lupattelli, A., Koren, G., & Nordeng, H. (2016). Safety classification of herbal medicines used in pregnancy in a multinational study. *BMC Complementary and Alternative Medicine, 16*, 102. https://doi.org/10.1186/s12906-016-1079-z

Kiernan, E., & Jones, K. L. (2019). Medications that cause fetal anomalies and possible prevention strategies. *Clinics in Perinatology, 46*, 203–213.

Kilpatrick, S. J. (2017). Trauma in pregnancy: An underappreciated cause of maternal death. *American Journal of Obstetrics and Gynecology, 217*, 499–500.

Korzeniewski, S. J., Slaughter, J., Lenski, M., Haak, P., & Paneth, N. (2019). The complex aetiology of cerebral palsy. *Nature Reviews Neurology, 14*, 528–543.

Kwak, M., Yum, M.-S., Yeh, H.-R., Kim, H.-J., & Ko, T.-S. (2018). Brain magnetic resonance imaging findings of congenital cytomegalovirus infection as a prognostic factor for neurological outcome. *Pediatric Neurology, 83*, 14–18.

Lee, S. Y., Cabral, H. J., Aschengrau, A., & Pearce, E. (2020). Associations between maternal thyroid function in pregnancy and obstetric and perinatal outcomes. *Journal of Clinical Endocrinology and Metabolism, 105*, e2015–e2023.

Leijser, L. M., & de Vries, L. S. (2019). Preterm brain injury: Germinal matrix–intraventricular hemorrhage and post-hemorrhagic ventricular dilatation. In de Vries, L. S., & Glass, H. C. (Eds.), *Handbook of clinical neurology* (Vol. 162, pp. 173–199). Elsevier.

Limperopoulos, C., du Plessis, A. J., & Volpe, J. J. (2018). Cerebellar hemorrhage. In Volpe, J. J., Inder, T. E., Darras, B. T., deVries, L. S., du Plessis, A. J., & Perlman, J. M. (Eds.), *Volpe's neurology of the newborn* (6th ed., pp. 623–636). Elsevier.

Mauricio La Rosa, M., Loaiza, S., Zambrano, M. A., & Escobar, M. F. (2020). Trauma in pregnancy, *Clinical Obstetrics and Gynecology, 63*, 447–454.

Medley, N., Vogel, J.P., Care, A., & Alfirevic, Z. (2018). Interventions during pregnancy to prevent preterm birth: An overview of cochrane systematic reviews. *Cochrane Database of Systematic Reviews, 11*(11), CD012505.

Monteiro, L. J., Norman, J. E., Rice, G. E., & Illanes, S. E. (2016). Fetal programming and gestational diabetes mellitus. *Placenta, 48*(Suppl. 1), S54–S60.

Moore, T. R., Hauguel-De Mouzon, S., & Catalanao, P. (2018). Diabetes in pregnancy. In Resnik, R., Lockwood, C. J., Moore, T. R., Greene, M. F., Copal, J. A., & Silver, R. M. (Eds.), *Creasy & resnik's maternal-fetal medicine: Principles and practice* (8th ed., pp. 1067–1097). Elsevier.

Nardozza, L. M., Caetano, A. C., Zamarian, A. C., Mazzola, J. B, Silva, C. P., Marçal, V. M., Lobo, T. F., Peixoto, A. B., & Araujo Júnior, E. (2017). Fetal growth restriction: Current knowledge. *Archives of Gynecology and Obstetrics, 295*, 1061–1077.

Natarajan, G., Laptook, A., & Shankaran, S. (2018). Therapeutic hypothermia: How can we optimize this therapy to further improve outcomes? *Clinics in Perinatology, 45*, 241–255.

National Center for Health Statistics. (2021). *Final natality data*. www.marchofdimes.org/peristats

Neil, J. J., & Volpe, J. J. (2018). Encephalopathy of prematurity: Clinical-neurological features, diagnosis, imaging, prognosis, therapy. In Volpe, J. J., Inder, T. E., Darras, B. T., deVries, L. S., du Plessis, A. J., & Perlman, J. M. (Eds.), *Volpe's neurology of the newborn* (6th ed., pp. 425–457). Elsevier.

Norman, J. E. (2020). Progesterone and preterm birth. *International Journal of Obstetrics and Gynecology, 150*, 24–30.

Ornoy, A., Weinstein-Fudin, L., & Ergaz, Z. (2017). Antidepressants, antipsychotics, and mood stabilizers in pregnancy: What do we know and how should we treat pregnant women with depression. Antidepressants, antipsychotics, and mood stabilizers in pregnancy. *Birth Defects Research, 109*, 933–956.

Palacios, C., Kostiuk, L. K., & Pena-Rosas, J. P. (2019). Vitamin D supplementation for women during pregnancy.*Cochrane Database of Systematic Reviews, 7*(7), CD008873.

Pearson, D. W., Kernaghan, D., Lee, R., & Penney, G. C. (2007). The relationship between pre-pregnancy care and early pregnancy loss, major congenital anomaly, or perinatal death. *BJOG: An International Journal of Obstetrics and Gynaecology, 114*, 104–107.

Prasad, M. R., & Jones, H. E. (2018). Substance abuse in pregnancy. In Resnik, R., Lockwood, C. J., Moore, T. R., Greene, M. F., Copal, J. A., & Silver, R. M. (Eds.), *Creasy & Resnik's maternal-fetal medicine: Principles and practice* (8th ed., pp. 539–548). Elsevier.

Rahmati, S., Azami, M., Badfar, G., Parizad, N., & Shayehmiri, K. (2020). The relationship between maternal anemia during pregnancy with preterm birth: A systematic review and meta-analysis, *Journal of Maternal-Fetal & Neonatal Medicine, 33*, 2679–2689.

Ramlakhan, K. P., Johnson, M. R., & Roos-Hesselink, W. (2020). Pregnancy and cardiovascular disease. *Nature Reviews Cardiology, 17*, 718–731.

Reefhuis, J., Devine, O., Friedman, J. M., Louik, C., Honein, M. A., & National Birth Defects Prevention Study. (2015). Specific SSRIs and birth defects: Bayesian analysis to interpret new data in the context of previous reports. *British Medical Journal, 351*, h3190. https://doi.org/10.1136/bmj.h3190

Roberts, D., Brown, J., Medley, N., & Dalziel, S. R. (2017). Antenatal corticosteroids for accelerating fetal lung maturation for women at risk of preterm birth. *Cochrane Database of Systematic Reviews, 3*(3), CD004454.

Romantsik, O., Calevo, M. G., & Bruschettini, M. (2020). Head midline position for preventing the occurrence or extension of germinal matrix-intraventricular haemorrhage in preterm infants. *Cochrane Database of Systematic Reviews, 7*(7), CD012362.

Roth, C. K. (2021). Diabetes in pregnancy. In Simpson, K. R., Creehand, P. A., O'Brien-Abel, N., Roth, C. K., & Rohan, A. J. (Eds.), *Perinatal nursing* (5th ed., pp. 182–198). Wolters Kluwer.

Rudd, K. M. (2021). Infectious diseases in the neonate. In Verklan, M. T., Walden, M., & Forest, S. (Eds.), *Core curriculum for neonatal intensive care* (6th ed., pp. 588–609). Elsevier.

Sabbagh, R., & Van den Veyver, I. B. (2020). The current and future impact of genome-wide sequencing on fetal precision medicine. *Human Genetics, 139*, 1121–1130.

Sakamoto, J., Michels, C., & Eisfelder, B. (2019). Trauma in pregnancy. *Emergency Medicine Clinics of North America, 37*, 317–338.

Schneider, J., & Miller, S. P. (2019). Preterm brain injury: White matter. In de Vries, L. S. & Glass, H. C. (Eds.), *Handbook of clinical neurology* (Vol. 162, pp. 155–178). Elsevier.

Shalish, W., Lakshminrusimha, S., Manzoni, P., Keszler, M., & Sant'Anna, G. M. (2020). COVID-19 and neonatal respiratory care: Current evidence and practical approach. *American Journal of Perinatology, 37*, 780–791.

Shepherd, E., Salam, R. A., Middleton, P., Makrides, S., McIntyre, S., Badawi, N., & Crowther, C. A. (2017). Antenatal and intrapartum interventions for preventing cerebral palsy: An overview of cochrane systematic reviews. *Cochrane Database of Systematic Reviews, 8*(8), CD012077.

Simpson, K. R. (2021). Perinatal patient safety and quality. In Simpson, K. R., Creehand, P. A., O'Brien-Abel, N., Roth, C. K., & Rohan, A. J. (Eds.), *Perinatal nursing* (5th ed., pp. 1–17). Wolters Kluwar.

Smid, M. C., Metz, T. D., & Gordon, A. J. (2019). Stimulant use in pregnancy – an under-recognized epidemic among pregnant women. *Clinical Obstetrics and Gynecology, 62*, 168–184.

Smith, L. M., & Santos, L. S. (2016). Prenatal Exposure: The effects of prenatal cocaine and methamphetamine exposure on the developing child. *Birth Defects Research (Part C), 108*, 142–146.

Smith, V., Seo, D., Warty, R., Payne, O., Salih, M., Chin, K. L., Ofori-Asenso, R., Krishnan, S., da Silva Costa, F., Vollenhoven, B., & Wallace, E. (2020). Maternal and neonatal outcomes associated with COVID-19 infection: A systematic review. *PLoS One, 15*(6), e0234187.

Sutter-Dallay, A. L., Bales, M., Pambrun, E., Glangeaud-Freudenthal, N. M., Wisner, K. L., & Verdoux, H. J (2015). Impact of prenatal exposure to psychotropic drugs on neonatal outcome in infants of mothers with serious psychiatric illnesses. *Clinical Psychiatry, 76*, 967–973.

Symes, A. (2016). Developmental outcomes. In MacDonald, M. G. & Seshia, M. M. (Eds.), *Avery's neonatology: Pathophysiology & management of the newborn* (7th ed., pp. 1157–1168). Wolters Kluwer.

Tailoi, C.-L., Gole, G. A., Quinn, G. E., Adamson, S. J., & Darlow, B. A. (2018). Pathophysiology, screening, and treatment of ROP: A multidisciplinary perspective. *Progress in Retinal and Eye Research, 62*, 77–119.

Tam, E. Y. W. (2018) Cerebellar injury in preterm infants. In Manto, M. & Huisman, T. A. G. (Eds.) *Handbook of clinical neurology* (Vol. 155, pp. 49–59). Elsevier.

Tam, W. H., Ma, R. C.W., Ozaki, R., Li, A. M., Chan, M. M., Yuen, L. Y., Lao, T. T. H., Yang, X., Ho, C. S., Tutino, G. E., & Chan, J. C. N. (2017). In utero exposure to maternal hyperglycemia increases childhood cardiometabolic risk in offspring. *Diabetes Care, 40*, 679–686.

Tappero, E. P., & Honeyfield, M. E. (2019). *Physical assessment of the newborn* (6th ed.). Springer.

Thadhani, R. I., & Young, B. (2018). Renal disorders. In Resnik, R., Lockwood, C. J., Moore, T. R., Greene, M. F., Copal, J. A., & Silver, R. M. (Eds.). *Creasy & resnik's maternal-fetal medicine: Principles and practice* (8th ed., pp. 1025–1044). Elsevier.

Umesawa, M., & Kobashi, G. (2017). Epidemiology of hypertensive disorders in pregnancy: Prevalence, risk factors, predictors, and prognosis. *Hypertension Research, 40*, 213–220.

Van den Bergh, B. R. H., van den Heuvel, M. I., Lahti, M., Braeken, M., de Rooij, S. R., Entringer, S., Hoyer, D., Roseboome, T., Räikkönen, K., King, S., & Schwab, M. (2020). Prenatal developmental origins of behavior and mental health: The influence of maternal stress in pregnancy. *Neuroscience and Biobehavioral Reviews, 117*, 26–64.

Vaughn, A., Reynolds, R., Zenge, J., & Marwan, A. I. (2020). Fetal surgery and NICU admissions, *Current Opinion in Pediatrics, 32*, 619–624.

Verani, J. R., McGee, L., Schrag, S. (2010). *Prevention of perinatal group B streptococcal disease--revised guidelines from CDC, 2010.*

Wastnedge, E. A. N., Reynolds, R. M., van Boeckel, S. R., Stock, S. J., Denison, F. C., Maybin, J. A, & Critchley, H. O. D. (2021). Pregnancy and COVID-19. *Physiological Reviews, 101*, 303–318.

Wedi, C. O., Kirtley, S., Hopewell, S., Corrigan, R., Kennedy, S. H., & Hemelaar, J. (2016). Perinatal outcomes associated with maternal HIV infection: A systematic review and meta-analysis. *Lancet HIV, 3*, e33–e48.

Wilson, J. G. (1977). Current status of teratology: General principles and mechanisms derived from animal studies. In Wilson, J. G. & Fraser, F. C. (Eds.). *Handbook of teratology: General principles and etiology.* Plenum.

Wojcik, M. H., Reimers, R., Poorvu, T., & Agrawal, P. B. (2020). Genetic diagnosis in the fetus. *Journal of Perinatology, 40*, 997–1006.

Wolf, H. T., Huusom, L. D., Henriksen, T. B., Hegaard, H. K., Brok, J., & Pinborg, A. (2020). Magnesium sulphate for fetal neuroprotection at imminent risk for preterm delivery: A systematic review with meta-analysis and trial sequential analysis. *BJOG: An Interatioal Journal for Obstetrics and Gynaecology, 127*, 1180–1188.

Xiong, T., Maheshwari, A., Neu, J., Ei-Saie, A., & Pammi, M. (2020). An overview of systematic reviews of randomized-controlled trials for preventing necrotizing enterocolitis in preterm infants. *Neonatology, 117*, 46–56.

Zhang, J., Li, J., Saucier, J. B., Feng, Y., Jiang, Y., Sinson, J., McCombs, A. K., Schmitt, E. S., Peacock, S., Chen, S., Dai, H., Ge, X., Wang, G., Shaw, C. A., Mei, H., Breman, A., Xia, F., Yang, Y., Purgason, A., … Eng, C. M. (2019). Noninvasive prenatal sequencing for multiple Mendelian monogenic disorders using circulating cell-free fetal DNA. *Nature Medicine, 25*, 439–447.

CHAPTER 11

Motor and Musculoskeletal Development of Neonates: A Dynamic Continuum

Teresa Gutierrez and Jane K. Sweeney

IFCDC Standard for Positioning and Touch

Standard 1: Positioning and Touch

- Babies in intensive care settings shall be positioned to support musculoskeletal, physiological, and behavioral stability.

Standard 2: Positioning and Touch

- Collaborative efforts among parents and intensive care unit (ICU) interprofessionals shall support optimal cranial shaping and prevent torticollis and skull deformity.

Standard 3: Positioning and Touch

- Body position shall be used as an ICU intervention for infants with gastrointestinal symptoms.

Standard 6: Systems thinking

- The interprofessional collaborative team should provide IFCDC through transition to home and continuing care for the baby and family to support the optimal physiologic and psychosocial health needs of the baby and family.

INTRODUCTION

Neonatal health professionals have a unique opportunity to observe early posture and movement in newborns and infants and to collaborate in promoting motor development and preventing or minimizing musculoskeletal deformity. In this chapter, the continuity of motor development is reviewed in the embryo, fetus, and neonate from the perspectives of musculoskeletal and tone maturation and movement patterns. Continuity and discontinuity are traced in the development of spontaneous movement, posture, and tone. The dynamic process of musculoskeletal shaping is analyzed, with clinical implications outlined for practitioners in neonatal developmental care and follow-up.

STRUCTURAL DEVELOPMENT

The chronology of musculoskeletal maturation is outlined from the structural perspective of skeletal, joint, and muscle development, followed by the functional perspective of posture, tone, and movement. These structural and functional elements create the foundation for coordinated motor behavior.

Skeleton

The skeletal system in the embryo is derived from mesoderm cells that, near the third week of gestation (day 20),
form *somites*, two blocks of mesoderm tissue located close to midline. The somites differentiate into sclerotome (vertebrae, ribs) and dermomyotome (skin, muscle) cells. The sclerotome has loosely organized mesenchymal (mesoderm) cells that further differentiate into the bone, cartilage, and connective tissue components of the skeletal system: fibroblasts, chondroblasts, osteoblasts, or myoblasts (Ditzenberger, 2018; Moore et al., 2020; Sadler, 2019).

Vertebrae and Ribs

The vertebral column is developed during the fourth week of gestation, when sclerotome cells in the somites migrate medially around the neural tube and notochord, forming the cartilaginous structures for vertebral arches and vertebral bodies. Mesenchymal costal processes on both sides of the thoracic vertebrae develop into ribs. Cartilaginous vertical bars form on the ends of the ribs, and rib pairs 1 to 7 fuse in midline to form the sternum. Fused vertebrae or ribs, hemivertebrae (Klippel–Feil syndrome), or defects in the vertebral arch (spina bifida) result from disrupted skeletal development in the fourth week of life (Moore et al., 2020; Sadler, 2019).

Limbs

In the fourth week of gestation, upper (day 26) and lower (day 28) limb buds appear when mesenchymal cells are activated and form a thick apical ectodermal ridge. The limb buds, initially resembling flippers, emerge into flatter hand and foot plates resembling paddles. In the fifth week the limbs elongate, with cartilage formation (chondrification) occurring in the sixth week. By the 12th week, primary ossification centers are present in the long bones, and at term the diaphysis (center shaft) usually is ossified, with the epiphyses (distal end) of bone remaining cartilaginous. At secondary ossification centers in the epiphyses, complete ossification varies and can extend through 20 to 30 years of age. Growth in thickness and density of the diaphysis is most rapid in the prenatal period, with spurts expected at 7 years of age and at puberty (Pax Lowes & Hay, 2017). During the fourth and fifth weeks of gestation, the following limb anomalies can occur: partial absence of limbs (meromelia, absence of radius), cleft hand or foot, polydactyly, syndactyly, and clubfoot deformities (Moore et al., 2020; Sadler, 2019). Bone growth and mineralization during gestation are dependent on the maternal supply of minerals, nitrogen, and vitamins. These factors contribute to rapid growth in length especially during the last trimester. In addition, the mechanical forces and bone loading from kicking movement against the uterine wall, resistance imposed by the amniotic fluid, and increase in muscle mass occurring during this period contribute to bone modeling and bone density in the fetus (Abrams & Tiosano, 2020; Ditzenberger, 2018; Eliakim et al., 2017; Hunter, 2010; Miller, 2003, 2005; Nowlan, 2015; Stalnaker & Poskey, 2016).

At birth, regardless of gestational age, the maternal supply of the nutrients needed for bone mineralization and strength is interrupted. An immediate drop in calcium appears within the first 24 to 48 hours as well as a change in mechanical forces requiring skeletal adaptation (Abrams & Tiosano, 2020; Ditzenberger, 2018; Rustico et al., 2014). In the full-term infant, gradual normalization of calcium levels occurs due to, among other factors, increased calcium intake with feedings (Abrams & Tiosano, 2020; Ditzenberger, 2018). The postnatal physiological hypocalcemia seen in full-term infants also takes place in the preterm infant and it relates inversely with birth weight and gestational age. Metabolic bone disease (MBD), also known as osteopenia of prematurity and neonatal rickets, is a common problem among low-birth-weight (LBW), very-low-birth-weight (VLBW), and extremely low-birth-weight (ELBW) infants. It is estimated that approximately 16% to 40% of VLBW infants and approximately 50% of ELBW infants develop MBD due to the abrupt interruption of maternal supply of calcium and other minerals as well as the placental hormones that support bone formation at a time when bone accretion is occurring at a fast pace in the prenatal environment. It is very difficult to maintain bone accretion at the same pace in the postnatal environment of the LBW, VLBW, and ELBW preterm infants (Abrams & Tiosano, 2020; Ditzenberger, 2018; El-Farrash et al., 2020; Eliakim et al., 2017; Sezer Efe et al., 2020).

In addition to the abrupt disruption of maternal nutritional support, preterm infants miss the mechanical forces and bone loading that occur in the last trimester resulting

from the physical activity against the resistance of the uterine wall and the amniotic fluid (Ditzenberger, 2018; Eliakim et al., 2017; Hunter, 2010; Miller, 2003, 2005; Stalnaker & Poskey, 2016). Immobility due to sedation during mechanical ventilation, exposure to medications that suppress or alter mineral levels including calcium, and often delayed establishment of enteral nutrition with fortified human milk or formula may contribute to MBD in the preterm infant (Abrams & Tiosano, 2020; Eliakim et al., 2017; Hunter, 2010; Rustico et al., 2014). As a result, preterm infants are at high risk for fracture of long bones and rib softening or fracture, which further increases the work of breathing and leads to prolonged mechanical ventilation. Great care is recommended when handling and repositioning this infant to prevent fractures (Abrams & Tiosano, 2020; Eliakim et al., 2017; Sezer Efe et al., 2020).

In term infants the most frequent neonatal fracture occurs at the clavicle with a reported incidence of 0.2% to 2.9% (Högberg et al., 2020) or 2 to 7 per 1,000 live births (Liu & Thompson, 2020). The most common cause is shoulder dystocia during delivery.

Lower-extremity fractures are less common in term infants and likely are related to underlying neuromuscular disorders that limit joint mobility (e.g., arthrogryposis multiplex congenita) or to bone and connective tissue disorders (e.g., osteogenesis imperfecta; Cardin, 2020). Some fractures inadvertently may be caused by stress and torque applied on bones during handling and positioning, especially when an underlying condition exists, such as osteogenesis imperfecta (Cardin, 2020).

Articular Structures

Derived from mesoderm and mesenchyme, joint structures develop in the sixth through the eighth week postmenstruation, when fibrous and cartilaginous connective tissue or synovial membranes develop between bones at articulation points. In joint capsules of extremities, mechanoreceptors are formed to assist in the perception of proprioception and in the direction and speed of movement. Joint molding is influenced by fetal movement, with continued shaping of joints occurring throughout childhood from forces of compression and movement (Cardin, 2020; Giorgi et al., 2014; Hepper, 2015; Moore et al., 2020; Nowlan, 2015; Pax Lowes & Hay, 2017; Verbruggen et al., 2018).

Development and alignment of limbs and joints can be altered by intrauterine conditions, including amniotic banding, irregular uterine shape, insufficient amniotic fluid, multiple gestation of more than twins, and breech presentation (Cardin, 2020; Liu & Thompson, 2020; Nowlan, 2015; Verbruggen et al., 2018). The presence of maturation-related hypotonia and ligamentous laxity predisposes the preterm infant to malalignment of the lower extremities during the neonatal period and may have an effect in the development of posture and movement over time (Teledevara et al., 2019; Vungarala & Rajeswari, 2018). Connective tissue elasticity may also predispose preterm infants to developing joint effusion or subluxation if vigorous passive range-of-motion maneuvers are administered (Sweeney, 2007).

Essential life support equipment used in the neonatal intensive care unit (NICU) can be a barrier to variability in positioning of fragile neonates and a limitation to their spontaneous movement. Preterm infants in the NICU may experience decreased variety of positions with prolonged pressure and compression on limbs, head, and trunk.

These positional dynamics can lead to changes in alignment and molding of the skeletal system, increasing the risk for positional deformities (Byrne & Garber, 2013; Danner-Bowman & Cardin, 2015; McManus et al., 2017; Ferrari et al., 2007).

Infants born at term have decreased extensibility and range of motion (ROM) in hip, knee, and elbow extension related to intrauterine crowding in the last trimester (Table 11-1). This transient decrease in passive ROM is considered normal in full-term infants, and it resolves spontaneously in the following sequence: knees and elbows within 3 months and hips within 6 to 12 months (Forero et al., 1989; Hoffer, 1980; Walker, 1992; Waugh et al., 1983). Joint mobility and passive ROM in infants born before the third trimester are typically much greater due to maturation-related hypotonia and lax ligaments (Allen & Capute, 1990; de Groot, 2000; Dubowitz & Dubowitz, 1999; Farmania et al., 2017; da Silva & Nunes, 2005; Teledevara et al., 2019; Vungarala & Rajeswari, 2018).

Muscle Tissue

Skeletal muscles emerge from myoblasts differentiated from mesoderm in the myotome area of somites. Myoblasts form elongated, multinucleated myotubes at 5 to 10 weeks and myofilaments (muscle fibers) at 10 to 20 weeks (Moore et al., 2020; Sadler, 2019). By 20 weeks postmenstrual age (PMA), muscle tissue differentiates into slow (type I) and fast (type II) twitch fibers (Grove, 1989; Sans, 1987. High-oxidative type I muscle fibers continue to develop while preterm infants are in NICUs but remain at decreased ratio to the low-oxidative type II fibers. Predisposition to muscular fatigue, particularly in respiratory muscles, may be related to this lower

ratio of high-oxidative type I fibers in preterm neonates. Low postural tone and difficulty sustaining postures may also be related in part to muscle fiber immaturity in preterm (compared with term) infants (Cardin, 2020; Teledevara et al., 2019). At term gestation, type I and type II muscle fibers are expected to be equal in number and to resemble the pattern in adult muscles (Dreyfus & Schapira, 1979; Dubowitz, 1965). Although overall numbers of muscle fibers continue to grow during the first year of life, muscle growth increases in length and diameter by addition of myofilaments. The eventual size of muscles is influenced by a combination of gender, genetics, nutrition, blood supply, innervation, and exercise throughout childhood (Pax Lowes & Hay 2017).

PRENATAL MOVEMENT

Observation and assessment of fetal movement and behavior were studied by early investigators who relied primarily on access to aborted fetuses or nonviable preterm newborn infants for analysis and documentation of fetal posture and tone (Gesell, 1945; Humphrey, 1978; Saint-Anne Dargassies, 1977). These early fetal and neonatal movement investigators were challenged by the absence of fetal ultrasound for prenatal observation and limitations of intensive care technology in the 1960s and 1970s to keep LBW infants alive. The comparatively limited neonatal physiologic support and higher neonatal morbidity and mortality in that era influenced the variability of posture, movement, and tone in the infants available for study (Albers & Jorch, 1994; Einspieler et al., 2008; Prechtl & Nolte, 1984; Towen, 1990). Advances in technology have created opportunities for researchers to observe, classify, and document the development of prenatal movement longitudinally (Brown et al., 1997; de Vries et al., 2001; de Vries et al., 1984; Einspieler et al., 2004; Einspieler et al., 2008; Hadders-Algra, 2008; Kozuma et al., 1997; Kurjak et al., 2012; Luchinger et al., 2008; Prechtl, 1984, 1989, 1997b; Roodenburg et al., 1991).

The earliest movements of the embryo are identified at 7 to 7.5 weeks PMA and are characterized by slow neck extension. Startles and general movements follow this motor activity. Startles are characterized by fast, phasic contraction of all limbs with secondary involvement of the neck and

	Forero et al. (1989)	Haas et al. (1973)	Hoffer (1980)	Waugh et al. (1983)
TABLE 11-1 Transient Range of Motion Limitation in Infants Born at Term				
Hip	17°–39°	10°–75°	50°–80°	21.7°–68.3°
Range	29.9°	27.9°	*	46.3°
Mean				
Knee	*	*	0°–35°	0°–43.3°
Range	*	*	*	15.3°
Mean				
Elbow	*	*	0°–30°	*
Range	*	*	*	*
Mean				

*Not reported.

trunk (Frudiger et al., 2021; Hadders-Algra, 2018; Hepper, 2015). General movements follow a distinct, complex pattern of whole-body involvement with fluid movement quality (Einspieler et al., 2004; Einspieler et al., 2008).

Einspieler et al., 2012; Frudiger et al., 2021; Hadders-Algra, 2008; Luchinger et al., 2008. The onset of general movements has been documented in the fetus at 9 weeks PMA, followed by rapid expansion of movement patterns and repertoire. Isolated movement of the extremities appears shortly after 9 weeks PMA, followed by a variety of head movements, including neck rotation and extension. Breathing movements begin between 10 and 12 weeks, accompanied by jaw opening and closing. By 13 weeks, suckling movements begin in rhythmic bursts, followed by swallowing. The rate of suckling and swallowing movements present at 14 weeks is believed to be similar to the rate present in term infants (de Vries et al., 1984; Ianniruberto & Tajani, 1981; Lu et al., 2016; Miller et al., 2003; Prechtl, 1997a). Fetal swallowing has an important functional role in regulating amniotic fluid volume (Miller, Sonies, & Macedonia, 2003; Prechtl, 1997a). Fetal movement during the first half of pregnancy has been well documented over the last 3 decades. Advances in real-time ultrasound and other technologies have made it possible to quantify and describe fetal movement during the second half of pregnancy (Amiel-Tison et al., 2006; Einspieler et al., 2012; Kozuma et al., 1997; Roodenburg et al., 1991; Sparling, 1993; Sparling et al., 1999). This process of clarifying and describing characteristics of fetal movement has led to discrete documentation of fetal movement sequences and assessment of fetal wellness through movement analysis (Kozuma et al., 1997; Lai et al., 2016; Sparling et al., 1999; Sparling & Wilhelm, 1993; Stanger et al., 2017).

The continuity of fetal and neonatal movement from prenatal to postnatal life has been amply documented by numerous investigators (de Vries et al., 1984; Einspieler et al., 2004; Einspieler et al., 2008; Hadders-Algra et al., 1997; Luchinger et al., 2008; Prechtl, 1984, 2001; Saint-Anne Dargassies, 1977; Stanojevic et al., 2012; Stanojevic et al., 2012). Prechtl led the way with a body of research inferring that spontaneous fetal movements are endogenously generated and have recognizable patterns that change over time, with qualitative features highly predictive of brain function (Hadders-Algra, 2018; Einspieler et al., 2012; Fagard et al., 2018; Kakebeeke et al., 1998; Prechtl, 1997a, 2001). The quality of general movements is altered by changes in brain function, and the continuity of motor development is disrupted (Amiel-Tison et al., 2006; Cioni et al., 1997; Einspieler et al., 2012; Einspieler et al., 2004; Einspieler et al., 1997; Lai et al., 2016; Prechtl, 1997a, 1997b, 2001).

The technology used in NICUs not only supports survival in preterm infants but also creates vulnerability because it disrupts motor development continuity (Stanojevic et al., 2012). These infants must cope unexpectedly with the effects of gravity, potential periods of sedation-related suppression of movement, and postural adaptation to respiratory and infusion equipment. In NICU environments, infant body and extremity alignment and the quantity, frequency, and intensity of spontaneous movement are disrupted intermittently (Ferrari et al., 2007; Stanojevic et al., 2012). Early use of developmental care practices in positioning, handling, and environmental modification provides critical support to the continuity and quality of movement in infants during intensive care (Eskandari et al., 2020; Ferrari et al., 2007; King & Norton, 2017; Kitase et al., 2017; Nakano et al., 2010; Ullenhag et al., 2009; Vaivre-Douret et al., 2004; Zahed et al., 2015).

DEVELOPMENT OF POSTURE, MOVEMENT, AND TONE

From the early development and continuity of fetal movement, infants have an innate repertoire of movement that evolves during a term pregnancy. The movement experience of a term infant differs from that of a preterm infant. The infant born at term has moved within a well-contained and stable environment, receiving a variety of proprioceptive and sensory inputs under ideal physiologic conditions. Term infants are equipped with effective muscle power, posture, tone, and movement to respond in dynamic interaction with the extrauterine environment. When birth occurs prematurely, muscle tone, posture, and movement continue to develop, but the infant now must adapt to the influence of gravity and tactile and proprioceptive stimuli from prolonged lying (weight bearing) on a mattress before the musculoskeletal system is equipped to deal with these forces (de Groot, 2000; de Groot et al., 1991, 1993; de Groot et al., 1992; Danner-Bowman & Cardin, 2015; Einspieler et al., 2004; Ferrari et al., 2007; Hadders-Algra, 2008; Luchinger et al., 2008; Prechtl & Nolte, 1984; Stanojevic et al., 2012). Muscle tone is viewed as passive tone and as active or postural tone. Passive tone is measured by the amount of resistance offered in response to passive movement (e.g., traction and recoil).

Pronounced, passive flexor tone in term infants is related to the mechanical constraint of uterine-wall resistance during fetal growth in the last trimester. At term, equivalent-age preterm infants do not reach the same level of flexion as infants born at term gestation (Dubowitz & Dubowitz, 1999; Pineda et al., 2013; Ricci et al., 2008). The biomechanical advantage of strong "physiologic" flexor tone at birth enhances head control, midline extremity posture, and suck–swallow proficiency. Postural or active tone involves sustained muscle contraction necessary for maintaining posture against gravity and is fluid, adaptive, and constantly changing in response to movement (Brown et al., 1997; de Groot, 2000).

The development of infant posture and tone has been an ongoing study topic (Hadders-Algra, 2018; Allen, 1996; Allen & Capute, 1990; Amiel-Tison & Grenier, 1983; de Groot et al., 1991; Dubowitz & Dubowitz, 1999; Dusing et al., 2014; Farmania et al., 2017; Grant-Beuttler et al., 2009; Hadders-Algra, 2008; Hadders-Algra, 2018; Pineda et al., 2013; Ricci et al., 2008; Saint-Anne Dargassies, 1977). The consensus is that preterm infants are hypotonic, and the subsequent development of flexor tone follows a caudad to cephalad progression. Dubowitz and Dubowitz reported a longitudinal investigation of the progression of flexor tone in 57 low-risk, preterm infants at 28 to 35 weeks PMA. They measured passive extremity tone by traction, recoil, and popliteal angles. Earlier assumptions were confirmed on the chronology of passive and active tone, including flexor tone progression in a caudad to cephalad direction. Allen and Capute documented the beginning of leg flexion at 29 to 32 weeks and arm flexion at 35 to 37 weeks. Because of this maturation-related hypotonia, caregivers play an important role in creating postural support for extremity flexion in legs (in infants <29 to 32 weeks PMA) and arms (in infants <35 to 37 weeks PMA). In a series of studies directed by de Groot et al. (1991, 1992, 1993), a distinction was made between active muscle power and passive tone during examination of posture and movement in preterm infants. The researchers concluded that preterm infants have low muscle tone, measured by resistance to traction or passive movement. Differences in muscle power between preterm and term infants were attributed to differences in weight and muscle mass. They noted that some preterm infants appeared to develop exaggerated, active muscle power specially along the paraspinals and the scapulae expressed by hyperextension of the trunk with scapular adduction When preterm infants were placed predominantly in the supine position they demonstrated imbalanced muscle power regulation resulting in hyperextension of the trunk and shoulders (de Groot et al., 1992; de Groot, 2000; Plantinga et al., 1997; Samson & de Groot, 2000; Sweeney & Gutierrez, 2002). Those motor behaviors are now minimized due to current practices in neonatal positioning, including nested containment and swaddling. (Eskandari et al., 2020; Ferrari et al., 2007; King & Norton, 2017; Kitase et al., 2017; Nakano et al., 2010; Vaivre-Douret et al., 2004; Zahed et al., 2015).

The stress induced by abrupt physiologic changes, pain, or discomfort from essential interventions often results in disorganized movement and posture (Altimier & Phillips, 2016; Ferrari et al., 2007; Stanojevic et al., 2012). Neonatal abstinence syndrome (NAS) and neonatal opioid withdrawal syndrome (NOWS) also have an effect on posture and movement specifically in full-term infants (Alloco et al., 2016). Restlessness, tremors, jerky movements, jitteriness, and hypertonicity are among the motor signs of NAS and NOWS reflecting transient central nervous system dysfunction (Alloco et al., 2016; D'Apolito, 2009; Finnegan et al., 1975; Hamdan, 2008; Hudak, 2020; Hudak et al., 2012; Mactier & Hamilton, 2020; McCarty et al., 2019). The stress induced by these symptoms affects the quality of spontaneous movement and disrupts continuity of motor development. Positioning and postural support throughout the withdrawal period are essential to minimize motor and behavioral disorganization. Swaddling, holding, skin-to-skin care and avoiding abrupt changes in an infant's environment are among the recommendations for nonpharmacological management of infants with signs and symptoms of NAS (Grisham et al., 2019; Hamdan, 2008; McCarty et al., 2019; Ryan et al., 2019; Wachman et al., 2018).

By the time preterm infants reach term equivalent age, they are expected to demonstrate the following posture and motor competencies (Dubowitz & Dubowitz, 1999):

- Maintain semiflexed extremity posture in supine and prone positions.
- Move head side to side in supine and prone positions.
- Lift head in prone and hold head erect momentarily in supported sitting.
- Maintain head in line with trunk during pull-to-sit maneuver.
- Bring hands toward midline intermittently (e.g., chest, mouth).
- Sustain rhythmic suck, swallow, and breathing sequence.
- Demonstrate movements that support behavioral state regulation (e.g., hand-to-mouth, foot-to-foot holding).

Although preterm infants may not demonstrate the same level of active, postural tone as term infants at 40 weeks' PMA, neonatal caregivers can create supportive environments to help them approach similar postural stability and midline movement. Ferrari et al. (2007) investigated the effects of nested containment on posture and spontaneous movement in 10 healthy infants observed at 30 to 33, 34 to 36, and 37 to 40 weeks PMA. A significant difference ($p < .05$) was found on the quality of spontaneous motor behavior in the infants placed in nested containment compared with infants not placed in nested containment. They concluded that this form of containment promotes flexion of the arms and legs with adduction of the shoulders and midline movements. In more recent studies, the consistent use of nested containment and swaddling have resulted in improved symmetry, flexed posture, and midline orientation (Eskandari et al., 2020; Kitase et al., 2017; Madlinger-Lewis et al., 2014).

CLINICAL IMPLICATIONS FOR NEONATAL CARE

Growth and plasticity of the musculoskeletal system is like a double-edged sword capable of positive or negative effects. Neonatal health professionals can use the rapid neonatal growth process and joint and tissue laxity not found in later childhood to promote musculoskeletal alignment and motor organization while infants remain in NICUs (Byrn & Garber, 2013; McManus et al., 2017; Sweeney & Gutierrez, 2002). This rapid growth, combined with inattention to body alignment, can contribute to striking positional deformities in the skull and extremities in a remarkably short amount of time.

Musculoskeletal Shaping

Shaping of the musculoskeletal system occurs during each body position experienced by infants in the NICU. Supporting skeletal integrity of LBW and ELBW infants is challenging amid multiple equipment obstacles and handling limits dictated by fluctuating physiologic stability. Skull deformity and extremity malalignment (Table 11-2) are not uncommon and result from the combination of maturation-related hypotonia and neonatal care procedures such as prolonged ventilation.

Positional deformities disrupt the continuity of musculoskeletal development begun in utero and shaped in the NICU environment, but they can be minimized. When a variety of recumbent positions and nesting are provided within the constraints of neonatal equipment, infants can experience varying forces, pressure, and varying somatosensory experiences for balanced muscle power regulation of the trunk and shoulders, coordination of movement, and organization of posture with flexion (Byrne & Garber, 2013; Danner-Bowman & Cardin, 2015; Eskandari et al., 2020; Ferrari et al., 2007; Madlinger-Lewis et al., 2014; Nakano et al., 2010; Sweeney & Gutierrez, 2002).

Current evidence and long-term outcomes support the consistent use of nested containment and loose swaddling to promote organized motor behaviors with extremity semiflexion and midline orientation. Neonatal positioning, a core measure of the Neonatal Integrative Developmental Care Model, also has physiological benefits including improved sleep patterns and stress reduction (Abdeyazdan et al., 2016; Altimier & Phillips, 2016; Kahraman et al., 2018; King & Norton, 2017; Reyhani et al., 2016; Valizadeh et al., 2016; Zahed et al., 2015.

Goals of positioning:

- Optimize alignment: neutral neck–trunk; semiflexed, midline extremity posture; hands together; neutral foot alignment.

- Support posture and movement within "containment boundaries" of rolls, swaddling blankets, or other positioning aids; avoid creating a barrier to spontaneous movement.

- Modify positioning and handling to promote regulation of behavioral states that enhance short-duration interaction and sleep states that promote growth.

- Offer positions that allow controlled, individualized exposure to proprioceptive, tactile, visual, or auditory stimuli

- Monitor for signs of behavioral stress from potential overstimulation.

Transition infant to back to sleep position as soon as infant is physiologically and developmentally ready in preparation for discharge (AAP Task Force on SIDS, 2016; AAP Committee on Fetus and Newborn, 2008; Altimier & Phillips, 2016; Bagwell, 2020; Browne et al., 2020; NANN, 2019; Spilker et al., 2016).

These goals can be achieved using swaddling, commercial or noncommercial postural devices, and caregiver hand support during procedures (Altimier & Phillips, 2016; Kahraman et al., 2018; Kitase et al., 2017).

The incidence of positional deformities such as dolichocephaly (also known as scaphocephaly), brachycephaly, and plagiocephaly is high among preterm infants at term equivalent age (Danner-Bowman & Cardin, 2015; Dunsirn et al., 2016; Ifflaender et al., 2013; McCarty et al., 2017; Nuysink et al., 2012, 2013; Yang et al., 2019). The essential medical care to support preterm infants in the NICU often requires limited positioning options. For infants under 32 weeks of gestation, side lying and prone are the preferred positions.

Current evidence supports the use of prone position to improve gastric emptying and oxygenation (Abdeyazdan et al., 2010; Ameri et al., 2018; Chen et al., 2013; Cheraghia et al., 2020; Ghorbani et al., 2013; Gouna et al., 2013; Jagadeeswari & Soniya, 2020; Khatony et al., 2019).

Bilateral flattening of the skull develops as a result of pressure from weight bearing and influence of gravity on a very pliable skull (Danner-Bowman & Cardin, 2015; Gouna et al., 2013; Ifflaender et al., 2013; McCarty et al., 2017; McCarty et al., 2018; Yang et al., 2019).

Prevention through careful positioning in the NICU has gained attention, and emerging evidence indicates that early intervention minimizes positional deformities (Byrne & Garber, 2013; Danner-Bowman & Cardin, 2015; Madlinger-Lewis et al., 2014; McCarty et al., 2018; Mehmood et al., 2020). Nevertheless, a positional preference and deformational plagiocephaly remain prevalent at term equivalent age (Danner-Bowman & Cardin, 2015; Ifflaender et al., 2014; McCarty et al., 2017; Nuysink et al., 2012, 2013; Yang et al., 2019).

Skull shaping continues to evolve after NICU discharge and can be influenced by caregiving practices at home. For example, overuse of infant seats and limited prone play activities can perpetuate positional deformities and warrant close follow-up of infant head shape following discharge (Danner-Bowman & Cardin, 2015; Ifflaender et al., 2014; McCarty et al., 2017; Rogers, 2011).

Infant and Family-Centered Developmental Care (IFCDC) calls for early and ongoing parental involvement in care of their infant, including components of positioning and touch (Browne et al., 2020; Roué et al., 2017). Teaching families the principles of optimal musculoskeletal alignment and positioning in the NICU allows them to practice under supervision to prepare for caregiving after discharge. Recommendations for positioning to support musculoskeletal integrity and motor development include the following:

- Vary the direction of the head turn for sleeping in supine to prevent plagiocephaly.

- Place and support infant's head in midline position with lateral thin blanket rolls (extending along the side of trunk) in car seats, "bouncy" seats, and swings.

- Limit use of the infant seat and replace with play on the floor in prone with a roll under the arms and upper chest to assist head lifting and weight support on arms.

- Discuss the value of playing on the floor including the prone play position for strengthening the neck, arms, and trunk in preparation for rolling, sitting, and standing.

- Warn of injury risk associated with infant walkers and their impact on development (Sims et al., 2018).

- Reinforce the importance of interdisciplinary follow-up for musculoskeletal and neurodevelopmental monitoring. Preterm infants are at risk for developmental delay and motor impairments that may lead to disability (AAP Committee on Fetus and Newborn, 2008; Bjorg & Bartlett, 2008; Brachio et al., 2020; Brown et al., 2020; Doyle et al., 2014; Purdy et al., 2015; Snider et al., 2008, 2009).

TABLE 11-2 Musculoskeletal Malalignment and Functional Limitations in Infants

Positional Deformity	Consequences	Functional Limitations
Plagiocephaly	Unilateral, flat, occipital region Head-turn preference High risk for torticollis	Limited visual orientation from asymmetric head position Delayed midline head control
Scaphocephaly or dolichocephaly	Bilateral, flat, parietal, and temporal regions	Difficulty developing active midline head control in supine from narrowing of occipital region
Brachycephaly	Flattening across the back of the head	Results from prolonged supine position and may interfere with head turning, visual following, and rolling
Hyperextended neck and retracted shoulders	Shortened neck extensor muscles Overstretched neck flexor muscles Excessive cervical lordosis Shortened scapular adductor muscles	Interferes with head centering and midline arm movement in supine Interferes with head control in prone and sitting Limited downward visual gaze
"Frog" legs	Shortened hip abductor muscles and iliotibial bands Increased external tibial torsion	Interferes with movement transitions in and out of sitting and prone positions Interferes with hip stability in four-point crawling Prolonged wide-based gait with excessive out-toeing
Everted feet	Overstretched ankle invertor muscles Altered foot alignment from muscle imbalance	Pronated foot position on standing Retained immature "foot flat" gait with potential delay in development of "heel-to-toe" gait pattern from excessive pronation

Adapted from Sweeney, J. K., & Gutierrez, T. (2002). "Musculoskeletal implications of preterm infant positioning in the NICU." *Journal of Perinatal and Neonatal Nursing, 16*(1), 58–70.

■ Advise expedient follow-up if parents notice signs of head flattening, persistent lateral head tilt, strong head-turn preference, or asymmetric arm use. Some infants require specific positioning recommendations from a physical therapist to optimize motor development after discharge and early management of plagiocephaly and muscular torticollis (Danner-Bowman & Cardin, 2015; Ifflaender et al., 2014; McCarty et al., 2017; Rogers, 2011; Sweeney & Gutierrez, 2002; van Vlimmeren et al., 2008).

EARLY INTERVENTION AND INTERDISCIPLINARY FOLLOW-UP

Preterm infants with LBW and ELBW are widely recognized to be at high risk for neurodevelopmental impairments and warrant early identification and follow-up. These impairments range from developmental coordination disorder to cerebral palsy (Adams-Chapman et al., 2018; Anderson et al., 2020; Cheong et al., 2020; Dannemiller et al., 2020; Doyle et al., 2014; Evensen et al., 2020; Litt et al., 2020; McGowan & Vohr, 2019; Rogers & Hintz, 2016). Early assessment is useful to plan follow-up and to identify infants at the highest risk for neurodevelopmental impairments so they can be appropriately referred for neonatal follow-up and early intervention. Many tools are available to assess all aspects of infant development including oral motor skills. The decision of when to assess the infant and which tool to use involves a collaboration with all members of the team including the parents and an understanding of the infant's maturity and readiness for assessment at any given time (Byrne & Campbell, 2013; Noble & Boyd, 2012).

Limited specific recommendations or guidelines are available for when and how to follow up LBW and ELBW infants after discharge. The American Academy of Pediatrics (AAP) issued a mandate for all level III nurseries to provide the means for discharge and follow-up for high-risk infants. Recommendations for timing and intervals were not specific, leaving the follow-up schedule design to each institution (AAP Committee on Fetus and Newborn, 2008). Doyle et al., 2014 recommend using the areas of development and outcomes to be assessed as a guide for defining the age, frequency, and intervals. Another important consideration is the setting in which the follow-up takes place. A well-staffed setting with good resources could provide comprehensive assessment addressing all areas of development. A busy primary medical practitioner may rely on screening tools and questionnaires available in an office setting (Doyle et al., 2014). Finally, family resources and the ability to comply with follow-up appointments must be considered.

Social disparities in income and education may be a barrier to follow-up. Targeting these families early during hospitalization and providing education are recommended to decrease the dropout rate (Ballantyne et al., 2012; Brachio et al., 2020; Craig et al., 2015; Hintz et al., 2019; Swearingen et al., 2020).

Follow-up clinics targeting specific age groups may be beneficial. A follow-up visit at 2, 4, 8, 12, and 18 months can offer opportunities to systematically monitor musculoskeletal alignment, growth, and neuromotor maturation as infants acquire and refine upright posture, movement through basic positions, stance, ambulation, and manipulative hand skills. Refer to Table 11-3 for signs of musculoskeletal or neuromotor abnormality that indicate the need for comprehensive examination by a pediatric physical therapist and possible

TABLE 11-3 Motor Impairment "Red Flags" During NICU Follow-Up

2 Months[a]	4 Months[a]	8 Months[a]	12 Months[a]
Persistent asymmetrical head position; risk for plagiocephaly and torticollis Absent midline orientation (even when visual stimulation is present) Jerky or stiff movements of extremities Excessive neck or trunk hyperextension in supine position	Poor midline head control in supine position Difficulty engaging hands at midline and in reaching for dangling toy Persistent fisting of hands. Difficulty lifting head and supporting weight on arms in prone position Trunk hypertonicity or hypotonicity; resistance to passive movement in extremities Persistent, dominant asymmetrical tonic neck reflex ("fencing" position of arms) Stiffly extended or "scissored" legs, with weight bearing on toes in supported standing	Inability to sit and roll independently Inability to transfer objects between hands Persistent asymmetry of extremities with differences in muscle tone and motor skill Hypertonicity of trunk or extremities	Inability to pull to stand, four-point crawl, walk around furniture Movement between basic positions Persistent asymmetry of control in extremities

[a]Ages corrected for prematurity.

referral for immediate intervention with a strong family teaching component.

Examining developmental performance in communication and cognition is critical to identify delays early so expedient referral for intervention services can occur. Sensitive management of family concerns and current levels of support (emotional, financial, knowledge) needed for ongoing complex care are important parts of the follow-up process. In addition to routine primary care needs, continuous medical management is required for specific conditions resulting from preterm birth such as feeding difficulty or cardiopulmonary sequelae. An interdisciplinary approach that uses a developmental care team is the ideal way to provide follow-up for an infant at risk for motor impairment (Doyle et al., 2014; Purdy et al., 2015). A pediatrician, nurse practitioner, nurse, physical therapist, or occupational therapist can coordinate initial care with a family. Social work, speech pathology, audiology, psychology, neurology, clinical nutrition, pediatric gastroenterology, and orthopedics may be indicated. Families are an integral part of the interdisciplinary team and may be the first caregivers to detect emerging functional difficulties in moving or positioning their infant during dressing, bathing, or feeding at home. The care team relies on family concerns and observations to prioritize the case management process.

Table 11-4 guides neonatal practitioners on care giving practices that support musculoskeletal integrity and motor organization.

TABLE 11-4 Practice Recommendations for Musculoskeletal Alignment

Type	Recommendation	Level of Evidence	References
Prevention	Change body position in infants to reduce risk for skull deformity, retracted shoulder/arm malalignment, and excessive hip external rotation (out-toe) posture	IV	Byrne & Garber, 2013; Danner-Bowman & Cardin, 2015; Davis et al., 1993; Georgieff & Bernbaum, 1986; Gorga et al., 1988; Hutchison et al., 2004; Madlinger-Lewis et al., 2014; McCarty et al., 2018; Mehmood et al., 2020
Intervention	Provide nested containment to support body posture and movement toward midline flexion Change head position to minimize skull deformity Place infants with reflux on left side or prone for the first hour after feeding; refer infants for pediatric physical therapy services at NICU discharge if asymmetrical positional preference of the head and neck is present	II, IV, IV III	Corvaglia et al., 2007; Downs et al., 1991; Ewer et al., 1999; Ferrari et al., 2007; Hutchison et al., 2004; McCarty et al., 2018; Tobin et al., 1997; van Vlimmeren et al., 2008

Note: Level II = evidence obtained from at least one well-designed RCT; level III = evidence obtained from well-designed controlled trials without randomization; level IV = evidence from well-designed case–control and cohort studies.

CONCLUSION

In this chapter, the chronology and continuity of motor development were discussed in relation to musculoskeletal maturation; prenatal movement sequences; and neonatal posture, tone, and movement competencies. Implications for care and interdisciplinary monitoring were reviewed and updated with current evidenced-based strategies for positioning and handling of infants at risk for musculoskeletal or motor impairment. Standards for infant and family-centered care were integrated highlighting the importance of early parent participation and education.

Each member of the multidisciplinary team caring for LBW and ELBW infants in the NICU brings their unique area of expertise to the care and management of these infants.

Collectively we have a unique window of opportunity to help shape the musculoskeletal system and motor organization of infants requiring intensive care and to monitor skeletal alignment and motor behavior during the first year of life. Neonatal nurses must take advantage of infant musculoskeletal plasticity through strategic positioning and handling to prevent or minimize deformity in LBW and VLBW infants. By looking for early signs of potential movement abnormalities nurses can advocate for individualized infant and family-centered developmentally appropriate intervention. Neonatal nurses and all members of the interdisciplinary team must make time for creative collaboration on interventions to advance, analyze, and refine neonatal practice including early parental participation and education for a successful transition from the NICU to home and beyond.

Potential Research Questions

Prevention

- More evidence is needed to document the effectiveness of positioning aids to prevent plagiocephaly:
  - What is the most effective positioning aid to prevent plagiocephaly?

Intervention

- More evidence is needed to document the effectiveness of commercially available products for gentle swaddling to promote behavioral and motor organization.
  - What differences are found with the use of standard blankets for swaddling compared with commercially available products in term and preterm infants?
- The evidence for nonpharmacological management (i.e., positioning, feeding) to decrease the frequency of gastroesophageal reflux disease (GERD) is inconclusive in the recent literature (Eichenwald, 2018; Gulati & Jadcherla, 2019).
  - What is the most effective positioning plan for infants with a confirmed diagnosis of GERD?
  - What is the most effective feeding plan for these infants?

Outcomes

- Long-term outcome studies are limited on infants with positional cranial deformities (dolichocephaly, brachycephaly, and plagiocephaly).
  - What are the long-term consequences of acquired positional cranial deformity?
  - What is the impact of cranial deformity on brain volume and shape?

REFERENCES

Abdeyazdan, Z., Mohammadian-Ghahfarokhi, M., Ghazavi, Z., & Mohammadizadeh, M. (2016). Effects of nesting and swaddling on the sleep duration of premature infants hospitalized in neonatal intensive care units. *Iranian Journal of Nursing and Midwifery Research, 21*(5), 552–556. https://doi.org/10.4103/1735-9066.193422

Abdeyazdan, Z., Nematollahi, M., Ghazavi, Z., & Mohhamadizadeh, M. (2010). The effects of supine and prone positions on oxygenation in premature infants undergoing mechanical ventilation. *Iranian Journal of Nursing and Midwifery Research, 15*(4), 229–233.

Abrams, A. S., & Tiosano, D. (2020). Disorders of calcium, phosphorus and magnesium metabolism in the neonate. In Martin, R. J., Fanaroff, A. A., & Walsh, M. C. (Eds.), *Fanaroff & Martin's neonatal-perinatal medicine: Diseases of the fetus and infant* (Vol. 2, 11th ed., pp. 1611–1642). Elsevier.

Adams-Chapman, I., Heyne, R. J., DeMauro, S. B., Duncan, A. F., Hintz, S. R., Pappas, A, Vohr, B. R., McDonald, S. A., Das, A., Newman, J. E., & Higgins, R. D. (2018). Neurodevelopmental impairment among extremely preterm infants in the Neonatal Research Network. *Pediatrics, 141*(5), e20173091.

Albers, S., & Jorch, G. (1994). Prognostic significance of spontaneous motility in very immature preterm infants under intensive care treatment. *Biology of the Neonate, 66*, 182–187.

Allen, M. C. (1996). Preterm development. In Capute, A. J. & Accardo, P. J. (Eds.), *Developmental disabilities in infancy and childhood: The spectrum of developmental disabilities* (Vol. 2, 2nd ed., pp. 31–47). Paul H. Brookes.

Allen, M. C., & Capute, A. J. (1990). Tone and reflex development before term. *Pediatrics, 85*(3 Pt. 2), 393–399.

Allocco, E., Melker, M., Rojas-Miguez, F., Bradley, C., Hahn, K. A., & Wachman, E. M. (2016). Comparison of Neonatal abstinence syndrome manifestations in preterm versus term opioid-exposed infants. *Advances in Neonatal Care: Official Journal of the National Association of Neonatal Nurses, 16*(5), 329–336. https://doi.org/10.1097/ANC.0000000000000320

Altimier, L., & Phillips, R. (2016). The neonatal integrative developmental care Model: Advanced clinical applications of the seven core measures for neuroprotective family-centered developmental care. *Newborn and Infant Nursing Reviews, 16*, pp. 230–244. https://doi.org/10.1053/j.nainr.2016.09.030

American Academy of Pediatrics Committee on Fetus and Newborn (2008). Hospital discharge of the high-risk neonate. *Pediatrics, 122*(5), 1119–1126. https://doi.org/10.1542/peds.2008-2174

Ameri, G., Rostami, S., Baniasadi, H., Aboli, B., & Ghorbani, F. (2018). The effect of prone position on gastric residuals in preterm infants. *Journal of Pharmaceutical Research International, 22*(2), 1–6. https://doi.org/10.9734/JPRI/2018/40433

Amiel-Tison, C., Gosselin, J. & Kurjak, A.. (2006). Neurosonography in the second half of fetal life: A neonatologist's point of view. *Journal of Perinatal Medicine, 34.* 437–446. https://doi.org/10.1515/JPM.2006.088

Amiel-Tison, C., & Grenier, A. (1983). *Neurologic evaluation of the newborn infant* (J. J. Steichen, P. Steichen-Asch, & C. Paxton Braun, Trans.). Masson Publishing.

Anderson, P. J., Treyvaud, K., & Spittle, A. J. (2020). Early developmental interventions for infants born very preterm - what works? *Seminars in Fetal & Neonatal Medicine, 25*(3), 101119. https://doi.org/10.1016/j.siny.2020.101119

Ballantyne, M., Stevens, B., Guttmann, A., Willan, A. R., & Rosenbaum, P. (2012). Transition to neonatal follow-up programs: Is attendance a problem? *The Journal of Perinatal & Neonatal Nursing, 26*(1), 90–98. https://doi.org/10.1097/JPN.0b013e31823f900b

Bagwell, G. A. (2020). NANN's guideline for safe sleep executive summary. *Advances in Neonatal Care: Official Journal of the National Association of Neonatal Nurses, 20*(2), 108. https://doi.org/10.1097/ANC.0000000000000722

Bjorg, F., & Bartlett, D. (2008). Postural control in children born preterm. In Hadders-Algra, M. & Brogren Carlberg, E. (Eds.), *Postural control: A key issue in developmental disorders. Clinics in developmental medicine* (Vol. 179, pp. 22–73). Mac Keith Press.

Brachio, S. S., Farkouh-Karoleski, C., Abreu, A., Zygmunt, A., Purugganan, O. & Garey, D. (2020). Improving neonatal follow-up: A quality improvement study analyzing in-hospital interventions and long-term show rates. *Pediatric Quality and Safety, 5*(6), e363. https://doi.org/10.1097/pq9.0000000000000363

Browne, J. V., Jaeger, C. B., Kenner, C., & on behalf of the Gravens Consensus Committee on Infant and Family Centered Developmental Care. (2020). Executive summary: Standards, competencies, and recommended best practices for infant-and family-centered developmental care in the intensive care unit. *Journal of Perinatology, 40,* 5–10. https://doi.org/10.1038/s41372-020-0767-1

Brown, K. J., Omar, T., & O'Regan, M. (1997). Brain development and the development of tone and movement. In Connolly, K. J., & Frosberg, H. (Eds.), *Neurophysiology & neuropsychology of motor development. Clinics in developmental medicine* (Vols. 143–144, pp. 42–53). Cambridge Press.

Byrne, E., & Campbell, S. K. (2013). Physical therapy observation and assessment in the neonatal intensive care unit. *Physical & Occupational Therapy in Pediatrics, 33*(1), 39–74. https://doi.org/10.3109/01942638.2012.754827

Byrne, E., & Garber, J. (2013). Physical therapy intervention in the neonatal intensive care unit. *Physical & Occupational Therapy in Pediatrics, 33*(1), 75–110. https://doi.org/10.3109/01942638.2012.750870

Cardin, A. D. (2020). Musculoskeletal system. In Kenner, C., Altimier, L. D., & Boykova, M. V. (Eds.), *Comprehensive neonatal care: A physiologic perspective* (6th ed., pp. 254–266). Springer Publishing Company.

Chen, S. S., Tzeng, Y. L., Gau, B. S., Kuo, P. C., & Chen, J. Y. (2013). Effects of prone and supine positioning on gastric residuals in preterm infants: A time series with cross-over study. *International Journal of Nursing Studies, 50*(11), 1459–1467. https://doi.org/10.1016/j.ijnurstu.2013.02.009

Cheong, J. L., Spittle, A. J., Burnett, A. C., Anderson, P. J., & Doyle, L. W. (2020). Have outcomes following extremely preterm birth improved over time? *Seminars in Fetal & Neonatal Medicine, 25*(3), 101114. https://doi.org/10.1016/j.siny.2020.101114

Cheraghia, F., Mahabadib, M., Sadeghianc, E., Tapakd, L., & Basirie, B. (2020). Physiological parameters of preterm infants in different postures: An observational study. *Journal of Neonatal Nursing, 26,* pp. 212–216.

Cioni, G., Prechtl, H. F. R., Ferrari, F., Paolicelli, P. B., Einspieler, C., & Roversi, M. F. (1997). Which better predicts later outcome in full-term infants: Quality of general movements or neurological examination? *Early Human Development, 50*(1), 71–85.

Corvaglia, L., Rotatori, R., Ferlini, M., Aceti, A., Ancora, G., & Faldella, G. (2007). Effect of body positioning on gastroesophageal reflux in premature infants: Evaluation by combined impedance and pH monitor-ing. *The Journal of Pediatrics, 151,* 591–596.

Craig, J. W., Glick, C., Phillips, R., Hall, S. L., Smith, J., & Browne, J. (2015). Recommendations for involving the family in developmental care of the NICU baby. *Journal of Perinatology: Official Journal of the California Perinatal Association, 35*(Suppl. 1), S5–S8.

Dannemiller, L., Mueller, M., Leitner, A., Iverson, E., & Kaplan, S. L. (2020). Physical therapy management of children with developmental coordination disorder: An evidence-based clinical practice guideline from the academy of pediatric physical therapy of the American physical therapy association. *Pediatric Physical Therapy: The Official Publication of the Section on Pediatrics of the American Physical Therapy Association, 32*(4), 278–313. https://doi.org/10.1097/PEP.0000000000000753

Danner-Bowman, K., & Cardin, A.D. (2015). Neuroprotective core measure 3: Positioning & handling—a look at preventing positional plagiocephaly. *Newborn and Infant Nursing Reviews, 15,* 111–113.

D'Apolito, K. (2009). Neonatal opiate withdrawal: Pharmacologic management. *Newborn and Infant Nursing Reviews, 9*(1), 62–69.

Davis, P. M., Robinson, R., Harris, L., & Cartlidge, P. H. (1993). Persistent mild hip deformation in preterm infants. *Archives of Disease in Childhood, 69*(5), 597–598.

Ditzenberger, G. R. (2018). Calcium and phosphorus metabolism. In Blackburn, S. T. (Ed.), *Maternal, fetal, neonatal physiology: A clinical perspective* (5th ed., pp. 571–588). Elsevier.

Downs, J. A., Edwards, A. D., McCormick, D. C., Roth, C., & Steward, A. L. (1991). Effect of intervention on development of hip posture in very preterm babies. *Archives of Disease in Childhood, 66,* 797–801.

Doyle, L. W., Anderson, P. J., Battin, M., Bowen, J. R., Brown, N., Callanan, C., Campbell, C., Chandler, S., Cheong, J., Darlow, B., Davis, P. G., DePaoli, T., French, N., McPhee, A., Morris, S., O'Callaghan, M., Rieger, I., Roberts, G., Spittle, A. J., … Woodward, L. J. (2014). Long term follow up of high risk children: Who, why and how? *BMC Pediatrics, 14,* 279. https://doi.org/10.1186/1471-2431-14-279

Dreyfus, C. J., & Schapira, F. (1979). Biochemistry of muscle development. In Stave, U. (Ed.), *Perinatal physiology* (pp. 239–252). Plenum.

Dubowitz, V. (1965). Enzyme histochemistry of skeletal muscle: Part 1. Developing animal muscle; Part 2 developing human muscle. *Journal of Neurology, Neurosurgery, & Psychiatry, 28,* 516–524.

Dubowitz, L. M. S., & Dubowitz, V. (1999). *The neurological assessment of the preterm and full-term newborn infant. Clinics in developmental medicine* (Vol. 148, 2nd ed.). J. B. Lippincott.

Dunsirn, S., Smyser, C., Liao, S., Inder, T., & Pineda, R. (2016). Defining the nature and implications of head turn preference in the preterm infant. *Early Human Development, 96,* 53–60. https://doi.org/10.1016/j.earlhumdev.2016.02.002

Dusing, S. C., Izzo, T. A., Thacker, L. R., & Galloway, J. C. (2014). Postural complexity differs between infant born full term and preterm during the development of early behaviors. *Early Human Development, 90*(3), 149–156. https://doi.org/10.1016/j.earlhumdev.2014.01.006

Eichenwald, E. C. (2018). Committee on fetus and newborn. *Pediatrics, 142*(1), 1–9. https://doi.org/10.1542/peds.2018-1061

Einspieler, C., Marschik, P. B., & Prechtl, H. F. R. (2008). Human motor behavior: Prenatal origin and early postnatal development. *Zeitschrift für Psychologie/Journal of Psychology, 216*(3), 147–153. https://doi.org/10.1027/0044-3409.216.3.147

Einspieler, C., Prayer, D., & Prechtl, H. F. R. (2012). *Fetal behaviour: A neurodevelopmental approach. Clinics in developmental medicine* (Vol. 189). Mac Keith Press.

Einspieler, C., Prechtl, H. F. R., Boss, A. F., Ferrari, F., & Cioni, G. (2004). *Prechtl's method on the qualitative assessment of general movements in pre-term, term and young infants. Clinics in Developmental Medicine* (Vol. 167). Mac Keith Press.

Einspieler, C., Prechtl, H. F. R., Ferrari, F., Cioni, G., & Bos, A. F. (1997). The qualitative assessment of general movements in preterm, term and young infants—review of the methodology. *Early Human Development, 50*(1), 47–60.

El-Farrash, R. A., Abo-Seif, S. I., El-Zohiery, A. K. Hamed, G. M. & Abulfadl, R. M. (2020). Passive range of motion exercise and bone mineralization in preterm infants: A randomized control trial. *American Journal of Perinatology, 37*(3), 313–321. https://doi.org/10.1055/s-0039-1678559

Eliakim, A., Litmanovitz, I., & Nemet, D. (2017). The role of exercise in prevention and treatment of osteopenia of prematurity: An update. *Pediatric Exercise Science, 29,* 450–455. https://doi.org/10.1123/pes.2017-0017

Eskandari, Z., Seyedfatemi, N., Haghani, H., Almasi-Hashiani, A., & Mohagheghi, P. (2020). Effect of nesting on extensor motor behaviors in preterm infants: A randomized clinical trial. *Iranian Journal of Neonatology*, *11*(3). https://doi.org/10.22038/ijn.2020.42355.1703

Evensen, K., Ustad, T., Tikanmäki, M., Haaramo, P., & Kajantie, E. (2020). Long-term motor outcomes of very preterm and/or very low birth weight individuals without cerebral palsy: A review of the current evidence. *Seminars in Fetal & Neonatal Medicine, 25*(3), 101116. https://doi.org/10.1016/j.siny.2020.101116

Ewer, A. K., James, M. E., & Tobin, J. M. (1999). Prone and left lateral positioning reduce gastro-oesophageal reflux in pre-term infants. *Archives of Disease in Childhood Fetal and Neonatal Edition, 81*, F201–F205.

Fagard, J., Esseily, R., Jacquey, L., O'Regan, K., & Somogyi, E. (2018). Fetal origin of sensorimotor behavior. *Frontiers in Neurorobotics, 12*. https://doi.org/10.3389/fnbot.2018.00023

Farmania, R., Sitaraman, S., & Das, R. R. (2017). Goniometric assessment of muscle tone of preterm infants and impact of gestational age on its maturation in Indian setting. *Journal of Neurosciences in Rural Practice, 8*(Suppl. 1), S44–S48. https://doi.org/10.4103/jnrp.jnrp_417_16

Ferrari, F., Bertoncelli, N., Gallo, C., Roversi, M. F., Guerra, M. P., Ranzi, A., & Hadders-Algra, M. (2007). Posture and movement in healthy preterm infants in supine position in and outside the nest. *Archives of Disease in Childhood Fetal and Neonatal Edition, 92*, 386–390.

Finnegan, L., Connaughton, J., Kron, R., & Emich, J. P. (1975). Neonatal abstinence syndrome: Assessment and management. *Addictive Diseases, 2*, 141–158.

Forero, N., Okamura, L. A., & Larson, M. A. (1989). Normal ranges of hip motion in neonates. *Journal of Pediatric Orthopaedics, 9*, 391–395.

Frudiger, A., Mulders, A., Rousian, M., Plasschaert, S., Koning, A., Willemsen, S. P., Steegers-Theunissen, R., de Vries, J., & Steegers, E. (2021). Evaluation of embryonic posture using four-dimensional ultrasound and virtual reality. *The Journal of Obstetrics and Gynaecology Research, 47*(1), 397–406.

Georgieff, M. K., & Bernbaum, J. C. (1986). Abnormal shoulder muscle tone in premature infants during their first 18 months of life. *Developmental and Behavioral Pediatrics, 6*, 327–333.

Ghorbani, F., Asadollahi, M., & Valizadeh, S. (2013). Comparison the effect of sleep positioning on cardiorespiratory rate in noninvasive ventilated premature infants. *Nursing and Midwifery Studies, 2*(2), 182–187. https://doi.org/10.5812/nms.10318

Giorgi, M., Carriero, A., Shefelbinea, S. J., & Nowlan, N. C. (2014). Mechanobiological simulations of prenatal joint morphogenesis. *Journal of Biomechanics, 47*, 989–995. http://dx.doi.org/10.1016/j.jbiomech.2014.01.002

Gorga, D., Stern, F. M., Ross, G., & Nagler, W. (1988). Neuromotor development of preterm and full-term infants. *Early Human Development, 18*, 137–149.

Gouna, G., Rakza, T., Kuissi, E., Pennaforte, T., Mur, S., & Storme, L. (2013). Positioning effects on lung function and breathing pattern in premature newborns. *The Journal of Pediatrics, 162*(6), 1133–1137.e1. https://doi.org/10.1016/j.jpeds.2012.11.036

Grant-Beuttler, M., Palisano, R. J., Miller, D. P., Wag-ner, B. R., Heriza, C. B., & Shewokis, P. A. (2009). Gastrocnemius-soleus muscle tendon unit changes over the first 12 weeks of adjusted age in infants born preterm. *Physical Therapy, 89*(2), 136–148.

Grisham, L. M., Stephen, M. M., Coykendall, M. R., Kane, M. F., Maurer, J. A., & Bader, M.Y. (2019). Eat, sleep, console approach, *Advances in Neonatal Care, 19*(2), 138–144. https://doi.org/10.1097/ANC.0000000000000581

de Groot, L. (2000). Posture and motility in preterm infants. *Developmental Medicine and Child Neurology, 42*(1), 65–68.

de Groot, L., Hopkins, B., & Touwen, B. C. L. (1991). A method to assess development of muscle power in preterms after term age. *Neuropediatrics, 23*, 172–179.

de Groot, L., vd Hoek, A. M., Hopkins, B., & Touwen, B. C. (1992). Development of the relationship between active and passive muscle power in preterms after term age. *Neuropediatrics, 23*, 298–305.

de Groot, L., vd Hoek, A. M., Hopkins, B., & Touwen, B. C. (1993). Development of muscle power in pre-term infants: Individual trajectories after term age. *Neuropediatrics, 24*, 68–73.

Gesell, A. (1945). *The embryology of behaviour: The beginnings of the human mind*. New York: Harper.

Grove, B. K. (1989). Muscle differentiation and the origin of muscle fiber diversity. *CRC Critical Reviews in Neurobiology, 4*, 201–234.

Gulati, I. K., & Jadcherla, S. R. (2019). Gastroesophageal reflux disease in the neonatal intensive care unit infant: Who needs to be treated and what approach is beneficial? *Pediatric Clinics of North America, 66*(2), 461–473. https://doi.org/10.1016/j.pcl.2018.12.012

Haas, S. S., Epps, C. H., & Adams, J. P. (1973). Normal ranges of hip motion in the newborn. *Clinical Orthopaedics and Related Research, 91*, 114–118.

Hadders-Algra, M. (2008). Development of postural control. In M. Hadders-Algra & E. Brogren Carlberg (Eds.), *Postural control: A key issue in developmental disorders. Clinics in developmental medicine* (Vol. 179, pp. 22–73). Mac Keith Press.

Hadders-Algra, M. (2018). Neural substrate and clinical significance of general movements: an update. *Developmental Medicine and Child Neurology, 60*(1), 39–46. https://doi.org/10.1111/dmcn.13540

Hadders-Algra, M., Klip-Van den Nieuwendijk, A. W., Martijn, A., & van Eykern, L. A. (1997). Assessment of general movements: Towards a better understanding of a sensitive method to evaluate brain function in young infants. *Developmental Medicine and Child Neurology, 39*(2), 88–98.

Hamdan, A. (2008). *Neonatal abstinence syndrome.* www.emedicine.com/ped/TOPIC2760.htm

Hepper, P. (2015). Behavior during the prenatal period: Adaptive for development and survival. *Child Development Perspectives, 9*(1), pp 38–43. https://doi.org/10.1111/cdep.12104

Hintz, S. R., Gould, J. B., Bennett, M. V., Lu, T., Gray, E. E., Jocson, M., Fuller, M. G., & Lee, H. C. (2019). Factors associated with successful first high-risk infant clinic visit for very low birth weight infants in California. *The Journal of Pediatrics, 210*, 91–98.e1. https://doi.org/10.1016/j.jpeds.2019.03.007

Hoffer, M. H. (1980). Joint motion limitation in newborns. *Clinical Orthopedics and Related Research, 148*, 94–96.

Högberg, U., Fellman, V., Thiblin, I., Karlsson, R., & Wester, K. (2020). Difficult birth is the main contributor to birth related fracture and accidents to other neonatal fractures. *Acta Pediatrica, 109*, 2040–2048. https://doi.org/10.1111/apa.15217

Hudak, M. L. (2020). Infants of substance abusing mothers. In Martin, R. J., Fanaroff, A. A., & Walsh, M. C. (Eds.), *Fanaroff & Martin's neonatal-perinatal medicine: Diseases of the fetus and infant* (Vol. 2, 11th ed., pp 735–750). Elsevier.

Hudak, M. L., Tan, R. C., Committee on Drugs, Committee on Fetus and Newborn, , & American Academy of Pediatrics, . (2012). Neonatal drug withdrawal. *Pediatrics, 129*(2), e540–e560. https://doi.org/10.1542/peds.2011-3212

Humphrey, T. (1978). Function of the nervous system during prenatal life. In Stave, U. (Ed.), *Physiology of the perinatal period* (Vol. 2, pp. 751–796). Plenum Medical.

Hunter, J. G. (2010). Therapeutic positioning: Neuromotor, physiologic and sleep implications. In Kenner, C. & McGrath, J. M. (Eds.), *Developmental care of newborns and infants: A guide for health professionals* (2nd ed., pp. 285–312). National Association of Neonatal Nurses.

Hutchison, L. B., Hutchison, L. A. D., Thompson, J. M. D., & Mitchell, E. A. (2004). Plagiocephaly and brachycephaly in the first two years of life: A prospective cohort study. *Pediatrics, 114*, 970–980.

Ianniruberto, A., & Tajani, E. (1981). Ultrasonographic study of fetal movements. *Seminars in Perinatology, 5*(2), 75–181.

Ifflaender, S., Rüdiger, M., Konstantelos, D., Lange, U., & Burkhardt, W. (2014). Individual course of cranial symmetry and proportion in preterm infants up to 6 months of corrected age. *Early Human Development, 90*(9), 511–515. https://doi.org/10.1016/j.earlhumdev.2014.03.008

Ifflaender, S., Rüdiger, M., Konstantelos, D., Wahls, K., & Burkhardt, W. (2013). Prevalence of head deformities in preterm infants at term equivalent age. *Early Human Development, 89*(12), 1041–1047. https://doi.org/10.1016/j.earlhumdev.2013.08.011

Jagadeeswari, J, & Soniya, R. (2020). Effectiveness of prone and supine position on respiratory pattern among neonates. *Drug Invention Today, 13*, 983–985.

Kahraman, A., Başbakkal, Z., Yalaz, M., & Sözmen, E. Y. (2018). The effect of nesting positions on pain, stress and comfort during heel lance in premature infants. *Pediatrics and Neonatology, 59*(4), 352–359. https://doi.org/10.1016/j.pedneo.2017.11.010

Kakebeeke, T. H., von Siebenthal, K., & Largo, R. H. (1998). Movement quality in preterm infants prior to term. *Biology of the Neonate, 73,* 145–154.

Khatony, A., Abdi, A., Karimi, B., Aghaei, A., & Brojeni, H. S. (2019). The effects of position on gastric residual volume of premature infants in NICU. *Italian Journal of Pediatrics, 45*(1), 6. https://doi.org/10.1186/s13052-018-0591-9

King, C., & Norton, D. (2017). Does therapeutic positioning of preterm infants impact upon optimal health outcomes? A literature review. *Journal of Neonatal Nursing, 23,* pp. 218–222. https://doi.org/10.1016/j.jnn.2017.03.004

Kitase, Y., Sato, Y., Takahashi, H., Shimizu, M., Ishikawa, C., Yamamoto, H., & Hayakawa, M. (2017). A new type of swaddling clothing improved development of preterm infants in neonatal intensive care units. *Early Human Development, 112,* 25–28. https://doi.org/10.1016/j.earlhumdev.2017.06.005

Kozuma, S., Okai, T., Nemoto, A., Kagawa, H., Sakai, M., Nishina, H., & Taketani, Y. (1997). Developmental sequence of human fetal body movements in the second half of pregnancy. *American Journal of Perinatolgy, 14*(3), 165–169.

Kurjak, A., Stanojević, M., Predojević, M., Laušin, I., & Salihagić Kadić, A. (2012). Neurobehavior in fetal life. *Seminars in Fetal & Neonatal Medicine, 17*(6), 319–323. https://doi.org/10.1016/j.siny.2012.06.005

Lai, J., Nowlan, N. C., Vaidyanathan, R., Shaw, C. J., & Lees, C. C. (2016). Fetal movements as a predictor of health. *Acta Obstetricia Gynecologica Scandinavica, 95,* 968–975.

Litt, J. S., Edwards, E. M., Lainwala, S., Mercier, C., Montgomery, A., O'Reilly, D., Rhein, L., Woythaler, M., & Hartman, T. (2020). Optimizing high-risk infant follow-up in nonresearch-based paradigms: The new England follow-up network. *Pediatric Quality & Safety, 5*(3), e287. https://doi.org/10.1097/pq9.0000000000000287

Liu, R.W., & Thompson, G. H. (2020). Musculoskeletal disorders in neonates. In Martin, R. J., Fanaroff, A. A., & Walsh, M.C. (Eds.), *Fanaroff & Martin's neonatal-perinatal medicine: Diseases of the fetus and infant* (Vol. 2, 11th ed., pp. 1611–1642). Elsevier.

Luchinger, A. B., Hadders-Algra, M., VanKan, C. M., & DeVries, J. I. P. (2008). Fetal onset of general movements. *Pediatric Research, 63*(2), 191–195.

Lu, Y., Yang, T., Luo, H., Deng, F., Cai, Q., Sun, W., & Song, H. (2016). Visualization and quantitation of fetal movements by real-time three-dimensional ultrasound with live xPlane imaging in the first trimester of pregnancy. *Croatian Medical Journal, 57*(5), 474–481. https://doi.org/10.3325/cmj.2016.57.474

Mactier, H., & Hamilton, R. (2020). Prenatal opioid exposure – Increasing evidence of harm. *Early Human Development, 150,* 105188. https://doi.org/10.1016/j.earlhumdev.2020.105188

Madlinger-Lewis, L., Reynolds, L., Zarem, C., Crapnell, T., Inder, T., & Pineda, R. (2014). The effects of alternative positioning on preterm infants in the neonatal intensive care unit: A randomized clinical trial. *Research in Developmental Disabilities, 35*(2), 490–497. https://doi.org/10.1016/j.ridd.2013.11.019

McCarty, D. B., O'Donnell, S., Goldstein, R. F., Smith, P. B., Fisher, K., & Malcolm, W. F. (2018). Use of a midliner positioning system for prevention of dolichocephaly in preterm infants. *Pediatric Physical Therapy: The Official Publication of the Section on Pediatrics of the American Physical Therapy Association, 30*(2), 126–134. https://doi.org/10.1097/PEP.0000000000000487

McCarty, D. B., Peat, J. R., Malcolm, W. F., Smith, P. B., Fisher, K., & Goldstein, R. F. (2017). Dolichocephaly in preterm infants: Prevalence, risk factors, and early motor outcomes. *American Journal of Perinatology, 34*(4), 372–378. https://doi.org/10.1055/s-0036-1592128

McCarty, D. B., Peat, J. R., O'Donnell, S., Graham, E., & Malcolm, W. F. (2019). "Choose physical therapy" for neonatal abstinence syndrome: Clinical management for infants affected by the opioid crisis. *Physical Therapy, 99*(6), 771–785. https://doi.org/10.1093/ptj/pzz039. PMID: 31155664.

McGowan, E. C., & Vohr, B. R. (2019). Neurodevelopmental follow-up of preterm infants: What is new?. *Pediatric Clinics of North America, 66*(2), 509–523. https://doi.org/10.1016/j.pcl.2018.12.015

McManus, B., Blanchard, Y & Dusing, S. (2017). The neonatal intensive care unit. In Campbell, S. (Ed.), *Physical therapy for children* (5th ed., pp. 672–696). W. B. Saunders.

Mehmood, N., Hasan, A., Nwanne, O., Saeed, H., Salazar, A., Berlioz, C., Cano, M., & Chong, E. (2020). Impact of the use of the beanie on the neurodevelopmental outcomes of preterm infants with plagiocephaly: A pilot study. *Cureus, 12*(6), e8716. https://doi.org/10.7759/cureus.8716

Miller, M. E. (2003). The bone disease of preterm birth: A biomechanical perspective. *Pediatric Research, 53*(1), 10–15.

Miller, M. E. (2005). Hypothesis: Fetal movement influences fetal and infant bone strength. *Medical Hypothesis, 65,* 880–886. https://doi.org/10.1016/j.mehy.2005.05.025

Miller, J. L., Sonies, B. C., & Macedonia, C. (2003). Emergence of oropharyngeal, laryngeal and swallowing activity in the developing fetal upper aerodigestive tract: an ultrasound evaluation. *Early Human Development, 71*(1), 61–87. https://doi.org/10.1016/s0378-3782(02)00110-x

Moore, K. L., Persaud, T. V. N., & Torchia, M. G. (2020). *The developing human: Clinically oriented embryology* (11th ed.). Elsevier.

Nakano, H., Kihara, H., Nakano, J., & Konishi, Y. (2010). The influence of positioning on spontaneous movements of preterm infants. *Journal of Physical Therapy Science, 22,* pp. 337–344. https://doi.org/10.1589/jpts.22.337

National Association of Neonatal Nurses. (2019). *Guideline newborn safe sleep.* National Association of Neonatal Nurses.

Noble, Y., & Boyd, R. (2012). Neonatal assessments for the preterm infant up to 4 months corrected age: A systematic review. *Developmental Medicine and Child Neurology, 54*(2), 129–139. https://doi.org/10.1111/j.1469-8749.2010.03903.x

Nowlan, N. C. (2015). Biomechanics foetal movement. *European Cells and Materials 29,* 1–21. https://doi.org/10.22203/ecm.v029a01

Nuysink, J., Eijsermans, M. J., van Haastert, I. C., Koopman-Esseboom, C., Helders, P. J., de Vries, L. S., & van der Net, J. (2013). Clinical course of asymmetric motor performance and deformational plagiocephaly in very preterm infants. *The Journal of Pediatrics, 163*(3), 658–665.e1. https://doi.org/10.1016/j.jpeds.2013.04.015

Nuysink, J., van Haastert, I. C., Eijsermans, M. J., Koopman-Esseboom, C., van der Net, J., de Vries, L. S., & Helders, P. J. (2012). Prevalence and predictors of idiopathic asymmetry in infants born preterm. *Early Human Development, 88*(6), 387–392. https://doi.org/10.1016/j.earlhumdev.2011.10.001

Pax Lowes, L., & Hay, K. (2017). Musculoskeletal development and adaptation. In Campbell, S. (Ed.), *Physical therapy for children* (5th ed., pp. 99–116). W. B. Saunders.

Pineda, R. G., Tjoeng, T. H., Vavasseur, C., Kidokoro, H., Neil, J. J., & Inder, T. (2013). Patterns of altered neurobehavior in preterm infants within the neonatal intensive care unit. *The Journal of Pediatrics, 162*(3), 470–476.e1. https://doi.org/10.1016/j.jpeds.2012.08.011

Plantinga, Y., Perdock, J., & de Groot, L. (1997). Hand function in low-risk preterm infants: Its relation to muscle power regulation. *Developmental Medicine & Child Neurology, 39,* 6–11.

Prechtl, H. F. R. (1984). Continuity and change in early neural development. In Prechtl, H. F. R. (Ed.), *Continuity of neural functions from prenatal to postnatal life* (pp. 1–15). Spastics International Medical Publications.

Prechtl, H. F. R. (1989). Fetal behavior. In Hill, A. & Volpe, J. J. (Eds.), *Fetal neurology, international review of child neurology series* (pp. 1–14). Raven Press.

Prechtl, H. F. R. (1997a). The importance of fetal movements. In Connolly, K. J. & Frosberg, H. (Eds.), *Neurophysiology and neuropsychology of motor development. Clinics in developmental medicine (143-144).* (pp. 42–53). Cambridge Press.

Prechtl, H. F. R. (1997b). Editorial: State of the art of a new functional assessment of the young nervous system. An early predictor of cerebral palsy. *Early Human Development, 50*(1), 1–11.

Prechtl, H. R. (2001). General movement assessment as a method of developmental neurology: New paradigms and their consequences. The 1999 Ronnie MacKeith lecture. *Developmental Medicine and Child Neurology, 43*(12), 836–842.

Prechtl, H. F. R., & Nolte, R. (1984). Motor behavior of preterm infants. In Prechtl, H. F. R. (Ed.), *Continuity of neural functions from prenatal to postnatal life* (pp. 79–92). Spastics International Medical Publications.

Purdy, I., Craig, J., & Zeanah, P. (2015). NICU discharge planning and beyond: Recommendations for parent psychosocial support. *Journal of Perinatology, 35*, S24–S28. https://doi.org/10.1038/jp.2015.146

Reyhani, T., Ramezani, S., Boskabadi, H., & Mazlom, S. (2016). Evaluation of the effect of nest posture on the sleep-wake state of premature infants. *Evidence Based Care, 6*(1), 29–36. https://doi.org/10.22038/ebcj.2016.6713

Ricci, D., Romeo, D. M., Haataja, L., van Haastert, I. C., Cesarini, L., Maunu, J., Pane, M., Gallini, F., Luciano, R., Romagnoli, C., de Vries, L. S., Cowan, F. M., & Mercuri, E. (2008). Neurological examination of preterm infants at term equivalent age. *Early Human Development, 84*(11), 751–761. https://doi.org/10.1016/j.earlhumdev.2008.05.007

Rogers, G. F. (2011). Deformational plagiocephaly, brachycephaly, and scaphocephaly. Part II: Prevention and treatment. *The Journal of Craniofacial Surgery, 22*(1), 17–23. https://doi.org/10.1097/SCS.0b013e3181f6c342

Rogers, E. E., & Hintz, S. R. (2016). Early neurodevelopmental outcomes of extremely preterm infants. *Seminars in Perinatology, 40*(8), 497–509. https://doi.org/10.1053/j.semperi.2016.09.002

Roodenburg, P. J., Wladimiroff, J. W., van Es, A., & Prechtl, H. F. R. (1991). Classification and quantitative aspects of fetal movements during the second half of normal pregnancy. *Early Human Development, 25*(1), 19–35.

Roué, J. M., Kuhn, P., Lopez Maestro, M., Maastrup, R. A., Mitanchez, D., Westrup, B., & Sizun, J. (2017). Eight principles for patient-centred and family-centred care for newborns in the neonatal intensive care unit. *Archives of Disease in Childhood Fetal and Neonatal Edition, 102*(4), F364–F368.

Rustico, S. E., Calabria, A. C., & Garber, S. J. (2014). Metabolic bone disease of prematurity. *Journal of Clinical & Translational Endocrinology 1*, 85–91. http://dx.doi.org/10.1016/j.jcte.2014.06.004

Ryan, G., Dooley, J., Gerber Finn, L., & Kelly, L. (2019). Nonpharmacological management of neonatal abstinence syndrome: A review of the literature. *J Matern Fetal Neonatal Med. 32*(10), pp. 1735–1740. https://doi.org/10.1080/14767058.2017.1414180

Sadler, T. W. (2019). *Langman's medical embryology* (14th ed.). Wolters/Kluwer, Lippincott, Williams, & Wilkins.

Saint-Anne Dargassies, S. (1977). *Neurological development in the full term and premature neonate.* Excerpta Medica.

Samsom, J. F., & de Groot, L. (2000). The influence of postural control on motility and hand function in a group of 'high risk' preterm infants at 1 year of age. *Early Human Development, 60*(2), 101–113. https://doi.org/10.1016/s0378-3782(00)00107-9

Sans, J. R. (1987). Cell lineage and the origin of muscle fiber types. *Trends in Neuroscience, 10*, 119–121.

Sezer Efe, Y. Erdem, E., & Güneş, T. (2020). The effect of daily exercise program on bone mineral density and cortisol level in preterm infants with very low birth weight: A randomized controlled trial. *Journal of Pediatric Nursing, 51*, e6–e12. https://doi.org/10.1016/j.pedn.2019.05.021

Sims, A., Chounthirath, T., Yang, J., Hodges, N. L., & Smith, G. A. (2018). Infant walker-related injuries in the United States. *Pediatrics, 142*(4), e20174332. https://doi.org/10.1542/peds.2017-4332

da Silva, E. S., & Nunes, M. L. (2005). The influence of gestational age and birth weight in the clinical assessment of the muscle tone of healthy term and preterm newborns. *Arquivos de Neuro-Psiquiatria, 63*(4), 956–962. https://doi.org/10.1590/s0004-282x2005000600010

Snider, L. M., Majnemer, A., Mazer, B., Campbell, S., & Bos, A. F. (2008). A comparison of the general movements assessment with traditional approaches to newborn and infant assessment: Concurrent validity. *Early Human Development, 84*, 297–303.

Snider, L., Majnemer, A., Mazer, B., Campbell, S., & Bos, A. F. (2009). Prediction of motor and functional outcomes in infants born preterm assessed at term. *Pediatric Physical Therapy: The Official Publication of the Section on Pediatrics of the American Physical Therapy Association, 21*(1), 2–11. https://doi.org/10.1097/PEP.0b013e3181957bdc

Sparling, J. W. (Ed.). (1993). Concepts in fetal movement research. *Physical and Occupational Therapy in Pediatrics, 12*(2–3), 1–18.

Sparling, J. W., van Tol, J., & Chescheir, N. C. (1999). Fetal and neonatal hand movement. *Physical Therapy, 79*(1), 24–39.

Sparling, J. W., & Wilhelm, I. J. (1993). Quantitative measurement of fetal movement: Fetal posture and movement assessment (F-PAM). *Physical and Occupational Therapy in Pediatrics, 12*(2–3), 97–114.

Spilker, A., Hill, C., & Rosenblum, R. (2016). The effectiveness of a standardised positioning tool and bedside education on the developmental positioning proficiency of NICU nurses. *Intensive & Critical Care Nursing, 35*, 10–15. https://doi.org/10.1016/j.iccn.2016.01.004

Stalnaker, K. A., & Poskey, G. A. (2016). Osteopenia of prematurity: Does physical activity improve bone mineralization in preterm infants? *Neonatal Network, 25*(2), 95–104. https://doi.org/10.1891/0730-0832.35.2.95

Stanger, J. J., Horey, D., Hooker, L., Jenkins, M. J., & Custovic, E. (2017). "Fetal movement measurement and technology: A narrative review." (Vol. 5, pp. 16747–16756). IEEE Access. https://doi.org/10.1109/ACCESS.2017.2716964

Stanojevic, M., Zaputovic, S., & Bosnjak, A. P. (2012). Continuity between fetal and neonatal neurobehavior. *Seminars in Fetal & Neonatal Medicine, 17*(6), 324–329. https://doi.org/10.1016/j.siny.2012.06.006

Swearingen, C., Simpson, P., Cabacungan, E., & Cohen, S. (2020). Social disparities negatively impact neonatal follow-up clinic attendance of premature infants discharged from the neonatal intensive care unit. *Journal of Perinatology, 40*, 790–797. https://doi.org/10.1038/s41372-020-0659-4

Sweeney, J. K. (2007). Neonates and infants at neurodevelopmental risk. In Umphred, D. (Ed.), *Neurological rehabilitation* (5th ed., pp. 303–356). Mosby.

Sweeney, J. K., & Gutierrez, T. (2002). Musculoskeletal implications of preterm infant positioning in the NICU. *Journal of Perinatal and Neonatal Nursing, 16*(1), 58–70.

Task Force on Sudden Infant Death Syndrome. (2016). SIDS and other sleep-related infant deaths: Updated 2016 recommendations for a safe infant sleeping environment. *Pediatrics, 138*(5), e20162938. https://doi.org/10.1542/peds.2016-2940

Teledevara, S., Rajeswari, M., Kumar, R. S., & Udayakumar, N. (2019). Factors associated with low muscle tone and impact of common musculoskeletal problems on motor development in preterm infants at one year of corrected age. *Journal of Clinical and Diagnostic Research, 13*(3), 12–16. http://dx.doi.org/10.7860/JCDR/2019/39551.12675

Tobin, J. M., McCloud, P., & Cameron, D. J. S. (1997). Posture and gastro-oesophageal reflux: A case for left lateral positioning. *Archives of Disease in Childhood, 76*, 254–258.

Towen, B. C. (1990). Variability and stereotyping of spontaneous motility as a predictor of neurological development of preterm infants. *Developmental Medicine and Child Neurology, 32*(6), 501–508.

Ullenhag, A., Perrson, K., & Nyqvist, K. H. (2009). Motor performance in very preterm infants before and after implementation of the newborn individualized care and assessment programme in a neonatal intensive care unit. *Acta Paediatrica, 98*, 947–952.

Vaivre-Douret, L., Ennouri, K., Jrad, I., Garrec, C., & Papiernik, E. (2004). Effect of positioning on the incidence of abnormalities of muscle tone in low-risk, preterm infants. *European Journal of Pediatric Neurology, 8*, 21–34.

Valizadeh, L., Ghahremani, G., Gharehbaghi, M. M., & Jafarabadi, M. A. (2016). The effects of flexed (fetal tucking) and extended (free body) postures on the daily sleep quantity of hospitalized premature infants: A randomized clinical trial. *Journal of Research in Medical Sciences: The Official Journal of Isfahan University of Medical Sciences, 21*, 124. https://doi.org/10.4103/1735-1995.196606

Verbruggen, S.W., Kainz, B., Shelmerdine, S. C., Hajnal, J. V., Rutherford, M. A., Arthurs, O. J., Phillips, A. T. M., & Nowlan, N. C. (2018). Stresses and strains on the human fetal skeleton during development. *Journal of the Royal Society Interface, 15*, 20170593. http://dx.doi.org/10.1098/rsif.2017.0593

van Vlimmeren, L. A., van der Graaf, Y., Boere-Boonekamp, M., L'Hoir, M. P., Helders, P. J., & En-gelbert, R. H. H. (2008). Effect of pediatric physical therapy on deformational plagiocephaly in children with positional preference: A randomized control trial. *Archives of Pediatrics & Adolescent Medicine, 162*(8), 712–718.

de Vries, J. I. P., Visser, G. H., & Prechtl, H. F. R. (1984). Fetal motility in the first half of pregnancy. In H. F. Prechtl (Ed.), *Continuity of neural functions from prenatal to postnatal life* (pp. 46–64). J. B. Lippincott.

de Vries, J. I., Wimmers, R. H., Ververs, I. A., Hopkins, B., Savelsbergh, G. J., & van Geijn, H. P. (2001). Fetal handedness and head position preference: A developmental study. *Developmental Psychobiology, 39*(3), 171–180.

Vungarala, P., & Rajeswari, M. (2018). Correlation of birth weight, gestational age and muscle tone with motor development of preterm infants. *International Journal of Physiotherapy, 5*(2), 63–68. https://doi. org/10.15621/ijphy/2018/v5i2/170744

Wachman, E. M., Grossman, M., Schiff, D. M., Philipp, B. L., Minear, S., Hutton, E., Saia, K., Nikita, F., Khattab, A., Nolin, A., Alvarez, C., Barry, K., Combs, G., Stickney, D., Driscoll, J., Humphreys, R., Burke, J., Farrell, C., Shrestha, H., & Whalen, B. L. (2018). Quality improvement initiative to improve inpatient outcomes for Neonatal Abstinence Syndrome. *Journal of Perinatology, 38*, 1114–1122. https://doi.org/10.1038/s41372-018-0109-8

Walker, J. (1992). Musculoskeletal development: A review. In Rothstein, J. M. (Ed.), *Pediatric orthopedics: An American physical therapy monograph.* Ameerican Physical Therapy Association.

Waugh, K. G., Minkel, J. L., Parker, R., & Coon, V. A. (1983). Measurement of selected hip, knee, and ankle joint motions in newborns. *Physical Therapy, 63*, 1616–1621.

Yang, W., Chen, J., Shen, W., Wang, C., Wu, Z., Chang, Q., Li, W., Lv, K., Pan, Q., Li, H., Ha, D., & Zhang, Y. (2019). Prevalence of positional skull deformities in 530 premature infants with a corrected age of up to 6 months: A multicenter study. *BMC Pediatrics, 19*(1), 520. https://doi.org/10.1186/s12887-019-1864-1

Zahed, M., Berbis, J., Brevaut-Malaty, V., Busuttil, M., Tosello, B., & Gire, C. (2015). Posture and movement in very preterm infants at term age in and outside the nest. *Child's Nervous System, 31*, 2333–2340. https://doi.org/10.1007/s00381-015-2905-1

CHAPTER 12

The NICU Sensory Environment

Roberta Pineda and Joan R. Smith

Standards in ICU Sensory Environment for Babies

Positioning and Touch

Standard 4, Positioning and Touch

- Babies in intensive care unit (ICU) settings shall experience human touch by family and caregivers.

Sleep and Arousal

Standard 1, Sleep and Arousal

- Intensive care units (ICUs) shall promote developmentally appropriate sleep and arousal states and sleep wake cycles.

Standard 2, Sleep and Arousal

- The ICU shall provide modifications to the physical environment and to caregiving routines that are specifically focused on optimization of sleep and arousal of ICU babies.

Standard 3, Sleep and Arousal

- The ICU shall encourage family presence at the baby's bedside and family participation in the care of their baby.

Skin-to-skin Contact (SSC) With Intimate Family Members

Standard 1, SSC

- Parents shall be encouraged and supported in early, frequent, and prolonged SSC with their babies.

INTRODUCTION

Theoretical Construction in Developmental Support and Its Relation to the Sensory Environment

Preterm and critically ill infants in the neonatal intensive care unit (NICU) are exposed to sensory stimulation that can disrupt both endogenous stimulation within the central nervous system (CNS) and exogenous stimulation (experience dependent) of the developing brain (Lickliter, 2011; Liu et al., 2007; Woodward et al., 2018). Normal sensory development proceeds without difficulty in the uterine environment because of the high degree of control over a fetus's sensory development and sensory stimulation. Prior to birth, the fetus is contained in an environment that provides developmentally timed auditory, tactile, olfactory, gustatory, and vestibular kinesthetic sensory exposures, while being shielded from visual stimuli. Early fetal environmental sensory exposures are modulated by the physical barrier of the womb, but sensory exposure can also result from maternal activity. In addition, the normal fetal progression of sensory development occurs in a sequential manner ((1) tactile, (2) vestibular, (3) olfactory/gustatory, (4) auditory, and then (5) visual) (Graven & Browne, 2008a), which correlates with experiences in the womb. These early timed sensory experiences are likely to be very important for optimal growth and health, yet are interrupted when an infant is born preterm and placed in the dynamic and unpredictable environment of the NICU, where sensory exposures are often unexpected, too intense, and poorly timed (AAP, 1997; Byers, 2003). Altered sensory exposures in the NICU environment, in addition to poorly timed and painful exposures, may be harmful to the developing sensory system (Field, 1990; Graven et al., 1992).

Outcomes of very preterm infants, requiring care in the NICU for several months after birth (Pineda et al., 2014), are influenced by multiple biologic (e.g., gestational age) (Boyle et al., 2012), clinical, (e.g., intraventricular hemorrhage) Bolisetty et al., 2014; Radic et al., 2015), and psychosocial (e.g., maternal depression) factors (Bozkurt et al., 2017). However, the NICU environment can also have significant effects on early brain structure and function (Pineda et al., 2014; Smith et al.,

2011). The time in the NICU is an important period when brain development is susceptible to external stimuli (Brown et al., 2009; Pineda et al., 2013). It is a time when the preterm infant should be in utero and experiencing multidimensional sensory exposures, and the full-term infant should be receiving constant parental nurturing at home. Instead, high-risk infants in the NICU are often exposed to invasive and painful medical interventions (Smith et al., 2011) and often lack adequate positive and consistent forms of sensory exposures (Lickliter, 2011), which are critical for optimizing development.

Although appropriate early sensory exposures are important for the developing infant in the NICU, parent interaction is also critical. The infant's need for human contact and nurturing has long been understood. Animal studies have identified that even brief periods of maternal separation can result in emotional disturbances and decreased motor activity among offspring (Sealy & Harlow, 1965; Seay et al., 1962). Clinical studies on early parent–infant interactions have also demonstrated positive effects of parent interaction on motor and attentional responses of the infant (Brazelton et al., 1975). Early deprivation of social and caregiver interaction has been shown to have lasting effects, with poor physical growth, developmental delay, increased emotional and neurocognitive difficulties, and abnormalities on magnetic resonance imaging among abandoned infants (Beurment et al., 2012; Daunhauer et al., 2007; Daunhauer et al., 2010; Govindan et al., 2010; Tottenham & Sheridan, 2009). Although the vulnerable critically ill infant differs from a child who has been institutionalized or deprived of caregiving attention after full-term birth, there are striking similarities to orphaned infants with altered temporal structures (Govindan et al., 2010) and higher risk of developmental impairment (Anderson & Doyle, 2008; Barre et al., 2011). However, parent involvement is an important and modifiable factor in the NICU, and infants whose parents are present and engaged in the NICU demonstrate more favorable outcomes (Pineda et al., 2018; Reynolds et al., 2013). Parental involvement is linked to the domains and standards found at the beginning of this chapter.

Research has demonstrated that the NICU is not as effective at supporting sensory development as the uterus (Atun-Einy & Scher, 2008; Behrman & Butler, 2007; Bustani, 2008; Hussey-Gardner & Famuyide, 2009; Liu et al., 2007; Martucci, 2004; Robinson, 2003; Symington & Pinelli, 2009). In addition to an altered sensory environment in the NICU, infants can be exposed to a significant number of stressful procedures, and higher exposure to stress can also alter early brain development (Smith et al., 2011). Furthermore, interruptions to sleep can also have lasting consequences on the infant in the NICU (Fumagalli et al., 2018). Finally, lack of parent engagement can impact early brain development as well as impact early parent–child relationships, which are critical foundations that are important throughout life (Klawetter et al., 2019; Lean et al., 2018; Pineda et al., 2018; Reynolds et al., 2013).

Although developmental problems (Anderson & Doyle, 2008; Anderson et al., 2003; Barre et al., 2011; Foulder-Huges & Cooke, 2003; Goldenberg et al., 2008; Goyen et al., 1998; Holsti et al., 2002; Maguire et al., 2009; Williams et al., 2010) as well as attachment disorders (Pedspan, 2004) and other social–emotional problems (Quesada et al., 2014) are common, infants hospitalized in the NICU also have a heightened risk of sensory processing challenges (Broring et al., 2017). Although sensory modulation disorders can correlate with brain injury, the potential influence of the early sensory environment is gaining increased attention (Broring et al., 2017). Researchers and healthcare professionals acknowledge that NICU stress has a significant impact on sensory development (Brummelte et al., 2012; Fumagalli et al., 2018; Sherman, 2019). Therefore, developmentally supportive care theories and practices have emerged over the last 40 years, which have improved the NICU environment and caregiving practices (About FiCAre, 2020; Als, 1982; Gibbins et al., 2008; Pineda et al., 2019). Altering the NICU environment by clustering care, positioning appropriately, and encouraging family involvement can positively impact the developing CNS. The Infant and Family-Centered Developmental Care principles stress the importance of supporting the family to engage in care and assist with the needs of the infant in the NICU through practices that include supportive positioning and touch, engaging in interventions to promote sleep and arousal, and providing SSC (Browne et al., 2020). Developmental care principles also include the implementation of strategies that mimic the intrauterine environment and provide developmentally appropriate stimuli tailored to the infant's state of arousal and behavioral responses (Gibbins et al., 2008). Further, optimal sensory neuromaturation is supported through interventions that engage the parents in care (Klawetter et al., 2019; Lean et al., 2018; Pineda et al., 2018; Reynolds et al., 2013). Appropriate sensory support in the NICU environment requires an understanding of how all sensory systems work together so infants can make sense of the world in which they reside and to equip parents with the tools to engage appropriately with their infants.

Why Are Sensory Experiences Important?

As theorized by A. Jean Ayres, "Sensory integration is the neurological process that organizes sensation from one's own body and the environment and makes it possible to use the body effectively within the environment" (Ayres, 2005, p. 5). The adaptive response is at the core of the sensory integration theory. Ayres defined an adaptive response as "…a purposeful, goal-directed response to a sensory experience. In an adaptive response, we master a challenge and learn something new. At the same time, the formation of an adaptive response helps the brain develop and organize itself" (Ayres, 2005, p. 7).

For most children, sensory integration occurs without any difficulty as a normal process of development and supports developmental skills acquisition and learning (Vergara & Bigsby, 2004). For some infants, the senses do not work together, and previous experience is not effectively organized into the brain. Furthermore, altered sensory development can occur with repetitive painful or stressful stimuli (Cabral et al., 2016; Ranger & Grunau, 2014; Vinall & Grunau, 2014). Infants born preterm and/or critically ill can also be at risk of sensory processing problems owing to the presentation of sensory stimulation outside the normal sequence, brain injury, and/or environmental excesses (Anderson & Doyle, 2008; Doyle & Saigal, 2009; Hack & Costello, 2008; Lickliter, 2011; Vergara & Bigsby, 2004). Consequently, infants with early alterations in sensory experiences may not understand how to process sensory stimulation (Ayres, 2005). This lack of understanding can cause difficulty in all areas of daily life, including academic tasks. Furthermore, optimal learning will not proceed without properly timed and age-appropriate sensory experiences (Lickliter, 2011). The type and timing of sensory exposure must match the level of maturity and be guided by infant cues (Vandenberg, 2007), yet the importance of positive, early sensory experiences is critical.

Developmental Care and Sensory Experiences

Theories/frameworks that support developmental care practices in the NICU include the sensory integration theory (Ayres, 2005), the synactive theory (Als, 1982), and the Infant and Family-Centered Developmental Care (IFCDC) in the Intensive Care Unit framework (Browne et al., 2019). In the sensory integration theory, Ayres (2005) postulates that sensory input to the neonate drives the learning process and CNS organization. In the synactive theory, Als (1982) interprets the developmental process to be based on subsystem interaction between a neonate's internal functioning, the environment, and caregivers. The IFCDC is a product of a multidisciplinary group of experts who compile evidence on neuroprotective strategies for high-risk NICU infants and define that the interaction and relationship between the parents and the infant are critical and should be the center of NICU care.

The synactive and sensory integration theories both uphold the idea that there needs to be a "match" between the demands of the sensory environment and the capacity of the child to process and make use of those sensory experiences for the child to develop adaptive skills and behaviors (Vinall & Grunau, 2014). Both theories look at the provision of sensory stimulation and its timing on a neonate's ability to process sensory information and integrate it into neurosensory processing. Both theories also identify the potential for sensory overload and its influence on sensory thresholds and processing (Als, 1982; Ayres, 2005; Lawhon & Hedlund, 2008).

The IFCDC focuses on the importance of supporting multiple aspects of developmental care with the focus on supporting the baby's behavioral communication and nurturing relationship of the parents being a critical element (Browne et al., 2019). There are six domains described in the IFCDC with standards underneath each that represent a safe, evidence-based expectation for best practice. The domains and standards that are specific to early sensory experiences include domain 2, standard 4: identifying that babies in ICU settings shall experience human touch by family and caregivers; domain 3, standard 2: the ICU shall provide modifications to the physical environment and to caregiving routines that are specifically focused on the optimization of sleep and arousal of ICU babies; domain 3, standard 3: the ICU shall encourage family presence at the baby's bedside and family participation in the care of their baby; and domain

4, standard 3: parents shall be encouraged and supported in frequent and prolonged SSC with their babies. The neonate's skin conducts the first sensory experiences (tactile) to the baby from the NICU environment. The epidermis of the skin and the neuronal cells of the CNS are closely linked, beginning in embryonic development, as they both originate from the ectoderm. Thus, it is crucial to recognize the paramount role of tactile experiences on neuronal development. In addition, careful attention to the sequence of sensory development can aid in timing of other sensory exposures such as auditory, visual, and olfactory stimuli. In order to address the infant's developmental needs, the NICU caregiver should take time to individualize patient care while considering the neonate's sensory environment (Gibbins et al., 2008). The aforementioned theories/frameworks embrace the concept that environmental and sensory interventions support the best developmental care (Ayres, 2005; Gibbins et al., 2008). Although most research on sensory integration theory and treatment has been completed with older children and adults, the NICU is an environment in which sensory integration and developmental care together support optimal sensory development for the high-risk infant population (Ayres, 2005; Rogers & Piecuch, 2009; Vergara & Bigsby, 2004).

THE NICU SENSORY ENVIRONMENT

Research on the NICU environment has demonstrated that stimuli can be too intense for the immature infant receiving care. Noise levels are high, especially for those who are critically ill receiving high-frequency oscillatory ventilation (Pineda et al., 2017). Furthermore, light exposure can also be too intense with such exposure occurring too early in the developmental trajectory (Lai & Bearer, 2008). Therefore, special attention to minimizing sensory exposures that are too intense or poorly timed are an important consideration when working with infants in the NICU. It has also been noted that poorly timed exposures in the NICU can disrupt sleep (Calciolari & Montirosso, 2011). However, developmentally appropriate and appropriately timed sensory exposures are important for brain development (McGrath et al., 2011; Woodward et al., 2018).

SENSORY SYSTEMS OVERVIEW

We perceive and interact with the world using our senses. It is important to define these senses (Milford & Zapalo, 2010) and then discern how to alter the NICU environment to support their optimal development. This brief overview of sensory systems in their developmental sequence provides a basis for the discussion of sensory integration.

Tactile System (Touch)

The tactile system comprises four different sensory modalities: touch, temperature, pain, and proprioception. Recognition of touch starts when a force acts on a mechanoreceptor or nociceptor in the skin. The receptor registers the force and converts the information to a neuronal signal.

Dorsal column sensory fibers carry the information via the spinal cord to the thalamus from where the information is further sent to the primary and secondary somatosensory cortexes within the parietal lobe where the touch in interpreted (Gazzaniga et al., 2014). Touch, temperature, and pain are perceived cutaneously with dedicated receptors for each modality present in the skin (Zimmerman et al., 2014). Proprioception is perceived by continuously using information from the skin and signals from muscles and joints to update the brain about the current position and movement of the limbs (Johnson et al., 2008). The tactile system is the first system to develop, with Merkel receptors developing at approximately 8 to 10 weeks in fetal development (Chu & Loomis, 2016) and becoming functional by 24 weeks' gestation. Because skin is the largest system, touch is the largest sensory system and plays a vital role in sensory development. Although it is challenging to discern between spontaneous and direct reactions to sensations by fetuses, it has been noted that reflexive reaction to touch occurs within the first trimester and purposeful directed movement of self-touch of highly innervated body areas occurs from 10 to 12 weeks (Fagard et al., 2018). Notable fetal behavioral responses to maternal touch of the abdomen have been recorded in fetuses between the 21st and 25th week of gestation (Marx & Nagy, 2015).

Touch establishes identity and security within the environment. It is a protective, as well as a discriminatory, system. Touch sensations can be negative, as in discomfort from having diaper rash. Touch sensations can be positive, as in the comfort of a gentle hand by the mother. When touch is provided in a negative or abnormal way, such as pulling adhesive tape off of the face, there is a complex reaction in the CNS (Boggini et al., 2021; Gursul et al., 2019). Infants undergoing painful medical interventions for long periods in the NICU demonstrate functional changes in pain perception (Chorna et al., 2014b; Slater et al., 2010). This can lead to tactile defensiveness, which is an overactive tactile protective response. Tactile defensiveness is common in high-risk infants in the NICU and often is present with other developmental challenges. Alternatively, positive tactile exposures are critical for optimizing brain development (Maitre et al., 2017), and evidence supports the positive impact of tactile exposures on long-term outcomes (Feldman et al., 2014). Of importance, positive sensory exposures, when used as supportive measures during painful interventions, can change the architecture of the brain and subsequent tactile responsivity (Gursul et al., 2019).

Gustatory System (Taste)

Gustatory is the system of taste and is classified as a *chemical sense*. Taste begins when a molecule is absorbed into a taste bud, which contains multiple receptor cells that are specialized for different flavors (Gravina et al., 2013). The receptors become excited by the chemical molecules and carry the action potential to the facial and glossopharyngeal nerve. These cranial nerves carry the signal through multiple areas of the brain before reaching the gustatory complex of the insula. There are approximately ten thousand taste buds between the tongue, soft palate, and upper throat (Khan et al., 2019). Taste cells begin forming around 7 weeks' gestation and are fully mature at 17 weeks' gestation (Lipchock et al., 2011). The gustatory system is interrelated with the olfactory system, and together they are functional by 24 weeks' gestation (Lipchock et al., 2011).

A fetus will begin swallowing amniotic fluid around 12 weeks' gestation (Lipchock et al., 2011) and will swallow approximately 750 mL of amniotic fluid daily by 34 weeks' gestation (Bloomfield et al., 2017). This early experience of taste has important developmental consequences. The formation of taste pathways and preferences before birth helps babies to respond positively to their mother's milk, as many of the flavors in amniotic fluid are also present in breast milk (Lipchock et al., 2011; Mennella et al., 2001). Developmentally, the sense of taste likely encourages oral play, hand-to-mouth exploration, and midline activities.

Olfactory System (Smell)

Olfaction, or smell, is also known as a *chemical sense*. Smell occurs when odor molecules are inhaled through the nostrils and come in contact with extensions of olfactory receptors called cilia (Pinto, 2011). This causes a series of action potentials across nerves to the olfactory bulb and through the olfactory nerve, which travels to the primary olfactory cortex.

The olfaction pathway begins to develop by 8 weeks' gestation (Lipchock et al., 2011), and the olfactory system appears to be well developed by 24 weeks' gestation (Schaal et al., 2004). During fetal development, amniotic fluid passes through the fetus' nasal cavity and exposes it to strong odors from its mother's food (Sarnat et al., 2017). These odors can influence neonatal behavior, as seen by changes in movement and respiratory patterns on ultrasound imaging (Sarnat et al., 2017). Once born, the infant is exposed to many novel odors that will impact behavior during infancy (Bartocci et al., 2000). Research has demonstrated that a mother's scent can facilitate state regulation and optimal feeding experiences (Schaal et al., 2004). Alternatively, lack of maternal odor and exposures to nonnatural smells (such as rubbing alcohol or Betadine) can impact attachment and impact sensory-system development (Schaal et al., 2004; Winberg & Porter, 1998).

Auditory System (Hearing)

Hearing begins when sound passes through the ear canal to the eardrum, which creates vibrations or sound waves that cause fluid in the cochlea to ripple (Musiek & Baran, 2018). Hair cells in the cochlea bend, which release chemicals and create an electrical signal (Musiek & Baran, 2018). The auditory nerve carries the signal through numerous brainstem sites before making its way to the auditory cortex. The auditory system works closely with the vestibular system, which also receives information from hair cells in the inner ear (Moller, 2002) and informs the infant about movement in space.

There are marked changes in the auditory system from preterm birth until term equivalent age, or during fetal development in the 2nd and 3rd trimester (Weitzman et al., 1967). The connections between the cochlea and the brainstem are established by 24 to 25 weeks' gestation and between the temporal lobe and the auditory cortex (nonprimary) by as early as 30 to 31 weeks' gestation (Weitzman et al., 1967). Auditory-evoked potentials are evident by the 28th week of gestation, and there is a marked reduction in response as neural pathways mature from 28 through 34 weeks' gestation (Starr et al., 1977). Critical development of the neurosensory part of the auditory system occurs from 25 weeks' gestation to 5 to 6 months corrected age, requiring outside stimulation (e.g., speech, music, meaningful sounds) for the development of the ability to receive signals of specific frequencies and intensities (Graven & Browne, 2008b).

Prior to full-term birth, infants demonstrate auditory responses, and it is believed that the pitch, intensity, and pattern of *in utero* auditory exposures activate the system and stimulate associations between the cortex and cochlea. The *in utero* environment, which filters out high-frequency noise, is also believed to facilitate speech and language acquisition, and it has been suggested that human speech is perceived and learned by the fetus between 31 and 40 weeks of gestation (Hepper & Shahidullah, 1994). This is supported by research demonstrating that the fetus responds to extrauterine noise and can discriminate the mother's voice by term gestation. It has been proposed that experiencing mother's voice prior to birth is critical for typical brain development (DeCasper & Spence, 1985; Fifer & Moon, 1994) and that the timed auditory input of low-frequency sounds experienced *in utero* followed by the addition of higher-frequency sounds experienced *ex utero* is important for normal auditory development (Gottlieb, 1971). Hearing is important for attention and learning, essential for recognition, motivating for alerting and orientation behaviors, and essential for basic language development (Ayres, 2005).

Visual System

Vision, or seeing, is perceived through the eyes. Light hits the retina, at the back of the eye, which creates electrical signals that travel through the optic nerve to the brain. The brain then turns the signals into images or perceptions that are perceived and understood (Moller, 2002). Compared with the other senses, vision is primitive at the time of birth: visual functioning is not necessary for the fetus, and most of the system develops postnatally (Graven & Browne, 2008c). The brain devotes more of its territory to vision than to all the other senses combined (Sherman, 2019). With that increased territory and complexity, the visual system takes more time

to develop and organize during the first years of life (Graven & Browne, 2008c). The visual system supports recognition of caregivers and objects in the environment as well as visual perception of self in space and eventually facilitates academic learning, skills, and function (Ayres, 2005).

Research has demonstrated that preterm infants can visually fixate at short distances of approximately 10 to 12 inches (Liu et al., 2007). By 6 months of age, primary visual abilities have emerged: depth perception, color vision, fine acuity, and well-controlled eye movements (Graven & Browne, 2008c). By 1 year of age, the visual system is well developed. However, the right amount of stimulation at the right time is essential for proper development of the brain circuitry underlying the visual system (Madan et al., 2005). Of importance, introducing visual stimuli too early when infants are born preterm can result in negative outcomes (O'Connor et al., 2007). Exogenous light stimulation is not recommended for infants prior to term equivalent age, as it disrupts sleep. It is believed that avoiding this type of visual stimulation is protective of sleep and thus crucial for visual neural architecture development (Liu et al., 2007). Maintaining a dim environment has been a care standard to protect the developing visual system (Glass, 1990). However, circadian rhythms, important for quality sleep, are impacted by changes in the light environment (Guyer et al., 2015). Subsequently, the use of cycled light has been associated with better outcomes, including increased weight gain and shorted hospital stay (Vasquez-Ruiz et al., 2014). Thus, a blend of low light levels, cycling, and protection from bright lights is important. Furthermore, introducing complex visual stimuli too early (when infants are born preterm) can be problematic and is not recommended until closer to term gestation (Madan et al., 2005).

Sensory Integration

Although basic structures are critical for sensory perception, complex integration occurs in the brain that enable the infant to perceive, understand, and respond to the world. Furthermore, preterm birth disrupts normal sensory development, with the timing and intensity being altered. When sensory experiences and sensory processing do not proceed as expected, dysfunction occurs. This dysfunction is defined as a problem in processing sensory stimulation and results in difficulty with discrimination, modulation, and integration of stimuli to adaptively function in daily life (Ayres, 2005; Vergara & Bigsby, 2004). Behaviors that are observed in children with sensory integration dysfunction include being overly sensitive to touch, movements, noise, or sights; being underreactive to sensory stimulation; being hyperactive or hypoactive; having disorganized behavior; having poor self-concept; or experiencing delays in developmental milestones and academics (Miller et al., 2007). Preterm infants have significantly higher risk of developing sensory processing problems, compared with their full-term peers (Crozier et al., 2016). Although treatment is available, sensory dysfunction is a significant disability that interferes with daily living and academic skills (Romero-Ayuso, 2020). Of importance, sensory responses affect motor, cognitive, and behavioral systems (Lane et al., 2019; Parham & Cosbey, 2002). Families can struggle to support children with sensory processing problems, and the financial costs can be high. Occupational therapists address sensory processing challenges in young children (Lane et al., 2019; Schaaf et al., 2018), but the therapeutic process can be a long one. The interventions outlined in this chapter can support appropriate sensory experiences to potentially decrease the incidence of sensory dysfunction in the NICU graduate population.

PARENTS AS AN INTEGRAL PART OF THE NICU SENSORY ENVIRONMENT

Hospitalization in the NICU affects parents, as they spend the first months of their child's life often deferring to healthcare providers in the NICU (Bouet et al., 2012) and may experience challenges related to interacting with their infant. Subsequently, parents of preterm infants have a heightened risk of stress (Howe et al., 2014; Singer et al., 1999; Wright et al., 2015), depression (Miles et al., 2007), anxiety (Zelkowitz et al., 2011), and posttraumatic stress (Holditch-Davis et al., 2003). Limited engagement in the infant's care can further exacerbate anxiety and stress, prompting coping through withdrawal or avoiding participation in care (Heinemann et al., 2013). Poor parental mental health outcomes can lead to a parent's inability to interact effectively with the infant (O'Hara & McCabe, 2013; Park et al., 2016; Zelkowitz et al., 2011). Alterations in parent–infant interaction can lead to poor child social–emotional development, attachment insecurity (Shah et al., 2011), and maternal mental health issues (Gray et al., 2004; Nomura et al., 2002; Woodward et al., 2014). The importance of early parent–child interactions and early sensory exposures also relate to the infant's developmental skill acquisition (Caskey et al., 2011). Therefore, interventions that foster and support parent engagement can improve parent–infant outcomes (Athanasopoulou & Fox, 2014; White-Traut et al., 2013) as well as infant development. Making the parent–child dyad the center of care and mobilizing parents to engage and provide appropriate positive sensory exposures to their infants can have a lifelong impact.

Sensory stimulation: The intrauterine environment provides the fetus with developmentally timed sensory exposures, modulated by protective physical barriers and maternal activity, that are replaced by procedural touch/handling, movement, smell, sound, light, frequent nociceptive pain, and disruption of sleep (Graven et al., 1992). Exposures in the NICU environment may be harmful to the developing sensory system (Field, 1990; Graven et al., 2008). Further compounding the preterm infant's altered sensory experiences is a recent change in NICU design to private rooms, which can provide protection from NICU environmental stress and also can significantly reduce other positive sensory exposures (Pineda et al., 2017), especially when parents are

not able to engage in care. Subsequently, it is possible for the infant to spend significant amounts of time in a dark, quiet environment in the NICU private room. Even when they are present, parents may still not engage with their infant, not knowing how or when to interact (Reynolds et al., 2013). The result can be months of hospitalization in a sensory-deprived environment, which can alter the long-term developmental trajectory of the infant (Graven & Browne, 2008a). Therefore, there are rich opportunities for the clinician to intentionally foster positive sensory exposures to the infant through education and support of the parents.

TIMING OF PARENT ENGAGEMENT WITH THE INFANT AND TIMING OF DIFFERENT EXPOSURES

The NICU schedule enables structure to the daily routine and ensures infants receive appropriate monitoring, daily needs, and nutrition. Many NICUs establish a care schedule that supports the infant having periods of uninterrupted sleep with cares occurring during periods when the infant would be anticipated to be awake. However, this schedule may or may not correlate with the infant's arousal and sleep patterns. Some sensory exposures may increase arousal and should be clustered or reserved for times when the infant is anticipated to be awake or receiving other cares. Other sensory exposures may promote sleep and can be conducted to aid the infant into long periods of sleep in between cares (Liao et al., 2018; Park, 2020).

EVIDENCE AND SUPPORT OF BEST-PRACTICE STANDARDS TO SUPPORT THE NICU SENSORY ENVIRONMENT

Because NICU neonates are at high risk for sensory dysfunction based on immaturity or critical illness, it is essential that neonatal caregivers understand sensory development, the parents as an agent to providing appropriate and positive sensory experiences, and ways to support a healthy sensory system (Ayres, 2005; Doyle, 2009; Vergara & Bigsby, 2004). Delineating best practice standards through research in each area of sensory development supports a plan for intervention and holistic care.

Touch

Research conducted during the last 20 to 30 years has investigated four tactile interventions: gentle touch, infant massage, holding, and SSC (skin-to-skin, kangaroo mother care or KMC). See Chapter 16 on infant touch for more details.

Gentle touch is accomplished by placing adult hands on an infant with firm touch, usually applied to the head and trunk. Variations include containing the infant in a flexed position, supporting the arms across midline, or allowing the infant to grasp with the hands and brace against boundaries with the feet. This intervention has been found to lower levels of active sleep, motor agitation, and behavioral indicators of stress (Liu et al., 2007; Whitley & Rich, 2008). It appears to be appropriate for the most immature infants and does not necessitate moving the infant out of the bed/incubator. Firm, static touch has been demonstrated to be better tolerated than light or moving touch (Field et al., 2010). This technique can be taught to family members upon an infant's admission to the NICU. Family members can support their infant with touch. Parents' confidence in their ability to care for their infants can increase quickly as they learn how to calm their infants with this technique (Liu et al., 2007; Whitley & Rich, 2008).

Infant massage has been found to improve weight gain, decrease length of stay, improve behavioral responses, and improve parent–infant interaction and neurodevelopment while decreasing maternal mental health challenges (Alvarez et al., 2019; Baniasadi et al., 2019; Choi et al., 2016; Chen et al., 2008; Ferber et al., 2002; Ferber et al., 2005; Gonzalez et al., 2009; Liu et al., 2007). There are varying reports on appropriate timing of massage, but the majority of research and subsequent clinical guidelines indicate that massage is initiated no earlier than 32 weeks, postmenstrual age (Alvarez et al., 2017; Chan, 2015; Niemi, 2017). The benefits of massage are evident when parents provide it (Alvarez et al., 2019; Baniasadi et al., 2019; Chen et al., 2008; Choi et al., 2016; Feber et al., 2005; Feber et al., 2002; Gozalez et al., 2009). Teaching families specific infant massage techniques supports infant growth and development and parents' attachment to their infant and confidence in their ability to calm and support their infant.

Holding in arms is another intervention identified in the literature. Care must be taken when removing an immature infant from the incubator to hold in arms, as temperature instability can occur. Holding has been related to better infant reflex development (Pineda et al., 2018).

Of all the touch interventions, SSC has the most evidence. SSC is accomplished by placing the diapered infant on the skin of the mother or father's chest. In addition to supporting parental attachment to the infant, research has documented that this technique improves neurobehavioral development, leads to improved weight gain and decreased apnea, reduces maternal stress, and leads to improved rates of successful breastfeeding (Cho et al., 2016; Coskun & Gunay, 2020; El-Farrash et al., 2020; Kurt et al., 2020; Ludington-Hoe et al., 2008; Shattnawi et al., 2019). Research has established that SSC can be conducted with the most medically fragile and immature infants (Liu et al., 2007; Ludington-Hoe et al., 2008). However, care must be taken with the transfer from bed to parent's chest, as infant stress, changes in physiology, and temperature fluctuation have been observed (Bauer et al., 1998; Bohnhorst et al., 2001; Heimann et al., 2014). A nursing readiness assessment for SSC can aid in understanding if an infant may tolerate SSC, and SSC protocols have been published (Ludington-Hoe et al., 2008). See Chapter 16 on skin-to-skin holding for more details.

Touch intervention for infants between 23 weeks postmenstrual age and discharge should be implemented as detailed in Table 12-1. See Table 12-2 for details about touch intervention for infants starting at 32 weeks, postmenstrual age.

TABLE 12-1 Touch–Practice Recommendations for Sensory Experiences From 23 to 32 Weeks' Postmenstrual Age

Type	Recommendation	Level of Evidence	References
Prevention	Staff and families provide firm touch to organize neonate	IV, II	Field et al. (2010) Field et al. (2006)
	Apply tactile interventions to aid sleep in between cares	I	van den Hoogen et al. (2017)
	Avoid disruption of sleep	I	van den Hoogen et al. (2017)
	Encourage family presence and engagement with infant early and often	IV, IV	Klawetter et al. (2019) Pineda et al. (2018)
Treatment/ Prevention	Parents/caregivers provide skin-to-skin care to infants early, frequently, and for long periods of time among infants who are determined appropriate as assessed by medical/nursing/therapy staff	I, II, I	Charpak et al. (2021) Charpak et al. (2017) Ghojazadeh et al. (2019)
Treatment	Staff and families provide gentle touch intervention	I, II, II	van den Hoogen et al. (2017) Dur et al. (2020) Bijari et al. (2012)

Note: Level I, evidence from a systematic review or meta-analysis of all relevant randomized controlled trials (RCTs) or evidence-based clinical practice guidelines based on systematic reviews of RCTs; level II, evidence obtained from at least one well-designed RCT; level III, evidence obtained from well-designed controlled trials without randomization; level IV, evidence from well-designed case–control and cohort studies; level V, evidence from systematic reviews of descriptive and qualitative studies; level VI, evidence from a single descriptive or qualitative study; level VII, evidence from the opinion of authorities and/or reports of expert committees.

TABLE 12-2 Touch–Practice Recommendations for Sensory Experiences From 32 Weeks' Postmenstrual Age to Discharge

Type	Recommendation	Level of Evidence	References
Treatment/ Prevention	Continue with recommendations in Table 14-1, which includes gentle touch and skin-to-skin holding		
	Assess readiness for infant massage. Trained parents may provide massage as tolerated by the infant	I, V, I, V	Field et al. (2010) Juneau et al. (2015) Alvarez et al. (2017) Smith (2012)

Chemosensory: Taste

A neonate's ability to discriminate taste is developed by 24 weeks' gestation. Sweet taste elicits sucking reflexes and supports initiation of feeding. Sour and bitter tastes decrease sucking, and a neonate may attempt to withdraw from the stimuli (Liu et al., 2007; Vergara & Bigsby, 2004). Offering tastes of breast milk to preterm infants has been related to pain relief as well as improved weight gain (Beker et al., 2017; Collados-Gomez et al., 2018).Taste interventions that should be included in the NICU are featured in Table 12-3.

Chemosensory: Smell

The olfactory system has been noted in the literature to be functional by 28 weeks' gestation (Liu et al., 2007; Schaal et al., 2004). Schaal et al. (2004) reported that the mother's scent provides the first olfactory discrimination for feeding, which can aid digestion and prefeeding readiness. Noxious stimuli in the NICU are believed to interfere with the development of appropriate olfactory preferences, which in turn could interfere with feeding and attachment to the mother (Liu et al., 2007). Olfaction is important for both healthy and high-risk infants (Schaal et al., 2004).

The emotional impact of odors can be altered by the length of time of exposure and/or by the pairings of the odor with other stimuli and with reinforcers provided by caregivers. This effect can be used to generate substitutive neonatal odor expectations to the benefit of infants facing atypical developmental conditions caused by prolonged isolation in an incubator, nonoral feeding, or pain and procedural distress. As the NICU environment can be fraught with smells of alcohol or cleaners, it is important to keep these smells out of the infant's microenvironment. Mother's scent or the scent of breast milk have been related to better outcomes (Liu et al., 2007; Schaal et al., 2004; Laudert et al., 2007; Fitri et al., 2020). Emerging literature indicates potential benefits of aromatherapy for both healthy and high-risk infants, including reduced length of stay, decreased pain and stress, improved oxygen saturation rate, and decreased heart rate variability (Fitri et al., 2020; Daniel et al., 2020; Razaghi et al., 2020).

Based on the current literature, NICU interventions support olfactory neuromaturation among all postmenstrual ages (see Table 12-4).

Auditory

NICU noise levels have been investigated for the last 30 years. This research has demonstrated that NICU noise levels can be unpredictable, excessive, and loud. These noise levels can lead to noise-induced habituation difficulties and disrupted sleep (Behrman & Butler, 2007; Brown, 2009; Goines, 2008; Liu et al., 2007). However, the auditory environment must be considered in the context of whether the infant is in a louder open ward or in a quiet, private NICU room (Liszka

TABLE 12-3 Taste–Practice Recommendations for Sensory Experiences

Type	Recommendation	Level of Evidence	References
	Staff encourages mothers to have infants nuzzle at the breast during skin-to-skin contact to facilitate taste of breast and breast milk	II, VII, VII	Sullivan and Toubas (1998) Nye (2008) Lemons (2001)
Treatment/ Prevention	Nurses provide oral care using swabs that have sterile water or breast milk	VII, II	Digal et al. (2020) Lee et al. (2015)
	Provide tastes of breast milk	II	Muelbert et al. (2019)

TABLE 12-4 Smell–Practice Recommendations for Sensory Exposures

Type	Recommendation	Level of Evidence	References
Prevention	Staff encourages mothers to have infants nuzzle at the breast during SSC to support discrimination of maternal breast scent and breast milk scent	II, II	Muelbert et al. (2019) Cakirli and Acikgoz (2021)
	Cleaning products used in the NICU should be unscented. Staff does not wear perfume or aftershave in the NICU. Laundry services should use unscented products	V, VII	Bartocci et al. (2001) Laudert et al. (2007)
	Keep unnatural odors out of the infant's microenvironment	V	Bartocci et al. (2001)
Treatment/ Prevention	Mother provides cloth with maternal scent to place in infant's bed	II, VII	Ozdemir and Tufekci (2014) Laudert et al. (2007)
	Encourage close contact with parents	IV, IV, V	Pineda et al. (2018) Renolds et al. (2013) Klawetter et al. (2019)

et al., 2019). Since its inception, developmental care has addressed the issues of auditory stimulation. The recommendations have varied little in recent years (Goines, 2008). The American Academy of Pediatrics recommends that average NICU noise levels not exceed 45 dB. Exposure to parental voices speaking quietly, especially the mother, supports learning of human speech patterns that usually develop in utero between 31 and 40 weeks' gestation (Liu et al., 2007). Over the past several years, there has been more research emerging on the use of appropriate, positive forms of auditory exposure. The auditory exposures supported in the literature include reading to or singing to the infant and playing music or other recorded sounds. Language exposure during NICU hospitalization has been related to positive outcomes (Caskey et al., 2014; Chorna et al., 2014; Doheny et al., 2012;

Flippa et al., 2013; Krueger et al., 2010; Scala et al., 2018). Owing to the reciprocal nature of human interaction during auditory exposures, use of recorded sounds for immature infants <32 weeks may be inappropriate.

To support appropriate auditory development, see Table 12-5 for recommendations for infants between 23 and 32 weeks', postmenstrual age. See Table 12-6 for auditory recommendations for infants who are older than 32 weeks' postmenstrual age.

Visual

The visual system does not require external stimulation before 40 weeks' postmenstrual age (Liu et al., 2007). Preterm infants do not have a competent pupillary reflex

TABLE 12-5 Auditory–Practice Recommendations for Sensory Exposures at 23 to 32 Weeks' Postmenstrual Age

Type	Recommendation	Level of Evidence	References
Prevention	Staff and families keep ambient noise to <45 dB	V	Casavant et al. (2017)
	Monitor sound levels	I	Almadhoob and Ohlsson (2020)
	Staff models and educates families to use quiet voices in the NICU	IV	Scala et al. (2018)
Treatment/ Prevention	Quiet conversations at the bedside	VI, IV	Scala et al. (2020) Chorna et al. (2014b)
	Families may begin reading simple children's books to the infant after 28 weeks' postmenstrual age; increase parent talking to infant as postmenstrual age advances	IV, V	Caskey et al. (2011) Pineda et al. (2019)

TABLE 12-6 Auditory–Practice Recommendations for Sensory Experiences From 32 Weeks' Postmenstrual Age to Discharge

Type	Recommendation	Level of Evidence	References
Prevention	Continue with recommendations in Table 14-5		
	After 32 weeks' postmenstrual age, families may provide recorded music or sounds. Staff monitors appropriateness and volume of <45 dB	I, V, V	van der Heijden et al. (2016) Williamson and McGrath (2019)
	Staff models and educates families to use quiet voices when interacting with the infant	IV	Scala et al. (2020)

until 35 weeks' gestation. Because external stimulation is not necessary and the infant's visual system is immature until term age, promoting focusing and following of inanimate objects is not encouraged. However, owing to parent–child interaction being important and early interaction relating to parent–child visual interaction, use of parents faces to encourage focus and follow can be encouraged once the infant is able to demonstrate arousal for sustained periods of time without significant stress signs. See Table 12-7 for recommendations for infants between 23 and 35 weeks' postmenstrual age. See Table 12-8 for visual recommendations for infants who are at least 36 weeks' postmenstrual age.

To protect the developing visual system, it is recommended that ambient lighting levels in infant spaces within the NICU should be adjustable through a range of at least 10 to no more than 600 lux (~1 to 60 foot-candles) (White, & on behalf of the Consensus Committee, 2019). Cycled lighting that follows circadian rhythms (<30 lux during the night, maximum of 300 to 580 lux during the day) is recommended, with implementation of cycled lighting leading to improved growth rates and decreased length of stay (Morag & Ohlsson, 2016).

Sensory Experiences in the NICU

Implementing practices that support the integration of the early sensory systems will improve the neonate's development of adaptive responses to the environment (Aylward, 2005; Ayres, 2005; Bonnier, 2008). Each system is important, reliant on the others, and necessitates attention and intention. The Supporting and Enhancing NICU Sensory Experiences (SENSE) program is a detailed strategy aimed at providing appropriate timing and amounts of developmentally appropriate stimuli across the senses (Pineda et al., 2019). Developmental care practices that support sensory experiences based on postmenstrual age and neuromaturation are neuroprotective in that these techniques promote appropriate brain development and decrease the incidence of neurodevelopmental delays (Bonnier, 2008). This neuroprotection is of critical importance in the NICU population at high risk for developmental delays based on immaturity and/or critical illness. Appropriate early sensory experiences protect and support optimal long-term outcome by facilitating adaptive response development (Ayres, 2005; Vergara & Bigsby, 2004).

TABLE 12-7 Visual–Practice Recommendations for Sensory Experiences at 23 to 37 Weeks' Postmenstrual Age

Type	Recommendation	Level of Evidence	References
Prevention	Staff protect the infant from direct lighting. When procedures require overhead lighting, staff protect the infant's eyes from direct light	V	White et al. (2019)
	There is insufficient evidence to support the use of visual stimulation prior to term age; however, enface interactions can foster parent-infant interaction once the infant is mature enough to tolerate it	I	Evans et al. (2014)
	Lighting in the room should be controlled to support appropriate sleep patterns	VII, VI	Laudert et al. (2007) Zores et al. (2018)

TABLE 12-8 Visual–Practice Recommendations for Sensory Experiences From 37 Weeks' Postmenstrual Age to Discharge

Type	Recommendation	Level of Evidence	References
Treatment/ Prevention	Continue with recommendations in Table 12-7		
	Staff encourages development of circadian rhythm, providing day/night cycling of light once the infant is mature (approximately 32 weeks)	I	Morag and Ohlsson (2016)

TABLE 12-9 Practice Recommendations for Sensory Experiences at Discharge

Type	Recommendation	Level of Evidence	References
Treatment/ Prevention	Staff educate parents that television should be avoided in infancy	I	Kostyrka-Allchorne et al. (2017)
	NICU staff refers infant to therapy programming (OT, PT, SLP) and other needed medical services. After discharge, developmental specialists in family's residential proximity will work with family to form appropriate goals, educate on therapeutic interventions, and monitor infant's development. Extra support may be needed to help families access services in a timely manner	IV, VII	Nwabara et al. (2017) Goldstein and Malcolm (2019)
	Staff models and explains that infants need to be held and cuddled, have age-appropriate sensory exposures, and engage in age-appropriate interaction and play		

OT, occupational therapy; PT, physical therapy; SPT, speech and language pathology.

SENSORY PROCESSING SUPPORT IN THE TRANSITION TO HOME

Developmental care must continue into the home environment over the first several months and throughout the first years of life. During this critical time of sensory development, parental understanding and engagement in sensory supportive activities is essential. Although discharge education may include the recommendations found in Table 12-9, referral to therapy programming (physical therapy, occupational therapy, and speech and language pathology) will aid in an individualized approach as the infant enters each new stage of development.

CONCLUSION

Sensory experiences are the building blocks of skill development and are critical for the infant to interact with the environment in a competent manner (Ayres, 2005). For infants born preterm and/or critically ill, optimal early sensory experiences require the support of healthcare professionals in the NICU and family members. Developmental care facilitates sensory processing through a combination of sensory protection techniques and appropriately timed sensory stimulation

approaches. Both of these aspects of practice support infants in developing adaptive responses to the environment and caregivers. In addition, these practices facilitate the early parent–child relationship and are foundational for fostering parental confidence in their abilities to care for their infant.

Ayres (2005) elegantly stated, "The brain must organize all of our sensations if a person is to move and learn and behave in a productive manner" (p. 5). Developmental care provides the neonatal brain with the opportunity to integrate sensory stimulation into appropriately processed information to support ongoing development. Knowledge of developmental care practices and sensory integration theory provides NICU professionals with the ability to influence optimal developmental outcomes and optimal parental attachment and confidence in caregiving abilities.

ACKNOWLEDGMENTS

The authors wish to thank Rebecca Guth and Audrey Gronemeyer for their time and dedication in searching the evidence on sensory interventions in the NICU. The authors also wish to thank Polly Kellner, Marinthea Richter, Prutha Saptute, Alexis Killam, Julia Lisle, and Brittany Ngo for their editing support.

Potential Research Questions

Prevention

- What is the effect of positive sensory experiences applied every day of NICU hospitalization?
- What is the impact of positive sensory exposures in the NICU in extremely preterm infants?
- What are the unique contributions of parent-delivered positive sensory exposures, compared with sensory experiences provided by a non-parent?
- How does the amount and intensity of one type of sensory exposure impact the effect of others?
- What is the correct combination of sensory exposures to optimize outcomes?

Confirmation

- Can a universal tool guide the clinician to understand when infants are and are not ready for sensory exposures?
- What are the immediate and long-term effects of positive sensory experiences on the infant and family?

Treatment

- Which sensory exposures foster sleep? Arousal?
- Would family perspective on the NICU experience be altered by a parent feeling confident in providing sensory experiences of their high-risk infant in the NICU?

REFERENCES

About FiCare. (2020). http://familyintegratedcare.com/about-ficare/

Almadhoob, A., & Ohlsson, A. (2020). Sound reduction management in the neonatal intensive care unit for preterm or very low birth weight infants. *Cochrane Database of Systematic Reviews, 1*(1), CD010333. https://doi.org/10.1002/14651858.CD010333.pub3. PMID: 31986231 Free PMC article.

Als, H. (1982). Toward a synactive theory of development: Promise for the assessment and support of infant individuality. *Infant Mental Health Journal, 34*(4), 229–243.

Alvarez, M. J., Fernández, D., Gómez-Salgado, J., Rodríguez-González, D., Rosón, M., & Lapeña, S. (2017). The effects of massage therapy in hospitalized preterm neonates: A systematic review. *International Journal of Nursing Studies, 69*, 119–136.

Alvarez, M. J., Rodriguez-Gonzalez, D., Roson, M., Lapena, S., Gomez-Salgado, J., & Fernandez-Garcia, D. (2019). Effects of massage therapy and kinesitherapy to develop hospitalized preterm infant's anthropometry: A quasi-experimental study. *Journal of Pediatric Nursing, 46*, E86–E91.

American Academy of Pediatrics (AAP) Committee on Environmental Health. (1997). Noise: A hazard for the fetus and newborn. *Pediatrics, 100*(4), 724–727.

Anderson, P. J., & Doyle, L. W. (2008). Cognitive and educational deficits in children born extremely preterm. *Seminars in Perinatology, 32*(1), 51–58.

Anderson, P., Doyle, L. W., & Victorian Infant Collaborative Study Group, . (2003). Neurobehavioral outcomes of school-age children born extremely low birth weight or very preterm in the 1990s. *The Journal of the American Medical Association, 289*(24), 3264–3272.

Athanasopoulou, E., & Fox, J. R. (2014). Effects of kangaroo mother care on maternal mood and interaction patterns between parents and their preterm, low birth weight infants: A systematic review. *Infant Mental Health Journal, 35*(3), 245–262.

Atun-Einy, O., & Scher, A. (2008). Measuring developmentally appropriate practice in neonatal intensive care units. *Journal of Perinatology, 28*(3), 218–225.

Aylward, G. P. (2005). Neurodevelopmental outcomes of infants born prematurely. *Journal of Development & Behavior in Pediatrics, 26*(6), 427–440.

Ayres, A. J. (2005). *Sensory integration and the child: 25th anniversary edition*. Western Psychological Services.

Baniasadi, H., Hosseini, S. S., Abdollahyar, A., Sheikhbardsiri, H. (2019). Effect of massage on behavioural responses of preterm infants in an educational hospital in Iran. *Journal of Reproductive & Infant Psychology, 37*(3), 302–310.

Barre, N., Morgan, A., Doyle, L. W., & Anderson, P. J. (2011). Language abilities in children who were very preterm and/or very low birth weight: A meta-analysis. *Journal of Pediatrics, 158*(5), 766–777.

Bartocci, M., Winberg, J., Papendieck, G., Mustica, T., Serra, G., & Lagercrantz, H. (2001). Cerebral hemodynamic response to unpleasant odors in the preterm newborn measured by near-infrared spectroscopy. *Pediatric Research, 50*, 324–330. https://doi.org/10.1203/00006450-200109000-00006

Bartocci, M., Winberg, J., Ruggiero, C., Bergqvist, L. L., Serra, G., & Lagercrantz, H. (2000). Activation of olfactory cortex in newborn infants after odor stimulation: A functional near-infrared spectroscopy study. *Pediatric Research, 48*, 13–23.

Bauer, K., Pyper, A., Perling, P., Uhrig, C., & Versmold, H. (1998). Effects of gestational and postnatal age on body temperature, oxygen consumption, and activity during early skin-to-skin contact between preterm infants of 25-30-week gestation and their mothers. *Pediatric Research, 44*(2), 247–251.

Behrman, R. E., & Butler, A. S. (2007). *Preterm birth: Causes, consequences, and prevention. Institute of medicine (IOM) committee on understanding preterm birth and assuring healthy outcomes.* The National Academies Collection.

Beker, F., Opie, G., Noble, E., Jiang, Y., & Bloomfield, F. H. (2017). Smell and taste to improve nutrition in very preterm infants: A randomized controlled pilot trial. *Neonatology, 111*(3), 260–266.

Berument, S. K., Sonmez, D., & Eyupoglu, H. (2012). Supporting language and cognitive development of infants and young children living in children's homes in Turkey. *Child Care Health Development, 38*(5), 743–752.

Bijari, B. B., Iranmanesh, S., Eshghi, F., & Baneshi, M. R. (2012). Gentle Human Touch and Yakson: The effect on preterm's behavioral reactions. *International Scholarly Research Notices (ISRN) Nursing, 2012*, 750363. https://doi.org/10.5402/2012/750363

Bloomfield, E. H., Alexander, T., Muelbert, M., & Beker, F. (2017). Smell and taste in the preterm infant. *Early Human Development, 114*, 31–34.

Boggini, T., Pozzoli, S., Schiavolin, P., Erario, R., Mosca, F., Brambilla, P., & Fumagalli, M. (2021). Cumulative procedural pain and brain development in very preterm infants: A systematic review of clinical and preclinical studies. *Neuroscience & Biobehavioral Reviews. 123*, 320–336.

Bohnhorst, B., Heyne, T., Peter, C. S., & Poets, C. F. (2001). Skin-to-skin (kangaroo) care, respiratory control, and thermoregulation. *Journal of Pediatrics, 138*(2), 193–197.

Bolisetty, S., Dhawan, A., Abdel-Latif, M., Bajuk, B., Stack, J., & Lui, K. (2014). Intraventricular hemorrhage and neurodevelopmental outcomes in extreme preterm infants. *Pediatrics, 133*(1), 55–62.

Bonnier, C. (2008). Evaluation of early stimulation programs for enhancing brain development. *Acta Paediatrica, 97*(7), 853–858.

Bouet, K. M., Claudio, N., Ramirez, V., & Garcia-Fragoso, L. (2012). Loss of parental role as a cause of stress in the neonatal intensive care unit. *Boletin de la Asociacion Medica de Puerto Rico, 104*(1), 8–11.

Boyle, E. M., Field, D. J., Wolke, D., & Alfirevic, Z. (2012). Effects of gestational age at birth on health outcomes at 3 and 5 years of age: Population based cohort study. *British Medical Journal, 344*, e896.

Bozkurt, O., Eras, Z., Sari, F. N., Dizdar, E. A., Uras, N., Canpolat, F. E., & Oguz, S. S. (2017). Does maternal psychological distress affect neurodevelopmental outcomes of preterm infants at a gestational age of ≤32 weeks. *Early Human Developmental, 104*, 27–31.

Brazelton, T. B., Tronick, E., Adamson, L., Als, H., & Wise, S. (1975). Early mother-infant reciprocity. *Ciba Foundation Symposium, 33*, 137–154.

Broring, T., Oostrom, K. J., Lafeber, H. N., Jansma, E. P., & Ooosterlaan, J. (2017). Sensory modulation in preterm children: Theoretical perspective and systematic review. *PLoS One, 12*(2) https://doi.org/10.1371/journal.pone.0170828

Brown, G. (2009). NICU noise and the preterm infant. *Neonatal Network, 28*(3), 165–173.

Browne, J. V., Jaeger, C. B., & Kenner, C. (2020). Executive summary: Standards, competencies, and recommended best practices for infant-and family-centered developmental care in the intensive care unit. *Journal of Perinatology, 40*(Suppl. 1), 5–10.

Browne, J. V., Jaeger, C. B., & on behalf of the Consensus Committee of the Standards, Competencies, and Best Practices for Infant and Family-Centered Developmental Care in the Intensive Care Unit, . (2019). *Report of the first consensus conference on standards, competencies and best practices for infant and family-centered developmental care in the intensive care unit.* https://nicudesign.nd.edu/nicu-care-standards/

Brown, N. C., Inder, T. E., Bear, M. J., Hunt, R. W., Anderson, P. J., & Doyle, L. W. (2009). Neurobehavior at term and white and gray matter abnormalities in very preterm infants. *Journal of Pediatrics, 155*(1), 32–39.

Brummelte, S., Grunau, R. E., Chau, V., Poskitt, K. J., Brant, R., Vinall, J., Gover, A., Synnes, A. R., & Miller, S.P. (2012). Procedural pain and brain development in premature newborns. *Annuals of Neurology, 71*(3), 385–296.

Bustani, P. C. (2008). Developmental care: Does it make a difference? Archives of disease in childhood. *Fetal and Neonatal Edition, 93*(4), F317–F321.

Byers, J. F. (2003). Components of developmental care and the evidence for their use in the NICU. *MCN American Journal of Maternal Child Nursing, 28*(3), 174–190; quiz 181–182.

Cabral, T. I., da Silva, L. G. P., Martinez, C. M. S., & Tudella, E. (2016). Analysis of sensory processing in preterm infants. *Early Human Development, 103*, 77–81.

Cakirli, M., & Acikgoz, A. (2021). A randomized controlled trial: The effect of own mother's breast milk odor and another mother's breast milk odor on pain level of newborn infants. *Breastfeeding Medicine, 16*(1), https://doi.org/10.1089/bfm.2020.0222

Calciolari, G., & Montirosso, R. (2011). The sleep protection in the preterm infants. *Journal of Maternal Fetal Neonatal Medicine, 24*(Suppl. 10), 12–14.

Casavant, S.G., Bernier, K., Andrews, S., & Bourgoin, A. (2017). Noise in the neonatal intensive care unit: What does the evidence tell us? *Adances in Neonatal Care, 17*(4), 265–273.

Caskey, M., Stephens, B., Rucker, R., & Vohr, B. (2014). Adult talk in the nICU with preterm infants and developmental outcomes. *Pediatrics, 133*(3), e578–e584.

Caskey, M., Stephens, B., Tucker, R., & Vohr, B. (2011). Importance of parent talk on the development of preterm infant vocalizations. *Pediatrics, 128*(5), 910–916.

Chan, W. K. (2015). Development of an evidence-based guideline for preterm infant massage by parents. *International Journal of Complementary and Alternative Medicine, 2*, 191–197.

Charpak, N., Montealegre-Pomar, A., & Bohorquez, A. (2021). Systematic review and meta-analysis suggest that the duration of kangaroo mother care has a direct impact on neonatal growth. *Acta Paediatrica, 110*, 45–59.

Charpak, N., Tessier, R., Ruiz, J. G., Hernandez, J. T., Uriza, F., Villegas, J., Nadeau, L., Mercier, C., Maheu, F., Marin, J., Cortes, D., Gallego, J. M., & Maldonado, D. (2017). Twenty-year follow-up of kangaroo mother care versus traditional care. *Pediatrics, 139*(10, e20162063.

Chen, L. L., Su, S. Y., Lin, C. H., & Kuo, H. C., (2008). Acupressure and meridian massage: Combined effects on increasing body weight in premature infants. *Journal of Clinical Nursing, 17*, 1174–1181.

Choi, H. J., Kim, S.-J. Oh, J., Lee, M.-N., Kim, S. H., & Kang, K.-A. (2016). The effects of massage therapy on physical growth and gastrointestinal function in premature infants: A pilot study. *Journal of Child Health Care, 20*(3), 394–404.

Cho, E. S., Kim, S.-J., Kwon, M. S., Cho, H., Kim, E. H., Jun, E. M., & Lee, S. (2016). The effects of kangaroo care in the neonatal intensive care unit on the physiological functions of preterm infants, maternal-infant attachment, and maternal stress. *Journal of Pediatric Nursing 31*(40), 430–438.

Chorna, O. D., Slaughter, J. C., Wang, L., Stark, A. R., & Maitre, N. L. (2014a). A pacifier-activated music player with mother's voice improves oral feeding in preterm infants. *Pediatrics, 133*(3), 462–468.

Chorna, O., Solomon, J. E., Slaughter, J. C., Stark, A. R., & Maitre, N. L. (2014b). Abnormal sensory reactivity in preterm infants during the first year correlates with adverse neurodevelopmental outcomes at 2 years of age. *Archives of Disease in Childhood: Fetal Neonatal Edition, 99*(6), F475–F479.

Chu, D. H., & Loomis, C. A. (2016). Structure and development of the skin and cutaneous appendages. In Polin, R. A., Abman, S. H., Rowitch, D. H., Benitz, W. E., & Fox, W. W. (Eds.). *Fetal and neonatal physiology* (5th ed., pp. 490–497). Elsevier.

Collados-Gomez, L., Ferrera-Camacho, P., Fernandez-Serrano, E., Camacho-Vicente, V., Flores-Herrero, C., Garcia-Pozo, A. M., & Jimenez-Garcia, R. (2018). Randomised crossover trial showed that using breast milk or sucrose provided the same analgesic effect in preterm infants of at least 28 weeks. *Acta Paediatrica, 107*(3), 436–441.

Coskun, D., & Gunay, U. (2020). The effects of kangaroo care applied by Turkish mothers who have premature babies and cannot breastfeed on their stress levels and amount of milk production. *Journal of Pediatric Nursing, 50*, e26–e32.

Crozier, S. C., Goodson, J. Z., Mackay, M. L., Synnes, A. R., Grunau, R. E., Miller, S. P., & Zwicker, J. G. (2016). Sensory processing patterns in children born very preterm. *The American Journal of Occupational Therapy, 70*(10), 7001220050p1–7001220050p7. https://doi.org/10.5014/ajot.2016.018747

Daniel, J. M., Davidson, L. N., Havens, J. R., Bauer, J. A., & Shook, L. A. (2020). Aromatherapy as an adjunctive therapy for neonatal abstinence syndrome: A pilot study. *Journal of Opioid Management, 16*(2), 119–125.

Daunhauer, L. A., Coster, W. J., Tickle-Degnen, L., & Cermak, S. A. (2007). Effects of caregiver-child interactions on play occupations among young children institutionalized in Eastern Europe. *American Journal of Occupational Therapy, 61*(4), 429–440.

Daunhauer, L. A., Coster, W. J., Tickle-Degnen, L., & Cermak, S. A. (2010). Play and cognition among young children roared in an institution. *Physical and Occupational Therapy in Pediatrics, 30*(2), 83–97.

DeCasper, A., & Spence, M. (1985). Prenatal maternal speech influences newborns' perception of speech sounds. *Infant Behavior and Development, 9*, 133–150.

Digal, K. C., Upadhyay, J., Singh, P., Shubham, S., Grover, R., & Basu, S. (2020). Oral care with mother's own milk in sick and preterm neonates: A quality improvement initiative. *The Indian Journal of Pediatrics, 88*(1). https://doi.org/10.1007/s12098-0202-03434-5

Doheny, L., Hurwitz, S., Insoft, R., Ringer, S., & Lahav, A. (2012). Exposure to biological maternal sounds improves cardiorespiratory regulation in extremely preterm infants. *Journal of Maternal Fetal & Neonatal Medicine, 25*(9), 1591–1594.

Doyle, L. W., & Saigal, S. (2009). Long-term outcomes of very preterm or tiny infants. *NeoReviews, 10*, e130–e137.

Dur, S., Caglar, S., Uildiz, U., Dogan, P., Varnal, I. G. (2020). The effect of Yakson and gentle human touch methods on pain and physiological parameters in preterm infants during heel lancing. *Intensive Critcal Care Nursing, 61*, 102886. https://doi.org/10.1016/j.iccn.2020.102886

El-Farrash, R. A., Shinkar, D. M., Ragab, D. A., Salem, R. M., Saad, W. E., Farag, A. S., Salama, D. H., & Sakr, M. F. (2020). Longer duration of kangaroo care improves neurobehavioral performance and feeding in preterm infants: A randomized controlled trial. *Pediatric Research, 87*(4), 683–688.

Evans, T., Whittingham, K., Sanders, M., Colditz, P., & Boyd, R. N. (2014). Are parenting interventions effective in improving the relationship between mothers nad their preterm infants? *Infant Behavior & Development, 37*(2), 131–154.

Fagard, J., Esseily, R., Jacquey, L., O'Regan, K., & Somogyi, E. (2018). Fetal origin of sensorimotor behavior. *Fontiers in Neurorobotics, 12*(23), https://doi.org/10.3389/fnbot.2018.00023

Feldman, R., Rosenthal, Z., & Eidelman, A. I. (2014). Maternal-preterm skin-to-skin contact enhances child physiologic organization and cognitive control across the first 10 years of life. *Biological Psychiatry, 75*(1), 56–64.

Ferber, S. G., Kohelet, F. R., Kuint, J., Dollberg, S., Arbel, E., & Weller, A. (2005). Massage therapy facilitates mother-infant interaction in premature infants. *Infant Behavior & Development, 28*, 74–81.

Ferber, S. G., Kuint, J., Weller, A., Feldman, R., Dollberg, S., Arbel, E., & Kohelet, D. (2002). Massage therapy by mothers and trained professionals enhances weight gain in preterm infants. *Early Human Development, 67*(1–2), 37–45.

Field, T. (1990). Alleviating stress in newborn infants in the intensive care unit. *Clinical in Perinatology, 17*(1), 1–9.

Field, T., Diego, M., & Hernandez-Reif, M. (2010). Preterm infant massage therapy research: A review. *Infant Behavior & Development, 33*(2), 115–124.

Field, T., Diego, M. A., Hernandez-Reif, M., Deeds, O., & Figuereido, B. (2006). Moderate versus light pressure massage therapy leads to greater weight gain in preterm infants. *Infant Behavior & Development, 29*(4), 574–578.

Fifer, W. P., & Moon, C. M. (1994). The role of mother's voice in the organization of brain function in the newborn. *Acta Paediatrica, 83*(Suppl. 397), 86–93.

Fitri, S. Y. R., Wardhani, V., Rakhmawati, W., Pahria, T., & Hendrawati, S. (2020). Culturally based practice in neonatal procedural pain management: A mini review. *Frontiers in Pediatrics, 8*, 540. https://doi.org/10.3389/fped.2020.00540

Flippa, M., Devouche, E., Arioni, C., Imberty, M., & Gratier, M. (2013). Live maternal speech and singing have beneficial effects on hospitalized preterm infants. *Acta Paediatrica, 102*(10), 1017–1020.

Foulder-Hughes, L. A., & Cooke, R. W. (2003). Motor, cognitive, and behavioural disorders in children born very preterm. *Developmental Medicine & Child Neurology, 45*(2), 97–103.

Fumagalli, M., Provenzi, L., De Caroli, P., Dessimone, F., Sirgiovanni, I., Giorda, R., Cinnante, C., Squarcina, L., Pozzoli, U., Triulzi, F., Brambilla, P., Borgatti, R., Mosca, F., & Montirosso, R. (2018). From early stress to 12-month development in very preterm infants: Preliminary findings on epigenetic mechanisms and brain growth. *PLoS One, 13*(1), e0190602.

Gazzaniga, M. S., Irvry, R. B., & Mangun, R. G. (2014). Perception and sensation. . In Javsicas, A. & Snavely, S. (Eds.). *Cognitive neuroscience: The biology of the mind* (pp. 162–217). W.W. Norton.

Ghojazadeh, M., Hajebrahimi, S., Pournaghi-Azar, F., Mohseni, M., Derakhshani, N., & Azami-Aghdash, S. (2019). Effect of kangaroo mother care on successful breastfeeding: A systematic review and meta-analysis of randomized controlled trials. *Reviews of Recent Clinical Trials, 14*(1), 31–40.

Gibbons, S., Hoath, S. B., Coughlin, M., Gibbins, A., & Franck, L. (2008). The universe of developmental care: A new conceptual model for application in the neonatal intensive care unit. *Advanced in Neonatal Care, 8*(3), 141–147.

Glass, P. (1990). Light and the developing retina. *Documenta Ophthalmologica, 74*(3), 195–203.

Goines, L. (2008). The importance of quiet in the home: Teaching noise awareness to parents before the infant is discharged from the NICU. *Neonatal Network, 37*(3), 171–176.

Goldenberg, R. L., Culhane, J. F., Iams, J. D., & Romero, R. (2008). Epidemiology and causes of preterm birth. *Lancet, 371*(9606), 75–84.

Goldstein, R. F., & Malcolm, W. F. (2019). Care of the neonatal intensive care unit graduate after discharge. *Pediatric Clinics of North American, 66*(2), 489–508.

Gonzalez, A. P., Vasquez-Mendoza, G., Garcia-Vela, A., Guzman-Ramirez, A., Salazar-Torres, M., & Romero-Gutierrez, G. (2009). Weight gain in preterm infants following parent-administered vimala massage: A randomized controlled trial. *American Journal of Perinatology, 26*(4), 247–252.

Gottlieb, G. (1971). Ontogenesis of sensory function in birds and mammals. In Tobach, E., Aronson, L., & Shaw, E. (Eds.), *The biopsychology of development* (pp. 66–182). Academic Press.

Govindan, R. M., Behen, M. E., Helder, E., Makki, M. I., & Chugani, H. T. (2010). Altered water diffusivity in cortical association tracts in children with early deprivation identified with tract-based spatial statistics (TBSS). *Cerebral Cortex, 20*(3), 561–569.

Goyen, T. A., Lui, K., & Woods, R. (1998). Visual-motor, visual-perceptual, and fine motor outcomes in very-low-birthweight children at 5 years. *Developmental Medicine & Child Neurology, 40*(2), 76–81.

Graven, S. N., Bowen, F. W., Jr, Brooten, D., Eaton, A., Graven, M. N., Hack, M., Hall, L. A., Hansen, N., Hurt, H., & Kavalhuna, R., (1992). The high-risk infant environment. Part 1. The role of the neonatal intensive care unit in the outcome of high-risk infants. *Journal of Perinatology, 12*(2), 164–172.

Graven, S. N., & Browne, J. V. (2008a). Sensory development in the fetus, neonate, and infant: Introduction and overview. *Newborn and Infant Nursing Reviews, 8*(4), 169–172.

Graven, S. N., & Browne, J. V. (2008b). Auditory development in the fetus and infant. *Newborn and Infant Nursing Reviews, 8*(4), 187–193.

Graven, S. N., & Browne, J. V. (2008c). Visual development in the human fetus, infant, and young child. *Newborn and Infant Nursing Reviews, 8*(4), 194–201.

Gravina, S. A., Yep, G. L., & Khan, M. (2013). Human biologic of taste. *Annals of Saudi Medicine, 33*(3), 217–222.

Gray, R. F., Indurkhya, A., & McCormick, M. C. (2004). Prevalence, stability, and predictors of clinically significant behavior problems in low birth weight children at 3, 5, and 8 years of age. *Pediatrics* 114(3), 736–743.

Gursul, D., Harley, C., & Slater, R. (2019). Nociception and the neonatal brain. *Seminars in Fetal and Neonatal Medicine, 24*(4), 101016.

Guyer, C., Huber, R., Fontijn, J., Bucher, H. U., Nicolai, H., Werner, H., Molinari, L., Latal, B., & Jenni, O. G. (2015). Very preterm infants show earlier emergence of 24-hour sleep-wake rhythms compared to term infants. *Early Human Development, 91*(1), 37042.

Hack, M., & Costello, D. W. (2008). Trends in the rates of cerebral palsy associated with neonatal intensive care of preterm children. *Clinics in Obstetrics & Gynecology, 51*(4), 763–774.

van der Heijden, M. J. E., Araghi, S. O., Jeekel, J., Reiss, I. K. M., Hunink, M. G. M., & van Dijk, M. (2016). Do hospitalized premature infants benefit from music interventions? A systematic review of randomized controlled trials. *PLoS One, 11*(9), e0161848. https://doi.org/10.1371/journal.pone.0161848

Heimann, K., Ebert, A. M., Abbas, A. K., Heussen, N., Leohardt, S., & Orlikowsky, T. (2014). Thermoregulation of premature infants during and after skin-to-skin care. *Z Geburtshilfe Neonatology, 217*(6), 220–224.

Heinemann, A. B., Hellstrom-Westas, L., & Nyqvist, K. H. (2013). Factors affecting parents' presence with their extremely preterm infants in a neonatal intensive care room. *Acta Paediatrica, 102*(7), 695–702.

Hepper, P. G., & Shahidullah, B. S. (1994). Development of fetal hearing. *Archives of Disease in Children, 71*(2), F81–F87.

Holditch-Davis, D., Barlett, T. R., Blickman, A. L., & Miles, M. S. (2003). Posttraumatic stress symptoms in mothers of premature infants. *Journal of Obstetrics, Gynecology, & Neonatal Nursing (JOGNN), 32*(2), 161–171.

Holsti, L., Grunau, R. V., & Whitfield, M. F. (2002). Developmental coordination disorder in extremely low birth weight children at nine years. *Journal of Developmental & Behavioral Pediatrics, 23*(1), 9–15.

van den Hoogen, A., Teunis, C. J., Shellhaas, R. A., Pillen, S., Benders, M., & Dudink, J. (2017). How to improve sleep in a neonatal intensive care unit: A systematic review. *Early Human Development, 113*, 78–86.

Howe, T.-H., Sheu, C.-F., Wang, T.-N., & Hsu, Y.-W. (2014). Parenting stress in families with very low birth weight preterm infants in early infancy. *Research in Developmental Disabilities, 35*(7), 1748–1756.

Hussey-Gardner, B., & Famuyide, M. (2009). Developmental interventions in the NICU: What are the developmental benefits? *NeoReviews, 10*(3), e113–e119.

Johnson, E. O., Babis, G. C., Soultanis, K. C., & Soucacos, P. N. (2008). Functional neuroanatomy of proprioception. *Journal of Surgical Orthopaedic Advances, 17*(3), 159–164.

Juneau, A. L., Aita, M., & Heon, M. (2015). Review and critical analysis of massage studies for term and preterm infants. *Neonatal Network, 34*(3), 165–177.

Khan, A. M., Ali, S., Jameela, R. V., Muhamood, M., & Haqh, M. F. (2019). Impact of fungiform papillae count on taste perception and different methods of taste assessment and their clinical applications. *Sultan Qaboos University Medical Journal, 19*(3), e184–e191.

Klawetter, S., Greenfield, J. C., Speer, S. R., Brown, K., & Hwang, S. S. (2019). An integrative review: Maternal engagement in the neonatal intensive care unit and health outcomes for U.S.-born preterm infants and their parents. *AIMS Public Health, 6*(2), 160–183.

Kostyrka-Allchorne, K., Cooper, N. R., & Simpson, A. (2017). The relationship between television exposure and children's cognition and behavior: A systematic review. *Developmental Review, 44*, 19–58.

Krueger, X., Parker, L., Chiu, S.-H., & Theriaque, D. (2010). Maternal voice and short-term outcomes in preterm infants. *Developmental Psychobiology, 52*(2), 205–212.

Kurt, F. Y., Kucukoglu, S., Ozdemir, A. A., & Ozcan, Z. (2020). The effect of kangaroo care on maternal attachment in preterm infants. *Niger Journal of Clinical Practice, 23*(1), 26–32.

Lai, T. T., & Bearer, C. F. (2008). Iatrogenic environmental hazards in the neonatal intensive care unit. *Clinics in Perinatology, 35*(1), 163–181.

Lane, S. J., Mailloux, Z., Schoen, S., Bundy, A., May-Benson, T. A., Parham, L. D., Roley, S. S., & Schaar, R. C. (2019). Neural foundations of Ayres sensory Integration˙. *Brain Science, 9*(7), 153.

Laudert, S., Liu, W. F., Blackington, S., Perkins, B., Martin, S., Macmillian-York, E., Graven, S., Handyside, J., & NIC/Q 2005 Physical Environment Exploratory Group. (2007). Implementing potentially better practices to support the neurodevelopment of infants in the NICU. *Journal of Perinatology, 27*(Suppl. 2), S75–S93.

Lawhon, G., & Hedlund, R. E. (2008). Newborn individualized developmental care and assessment program training and education. *Journal of Perinatal & Neonatal Nursing, 22*(2), 133–144; quiz 145–146.

Lean, R. E., Rogers, C. E., Paul, R. A., & Gerstein, E. D. (2018). NICU hospitalization: Long-term implication on parenting and child behaviors. *Current Treatment Options in Pediatrics, 4*(1), 49–69.

Lee, J., Kim, H.-S., Jung, Y. H., Choi, K. Y., Shin, S. H., Kim, E.-K., & Choi, J.-H. (2015). Oropharyngeal colostrum administration in extremely premature infants: An RCT. *Pediatrics, 135*(2), e357–e366.

Lemons, P. K. (2001). Breast milk and the hospitalized infant: Guideline for practice. *Neonatal Network, 20*(7), 47–52.

Liao, J.-H., Hu, R.-F., Su, L.-J., Wang, S., Xu, Q., Qian, X.-F., & He, H.-G. (2018). Nonpharmacological interventions for sleep promotion on preterm infants in neonatal intensive care unit: A systematic review. *Worldviews on Evidence-Based Nursing, 15*(5), 386–293.

Lickliter, R. (2011). The integrated development of sensory organization. *Clinical Perinatology, 38*(40, 591–603.

Lipchock, S. V., Reed, D. R., & Mennella, J. A. (2011). The gustatory and olfactory systems during infancy: Implications for development of feeding behaviors in the high-risk neonate. *Clinics in Perinatology, 38*(4), 627–641.

Liszka, L., Smith, J., Mathur, A., Schlaggar, B.L., Colditz, G., & Pineda, R. (2019). Differences in early auditory exposure across neonatal environments. *Early Human Development, 136*, 27–32.

Liu, W. F., Laudert, S., Perkins, E., Macmillian-York, E., Martin, S., Graven, S., & the NIC/Q 2005 Physical Environment Exploratory Group, . (2007). The development of potentially better practices to support the neurodevelopment of infants in the NICU. *Journal of Perinatology, 27*(Suppl. 2), S48–S74.

Ludington-Hoe, S. M., Morgan, K., & Abouelfettoh, A. (2008). A clinical guideline for implementation of kangaroo care with premature infants of 30 or more weeks postmenstrual age. *Advances in Neonatal Care, 8*(3), S3–S23.

Madan, A., Jan, J. E., & Good, W. V. (2005). Visual development in preterm infants. *Developmental Medicine in Child Neurology, 47*(4), 276–280.

Maguire, C. M., Walter, F. J., van Zwieten, P. H. T., Le Cessie, S., Wit, J. M., & Veen, S. (2009). Follow-up outcomes at 1 and 2 years of infants born less than 32 weeks after newborn individualized developmental care and assessment program. *Pediatrics, 132*(4), 108–1087.

Maitre, N. L., Key, A. P., Chorna, O. D., Slaughter, J. C., Matusz, P. J., Wallace, M. T., & Murray, M. M. (2017). The dual nature of early-life experience on somatosensory processing in the human infant brain. *Current Biology, 27*(7), 1048–1054.

Martucci, M. (2004). Considerations in planning a newborn developmental care program in a community hospital setting. *Advances in Neonatal Care, 4*(2), 59–66.

Marx, V., & Nagy, E. (2015). Fetal behavioural responses to maternal voice and touch. *PLoS One, 10*(6), e0129118. https://journals.plos.org/plosone/article?id=10.1371/journal.pone.0129118

McGrath, J. M., Cone, S., & Samra, H. A. (2011). Neuroprotection in the preterm infant: Further understanding of the short-and long-term implications for brain development. *Newborn and Infant Nursing Reviews, 11*, 109–112.

Mennella, J. A., Jagnow, C. P., & Beauchamp, G. K. (2001). Prenatal and postnatal flavor learning by human infants. *Pediatrics, 107*(6), E88.

Miles, M. S., Holditch-Davis, D., Schwartz, T. A., & Scher, M. (2007). Depressive symptoms in mothers of prematurely born infants. *Journal of Developmental & Behavioral Pediatrics, 28*(1), 36–44.

Milford, C. A., & Zapalo, B. J. (2010). The NICU experience and its relationship to sensory integration. In Kenner, C. & McGrath, J. M. (Eds.). *Developmental care of newborns and infants: A guide for health professionals* (2nd ed.). National Association of Neonatal Nurses (NANN).

Miller, L. J., Anzalone, M. E., Lane, S. J., Cermak, S. A., & Osten, E. T. (2007). Concept evolution in sensory integration: A proposed nosology for diagnosis. *The American Journal of Occupational Therapy, 61*(2), 135–140.

Moller, A. R. (2002). *Sensory systems: Anatomy, physiology, and pathophysiology.* Academic Press.

Morag, I., & Ohlsson, A. (2016). Cycled light in the intensive care unit for preterm and low birth weight infants. *Cochrane Library, 8*, https://doi.org/10.1002/14651858.CD006982.pub4

Muelbert, M., Lin, L., Bloomfield, F. H., & Harding, J. E. (2019). Exposure to the smell and taste of milk to accelerate feeding in preterm infants. *Cochrane Database Systematic Reviews, 7*(7), CD013038. https://doi.org/10.1002/14651858.CD013038.pub2

Musiek, F. E., & Baran, J. A. (2018). *The auditory system: Anatomy, physiology, and clinical correlates* (2nd ed.). Plural Publishing.

Niemi, A. K. (2017). Review of randomized controlled trials of massage in preterm infants. *Children (Basil), 4*(4), 21.

Nomura, Y., Wickramaratne, P. J., Warner, V., Mufson, L., & Weissman, M. M. (2002). Family discord, parental depression, and psychopathology in offspring: Ten-year follow-up. *Journal of the American Academy of Child and Adolescent Psychiatry, 41*(4), 402–409.

Nwabara, O., Rogers, C., Inder, T., & Pineda, R. (2017). Early therapy services following neonatal intensive care unit discharge. *Physical & Occupational Therapy in Pediatrics, 37*(4), 414–424.

Nye, C. (2008). Transitioning premature infants from gavage to breast. *Neonatal Network, 27*(1), 7–43.

O'Connor, A. R., Wilson, C. M., & Fielder, A. R. (2007). Ophthalmological problems associated with preterm birth. *Eye (London), 21*(10, 1254–1260.

O'Hara, M. W., & McCabe, J. E. (2013). Postpartum depression: Current status and future directions. *Annual Reviews of Clinical Psychology, 9*, 379–407.

Ozdemir, F. K., & Tufekci, F. G. (2014). The effect of individualized developmental care practices on the growth and hospitalization duration of premature infants: The effect of mother's scent and flexion position. *Journal of Clinical Nursing, 23*(21–22), 3026–3044.

Parham, L.D., & Cosbey, J. (2002). Sensory integration in everyday life. In Bundy, A.C., Lane, S. L., Mulligan, S., & Reynolds, S. (Eds.). *Sensory integration: Theory and practice* (3rd ed., pp. 21–39). F.A. Davis.

Park, J. (2020). Sleep promotion for preterm infants in the NICU. *Nursing for Women's Health, 24*(1), 24–35.

Park, J., Thoyre, S., Estrem, H., Pados, B. F., Knafl, G. J., & Brandon, D. (2016). Mothers' psychological distress and feeding of their preterm infants. *MCN American Journal of Maternal Child Nursing, 41*(1), 221–229.

Pedespan, L. (2004). Attachment and prematurity. Gynecology. *Obstertrics & Fertility, 32*(9), 716–720.

Pineda, R., Bender, J., Gall, B., Shabosky, L., Annecca, A., & Smith, J. (2018). Parent participation in the neonatal intensive care unit: Predictors and relationships to neurobehavior and developmental outcomes. *Early Human Development, 117*, 32–38.

Pineda, R., Durant, P., Mathur, A, Inder, T., Wallendorf, M., & Schlaggar, B. L. (2017). Auditory exposure in the neonatal intensive care unit: Room type and other predictors. *Journal of Pediatrics, 183*, 56–66.

Pineda, R. G., Neil, J., Dierker, D., Smyser, C. D., Wallendorf, M., Kidokoro, H., Reynolds, L. C., Walker, S., Rogers, C., Mathur, A. M., Van Essen, D. C., & Inder, T. (2014). Alterations in brain structure and neurodevelopmental outcome in preterm infants hospitalized in different neonatal intensive care unit environments. *Journal of Pediatrics, 164*(1), 52–60.

Pineda, R., Raney, M., & Smith, J. (2019). Supporting and enhancing NICU sensory experience (SENSE): Defining developmentally-appropriate sensory exposures for high-risk infants. *Early Human Development, 133*, 29–35.

Pineda, R. G., Tjoeng, T. H., Vavasseur, C., Kidokoro, H., Neil, J. J., & Inder, T. (2013). Patterns of altered neurobehavior in preterm infants within the neonatal intensive care unit. *Journal of Pediatrics, 162*(3), 470–476.

Pinto, J. M. (2011). Olfaction. *Proceeding of the American Thoracic Society, 8*(1), 46–52.

Quesada, A. A., Tristao, R. M., Pratesi, R., & Wolf, O. T. (2014). Hyper-responsiveness to acute stress, emotional problems and poorer memory in former preterm children. *Stress, 17*(5), 389–399.

Radic, J. A., Vincer, M., & McNeely, P. D. (2015). Outcomes of intraventricular hemorrhage and posthemorrhagic hydrocephalus in a population-based cohort of very preterm infants born to residents of Nova Scotia from 1993 to 2010. *Journal of Neurosurgery: Pediatrics.* 15(6). 580–588.

Ranger, M., & Grunau, R. E. (2014). Early repetitive pain in preterm infants in relation to the developing brain. *Pain Management, 4*(1), 57–67.

Razaghi, N., Aemmi, S. Z., Hoseini, A. S. S., Boskabadi, H., Mohebbi, T., & Ramezani, M. (2020). The effectiveness of familiar olfactory stimulation with lavender scent and glucose on the pain of blood sampling in term neonates: A randomized controlled clinical trial. *Complementary Therapy Medicine, 49*, 102289. https://doi.org/10.1016/j.ctim.2019.102289

Reynolds, L. C., Duncan, M. M., Smith, G. C., Mathur, A., Neil, J., Inder, T., & Pineda, R. G. (2013). Parental presence and holding in the neonatal intensive care unit and associations with early neurobehavior. *Journal of Perinatology, 33*(8), 636–641.

Robison, L. D. (2003). An organizational guide for an effective developmental care program in the NICU. *Journal of Obstetrics & Gynecology, and Neonatal Nursing (JOGNN), 32*(3), 379–386.

Rogers, E. E., & Piecuch, R. E. (2009). Neurodevelopmental outcomes of infants who experience intrauterine growth restriction. *NeoReviews, 10*(3), e100–e112.

Romero-Ayuso, T. (2020). Assessment of sensory processing and executive functions at the school: Development, reliability, and validity of EPYFEI-Escolar. *Frontiers in Pediatrics, 8*, 275. https://doi.org/10.3389/fped.2020.00275

Sarnat, H. B., Flores-Sarnat, L., & Wei, X. C. (2017). Olfactory development, part 1; Function, from fetal perception to adult wine-tasting. *Journal of Child Neurology, 32*(6), 566–578.

Scala, M. L., Marchman, V. A., Godenzi, C., Gao, C., & Travis, K. E. (2020). Assessing speech exposure in the NICU: Implications for speech enrichment for preterm infants. *Journal of Perinatology, 40*(10), 1537–1545.

Scala, M., Seo, S., Lee-Park, J., McClure, C., Scala, M., Palafoutas, J. J., & Abubakar, K. (2018). Effect of reading to preterm infants on measures of cardiorespiratory stability in the neonatal intensive care unit. *Journal of Perinatology, 38*(11).1536–1541.

Schaaf, R. C., Dumont, R. L., Arbesman, M., & May-Benson, T. A. (2018). Efficacy of occupational therapy using Ayres sensory Integration®: A systematic review. *The American Journal of Occupational Therapy, 72*(1), 7201190010p1–7201190010p10. https://doi.org/10.5014/ajot.2018.028431

Schaal, B., Hummel, T., & Soussignan, R. (2004). Olfaction in the fetal and premature infant: Functional status and clinical implications. *Clinics in Perinatology, 32*(2), 261–285.

Sealy, B., Hansen, E., & Harlow, H. F. (1962). Mother-infant separation in monkeys. *Journal of Child Psychology and Psychiatry, 3*, 123–132.

Sealy, B., & Harlow, H. F. (1965). Maternal separation in the rhesus monkey. *Journal of Nervous and Mental Disease, 140*(6), 434–441.

Shah, P. E. Clements, M., & Poehlmann, J. (2011). Maternal resolution of grief after preterm birth: Implications for infant attachment security. *Pediatrics, 127*(2), 284–292.

Shattnawi, K. K., Al-Ali, N., & Alnuaimi, K. (2019). Neonatal nurses' knowledge and beliefs about kangaroo mother care in neonatal intensive care units: A descriptive cross-sectional study. *Nursing & Health Science, 21*(3), 352–358.

Sherman, C. (2019). *The senses: Vision.* https://www.dana.org/article/the-senses-vision/

Singer, L. T., Salvator, A., Guo, S., Collin, M., Lilien, L., & Baley, J. (1999). Maternal psychological distress and parenting stress after the birth of a very low-birth-weight infant. *Journal of the American Medical Association (JAMA), 281*(9), 799–805.

Slater, R., Fabrizi, L., Worley, A., Meek, J., Boyd, S., & Fitzgerald, M. (2010). Premature infants display increased noxious-evoked neuronal activity in the brain compared to healthy age-matched term-born infants. *Neuroimage, 52*(2), 583–589.

Smith, J. R. (2012). Comforting touch in the very preterm hospitalized infant: An integrative review. *Advances in Neonatal Care, 12*(6), 349–365.

Smith, G. C., Gutovich, J., Smyser, C., Pineda, R., Newnham, C., Tjoeng, T. H., Vavasseur, C., Wllendorf, M., Neil, J., & Inder, T. (2011). Neonatal intensive care unit stress is associated with brain developmental in preterm infants. *Annals of Neurology, 70*(4), 541–549.

Starr, A., Amlie, R. N., Martin, W. H., & Sanders, S. (1977). Development of auditory function in newborn infants revealed by auditory brainstem potentials. *Pediatrics, 6*096), 831–839.

Sullivan, R. M., & Toubas, P. (1998). Clinical usefulness of maternal odor in newborns: Soothing and feeding preparatory responses. *Biology of Neonate, 74*(6), 402–408.

Symington, A., & Pinelli, J. (2009). Developmental care for promoting developmental and preventing morbidity in preterm infants (review). *The Cochrane Database of Systematic Reviews, 1*, 1–50.

Tottenham, N., & Sheridan, M. A. (2009). A review of adversity, the amygdalia and the hippocampus: A consideration of developmental timing. *Frontiers in Human Neuroscience, 3*, 68.

Vandenberg, K. A. (2007). Individualized developmental care for high risk newborns in the NICU: A practice guideline. *Early Human Development, 83*(7), 433–442.

Vasquez-Ruiz, S., Maya-Barrios, J. A., Torres-Narvaez, P., Bega-Martinez, B. R., Rojas-Granados, A., Escobar, C., & Angeles-Castellanos, M. (2014). A light/dark cycle in the NICU accelerates body weight gain and shortens time to discharge in preterm infants. *Early Human Development, 90*(9), 535–540.

Vergara, E. R., & Bigsby, R. (2004). *Developmental and therapeutic interventions in the NICU.* Aul H. Brookes Publishing Company.

Vinall, J., & Grunau, R. E. (2014). Impact of repeated procedural pain-related stress in infants born very preterm. *Pediatric Research, 75*(5), 584–587.

Weitzman, L., Graziani, L., & Duhamel, L. (1967). Maturation and topography of the auditory evoked response of the prematurely born infant. *Electroencephalography Clinics of Neurophysiology, 23*(1), 82–83.

White-Traut, R., Norr, K. F., Fabiyi, C., Rankin, K. M., Li, Z., & Liu, L. (2013). Mother-infant interaction improves with a developmental intervention for mother-preterm infant dyads. *Infant Behavior & Development, 36*(4), 694–706.

White, R. D., & on behalf of the Consensus Committee. (2019). *NICU Recommended Standards for newborn ICU design* (9th ed.). https://nicu-design.nd.edu/nicu-standards/

Whitley, J. A., & Rich, B. L. (2008). A double-blind randomized controlled pilot trial examining the safety and efficacy of therapeutic touch in premature infants. *Advances in Neonatal Care, 8*(6), 315–333.

Williams, J., Lee, K. J., & Anderson, P. J. (2010). Prevalence of motor-skill impairment in preterm children who do not develop cerebral palsy: A systematic review. *Developmental Medicine in Child Neurology, 52*(3), 232–237.

Williamson, S., & McGrath, J. M. (2019). What are the effects of the maternal voice on preterm infants in the NICU? *Advanced in Neonatal Nursing, 19*(4), 294–310.

Winberg, J., & Porter, R. H. (1998). Olfaction and human neonatal behavior: Clinical implications. *Acta Paediatrica, 87*(1), 6–10.

Woodward, L. J., Bora, S., Clark, C. A. C., Montgomery-Honger, A., Pritchard, V. E., Spencer, C., & Austin, N. C. (2014). Very preterm birth: Maternal experiences of the neonatal intensive care environment. *Journal of Perinatology, 34*(7), 555–561.

Woodward, L. J., McPherson, C. C., & Volpe, J. J. (2018). Passive addiction and teratogenic effects. In Volpe, J., Inder, T., Darras, B., de Vries, L. S., du Plessis, A., Neil, J., & Perlman, J (Eds.). *Volpe's neurology of the newborn* (6th ed., pp. 1149–1240). Elsevier.

Wraight, C. L., McCoy, J., & Meadow, W. (2015). Beyond stress: Describing the experiences of families during neonatal intensive care. *Acta Paediatrica, 104*(10), 1012–1017.

Zelkowitz, P., Na, S., Wang, T., Bardin, C., & Papageorgiou, A. (2011). Early maternal anxiety predicts cognitive and behavioural outcomes of VLBW children at 24 months corrected age. *Acta Paediatrica, 100*(5), 700–704.

Zimmerman, A., Bai, L., & Ginty, D. D. (2014). The gentle touch receptors of mammalian skin. *Science, 346*(6212), 950–954.

Zores, C., Dugour, A., Pebayle, T., Dahan, I., Astruc, D., & Kuhn, P. (2018). Observational study found that even small variations in light can wake up very preterm infants in a neonatal intensive care unit. *Acta Paediatrica, 107*(7), 1191–1197.

CHAPTER 13

Infant Sleep and Arousal

Amy L. Salisbury and Kathleen S. S. Kolberg

Standards in Infant Sleep and Arousal States

Standard 1: Promote developmentally appropriate sleep and arousal states
Standard 2: Optimize physical environment and caregiving routines to promote safe sleep and arousal
Standard 3: Encourage family presence and participation in care of their baby
Standard 4: Document and review infant sleep and arousal states to enhance care planning

---

INTRODUCTION

Sleep, the seemingly simple state of not being awake, is far more complex and critical to sustaining health than previously imagined. Discoveries over the past several decades revealed that sleep is the observable result of coordinated neurological and physiological processes, each contributing to stages within the sleep state. These interrelated processes begin to emerge before birth and play a central role in the generation of sleep–wake cycles as well as state cycling patterns. The coordinated cycling of states within sleep and between sleep and wake, or "sleep state organization," is a central index of brain maturation (Kostović et al., 2019; Scher et al., 1995), exhibits individual consistency and stability over time (Thoman et al., 1987), and predicts neurodevelopmental outcome in premature as well as full-term infants (Bennet et al., 2018; Gogou et al., 2019; Holditch-Davis & Edwards, 1998). Understanding the typical vs. atypical patterning of sleep state organization is an important step toward a complete assessment of the preterm and at-risk infant as well as support for optimal developmental outcomes. Regardless of gestational age, many physiologically compromised infants benefit from strategies to promote developmentally appropriate sleep and arousal states. These strategies often include supportive positioning and care practices. It is imperative to support infant sleep development and educate caregivers about the role that sleep plays in neurodevelopment. This includes preparing well in advance of discharge for the sleep patterns, disruptions, and situations infants and their parents will experience in their home setting.

In this chapter, we will provide a brief review on what is known about the emergence of sleep and wake states in infancy and their importance to health and development. This includes information about alterations in typical sleep patterns due to preterm birth, medical complications, environmental conditions, and treatment in the intensive care unit (ICU). This is followed by a review of evidenced-based care standards for the incorporation of sleep and arousal assessment into the ICU environment. Finally, we will discuss the current understanding of safe sleep practices in the ICU and for the transition home to prevent sudden infant death syndrome (SIDS). We will consider the issues associated with integrating the American Academy of Pediatrics (AAP) recommendations for safe infant sleep and developmentally supportive care.

SLEEP DEVELOPMENT OF PRETERM AND TERM BABIES

Fetal Sleep State Development

Sleep and wake states emerge throughout fetal gestation commensurate with neuronal development (Kostović et al., 2019). Like most newborn behaviors that are required for survival, such as swallowing and elimination, the development of stable behavioral states is experience dependent with a reciprocal neural–behavioral progression. Following a period of relatively low motor activity in the first 7 weeks of the human embryonic period, reflexive and spontaneous movement patterns emerge as neuronal migration and corticospinal connections are formed (Kostović et al., 2019; Krsnik et al., 2017). By the 15th gestational week, larger, whole-body movements become more frequent with nearly continuous motor activity. Neuronal maturation proceeds from spinal to cortical structures with the beginning stages of myelination (Kostović et al., 2019). During this time, brief periods of motor quiescence occur and lead to cyclical rest–activity patterns that lengthen throughout the second gestational trimester (Pillai et al., 1992; Arduini et al., 1986). Rest–activity patterns gradually become more organized and coincident with fetal heart rate variability patterns and eye movements in late gestation, representing the emergence of more organized fetal behavioral states (Timor-Tritsch, Dierker, Hertz, et al., 1978). By 36 weeks of gestation, periods with these co-occurring behaviors and physiology become more stable, typically moving from large periods of "indeterminant states" to increasing time spent in stable co-occurrence of sleep state behaviors and physiology (Junge, 1979, 1980; Martin, 1981; Nijhuis et al., 1982; Timor-Tritsch, Dierker, Hertz, et al., 1978). The primary sleep states include fetal active sleep (an immature precursor to rapid eye movement or REM sleep) and quiet sleep (an immature form of non-REM [NREM] sleep). Active sleep periods are defined by intermittent motor activity that is coincident with fetal heart rate accelerations and, intermittently, with eye movements. Quiet sleep periods are marked by a relative lack of motor activity and eye movements, low heart rate variability, and heart rate at or below the baseline level. Most of late fetal gestation is spent in active sleep, with brief and increasing periods of quiet sleep through the newborn period (Martin, 1981; Nijhuis et al., 1982; van Geijn et al., 1980). Fetal arousal behaviors include yawning, stretching, and kicking and are frequently observed in the transition from active sleep to arousal periods, characterized by high motor activity coincident with prolonged fetal heart rate accelerations (Walusinski, 2010).

Preterm and Term Infant Sleep

When considering sleep in the preterm infant, we must understand the implications of a drastically altered environment from the intrauterine milieu. Sleep state development no longer occurs without the influence of demands to breathe air, tolerate new levels of sensory input, and absorb nutrients from external sources. These changes may in fact accelerate or derail the maturation of sleep–wake organization. As term age approaches, the regulation of arousal, and the ability to successfully emerge from sleep to maintain wakeful states, becomes a necessity for the preterm infant, who now needs to be able to take in nutrition for continued growth. The term newborn enjoys a gradual lengthening of wake periods from brief periods at birth to longer, more organized periods over the first three postnatal months, whereas the preterm infant may develop longer wake periods far in advance of term age. Circadian rhythmicity, or the entrainment of sleep and physiological processes to environmental cues may also emerge earlier for the preterm infant compared with the full-term infant over the first six postnatal months (Bonan et al., 2015; Cirelli & Tononi, 2015; Dereymaeker et al., 2017; Franco et al., 2010; Grigg-Damberger, 2016; Guyer et al., 2015; Holditch-Davis & Edwards, 1998; Scher, Johnson & Holditch-Davis, 2005).

However, the potential early emergence of sleep state cycling may not translate into stable sleep state organization. The ability to transition smoothly between states of sleep and wakefulness and to regulate the transition between states of alertness reflects neurodevelopmental maturation, including predictable cortical and subcortical brain activation patterns, which may be disrupted or delayed by preterm birth, or other insults to typical development as discussed below (Anders & Keener, 1985; Bennet et al., 2018; Chu et al., 2014; Kostović et al., 2019).

Functions of Sleep in Neurodevelopment

The confluence of developmental processes is evident in state organization, as stability of states also facilitates central nervous system plasticity through enhanced production of the structures involved in building neuronal circuitry (Bennet et al., 2018; Bourel-Ponchel et al., 2021). In contrast, alterations in typical sleep development and poor sleep state organization may be deleterious to neurodevelopment. Poor sleep patterns in humans predict abnormal neurodevelopment and behavior problems (Hiscock et al., 2008; Lam et al., 2003; Matthey & Speyer, 2008; Whitney & Thoman, 1993), whereas less fragmented sleep is related to higher cognitive scores in infants, toddlers, and school-aged children (Scher, 2005); therefore, sleep state architecture not only is a potential measure of current neurological and physiological stability but may also be a potential mechanism contributing adverse outcomes for at-risk infants. Thus, organized sleep can be considered a clinical marker and facilitator of normal neurodevelopment (Geva et al., 2016; Takenouchi et al., 2011).

Alterations in brain development and stability of physiological systems may change observed infant sleep and arousal patterns. Some of these alterations have been related to specific changes in sleep and arousal patterns such as hypoxic–ischemic encephalopathy, congenital heart disease, neonatal abstinence syndrome, errors of metabolism, and chronic lung disease (Barbeau & Weiss, 2017; Shellhaas et al., 2018). Moreover, low arousal at term age is a risk factor for sudden infant death syndrome (SIDS) (Franco et al., 2010).

The heightened risk of poor sleep to long-term outcomes may be, at least in part, due to the intrinsic interrelated nature of sleep to physiologic functions, such as body temperature (Barcat et al., 2017), breathing, heart rate (Lehtonen & Martin, 2004), and digestion, including gastroesophageal reflux events (Qureshi et al., 2015) For example, persistence of sleep-disordered breathing has been demonstrated among preterm babies born at <32 weeks, with associated lower IQ, memory, and visual–spatial performance at school age, compared with term-born peers (Hagmann-von Arx et al., 2014). Regulation of states of arousal also has the potential to impact participation in feeding (Bueno & Menna-Barreto, 2016) and social interaction and has been shown to predict neurobehavioral development later in infancy, at school age, and in adolescence (Arditi-Babchuk et al., 2009; El-Dib et al., 2014; Weisman et al., 2011).

SLEEP CONCERNS IN THE HOSPITALIZED INFANT

It is increasingly clear that it is critical to support optimal sleep and state organization in early development. This is particularly important, and challenging, in the preterm or hospitalized infant given the often-chaotic environment of the neonatal ICU. The importance of sleep for energy conservation, growth, and healing of babies in the ICU is widely acknowledged, and support of babies' sleep is a critical component of developmentally supportive care. Sleep state and level of arousal during routine care may influence baby's responses to care and readiness for feeding. For example, preterm babies desaturated more frequently when handled during active sleep compared with handling in quiet sleep or wake states (Levy et al., 2017). Handling techniques and positioning also have a significant influence on sleep and wake states (Edraki et al., 2014; Liaw et al., 2012).

Any stress to the physiological system may be associated with changes in the sleep state architecture. Fever, infection, excessive handling, and prolonged periods of wakefulness may result in decreases in active sleep and or increases in quiet sleep in the subsequent sleep periods. Prone positioning and elevated room temperatures have been associated with increases in quiet sleep. Medications may also influence sleep state architecture by inhibiting one or more sleep state processes. For example, opioid medications inhibit quiet/NREM sleep and is linked to significant alterations in sleep state organization in adults and children (Staedt et al., 1996). Prenatal opioid exposure results in significant reductions in infant quiet sleep and increased active sleep during the immediate postnatal period, which may be dose dependent (Dinges et al., 1980; O'Brien & Jeffery, 2002; Pinto et al., 1988).

These studies support the importance of including an adequate assessment of infant arousal and sleep states as a standard of care in the newborn ICU, with appropriate training provided to care providers and parents (Jeanson, 2013; Mahmoodi et al., 2015). The care provider's goal should be to help parents understand their infants' sleep development, importance for future health, and strategies to support adequate amounts and quality of sleep through the transition home. This should include specific information and teaching about safe infant sleep practices, which we will discuss in subsequent sections.

Ways to Support Sleep and Arousal States in the Hospital

The previous paragraphs provided a brief overview of the importance and benefits of assessing the baby's sleep state organization as well as the arousal state before, during, and after care and handling. It is also important to incorporate interventions or practices that may reduce unnecessary

stress. Table 13-1 summarizes the key recommendations for supporting optimal sleep and arousal development in the acute hospital environment. The first recommendation is to routinely assess infant sleep and wake states. Guidelines for valid criteria for determining states of sleep and arousal in preterm and term infants have been established for both direct observation and physiologic methodologies. A combination of observed behaviors (rapid eye movements, facial movements, gross body movements) and physiologic parameters (respiration and/or heart rate variability) provides a structured approach for determining states of sleep and arousal that can be incorporated into routine assessment by ICU staff (Anders, 1976; Anders et al., 1985; Grigg-Damberger, 2016; Holditch-Davis et al., 2003; Davis & Thoman, 1987; Lacina et al., 2015). Table 13-2 summarizes the observed parameters for each sleep or wake state. Electroencephalography (EEG) is the gold standard for the measurement of sleep states, but it is more invasive and challenging to use routinely. However, use of two-channel EEG systems in the neonatal intensive care unit (NICU) may facilitate an objective, streamlined assessment of infant sleep state organization into routine care. Newer measures of the parameters of state are emerging and may facilitate objective and unobtrusive sleep state measurement (Werth et al., 2017).

Cultural buy-in among ICU staff occurs more readily when training and evaluation experiences incorporate peer participation, and when care practices are included in routine documentation according to a defined standard of care (Jeanson, 2013). Information about the infant's sleep and arousal patterns contributes to an accurate assessment of the infant's readiness for interactions and feeding. A contextual approach, incorporating documentation of routine observations of the baby's states of arousal before, during, and after care; presence and level of participation of family members in care; and features of the environment, has the potential to inform the team regarding the baby's ability to tolerate/participate in developmentally appropriate activities of daily living such as routine handling during care, feeding, being held, and obtaining adequate sleep. Providing the infant with adequate uninterrupted time and environmental conditions also support sleep cycle development (e.g., lighting, temperature, cycled care) (Bastani et al., 2017; Levy et al., 2017; Milgrom et al., 2010; Morag & Ohlsson, 2016; Rivkees et al., 2004).

Documentation enhances compliance with a higher standard of care and provides objective data to inform

TABLE 13-1 Support Infant Sleep and Arousal Development

- Assess infant sleep and wake states routinely: duration, quality, and transitions
- Assess readiness for interaction and feeding
- Provide adequate time and environment to promote sleep development
- Provide caregiver education and guidance to support safe infant sleep throughout early development
- Document infant sleep and arousal states as part of the routine assessment

TABLE 13-2 Sleep and Arousal States: Definitions by Observed Behaviors and Respiration

Indicator	Sleep States		Transition		Wakefulness		
	1	2	3		4	5	6
	Quiet Sleep (QS or NREM)	Active Sleep (AS or REM)	Sleep–Wake Transition	Drowse (Nonalert)	Quiet Awake	Active Awake	Cry
Eye movement	None; eyes closed	Intermittent or steady	Brief or none	Eyes opening and closing	Eyes open, eye blinks, may scan or pursue visual targets	Eyes open, scanning, (unless crying)	Eyes closed, variable
Motor activity	Little or none	Intermittent	Continuous	Little or none	Little or none	Large, sustained	Continuous
Behaviors	Occasional startles, rhythmic mouthing	Mouthe, startle, intermittent limb, head	Stretch, yawn, large body movements	Rare	Startles, small limb, sucking	Stretch, startle, large movements	Sustained cry vocalizations
Respiration	Regular	Irregular	Irregular	Irregular	Irregular	Irregular	Irregular

decisions made by the ICU medical team, as well as family members, to optimize the plan of care. This documentation, as part of the electronic medical record, also provides data for quality improvement measures (Bakermans-Kranenburg & van IJzendoorn, 2017; Pierrat et al., 2007).

SAFE INFANT SLEEP ENVIRONMENT

For almost 30 years, a great deal of attention surrounding infant sleep was directed toward the vital work of reducing sleep-related infant deaths. Sudden unexpected infant death (SIUD) or sudden unexpected death in infancy (SUDI) describe unexpected death, explained or unexplained, that occurs suddenly during the first year of life (AAP Task Force on Sudden Infant Death Syndrome, 2016). Some of these cases can be attributed to suffocation, entrapment, trauma, arrhythmias, metabolic diseases, infection, or ingestion. SIDS is a subcategory of SUID that cannot be explained after a thorough investigation, including autopsy, scene investigation, and a review of clinical history. Sleep-related infant deaths include SUIDs that occur during an unobserved period of sleep (AAP, 2016). Each year in the United States, there are ~3,500 SIUD s; approximately 1,350 are attributed to SIDS, 850 are attributed to accidental suffocation strangulation, and almost 1,300 are of unknown or other causes (CDC, 2020). SUID is currently 91/100,000 live births in the United States, with rates ranging from 49.5/100,000 in California to 178/100,000 in Alabama. Rates also differ among racial and ethnic groups, with the lowest rates in the United States among Asian/Pacific islanders and Hispanic infants (34/100,000 and 54/100,000) and the highest among American Indian/Alaskan Native and non-Hispanic black infants (212/100,000 and 187/100,000). Low socioeconomic status is also related to an increased risk of SUID (CDC, 2020). The United States has the world's highest prevalence of SUID/SIDS with lower-risk group rates in the United

States similar to the rates of high-risk populations in Europe and Australia (Bartick & Tomori, 2019). Being born preterm or small for gestational age also significantly increases the risk of SIDS/SUID making it a critical matter of interest in the NICU (Moon & AAP, 2016).

Research into the causes and modifiable risk factors of SIDS motivated the AAP to release its first recommendations against prone sleeping, which was the most common sleep position used in the United States at the time (AAP, 1992). This recommendation encouraging nonprone positions in healthy infants and an accompanying "Back to Sleep" public health campaign initiated in 1994 by the National Institute of Child Health and Human Development led to a 53% reduction of SIDS in the first 10 years and then plateaued (AAP, 2011). Other sleep-related infant deaths such as suffocation and entrapment increased by 10% between 1994 and 1999, leading to an expansion of recommendations to reduce modifiable risk. The AAP expanded their recommendations in the policy statements to include details about the sleep environment and call for only supine sleep positions in 2005. The US rate of SIDS then declined from 54 per 100,000 live births in 2009 to 40 per 100,000 in 2013. Despite the expansions and improvements, SIDS remains the leading cause of postneonatal mortality (28 days to 1 year). The AAP Task Force expanded their recommendations based on additional research in 2011 and 2016 with attention to both SIDS and unintentional suffocation. The two most recent sets of recommendations for a safe infant sleeping environment specifically called upon newborn ICUs to endorse and model SIDS/SUID reduction recommendations (AAP, 2016). This emphasis is justified by the extended time NICU nursing staff spends with families and the increased risk for preterm and special care needs children for sleep-related death (Moon & AAP Task Force, 2016). Incorporating these recommendations into unit policies, protocols, and assessment is a vital part of evidence-based practice.

Neonatal nurses must acknowledge that they serve as the first professional role models for new parents. Sleep positions and sleep environments at home are critical components for reducing infant mortality, and neonatal nurses play an important role in modeling sleep environments after discharge. The AAP policy statement advocates sleep in a supine position, alone, on firm surfaces without soft or loose bedding (AAP, 2016). Because these recommendations were designed to decrease the risk of SIDS/SUID in the general population, they might not seem to apply in an NICU, but it is imperative to prepare well in advance of discharge for the sleep situations that NICU graduates will encounter in their home setting. Regardless of how a critically ill infant is positioned for sleep in the NICU for ventilatory support, physiological stability, postsurgical care, and developmental positioning, almost all infants will be expected to sleep supine without supportive containment at home. For this reason, it is critical to transition as rapidly as possible from infant care practices that may be appropriate in the hospital setting but high risk at home. Parents are watching everything the nurse does with their infant, and this care is highly regarded often to the point of mirroring the caregiving received in the NICU after discharge even when that care may not be appropriate in the home environment.

This section considers the issues associated with integrating AAP recommendations for safe infant sleep and developmentally supportive care.

- The transition process is interpreted in the framework of a developmental continuum. The infant progresses from "ill" status to "healthy" status and from supported prone or side-lying to unsupported supine positioning.
- NICU care providers' transfer of information and modeling of safe sleep practices provides families with the foundation to reduce SIDS/SUID risk while supporting developmentally appropriate sleep states.

SIDS and Infant Sleep Position: Historical Perspectives on the International and US Experience

Through the centuries, SIUDs related to sleep were commonly described as overlaying or accidental smothering (Wright, 2017). An 1,893 review of 399 infants found dead in bed with parents in Dundee, Scotland, suggested a mandate for infants to sleep separately from their parents. The theory of overlaying lost credibility when the use of cribs did not substantially decrease the rates of infant death. In the mid-20th century, pathologists published a series of papers on sudden apparently unexplained deaths during infancy, and the term SIDS was proposed in 1969 (Wright, 2017).

Researchers have long speculated that infant sleep positions may be related to unexpected death during sleep. An association between SIDS and infant sleep position was established when the incidence of SIDS nearly tripled in the late 1980s following a media campaign that advocated a change from supine to prone sleep positioning in Holland. The SIDS rate declined rapidly after a subsequent campaign

discouraged prone sleep positioning (AAP Task Force on Infant Positioning and SIDS, 1992; Obladen, 2018). No increase in adverse outcomes, such as aspiration or acute life-threatening events (ALTEs), was noted in conjunction with the change to predominantly supine sleep.

Between 1992 and 2016, the AAP Task Force on Sudden Infant Death Syndrome released numerous policy statements to disseminate emerging information on SIDS, sleep position, and sleep environment (AAP Task Force on Infant Positioning and SIDS, 1992, 2000, 2011, 2016; Barsman et al., 2015). As of this writing, the most recent AAP statement on SIDS and infant sleep was released in November 2016 (AAP, 2016). Readers are encouraged to review the literature for subsequent updates because AAP policy statements are reaffirmed or updated 5 years after publication unless formally reaffirmed, amended, or canceled before that time (AAP, 2016).

Several hypotheses were identified that might explain this link (AAP, 1992). The "triple-risk theory," originally proposed by Filiano and Kinney (1994), remains a reasonable model that may help to explain SIDS. According to this premise, an unfortunate interaction of three conditions may culminate in death (Figure 13-1). The first element is a vulnerable infant with an undetected underlying anomaly (e.g., brainstem abnormalities that control respiration and heart rate). The second element is a critical developmental period. The first 6 months of life are a period of rapid growth and development, leading to occasional periods of instability in homeostatic control over heart rate, respiration, thermoregulation, and blood pressure. The third element involves an external stressor that is easily overcome by a healthy, stable infant but not by a vulnerable infant experiencing homeostatic instability. External stressors include prone sleep

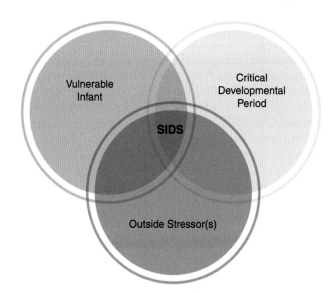

FIGURE 13-1. The triple risk model. [From Eunice Kennedy Shriver National Institute of Child Health and Human Development, NIH, DHHS. (2006). *Curriculum for nurses: Continuing education program on SIDS risk reduction* [06-6005; p. 9]. U.S. Government Printing Office.]

position, overheating, secondhand tobacco smoke, and upper-respiratory infections. There currently is no means to identify vulnerable infants or prevent critical developmental periods, so eliminating the third element created by external stressors may be the best tactic to reduce the risk of SIDS (Filiano & Kinney, 1994; National Institute of Child Health and Human Development, 2020c). The AAP task force recommendations focus on reducing exposure to external stressors that could serve as the third risk factor.

The initial AAP statement was met with skepticism, and adherence to the new recommendations was inconsistent early on in the United States. By 1994, the international experience with SIDS and sleep positions provided enough evidence that several US federal agencies and the AAP joined forces to implement an aggressive Back to Sleep public health campaign directed against prone sleep positioning during infancy (Table 13-3). The AAP reaffirmed its previous recommendations and discouraged soft surfaces and gas-trapping objects within the sleep environment, consistent with a safety alert published that same year by the Consumer Product Safety Commission (Moon & AAP, 2016; NICHD, 2020b). The incidence of SIDS in the United States fell 15% to 20% by 1996. At this time, the AAP Task Force updated its recommendations to clarify areas of confusion over exceptions to prone positioning, specifically regarding preterm infants. The updated recommendations were more clearly directed toward healthy infants, regardless of gestational age. They provided specific directives to minimize supine sleep complications, such as positional plagiocephaly (AAP Task Force on Infant Positioning and SIDS, 1996). The AAP Task Force on Infant Sleep Position and Sudden Infant Death Syndrome in 2000 identified risk factors associated with a higher risk for SIDS, including prone sleep position, soft sleep surfaces, bed-sharing, overheating, maternal smoking during pregnancy, limited prenatal care, prematurity, low birth weight, and infant male gender. Back to Sleep training for parents should be part of the discharge planning significantly before the anticipated day of discharge. The 2011 and 2016 recommendations specifically called out staff in NICUs to model and implement all SIDS reduction recommendations as soon as the infant is medically stable and well in advance of discharge.

The 2016 recommendations continued to refine and expand advice based on recent evidence. They also clarify that these recommendations are to prevent SIDS and other sleep-related infant deaths by acting upon modifiable risk factors (AAP, 2016). The accompanying technical report provides detailed evidence from both human and animal studies regarding the pathophysiology and genetics of SIDS, epidemiological evidence regarding risk factors, racial and ethnic disparities, and age at death. The authors encourage healthcare providers to have nonjudgmental conversations with families about sleep practices to facilitate the most effective safe sleep education. The report also states that individual medical conditions may warrant modifications after weighing relative risk and benefit. The technical report also provides evidence and a bibliography for each recommendation

(Moon & AAP, 2016). The following section reviews recommendations (1-6, 9, 11-14, 16-17, and 19) of most interest to NICU staff.

Recommendation 1. Back to sleep for every sleep

Back to sleep has been one of the most effective and successful components of safe sleep campaigns since the initial National Institute of Child Health and Human Development (NICHD) back to sleep public education campaign in 1994 (NICHD, 2020a).

Infants should be placed in a fully supine position, entirely on their back, for every sleep by every caregiver until the child reaches 1 year of age. Consistently placing infants supine for naps and nighttime sleep may be the single most effective step to reduce the risk of SIDS (National Institute of Child Health and Human Development (NICHD), 2020a). There is sufficient evidence that side sleeping is not safe. While it is established that the prone position increases the odds ratio (OR) of SIDS by up to 13.1 times, it has become increasingly clear that side lying is an unstable position with an OR of 2.0 to 8.7 (Moon & AAP, 2016). Prone position has been shown to alter the cardiovascular system's autonomic control and may decrease cerebral oxygenation in both term and preterm infants (Shepherd et al., 2019; Wong et al., 2011). As discussed earlier, prone positioning may also increase the amount of quiet sleep beyond what is developmentally appropriate. Although the exact mechanism for increased vulnerability in the prone position remains unknown, it is plausible that the nature of quiet sleep combined with the prone position may increase vulnerability to occlusion from soft bedding or other objects (discussed in next sections). Infants who are stressed, have fever, or have been deprived of adequate sleep may also have higher amounts of quiet sleep.

Because infants who usually sleep supine are at exceptionally high risk for SIDS if they are placed prone for sleep, supine positioning for every single sleep episode is essential, and it is also important that all caregivers comply (AAP Task Force on Infant Positioning and SIDS, 2016; Moon et al., 2005). Multiple studies have found that one reason parents have cited for not using the supine sleep position is that the infant does not sleep well or seems uncomfortable. Parent education should emphasize that normal infant sleep involves frequent arousal as a protective factor (Moon & AAP, 2016).

Special application in NICU: Preterm infants should be placed supine as soon as their clinical status is stabilized and significantly before discharge, with a target of supine sleep at least 32 weeks' postmenstrual age (PMA) and onward (Moon & AAP, 2016; American Academy of Pediatrics & American College of Obstetricians and Gynecologists, 2017).

Patients cared for in the NICU present a dilemma with regard to AAP recommendations on sleep positioning. On the surface, it seems easy to accept the premise that NICU patients are different from healthy full-term infants, and the information does not apply. Infants in the NICU are often attached to physiologic monitors and life-support devices.

TABLE 13-3 Practice Recommendation Evidence

Type	Practice Recommendation	Level of Recommendation	References
Sleep and Arousal Developmental Care			
Standard 1	**Promote developmentally appropriate sleep and arousal states**	II, III	Arditi-Babchuk et al., 2009; Bennet et al., 2018; Gogou et al., 2019; Geva et al., 2016; Holditch-Davis & Edwards, 1998; Thoman et al., 1987
Standard 2:	**Optimize physical environment and caregiving routines to promote safe sleep and arousal**	II, III	Edraki et al., 2014; Liaw et al., 2013; Levy et al., 2017
Standard 3:	**Encourage family presence and participation in care of their baby**	II, III	Edraki et al., 2014, p. 84; Bastani et al., 2017; Milgrom et al., 2010
Standard 4:	**Document and review infant sleep and arousal states to enhance care planning**	IV, V	Naugler and DiCarlo, 2018; Pierrat et al., 2007
AAP Standards to Prevent SIDS			
Sleep position	Back to sleep for every sleep by every caregiver up to 1 year of age. Prone and side positioning are not safe and not advised	I	AAP Task Force on Sudden Infant Death Syndrome, 2016; Moon & AAP Task Force on Sudden Infant Death Syndrome, 2016
Sleep surface	Use a firm sleep surface that meets Consumer Product Safety Commission standards covered by a fitted sheet	I	Moon & AAP Task Force on Sudden Infant Death Syndrome, 2016
Breastfeeding	Protective effects of breastmilk increase with exclusivity; any breastfeeding is more protective than no breastfeeding	I	Moon & AAP Task Force on Sudden Infant Death Syndrome, 2016
Sleep location	Room sharing with the infant on a separate sleep surface close to the parent's bed is recommended, ideally for 1 year, but at least for the first 6 months post term. Sleeping in chairs and sofas carries additional risk	I, II	Moon & AAP Task Force on Sudden Infant Death Syndrome, 2016; Tappin, Ecob, & Brooke, 2005
Bedding and soft objects	Keep soft objects such as a pillow, toys, and loose bedding away from infant sleep. Avoid overheating	I, II	Moon & AAP Task Force on Sudden Infant Death Syndrome, 2016; Schlaud et al., 2010
Smoking	Do not smoke during pregnancy. Avoid infant or pregnant woman exposure to secondhand smoke	I, II	Anderson et al., 2019; Moon & AAP Task Force on Sudden Infant Death Syndrome, 2016
Alcohol and illicit drug use	Avoid alcohol and illicit drug exposure during pregnancy and after birth	I, II	Moon & AAP Task Force on Sudden Infant Death Syndrome, 2016; O'Leary et al., 2013
Pacifiers	Consider offering a pacifier at nap and bedtime through the first year of life	I, II	Hauck et al., 2005; Moon & AAP Task Force on Sudden Infant Death Syndrome, 2016; Moon et al., 2012

(Continued)

TABLE 13-3 Practice Recommendation Evidence (Continued)

Type	Practice Recommendation	Level of Recommendation	References
Immunizations	Infants should be immunized according to AAP and CDC schedule	I, II	AAP, 2018; Moon & AAP Task Force on Sudden Infant Death Syndrome, 2016; Vennemann et al., 2007
NICU and nursery staff	Healthcare providers in newborn nurseries and NICUs should endorse and model SIDS reduction strategies from birth	I, II	Dowling et al., 2018; Hannen et al., 2020; Moon & AAP Task Force on Sudden Infant Death Syndrome, 2016
Home monitoring	Avoid home monitoring as a strategy to prevent SIDS	I, II	Moon & AAP Task Force on Sudden Infant *Death* Syndrome, 2016; Ramanthan et al., 2001
Positional plagiocephaly	Provide infant with regular periods of holding and awake "tummy time"	II, III	Ditthakasem & Kolar, 2017; Hewitt et al., 2020; van Vlimmeren et al., 2007
Safe sleep campaigns	Healthcare providers should participate in ongoing SIDS risk-reduction campaigns	III, IV	Moon & AAP Task Force on Sudden Infant Death Syndrome, 2016
Commercial sleep products	Avoid the use of commercial at-home positioning devices not consistent with safe sleep recommendations	I	CDC, 2012; Moon & AAP Task Force on Sudden Infant Death Syndrome, 2016
Sleep sacks	Consider using a sleep sack for infant sleep clothing to improve adherence to safe sleep practices	II	Geyer et al., 2016
Media	Media should follow safe sleep guidelines in messages and advertising	II	Goodstein et al., 2018; Joyner et al., 2009
Prone positioning for defined special cases	Prone positioning may optimize the respiratory function of hospitalized infants with acute respiratory or hemodynamic distress and is required for certain congenital anomalies	II, III	Rivas-Fernandez et al., 2016; Shepherd et al., 2020; Utario et al., 2017
Staff training program	SIDS training for nurses improves knowledge and beliefs regarding the Back to Sleep campaign. Training curriculum for nursing staff	I, II	Leong et al., 2019; Leong et al., 2020; McMullen et al., 2016; National Institute of Child Health & Human Development (NICHD), 2014; NICHD, 2020a, 2020b; Naugler & DiCarlo, 2018; Salm Ward & Balfour, 2016; Zachritz et al., 2016
Parent training programs and role modeling	Nurses serve as models and educators for SIDS-reduction behaviors	II	Dowling et al., 2018; Hannen et al., 2020; Leong et al., 2019; McMullen, Lipke, & LeMura, 2009; Naugler & DiCarlo, 2018
Implementation	Successful implementation and sustained adoption of innovation in health service delivery are based on a systems approach	I, II	Dowling et al., 2018; Kenner & Jaeger, 2020; McMullen et al., 2016; Naugler & DiCarlo, 2018; Zachritz et al., 2016

Note: Level I, evidence from a systematic review or meta-analysis of all relevant randomized controlled trials (RCTs), or evidence-based clinical practice guidelines based on systematic reviews of RCTs; level II, evidence obtained from at least one well-designed RCT; level III, evidence obtained from well-designed controlled trials without randomization; level IV, evidence from well-designed case-control and cohort studies; level V, evidence from systematic reviews of descriptive and qualitative studies. CDC, Centers for Disease Control and Prevention.

They may be premature, have significant congenital anomalies, or require surgical intervention—any of which could preclude following the recommendation for supine sleeping, and currently, patients with these conditions are not indicated for inclusion in the AAP recommendations. For example, prone and quarter prone position may be appropriate for infants receiving ventilatory assistance, especially for very preterm infants (Rivas-Fernandez et al., 2016; Shepherd et al., 2020; Utario et al., 2017). Exceptions also include symptomatic preterm infants with known or suspected airway obstruction (such as Pierre Robin sequence), infants receiving phototherapy, and infants with certain congenital anomalies (e.g., neural tube defects) for whom the supine position would be contraindicated (McMullen et al., 2016; Voos et al., 2014). These infants should receive care in a closely monitored setting, typically with continuous physiologic and comprehensive physical assessment as a baseline.

Neuromotor, physiologic, and neurobehavioral stability of preterm infants are overarching goals of ongoing care and development. These commonly are supported through careful positioning—often prone or side lying and with external support described as containment. These important components of developmentally supportive nursing care for premature and ill infants are useful tools in care, and infant physiological and behavioral cues drive the type of support provided. Written protocols should include the transition from special positioning and external supports to unsupported supine sleep on a cleared surface. Thirty-two weeks' PMA has been mentioned in several studies as a rule of thumb for the transition to supine sleep, but individualized care may support an earlier transition once infants have achieved cardiovascular and respiratory stability. Determining a workable trigger or set of cues for the timing of an introduction to home sleep position and bedding practices is key for the successful adoption of practice change (Leong et al., 2020).

Although prone sleep has been linked with a higher risk of SIDS, many healthcare providers and parents have been reluctant to embrace supine sleep positioning. Concerns expressed since the initial AAP statement include adverse outcomes such as aspiration, positional plagiocephaly, gastric reflux, and developmental delay. The AAP Task Force has addressed these concerns, and it is clear that the protective benefits of supine sleep outweigh potential disadvantages (AAP, 2016). The most common objection has involved an increased potential for aspiration. In a study of neonatal nurses' beliefs, 53% of nurses cited a risk of reflux or aspiration for using a position other than supine (Barsman et al., 2015). In the years after the transition to supine sleep patterns, there has been no evidence of an increase in aspiration in Holland, the United States, and Australia (Byard & Beal, 2000). Infants may clear secretions more effectively when placed supine rather than prone. During supine sleep, the trachea is positioned above the esophagus (Figure 13-2). Refluxed or regurgitated fluids must work against gravity to be aspirated into the trachea. During prone sleep, however, the trachea lies below the esophagus (Figure 13-3). Fluids

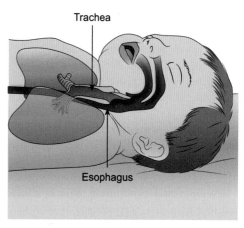

FIGURE 13-2. Supine anatomy illustration of trachea and esophagus. [From Eunice Kennedy Shriver National Institute of Child Health and Human Development, NIH, DHHS. (2007). *Infant sleep position and SIDS: Questions and answers for health care providers*. U.S. Government Printing Office.]

from the esophagus can easily collect above the trachea and be aspirated (National Institute of Child Health and Human Development, 2020b; National Institute of Child Health and Human Development, 2020e).

Recommendation 2. Use a firm sleep surface

Infants should be placed on a firm sleep surface such as a mattress that maintains its shape and will not indent or conform to the shape of the infant's head. The mattress should be covered by a fitted sheet without any soft or loose bedding present. Mattress toppers or sheepskin should not be placed under the fitted sheet (AAP, 2016).

For the transition to home, cribs, bassinets, and play yards should meet the safety standards of the Consumer Product Safety Commission (CPSC) (US CPSC, 2020). Bedside sleepers with a rigid frame secured to an adult bed were approved as a safe sleeping environment for newborns and infants by

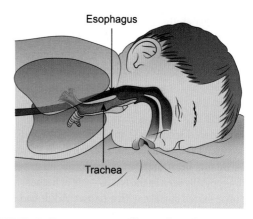

FIGURE 13-3. Prone anatomy illustration of trachea and esophagus. [From Eunice Kennedy Shriver National Institute of Child Health and Human Development, NIH, DHHS. (2007). *Infant sleep position and SIDS: Questions and answers for health care providers*. U.S. Government Printing Office.]

the CPSC. Still, the AAP Task Force on Sudden Infant Death Syndrome cannot recommend for or against bedside or in-bed sleepers owing to lack of evidence regarding their safety (Moon, 2020). In October 2019, the CPSC recalled all inclined sleep first with soft or plush surfaces, and incline of greater than 10° after 73 infant deaths were associated with inclined sleep products (US CPSC, 2020). It is an integral part of family education to discuss the current standards for sleep surfaces.

Special application in NICU: Preterm and ill infants may need to be placed on specialized surfaces for temperature control, prevention of skin breakdown, postsurgical care, and developmental positioning. Infants should be transitioned to a firm, flat sleep surface as soon as the concerns are alleviated and well in advance of discharge to decrease transition issues in the home for parents.

Recommendation 3. Breastfeeding is recommended.

Breastfeeding is associated with a reduced risk of SIDS. Mothers should breastfeed exclusively or feed with expressed milk for 6 months unless contraindicated. The protective effect of breastfeeding increases with exclusivity, but any breastfeeding is more protective against SIDS than no breastfeeding (Hauck et al., 2011; Thompson et al., 2017). Current NICU practice supports breastfeeding and the use of human breast milk.

4. It is recommended that infants sleep in the parent's room, close to the parents' bed, but on a separate surface designed for infants, ideally for the first year of life, but at least for the first 6 months.

SIDS risk is lessened by as much as 50% for infants sleeping in a crib, bassinet, or cradle within the same room as the parent(s) (Carpenter et al., 2004). Room sharing allows the parents easy access to the infant to facilitate observation and comfort; it also improves breastfeeding. Infants brought into bed for breastfeeding should be returned to their own sleep surface in a supine position when the parent is ready to return to sleep. The popular term of cosleeping has been used for both room sharing and bed-sharing, and the AAP encourages the use of separate terms for these conditions (Moon & AAP, 2016). Room sharing is protective, whereas epidemiologic studies show an increased risk of sleep-related death with bed-sharing. Based on extensive epidemiological evidence, the AAP recommends against bed-sharing. A meta-analysis of 11 studies showed that bed-sharing during sleep is considered to increase the risk of SIDS, suffocation, and entrapment (Venneman et al., 2012). Infants younger than 12 weeks, infants born preterm or with low birth weight—a population typically seen in the NICU—are at higher risk when sleeping on a shared surface with a parent. Adult bed surfaces in the United States do not conform to the firm sleep surfaces described in Recommendation 2. Certain factors increase the danger of bed-sharing. Among the highest risk are maternal smoking, parental use of sedating medications, soft surfaces, waterbeds, bed location against a wall, the use of bed rails, and the presence of pillows and blankets (Erck Lambert et al.,

2019). Recommendations 7 and 8 speak directly to the risk of smoking and other drug use as a significant risk, with maternal smoking responsible for 22% to 33% of SUID risk (AAP, 2016; Anderson et al., 2019; Elliott et al., 2020; Garrison-Desany et al., 2020) The SUID risk is particularly high when an infant bed shares with an adult smoker with an OR between 2.3 and 21.6. Sleeping on a couch or soft chair is particularly dangerous and carries a high risk of entrapment and suffocation.

Parents should be warned to be extra vigilant to their state of wakefulness during feedings, a common source of accidental cosleeping (Moon & AAP, 2016). It is less hazardous for parents to inadvertently fall asleep on a firm mattress than a chair or sofa, as sofas and soft chairs are very high-risk sleep environments with a high risk of entrapment and accidental suffocation. If there is a risk of parents falling asleep, blankets, top sheets, and pillows should be removed from the firm mattress bed. As soon as the parent rouses, they should place the infant back onto their separate sleep space (Moon & AAP, 2016; American Academy of Pediatrics & American College of Obstetricians and Gynecologists, 2017). Despite these recommendations, bed-sharing is common, with between 46% to 60% of parents reporting occasional bed-sharing and 13% commonly bed-sharing. Much of the occasional bed-sharing is reactive, in response to a problem and not planned (Mileva-Setiz et al., 2017). Bed-sharing is more common among certain ethnic groups, groups with strong family tradition, or in conditions where parents are concerned about environmental dangers such as vermin, especially among low-income mothers (Hauck et al., 2008; Joyner et al., 2010; Smith et al., 2016).

The topic of bed-sharing remains controversial, with some breastfeeding groups advocating bed-sharing as a method to increase the duration of breastfeeding. These studies' design does not allow the reader to ascertain whether mothers more likely to breastfeed longer are also more likely to bed-share or whether bed-sharing increases breastfeeding duration (Moon & AAP, 2016). There is also compelling electrophysiologic and careful observational research in the laboratory and in cross-cultural studies supporting bed-sharing while breastfeeding (Gettler & McKenna, 2011). This line of evidence also identifies high risk with parents who smoke or use alcohol or other sedating drugs, couch sleeping, or the infant sleeping with someone other than the parent. The AAP will continue to consider emerging evidence but finds the epidemiologically determined risk of bed-sharing through numerous studies over decades more compelling and has not determined safe parameters for bed-sharing, the use of in-bed sleep devices, or attached sleep surfaces (Moon & AAP, 2016).

Special application in NICU: Many NICUs currently have single-family rooms that models this recommendation throughout the stay. Units that still have open bays or pods will use rooms set aside for transitioning the parent(s) and infant to home care, where this behavior is modeled.

Recommendation 5. *Keep soft objects and loose bedding away from the infant sleep area to reduce the risk of SIDS, suffocation, entrapment, and strangulation.*

Soft objects and loose bedding can obstruct an infant's airway and increase the risk of suffocation, strangulation, rebreathing, and SIDS (Briker et al., 2019; Erck Lambert et al., 2019; Hauck et al., 2003). Pillows, quilts, sheepskins, and other soft bedding can be hazardous when placed under the infant or left in the infant's sleeping area. Bedding beyond a fitted sheet in the sleeping environment increases SIDS risk by 5× independent of sleep position and by 21× when the infant is placed prone (Hauck et al., 2003). Soft objects and loose bedding in the sleeping environment were associated with 69% of unintentional suffocation cases (Erck Lambert et al., 2019). Unintentional suffocation is the leading cause of injury death among infants less than 1 year of age in the United States, and 82% of these cases are attributed to accidental suffocation and strangulation in bed. Among soft bedding death, 49% occurred in an adult bed and 27% occurred in a crib or bassinet. Pillows caused airway obstruction twice as often among infants under 4 months old, and infants 5 to 11 months were more likely to have their airway obstructed by becoming entangled in the blankets. Parents should also be cautioned not to use bumper pads in the home crib (Moon & AAP, 2016). Swaddling, especially once an infant can turn, has not been shown to protect against SIDS/SUID and can prevent an infant from turning back to a supine position (Moon & AAP, 2016).

Special application in NICU: Near-term infants or those who do not require special positioning aids should be cared for on a firm sleep surface clear of objects. Ill or more premature infants who need positioning aids should only have those objects required for positioning in the bed. If deemed necessary, foot supports should be immobile, and side supports should be tightly rolled and maintained below the shoulder level. The infant should be dressed for warmth, although this may be difficult to achieve in the hospital setting when intravenous tubing, electrodes, and other required medical devices are present (Geyer et al., 2016; McMullen et al., 2016).

After determining that an infant meets the criteria for transition to supine sleeping, the recommendations regarding preventing microclimates and rebreathing should be initiated. These include placement on a firm, flat mattress covered with a single sheet and removal of additional bedding, linens, nesting supplies, and positioning supports. Some supportive-positioning devices may be required to support an infant's development early in transition. Transitioning an infant from an externally supported sleep position and bedding to healthy infant sleep expectations is best achieved gradually to encourage the infant to adapt to the changes. Similarly, removing bedding elements periodically over a few days may minimize infant stress and enhance the transition's success. An infant sleep sack can help maintain the infant's temperature while eliminating the chance of loose bedding covering the head (Geyer et al., 2016; McMullen et al., 2016). If initiated early enough before home readiness, it is possible to apply the home sleep and bedding recommendations over several days to weeks.

Removal of soft objects from the crib has been shown to provide a significant opportunity for improvement in modeling safe sleep environments for hospitalized infants. It is the most challenging goal to achieve 100% compliance with objects including spare clothing, diapers, stuffed toys, extra blankets, and medical equipment remaining when not in use (Leong et al., 2019; Leong et al., 2020; McMullen et al., 2016).

Recommendation 6. Consider offering a pacifier at nap time and bedtime.

Pacifier use appears to have a strong protective effect against SIDS according to data from case–control studies and meta-analyses (Hauck et al., 2005; Moon et al., 2012; Vennemann et al., 2009). The benefit is consistent between breastfeeding and formula-fed infants and seems to hold even when a pacifier falls from the mouth soon after the infant falls asleep. The mechanism of benefit remains unclear. The pacifiers should not be tethered to the infant's clothing, hung around the infant's neck, or attached to objects such as stuffed toys to avoid suffocation and strangulation. Concerns have been raised about the impact of pacifiers on breastfeeding, and the AAP Breastfeeding and Use of Human Milk Guidelines state that pacifiers can be used when infants are breastfed. Still, implementation should be delayed until breastfeeding is established if possible (AAP, 2012). NICU use of pacifiers is common, and so this method is modeled regularly.

Recommendation 9. Avoid overheating and head covering in infants.

The AAP recommends that infants be dressed appropriately for the environment with no more than one added layer over that an adult would wear. The incidence of SIDS has historically followed a noticeable seasonal pattern, with more deaths occurring during winter months in temperate climates such as the United States. The risk of SIDS appears to be related to environmental factors such as season and room temperature, as well as the amount of clothing or bedding (Moon & AAP, 2016). Studies have also shown increased SIDS incidence during heat waves (Auger et al., 2015; Jhun et al., 2017). Current guidelines no longer recommend the use of fans as a SIDS reduction strategy (Moon & AAP, 2016).

Recommendation 11. *Infants should be immunized in accordance with recommendations of the AAP and the Centers for Disease Control and Prevention.*

There is no evidence for a causal relationship between immunizations and SIDS, and case–control studies have shown a protective effect (Kuhnert et al., 2012; Vennemann et al., 2007).

Special application in NICU: Preterm infants who are medically stable and still in the hospital at 2 months of age should receive vaccinations on schedule. Discharge planning includes hand-off to community providers and a discussion of vaccine timelines with parents (AAP, 2018).

Recommendation 12. Avoid the use of commercial devices that are inconsistent with safe sleep recommendations.

Wedges and positioning devices used to maintain an infant in a side or supine position have been associated with suffocation deaths (CDC, 2012). Parents should be advised that, although such products may be available in stores and via the Internet, they should be avoided. Positioning devices used in the hospital for developmental care or physical therapy should be removed from the infant sleep area well before discharge to model safe sleep environments (Moon & AAP, 2016).

Special application in NICU: Parents, especially those whose baby required positioning devices, should receive guidance on commercial positioning devices for home use and how those are in opposition to Recommendation 5. A discussion about how infants have graduated from needing positioning devices can be helpful.

Recommendation 13. Do not use home monitors as a strategy to reduce the risk of SIDS.

There is no conclusive evidence that home cardiorespiratory monitoring reduces SIDS prevalence for infants who do not require monitoring for cardiovascular or respiratory conditions. In 2016, the AAP Subcommittee on Apparent Life-Threatening Events (ALTEs) recommended the replacement of ALTEs with BRUEs (Brief Resolved Unexplained Events) and stratification of high and low risk for repeated events or underlying disorders. It provided evidence-based management recommendations (Tieder et al., & AAP, 2016). BRUEs have a duration of less than 1 minute, and the patient returns to normal vital signs and appearance and baseline state of health. BRUEs are marked by pallor or central cyanosis, apnea, changes in tone, lethargy, or loss of consciousness. It excludes tachypnea, tachycardia, bradycardia, vomiting, petechia, noisy breathing, fever, choking, gagging, spasms, and seizure activity. These episodes generally peak between 6 and 10 weeks of age, occur while the infant is awake, and are not more common in small-for-gestational-age infants. Fewer than half of infants previously labeled as having ALTE will fit into the high- or low-risk BRUE. Low-risk BRUE patients appear to have lower risk of SIDS than the general population, and home cardiorespiratory monitoring should not be initiated (Benham-Terneus & Clemente, 2019; Ramgopal et al., 2019; Tieder et al., & AAP, 2016). Nuisance or false alarms, the complexity of technology in the home, and costs are negative aspects of home monitoring.

Special application in NICU: Much like positioning aids, parents become accustomed to monitoring systems when caring for their infant in the NICU and can be reluctant to transfer to home without the support of monitors. Single-family rooms or extended use of a transition room where parents and their infant spend nights together without monitoring help transition.

Recommendation 14. Supervised awake tummy time is recommended to facilitate development and to minimize development of positional plagiocephaly.

An increased incidence and awareness of occipital plagiocephaly (flattening of the head) without synostosis has been observed since full implementation of the AAP recommendations for exclusively supine sleep (Ditthakasem & Kolar, 2017; van Vlimmeren et al., 2007; Wittmeier & Mulder, 2017). The risk increases if the infant's head position is not varied; many infants prefer to have the right side of their head down when supine or side-lying, or they may prefer to face the activity in the room (NICHD, 2020d; Dunsirn et al., 2016). Risk increases if the infant spends little or no time in a week supervised tummy time, spends extended time in a car seat, and is not held in an upright position when not sleeping.

Forty percent of caregivers reported never putting their infant on their tummy to play but messaging can be successful in increasing tummy time and reducing deformational plagiocephaly (Wittmeier & Mulder, 2017). The NICHD recommends changing the infant's orientation in the crib, pointing the infant's feet toward one end of the crib for 1 week and the other end of the crib for the next week.

In addition to reducing risk for positional plagiocephaly, tummy time improves muscle development, head control, shoulder development, and progress to developmental milestones like crawling, sitting up, and walking (NICHD, 2020d). Along with education and role modeling of supine sleep positioning and appropriate bedding, nurses should ensure that families understand the importance of encouraging their infant to spend time in the prone position. Specific, concise information from nurses, therapists, and other members of the clinical team about the development of upper-body strength, normal progression of fine and gross-motor skills, and timely cognitive development will help parents understand the value of supervised prone positioning (Hewitt et al., 2020; Wittmeier & Mulder, 2017). This concept should be integrated into hospital practices, protocols, and education.

Special application in NICU: It may be a new way of thinking to consider introducing playtime in the NICU because many ill or premature infants do not have energy stores for activity beyond feeding and brief interactions. Skin-to-skin care with interaction during quiet alert states is an excellent transition to the concept of tummy time for play and interaction (Bastani et al., 2017). Families readily adopt the normative experience, and infants expect positive interactions associated with prone positioning. The collective behavior of nursing, parenting, and infant experiences makes adopting this new approach much more comfortable than a regimented authoritative change.

In "prone for play," the infant is meant to be awake and alert, and the parent or caregiver provides supervision and interaction. The duration of time can vary according to the infant's tolerance of the position, how the parent feels about the interaction, and other factors. The key is to give infants the opportunity for prone experiences regularly as a part of any transition within the hospital setting. The NICHD provides practical parent-teaching guides to supervised "tummy time."

Recommendation 16. *Healthcare professionals, staff in the newborn nurseries and NICUs, and childcare providers should endorse and model the SIDS risk reduction recommendations from birth.*

Staff in the NICU should model and implement all SIDS reduction recommendations as soon as the infant is medically stable and well in advance of discharge. All physicians, nurses, and other healthcare providers should receive up-to-date education on safe infant sleep. Hospital policy should be consistent with safe sleep recommendations. Families who do not have a safe sleep space for the infant should be provided with information about low-cost or free cribs or play yards from the hospital or community organizations before discharge (AAP, 2016).

Special application in NICU: NICU staff generally have extended time with families compared with labor and delivery or newborn nursery/mother–baby staff, providing an opportunity to engage in extended family education. Even for late preterm infants with shorter hospitalizations, NICU hospitalization was associated with a small but significant increase in breastfeeding initiation and the use of supine sleep position (Hannen et al., 2020).

Numerous studies have demonstrated that staff knowledge of safe sleep recommendations is often incomplete or outdated or that staff members do not consistently act upon the recommendations. Staff intervention aimed at knowledge of safe sleep practices alone is not sufficient for ensuring widespread use of the recommendations by NICU and other hospital staff (Barsman et al., 2015; De Luca & Hinde, 2016; Leong et al., 2019, 2020; McMullen et al., 2016; Naugler & DiCarlo, 2018; Newberry, 2019; Salm Ward & Balfour, 2016; Voos et al., 2014; Zachritz et al., 2016). Key portions of effective campaigns include written policies, audits of compliance with safe sleep recommendations, and multilevel messaging. Using system-based thinking increases the efficacy of policies, emphasizing leadership, collaborative practice, evidence-based practice, consideration of ethics, safety, efficiency, and cost-effectiveness (for competencies on systems thinking to improve best practices for infant and family center developmental care see Kenner & Jaeger, 2020).

Recommendation 17. *Media and manufacturer should follow safe sleep guidelines in their messaging and advertising.*

Media exposure in television, movies, magazines, websites, advertisements, social media, and store displays shapes individual behavior and influences attitudes and beliefs (AAP, 2016). Media messages in conflict with safe sleep recommendations create compelling misinformation about safe sleep practices. A survey of magazines aimed at expecting parents or parents of young children found that only 64% of pictures portraying sleeping infants, not being held, were in the supine position and only 36% of images displayed a safe sleep environment as recommended by the AAP (Joyner et al., 2009). Common problems included bumper pads, blankets, stuffed animals, evidence of smoking, and other people's presence on the same sleep surface. Of 17 pictures featuring celebrity parents, only two showed appropriate sleep environments.

Special application in NICU: In producing media for your unit or hospital, be aware of depicting safe sleep environments. Be particularly cautious about using stock photos; a survey of almost 2,000 stock photos showed only 5% complied with all the AAP sleep environment recommendations (Goodstein et al., 2018). The NICHD has provided numerous images as part of their SIDS Awareness Month Toolkit, including strategies for dealing with posted images in social media that violate safe sleep recommendations (NICHD, 2020a).

Recommendation 19. *Continue research and surveillance on the risk factors, causes, and pathophysiologic mechanisms of SIDS and other sleep-related infant deaths, with the ultimate goal of eliminating these deaths altogether.*

The basic science behind safe sleep recommendations, epidemiological information regarding SIDS/SUID, and the implementation science behind educational campaigns need to be encouraged and funded. Quality improvement projects surrounding safe sleep practices should be pursued and presented outside the organization at conferences and by publication.

Protocol Development: Nursing Education

Developing a unit or facility protocol for transitioning to AAP recommendations is a pivotal element in providing nurses with the information and reminders needed to implement these practices successfully. Hospitals with written protocols demonstrated increased nursing compliance with placing infants supine for sleep compared with hospitals without written protocols. Examples of such protocols are available in the literature and can be adapted to meet the unique needs of different neonatal care settings (Leong et al., 2020; McMullen et al., 2016; Naugler & DiCarlo, 2018; Voos et al., 2014). Leadership is required in making adherence to safe sleep protocols a yearly competency with education and review. Tools include educational modules with questions, case studies, peer reviews, and regular crib audits. Preparation for transition to a less acute or home setting should be the impetus for a re-evaluation of clinical and developmental status concerning possible inclusion at that time.

Family Education

Family education is critical to reducing SIDS risk, especially for the families of preterm infants. Families and extended families may already have integrated the recommendations for sleep position in older children. If this is the case, efforts should be targeted at explaining why or how preterm or ill infants may require additional support, with attention to when and how the transition to supine sleeping should occur. Many units and public health organizations use mnemonics as a reminder, such as the ABCs of safe sleep, which signify sleeping A-alone, B-on their back, and C-in a clear crib (Leong et al., 2019). The NICHD Safe to Sleep public education campaign provides many printable, shareable resources, videos, toolkits, sample campaigns, and events such as the

SIDS Awareness Month with weekly themes, Facebook Live block parties, checklists, and sample messages.

In addition to providing families with information and education, expected behaviors must be consistently established and reinforced in the hospital setting. The nurse, physician, or other healthcare provider is the model for parents and significantly influences parent beliefs and behaviors. Despite exposure to published or presented information such as Back to Sleep recommendations, families will continue to demonstrate behaviors and techniques seen in the hospital setting. Families must be aware that the differences in sleep practices for hospitalized ill or severely premature infants are designed to be temporary. Share with families information about timing and techniques for transition early on and throughout an infant's hospital stay. Families need encouragement from trusted individuals that reinforce their infant's progress along the developmental continuum and meet criteria to transition to healthy sleep behaviors and eventual discharge. Achieving a healthy infant sleep position is considered a developmental milestone in line with achieving full oral feedings and weaning from other medical devices (Dowling et al., 2018).

Neonatal nurses and caregivers critically influence the outcomes of their patients in all aspects of care. The use of a developmental continuum as a framework for introducing and applying the recommendations achieves the goals set forth by the AAP and resolves the perceived conflict between Back to Sleep and principles of developmentally supportive care. Successful transitioning of high-risk, critically ill, and premature infants to recommended sleep positions and behaviors is an expectation of care. Practitioners, families, and the community share accountability for reducing the risk for SIDS.

Conclusion

The importance of protecting sleep is a vital part of physiologic and developmentally supportive care. The quantity and quality of sleep essential for normal growth and development requires staff and families to understand the value of sleep–wake states and documentation of sleep–wake patterns. Effective support of infant sleep requires modification to the physical environment and caregiving routines. Quality sleep–wake cycles are supported by uninterrupted and extended time during parental skin-to-skin care. An understanding of sleep and arousal states are part of optimal care for feeding and interaction. Positioning strategies that support premature infant sleep should include practices and parent education that comply with the AAP safe sleep recommendations well in advance of discharge. SIDS risk reduction efforts should utilize a developmental continuum that optimizes each infant's capacities and works in partnership with families. Neonatal healthcare providers must rise to the challenges created by these recommendations during infant hospitalization to minimize the risk of SIDS after infants are discharged to home. Embracing change through systems-based innovation adoption processes will provide the necessary behaviors and modeling in the NICU to support and sustain SIDS risk reduction for all infants regardless of care needs early in development.

Potential Research Questions

- What is the long-term impact of skin-to-skin care on infant sleep development?
- What is the impact of developmentally supported sleep in the ICU on long-term neurodevelopmental outcomes?
- What are the maturational signs of readiness for unsupported supine sleep positioning in premature infants?
- What factors affect translation of evidence regarding SIDS risk reduction and NICU staff implementation of safe sleep protocols at this time?
- How does an intervention, including structured and supervised "tummy time" offered in the NICU and home setting, affect physical outcomes such as plagiocephaly, brachycephaly, and shoulder girdle strength/mobility?

REFERENCES

AAP Section on Breastfeeding. (2012). Policy Statement on breast-feeding and the use of human milk. *Pediatrics, 129*(3), e827–e841.

AAP Task Force on Sudden Infant Death Syndrome. (2011). SIDS and other sleep-related infant death. Expansion of recommendations for a safe sleeping environment technical report. *Pediatrics, 128*(5), e1341–e1367.

AAP Task Force on Sudden Infant Death Syndrome. (2016). SIDS and other sleep-related infant deaths. Updated 2016 recommendations for a safe sleeping environment. *Pediatrics, 138*(5), e20162938.

AAP Task Force on Infant Positioning and SIDS. (1992). Positioning and SIDS. *Pediatrics, 89*(6), 1122–1126.

AAP Task Force on Infant Positioning and SIDS. (1996). Positioning and sudden infant death syndrome (SIDS): Update. *Pediatrics, 98*(6), 1216–1218.

AAP Task Force on Infant Sleep Position and Sudden Infant Death Syndrome, (2000). Changing concepts of sudden infant death syndrome: Implications for infant sleeping environment and sleep position. *Pediatrics, 105*(3), 650–656.

American Academy of Pediatrics. (2018). Immunization in preterm and low birth weight infants. In Kimberlin, D. W., Brady, M. T., Jackson, M. A., & Long, S. S. (Eds.), *Red book 2018 of the committee on infectious diseases* (31st ed., pp. 67–68). American Academy of Pediatrics.

American Academy of Pediatrics (AAP) & American College of Obstetricians and Gynecologists (ACOG). (2017). *Guidelines for perinatal care* (8th ed.). AAP.

Anders, T. F. (1976). Maturation of sleep patterns in the newborn infant. In Weitzman, E. D. (Ed.), *Advances in sleep research* (Vol. 2, pp. 43–66). Spectrum Publications, Inc.

Anders, T. F., & Keener, M. (1985). Developmental course of nighttime sleep-wake patterns in full-term and premature infants during the first year of life. I. *Sleep, 8*(3), 173–192.

Anders, T. F., Keener, M. A., & Kraemer, H. (1985). Sleep-wake state organization, neonatal assessment and development in premature infants during the first year of life. II. *Sleep, 8*(3), 193–206.

Anderson, T. M., Lavista Ferres, J. M., Ren, S. Y., Moon, R. Y., Goldstein, R. D., Ramirez, J. M., & Mitchell, E. A. (2019). Maternal smoking before and during pregnancy and the risk of sudden unexpected infant death. *Pediatrics, 143*(4), e20183325.

Arditi-Babchuk, H., Feldman, R., & Eidelman, A. I. (2009). Rapid eye movement (REM) in premature neonates and developmental outcome at 6 months. *Infant Behavior & Development, 32*(1), 27–32. https://doi.org/10.1016/j.infbeh.2008.09.001

Arduini, D., Rizzo, G., Giorlandino, C., Valensise, H., Dell'Acqua, S., & Romanini, C. (1986). The development of fetal behavioural states: A longitudinal study. *Prenatal Diagnosis, 6*(2), 117–124.

Auger, N., Fraser, W. D., Simargiassi, A. & Kosatsky, T. (2015). Ambient heat and sudden infant death: The case-crossover study spanning thirty years in Montréal, Canada. *Environmental Health Perspectives, 123*, 712–716.

Bakermans-Kranenburg, M. J., & van IJzendoorn, M. H. (2017). Protective parenting: Neurobiological and behavioral dimensions. *Current Opinion in Psychology, 15*, 45–49. https://doi.org/10.1016/j.copsyc.2017.02.001

Barbeau, D. Y., & Weiss, M. D. (2017). Sleep disturbances in newborns. *Children, 4*(10), 90. https://doi.org/10.3390/children4100090

Barcat, L., Decima, P., Bodin, E., Delanaud, S., Stephan-Blanchard, E., Leke, A., Libert, J. P., Tourneux, P., & Bach, V. (2017). Distal skin vasodilation promotes rapid sleep onset in preterm neonates. *Journal of Sleep Research, 26*(5), 572–577. https://doi.org/10.1111/jsr.12514

Barsman, S. G., Dowling, D. A., Dmamato, E. G. & Czeck, P. (2015). Neonatal nurses beliefs, knowledge, and practices in relation to sudden infant death syndrome risk—reduction recommendations. *Advances in Neonatal Care, 15*(3), 209–219.

Bartick, M., & Tomori, C. (2019).Sudden infant death and social justice: A syndemics approach. *Maternity & Child Nutrition, 15*(1), e12652.

Bastani, F., Rajai, N., Farsi, Z., & Als, H. (2017). The effects of kangaroo care on the sleep and wake states of preterm infants. *The Journal of Nursing Research, 25*(3), 231–239.

Benham-Terneus, M., & Clemente, M. (2019). SIDS, BRUE, and safe sleep guidelines. *Pediatrics in Review, 49*(9), 443–455.

Bennet, L., Walker, D. W., & Horne, R. S. C. (2018). Waking up too early – the consequences of preterm birth on sleep development. *J Physiol, 596*(23), 5687–5708. https://doi.org/10.1113/JP274950

Bonan, K. C., Pimentel Filho Jda, C., Tristao, R. M., Jesus, J. A., & Campos Junior, D. (2015). Sleep deprivation, pain and prematurity: A review study. *Arquivos de Neuro-Psiquiatria, 73*(2), 147–154. https://doi.org/10.1590/0004-282X20140214

Bourel-Ponchel, E., Hasaerts, D., Challamel, M. J., & Lamblin, M. D. (2021). Behavioral-state development and sleep-state differentiation during early ontogenesis. *Clinical Neurophysiology, 51*(1), 89–98. https://doi.org/10.1016/j.neucli.2020.10.003

Briker, A., McLone, S., Mason, M., Matoba, N., & Sheehan, K. (2019). Modifiable sleep-related risk factors in infants deaths in Cook County, Illinois. *Injury Epidemiology, 29* (6 Suppl. 1), 24.

Bueno, C., & Menna-Barreto, L. (2016). Development of sleep/wake, activity and temperature rhythms in newborns maintained in a neonatal intensive care unit and the impact of feeding schedules. *Infant Behavior and Development, 44*, 21–28. https://doi.org/10.1016/j.infbeh.2016.05.004

Byard, R. W., & Beal, S. M. (2000). Gastric aspiration and sleeping position in infancy and early childhood. *Journal of Paediatrics and Child Health, 36*(4), 403–405.

Carpenter, R. G., Irgens, L. M., Blair, P. S., England, P. D., Fleming, P., Huber, J., Jorch, G., & Schreuder, P. (2004). Sudden unexplained infant death in 20 regions in Europe: Case control study. *Lancet, 363*(9404), 185–191.

Centers for Disease Control and Prevention. (2012). Suffocation deaths associated with use of infant sleep positioners—United States, 1997–2011. *Morbidity and Mortality Weekly Report (MMWR), 61*(46),933–937.

Centers for Disease Control and Prevention. (2020). *Sudden unexpected infant death and sudden infant death syndrome data and statistics.* www.cdc.gov/sids/index.htm

Chu, C. J., Leahy, J., Pathmanathan, J., Kramer, M. A., & Cash, S. S. (2014). The maturation of cortical sleep rhythms and networks over early development. *Clinical Neurophysiology, 125*(7), 1360–1370. https://doi.org/10.1016/j.clinph.2013.11.028

Cirelli, C., & Tononi, G. (2015). Cortical development, electroencephalogram rhythms, and the sleep/wake cycle. *Biological Psychiatry, 77*(12), 1071–1078. https://doi.org/10.1016/j.biopsych.2014.12.017

Davis, D. H., & Thoman, E. B. (1987). Behavioral states of premature infants: Implications for neural and behavioral development. *Developmantal Psychobiology, 20*(1), 25–38.

De Luca, F., & Hinde, A. (2016). Effectiveness of back to sleep campaigns among health care professionals in the past twenty years: A systematic review. *BMJ Open, 6*, e011435.

Dereymaeker, A., Pillay, K., Vervisch, J., De Vos, M., Van Huffel, S., Jansen, K., & Naulaers, G. (2017). Review of sleep-EEG in preterm and term neonates. *Early Human Development, 113*, 87–103. https://doi.org/10.1016/j.earlhumdev.2017.07.003

Dinges, D. F., Davis, M. M. & Glass, P. (1980). Fetal exposure to narcotics: Neonatal sleep as a measure of nervous system disturbance. *Science, 209*(4456), 619–621.

Ditthakasem, K., & Kolar, J. C. (2017). Deformational plagiocephaly: A review. *Pediatric Nursing, 43*(2), 59–95.

Dowling, D. A., Barsman, S. G., Forsythe, P., & Damato, E. G. (2018). Caring about preemies safe sleep (CAPSS): An educational program to improve adherence to safe sleep recommendations by mothers of preterm infants. *The Journal of Perinatal and Neonatal Nursing, 32*(4), 366–372.

Dunsirn, S., Smyser, C., Liao, S., Inder, T., & Pineda, R. (2016). Defining the nature and implications of head turn preference in the preterm infant. *Early Human Development, 96*, 53–60. https://doi.org/10.1016/j.earlhumdev.2016.02.002

Edraki, M., Paran, M., Montaseri, S., Razavi Nejad, M., & Montaseri, Z. (2014). Comparing the effects of swaddled and conventional bathing methods on body temperature and crying duration in premature infants: A randomized clinical trial. *Journal of Caring Sciences, 3*(2), 83–91. https://doi.org/10.5681/jcs.2014.009

El-Dib, M., Massaro, A. N., Glass, P., & Aly, H. (2014). Sleep wake cycling and neurodevelopmental outcome in very low birth weight infants. *The Journal of Maternal-Fetal & Neonatal Medicine, 27*(9), 892–897. https://doi.org/10.3109/14767058.2013.845160

Elliott, A. J., Kinney, H. C., Haynes, R. L., Dempers, J. D., Wright, C., Fifer, W. P., Angal, J., Boyd, T. K., Burd, L., Burger, E., Folkerth, R. D., Groenwald, C., Hankins, G., Hereld, D., Hoffman, H. J., Holm, I. A., Myers, M. M., Nelsen, L. L., Odendaal, H. J., ... Dukes, K. A. (2020). Concurrent prenatal drinking and smoking increases risk for SIDS: Safe Passage Study report. *E Clinical Medicine, 20*(19), 100247.

Erck Lambert, A. B., Parks, S. E., Cottengim, C., Faulkner, M., Hauck, F. R., & Shapiro-Mendoza, C. K. (2019). Sleep-related infant suffocation deaths attributable to soft bedding, overlay, and wedging. *Pediatrics, 143*(5), e20183408.

Filiano, J. J., & Kinney, H. C. (1994). A perspective on neuropathologic findings in victims of the sudden infant death syndrome: The triple-risk model. *Biology of the Neonate, 65*(3–4),194–197.

Franco, P., Kato, I., Richardson, H. L., Yang, J. S., Montemitro, E., & Horne, R. S. (2010). Arousal from sleep mechanisms in infants. *Sleep Med, 11*(7), 603–614. https://doi.org/10.1016/j.sleep.2009.12.014

Garrison-Desany, H. M., Nawa, N., Kim, Y., Ji, Y., Susan Chang, H. Y., Hong, X., Wang, G., Pearson, C., Zuckerman, B. S., Wang, X., & Surkan, P. J. (2020). Polydrug use during pregnancy and preterm birth in a low-income, multiethnic birth cohort, Boston, 1998-2018. *Public Health Reports, 135*(3),383–392.

van Geijn, H. P., Jongsma, H. W., de Haan, J., Eskes, T. K., & Prechtl, H. F. (1980). Heart rate as an indicator of the behavioral state. Studies in the newborn infant and prospects for fetal heart rate monitoring. *American Journal of Obstetrics & Gynecology, 136*(8), 1061–1066.

Gettler, L. T., & McKenna, J. J. (2011). Evolutionary perspectives on mother-infant sleep proximity and breastfeeding in a laboratory setting. *American Journal of Physical Anthropology, 144*(3), 454–462.

Geva, R., Yaron, H., & Kuint, J. (2016). Neonatal sleep predicts attention orienting and distractibility. *Journal of Attention Disorders, 20*(2), 138–150. https://doi.org/10.1177/1087054713491493

Geyer, J. E., Smith, P. K., & Kair, L. R. (2016). Safe sleep for pediatric inpatients. *Journals for Specialists in Pediatric Nursing, 21*(3), 119–130.

Gogou, M., Haidopoulou, K., & Pavlou, E. (2019). Sleep and prematurity: Sleep outcomes in preterm children and influencing factors. *World Journal of Pediatrics, 15*(3), 209–218. https://doi.org/10.1007/s12519-019-00240-8

Goodstein, M. H., Lagon, E., Bell, T., Joyner, B. L., & Moon, R. Y.(2018). Stock photographs do not comply with infant safe sleep guidelines. *Clinical Pediatrics, 57*(4), 403–409.

Grigg-Damberger, M. M. (2016). The visual scoring of sleep in infants 0 to 2 Months of age. *Journal of Clinical Sleep Medicine, 12*(3), 429–445. https://doi.org/10.5664/jcsm.5600

Guyer, C., Huber, R., Fontijn, J., Bucher, H. U., Nicolai, H., Werner, H., Molinari, L., Latal, B., & Jenni, O. G. (2015). Very preterm infants show earlier emergence of 24-hour sleep-wake rhythms compared to term infants. *Early Human Development, 91*(1), 37–42. https://doi.org/10.1016/j.earlhumdev.2014.11.002

Hagmann-von Arx, P., Perkinson-Gloor, N., Brand, S., Albert, D., Hosboer-Trachsler, E., Grob, A., Weber, P., Lemola, S. (2014). In school-age children who were born very preterm sleep efficiency is associated with cognitive function. *Neuropsychobiology, 70*, 244–252.

Hannen, K. E., Smith, R. A., Barfield, W. D., & Hwang, S. S. (2020). Association between neonatal intensive care unit admission and supine positioning, breastfeeding, and postnatal smoking among mothers of late preterm infants. *The Journal of Pediatrics, 227*, 114–120.

Hauck, F. R., Herman, S. M., Donovan, M., Iyasu, S., Merrick Moore, C., Donoghue, E., Kirschner, R. H., & Willinger, M. (2003). Sleep environment and the risk of sudden infant death syndrome in an urban population: The chicago infant mortality study. *Pediatrics, 111*(5 Pt. 2), 1207–1214.

Hauck, F. R., Omojokun, O. O., & Siadaty, M. S. (2005).Do pacifiers reduce the risk of sudden infant death syndrome? A meta-analysis. *Pediatrics, 116*(5),e716–e723.

Hauck, F. R., Signore, C., Fein, S. B., & Raju, T. N. K. (2008). Infant sleeping arrangements and practices during the first year of life. *Pediatrics, 122*(Suppl. 2), S113–S120.

Hauck, F. R., Thompson, J. M., Tanabe, K. O., Moon, R. Y., & Vennemann, M. M. (2011).Breastfeeding and reduced risk of sudden infant death syndrome: A meta-analysis. *Pediatrics, 128*(1), 103–110.

Hewitt, L., Kerr, E., Stanley, R. M., & Okely, A. D.. (2020). Tummy time and infant health outcomes: A systematic review. *Pediatrics, 145*(6), e20192168.

Hiscock, H., Bayer, J. K., Hampton, A., Ukoumunne, O. C., & Wake, M. (2008). Long-term mother and child mental health effects of a population-based infant sleep intervention: Cluster-randomized, controlled trial. *Pediatrics, 122*(3), e621–e627. https://doi.org/10.1542/peds.2007-3783

Holditch-Davis, D., Brandon, D. H., & Schwartz, T. (2003). Development of behaviors in preterm infants: Relation to sleeping and waking. *Nursing Research, 52*(5), 307–317.

Holditch-Davis, D., & Edwards, L. J. (1998). Temporal organization of sleep-wake states in preterm infants. *Dev Psychobiol, 33*(3), 257–269.

Jeanson, E. (2013). One-to-One bedside nurse education as a means to improve positioning consistency. *Newborn & Infant Nursing Reviews, 13*, 27–30.

Jhun, I., Mata, D. A., Nordio, F., Lee, M., Schwartz, J., & Zanobeth, A. (2017). Ambient temperature and sudden infant death syndrome in the United States. *Epidemiology, 28*(5), 728–734.

Joyner, B. L., Gill-Bailey, C., Moon, R. Y. (2009). Infant sleep environments depicted in magazines targeted to women of childbearing age. *Pediatrics, 124*(3):e416–e422.

Joyner, B. L., Oden, R. P., Ajao, T. I., & Moon, R. Y. (2010). Where should my baby sleep: A qualitative study of African American infant sleep location decisions. *Journal of the National Medicine Association, 102*(10), 881–889.

Junge, H. D. (1979). Behavioral states and state related heart rate and motor activity patterns in the newborn infant and the fetus antepartum—a comparative study. I. Technique, illustration of recordings, and general results. *Journal of Perinatal Medicine, 7*(2), 85–107.

Junge, H. D. (1980). Behavioral states and state-related heart rate and motor activity patterns in the newborn infant and the fetus ante partum. A comparative study. III. Analysis of sleep state-related motor activity patterns. *European Journal of Obstetrics, Gynecology, & Reproductive Biology, 10*(4), 239–246.

Kenner, C & Jaeger, CB. (2020). *IFCDC—recommendation for best practices and systems thinking.* https://nicudesign.nd.edu/nicu-care-standards/ifcdc--recommendation-for-best-practices-in-systems-thinking/

Kostović, I., Sedmak, G., & Judaš, M. (2019). Neural histology and neurogenesis of the human fetal and infant brain. *NeuroImage, 188*, 743–773. https://doi.org/10.1016/j.neuroimage.2018.12.043

Krsnik, Z., Majic, V., Vasung, L., Huang, H., & Kostovic, I. (2017). Growth of thalamocortical fibers to the somatosensory cortex in the human fetal brain. *Frontiers in Neuroscience, 11*, 233. https://doi.org/10.3389/fnins.2017.00233

Kuhnert, R., Schlaud, M., Poethko-Müller, C., Vennemann, M., Fleming, P., Blair, P. S., Mitchell, E., Thompson, J., & Hecker, H. (2012). Reanalysis of case-control studies examining the temporal association between sudden infant death syndrome and vaccination. *Vaccine, 30*(13), 2349–2356.

Lacina, L., Casper, T., Dixon, M., Harmeyer, J., Haberman, B., Alberts, J. R., Simakajornboon, N., & Visscher, M. O. (2015). Behavioral observation differentiates the effects of an intervention to promote sleep in premature infants: A pilot study. *Advances in Neonatal Care, 15*(1), 70–76. https://doi.org/10.1097/ANC.0000000000000134

Lam, P., Hiscock, H., & Wake, M. (2003). Outcomes of infant sleep problems: A longitudinal study of sleep, behavior, and maternal well-being. *Pediatrics, 111*(3), e203–e207.

Lehtonen, L., & Martin, R. J. (2004). Ontogeny of sleep and awake states in relation to breathing in preterm infants. *Seminars in Neonatology, 9*(3), 229–238. https://doi.org/10.1016/j.siny.2003.09.002

Leong, T., Billaud, M., Agarwal, M., Miller, T., McFadden, T., Johnson, J., & Lazarus, S. G. (2019). As easy as ABC: Evaluation of safe sleep initiative on safe sleep compliance in a freestanding pediatric hospital. *Injury Epidemiology, 6*(Suppl. 1), 26.

Leong, T., Roome, K., Miller, T., Gorbatkin, O., Singleton, L., Agarwal, M., & Lazarus, S. G. (2020). Expansion of a multi-pronged safe sleep quality improvement initiative to three children's hospital campuses. *Injury Epidemiology, 7*(Suppl. 1), 32.

Levy, J., Hassan, F., Plegue, M. A., Sokoloff, M. D., Kushwaha, J. S., Chervin, R. D., Barks, J. D., & Shellhaas, R. A. (2017). Impact of hands-on care on infant sleep in the neonatal intensive care unit. *Pediatric Pulmonology, 52*(1), 84–90. https://doi.org/10.1002/ppul.23513

Liaw, J. J., Yang, L., Lo, C., Yuh, Y. S., Fan, H. C., Chang, Y. C., & Chao, S. C. (2012). Caregiving and positioning effects on preterm infant states over 24 hours in a neonatal unit in Taiwan. *Research in Nursing & Health, 35*(2), 132–145. https://doi.org/10.1002/nur.21458

Mahmoodi, N., Arbabisarjou, A., Rezaeipoor, M., & Pishkar Mofrad, Z. (2015). Nurses' awareness of preterm neonates' sleep in the NICU. *Global Journal of Health Science, 8*(6), 226–233. https://doi.org/10.5539/gjhs.v8n6p226

Martin, C. B., Jr. (1981). Behavioral states in the human fetus. *The Journal of Reproductive Medicine, 26*(8), 425–432.

Matthey, S., & Speyer, J. (2008). Changes in unsettled infant sleep and maternal mood following admission to a parentcraft residential unit. *Early Human Development, 84*(9), 623–629. https://doi.org/10.1016/j.earlhumdev.2008.04.003

McMullen, S. L., Fioravanti, I. S., Brown, K., & Carey, M. G.. (2016). Safe sleep for hospitalized infants. *MCN. The American Journal for Maternal Child Nursing, 41*(1), 43–50.

McMullen, S. L., Lipke, B., & LeMura, C. (2009). Sudden infant death syndrome prevention: a model program for NICUs. *Neonatal Network, 28*(1), 7–12.

Mileva-Seitz, V. R., Bakermans-Kranenburg, M. J., Battaini, C., & Luijk, M. P. (2017). Parent-child bed-sharing: The good, the bad, and the burden of evidence. *Sleep Medicine Reviews, 32*, 4–27.

Milgrom, J., Newnham, C., Anderson, P., Doyle, P., Gemmill, A., Lee, K., Hunt, R. W., Bear, M., & Inder, T. (2010). Early sensitivity training for parents of preterm infants: Impact on the developing brain. *Pediatric Research, 67*(3), 330–335.

Moon, R. Y. (2020). *How to keep your sleeping baby safe: AAP policy explained.* https://www.healthychildren.org/English/ages-stages/baby/sleep/Pages/A-Parents-Guide-to-Safe-Sleep.aspx

Moon, R. Y., & AAP Task Force on Sudden Infant Death Syndrome, . (2016). SIDS and other sleep-related infant deaths: Evidence base for 2016 updated recommendations for a safer sleeping environment. *Pediatrics, 138*(5), e20162940.

Moon, R. Y., Sprague, B. M., & Patel, K. M. (2005). Stable prevalence but changing risk factors for sudden infant death syndrome in child care settings in 2001. *Pediatrics, 116*(4),972–977.

Moon, R. Y., Tanabe, K. O., Yang, D. C., Young, H. A., & Hauck, F. R. (2012). Pacifier use and SIDS: Evidence for a consistently reduced risk. *Maternal and Child Health Journal, 16*(3), 609–614.

Morag, I., & Ohlsson, A. (2016). Cycled light in the intensive care unit for preterm and low birth weight infants. *Cochrane Database Systematic Reviews, 2016*(8), CD006982. https://doi.org/10.1002/14651858.CD006982.pub4

National Institute of Child Health & Human Development (NICHD). (2014). *Safe sleep for your baby.* National Institutes of Health https://www.nichd.nih.gov/sites/default/files/publications/pubs/Documents/Safe_Sleep_Baby_English.pdf

National Institute of Child Health and Human Development. (2020a). *2020 SIDS awareness month #SafeSleepSnap digital toolkit.* https://safetosleep.nichd.nih.gov/resources/sids-awareness-toolkit

National Institute of Child Health and Human Development. (2020b). *Safe to sleep.* https://safetosleep.nichd.nih.gov/

National Institute of Child Health and Human Development. (2020c). *Research on possible causes of SIDS: The triple risk model.* https://safetosleep.nichd.nih.gov/research/science/causes

National Institute of Child Health and Human Development. (2020d). *Safe to sleep: Babies need tummy time.* https://safetosleep.nichd.nih.gov/safesleepbasics/tummytime

National Institute of Child Health and Human Development. (2020e). *Safe to sleep: Baby's anatomy when on stomach and on back.* https://safetosleep.nichd.nih.gov/resources/providers/downloadable/baby_anatomy_image

Naugler, M. R., & DiCarlo, K.. (2018). Barriers to and interventions that increase nurses' and parents' compliance with safe sleep recommendations for preterm infants. *Nursing for Womens Health, 22*(1), 24–39.

Newberry, J. A. (2019). Creating a safe sleep environment for the infant: What the pediatric nurse needs to know. *Journal of Pediatric Nursing, 44*, 119–122.

Nijhuis, J. G., Prechtl, H. F., Martin, C. B., Jr, & Bots, R. S. (1982). Are there behavioural states in the human fetus? *Early Human Development, 6*(2), 177–195.

O'Brien, C. M., & Jeffery, H. E. (2002). Sleep deprivation, disorganization and fragmentation during opiate withdrawal in newborns. *Journal of Pediatrics and Child Health, 38*(1), 66–71.

Obladen, M. (2018). Cot death: History of an iatrogenic disaster. *Neonatology, 113*(2), 162–169.

O'Leary, C. M., Jacoby, P. J., Bartu, A., D'Antoine, H., & Bower, C. (2013). Maternal alcohol use and sudden infant death syndrome and infant mortality excluding SIDS. *Pediatrics, 131*(3), e770–e778.

Pierrat, V., Goubet, N., Peifer, K., & Sizun, J. (2007). How can we evaluate developmental care practices prior to their implementation in a neonatal intensive care unit? *Early Human Development, 83*, 415–418.

Pillai, M., James, D. K., & Parker, M. (1992). The development of ultradian rhythms in the human fetus. *American Journal of Obstetrics and Gynecology, 167*(1), 172–177.

Pinto, F., Torrioli, M. G., Casella, G., Tempesta, E., & Fundaro, C. (1988). Sleep in babies born to chronically heroin addicted mothers. A follow up study. *Drug and Alcohol Dependence, 21*(1), 43–47.

Qureshi, A., Malkar, M., Splaingard, M., Khuhro, A., & Jadcherla, S. (2015). The role of sleep in the modulation of gastroesophageal reflux and symptoms in NICU neonates. *Pediatric Neurology, 53*(3), 226–232. https://doi.org/10.1016/j.pediatrneurol.2015.05.012

Ramanathan, R., Corwin, M. J., Hunt, C. E., Lister, G., Tinsley, L. R., Baird, T., Silvestri, J. M., Crowell, D. H., Hufford, D., Martin, R. J., Neuman, M. R., Weese-Mayer, D. E., Cupples, L. A., Peucker, M., Willinger, M., & Keens, T. G.; Collaborative Home Infant Monitoring Evaluation (CHIME) Study Group. (2001). Cardiorespiratory events recorded on home monitors: comparison of healthy infants with those at increased risk for SIDS. *JAMA, 285*(17), 2199–2207.

Ramgopal, S., Soung, J., & Pitetti, R. D. (2019). Brief resolved unexplained events: Analysis of an apparent life threatening event database. *Academic Pediatrics, 19*(8), 963–968.

Rivas-Fernandez, M., Roqué I Figuls, M., Diez-Izquierdo, A., Escribano, J., & Balaguer, A. (2016). Infant position in neonates receiving mechanical ventilation. *Cochrane Database Systematic Review, 11*(11), CD003668.

Rivkees, S. A., Mayes, L., Jacobs, H., & Gross, I. (2004). Rest-activity patterns of premature infants are regulated by cycled lighting. *Pediatrics, 113*(4), 833–839.

Salm Ward, T. C., & Balfour, G. M. (2016). Infant sleep interventions, 1990–2015: A review. *J Community Health, 41*, 180–196.

Scher, A. (2005). Infant sleep at 10 months of age as a window to cognitive development. *Early Human Development, 81*(3), 289–292.

Scher, A., Johnson, M. W., & Holditch-Davis, D. (2005). Cyclicity of neonatal sleep behaviors at 25 to 30 weeks' postconceptual age. *Pediatric Research, 57*(6), 879–882.

Scher, M. S., Steppe, D. A., Banks, D. L., Guthrie, R. D., & Sclabassi, R. J. (1995). Maturational trends of EEG-Sleep measures in the healthy preterm neonate. *Pediatric Neurology, 12*(4), 314–322.

Schlaud, M., Dreier, M., Debertin, A. S., Jachau, K., Heide, S., Giebe, B., Sperhake, J. P., Poets, C. F., & Kleemann, W. J. (2010). The German case-control scene investigation study on SIDS: epidemiological approach and main results. *International Journal of Legal Medicine, 124*(1), 19–26.

Shellhaas, R. A., Kenia, P. V., Hassan, F., Barks, J. D. E., Kaciroti, N., & Chervin, R. D. (2018). Sleep-disordered breathing among newborns with myelomeningocele. *The Journal of Pediatrics, 194*, 244–247.e241. https://doi.org/10.1016/j.jpeds.2017.10.070

Shepherd, K. L., Yiallourou, S. R., Odoi, A., Brew, N., Yeomans, E., Willis, S., Horne, R. S. C., & Wong, F. Y. (2019). Effects of prone sleeping on cerebral oxygenation in preterm infants. *The Journal of Pediatrics, 204*, 103–110.

Shepherd, K. L., Yiallourou, S. R., Odoi, A., Yeomans, E., Willis, S., Horne, R. S. C., & Wong, F. Y. (2020). When does prone sleeping improve cardiorespiratory status in preterm infants in the NICU? *Sleep, 43*(4):zsz256.

Smith, L. A., Geller, N. L., Kellams, A. L., Colson, E. R., Rybin, D. V., Heeren, T., & Corwin, M. J. (2016). Infant sleep location and bbreastfeeding practices in the United States, 2011–2014. *Academic Pediatrics, 16*(6), 540–549.

Staedt, J., Wassmuth, F., Stoppe, G., Hajak, G., Rodenbeck, A., Poser, W., & Ruther, E. (1996). Effects of chronic treatment with methadone and naltrexone on sleep in addicts. *European Archives of Psychiatry and Clinical Neuroscience, 246*(6), 305–309.

Takenouchi, T., Rubens, E. O., Yap, V. L., Ross, G., Engel, M., & Perlman, J. M. (2011). Delayed onset of sleep-wake cycling with favorable outcome in hypothermic-treated neonates with encephalopathy. *The Journal of Pediatrics, 159*(2), 232–237. https://doi.org/10.1016/j.jpeds.2011.01.006

Tappin, D., Ecob, R., & Brooke, H. (2005). Bedsharing, room sharing, and sudden infant death syndrome in Scotland: A case-control study. *Journal of Pediatrics, 147*, 32–37.

Thoman, E., Davis, D., & Denenberg, V. (1987). The sleeping and waking states of infants: Correlations across time and person. *Physiology & Behavior, 41*(6), 531–537. https://doi.org/10.1016/0031-9384(87)90307-6

Thompson, J. M. D., Tanabe, K., Moon, R. Y., Mitchell, E. A., McGarvey, C., Tappin, D., Blair, P. S., & Hauck, F. R. (2017). Duration of breastfeeding and risk of SIDS: An individual participant data meta-analysis. *Pediatrics, 140*(5), e20171324.

Tieder, J. S., Bonkowsky, J. L., Enzel, R. A., Franklin, W. H., Gremse, D. A., Herman, B., Katz, E. S., Krilov, L. R., Merritt, J. L. II, Norlin, C., Percelay, J., Sapién, R. E., Shiffman, R. N., Smith, M. B., & AAP Subcommittee on Apparent Life Threatening Events. (2016). Brief resolved unexplained events (formerly apparent life-threatening events) and evaluation of lower-risk infants. *Pediatrics, 137*(5), e20160590.

Timor-Tritsch, I. E., Dierker, L. J., Hertz, R. H., Deagan, N. C., & Rosen, M. G. (1978). Studies of antepartum behavioral state in the human fetus at term. *American Journal of Obstetrics and Gynecology, 132*(5), 524–528.

United States Consumer Product Safety Commission. (2020). *Safe sleep—cribs and infant products information center.* https://cpsc.gov/SafeSleep

Utario, Y., Rustina, Y., & Waluyanti, F. T. (2017). The quarter prone position increases oxygen saturation in premature infants using continuous positive airway pressure. *Comprehensive Child and Adolescent Nursing, 40*(Suppl. 1), 95–101.

van Vlimmeren, L. A., van der Graaf, Y., Boere-Boonekamp, M. M., L'Hoir, M. P., Helders, P. J., & Engelbert, R. H. (2007). Risk factors for deformational plagiocephaly at birth and at 7 weeks of age: a prospective cohort study. *Pediatrics, 119*(2), e408–e418.

Vennemann, M. M., Bajanowski, T., Brinkmann, B., Jorch, G., Sauerland, C., Mitchell, E. A., & GeSID Study Group, .(2009). Sleep environment risk factors for sudden infant death syndrome: The German sudden infant death syndrome study. *Pediatrics, 123*(4), 1162–1170.

Vennemann, M. M., Hense, H. W., Bajanowski, T., Blair, P. S., Complojer, C., Moon, R. Y., & Kiechl-Kohlendorfer, U. (2012). Bed sharing and the risk of sudden infant death syndrome: Can we resolve the debate? *The Journal of Pediatrics, 160*(1), 44–48.

Vennemann, M. M., Höffgen, M., Bajanowski, T., Hense, H. W., & Mitchell, E. A. (2007). Do immunisations reduce the risk for SIDS? A meta-analysis. *Vaccine, 25*(26), 4875–4879.

van Vlimmeren, L. A., van der Graaf, Y., Boere-Boonekamp, M. M., L'Hoir, M. P., Helders, P. J., & Engelbert, R. H. (2007). Risk factors for deformational plagiocephaly at birth and at 7 weeks of age: A prospective cohort study. *Pediatrics, 119*(2), e408–e418.

Voos, K. C., Terreros, A., Larimore, P., Leick-Rude, M. K., & Park, N. (2014). Implementing safe sleep practices in a neonatal intensive care unit. *Journal of Maternal Fetal & Neonatal Medicine, 28*(14), 1637–1640.

Walusinski, O. (2010). Fetal yawning. *Frontiers of Neurology and Neuroscience, 28*, 32–41.

Weisman, O., Magori-Cohen, R., Louzoun, Y., Eidelman, A. I., & Feldman, R. (2011). Sleep-wake transitions in premature neonates predict early development. *Pediatrics, 128*(4), 706–714. https://doi.org/10.1542/peds.2011-0047

Werth, J., Atallah, L., Andriessen, P., Long, X., Zwartkruis-Pelgrim, E., & Aarts, R. M. (2017). Unobtrusive sleep state measurements in preterm infants—a review. *Sleep Medicine Reviews, 32*, 109–122. https://doi.org/10.1016/j.smrv.2016.03.005

Whitney, M. P., & Thoman, E. B. (1993). Early sleep patterns of premature infants are differentially related to later developmental disabilities. *Journal of Developmental and Behavioral Pediatrics, 14*(2), 71–80.

Wittmeier, K., & Mulder, K. (2017). Time to revisit tummy time: A commentary on plagiocephaly and development. *Paediatrics & Child Health, 22*(3), 159–161.

Wong, F. Y., Witcombe, N. B., Yiallourou, S. R., Yorkston, S., Dymowski, A. R., Krishnan, L., Walker, A. M., & Horne, R. S. (2011). Cerebral oxygenation is depressed during sleep in healthy term infants when they sleep prone. *Pediatrics, 127*(3), e558–e565.

Wright, J. R. (2017). A fresh look at the history of SIDS. *Academic Forensic Pathology, 7*(2), 146–162.

Zachritz, W., Fulmer, M., & Chaney, N. (2016). An evidence-based infant safe sleep program to reduce sudden unexplained infant deaths. *The American Journal of Nursing, 116*(11), 48–55.

CHAPTER 14

Collaborative Therapeutic Positioning: Multisystem and Behavioral Implications

Jane K. Sweeney and Jan McElroy

Standard 1: Positioning

- Babies in intensive care settings shall be positioned to support musculoskeletal, physiological, and behavioral stability.

Standard 2: Positioning

- Collaborative efforts among parents and intensive care unit (ICU) interprofessionals shall support optimal cranial shaping and prevent torticollis and skull deformity.

Standard 3: Positioning

- Body position shall be used as an ICU intervention for infants with gastrointestinal symptoms.

Standard 4: Touch

- Babies in neonatal intensive care unit (NICU) settings shall experience human touch by family and caregivers.

Standard 5: Systems Thinking

- The ICU shall provide a professionally competent interprofessional collaborative practice team to support the baby, parent, and family's holistic physical, developmental, and psychosocial needs from birth through the transition of hospital discharge to home and assure continuity to follow-up care.

INTRODUCTION

Body positioning is a critical care component for infant comfort and stability throughout hospitalization and transition to the home environment. All NICU team and family members involved in touching or moving infants influence (stabilize or destabilize) infants' multiple body systems and behavior. Interdisciplinary collaboration is required to create and teach optimum, individualized positioning strategies to accommodate lines, tubes, and equipment. Diligent monitoring of multisystem body positioning effects and ongoing competency training are essential for risk management and quality improvement.

Positioning of infants is an accepted, although inconsistently used, practice in NICUs worldwide. A greater understanding of the value of positioning to the infant's comfort, well-being, and development can contribute to increased implementation of positioning guidelines. Historically, the practice of neonatal positioning has been valued primarily for duplication of the temporary position of "physiological" flexion seen in full-term newborn infants. Although prioritized for protecting skin and supporting motor development, time constraints and conflicts with essential medical procedures and caregiving often minimized the importance and consistency in positioning. Current knowledge on the needs

and capabilities of infants born preterm has created a better understanding of the role positioning plays in supporting systems other than motor and integumentary systems alone and now encompasses interaction with behavioral and regulatory systems. Infant positioning in an expanded multisystem view has a therapeutic focus and is linked to body alignment, developmental postural support, NICU environmental factors, and individualized medical needs.

This chapter highlights body system and behavioral effects of therapeutic positioning. Evidence-based competencies on therapeutic positioning are reviewed, and positioning evaluation models are identified. Inherent in positioning interventions and comfort strategies is human touch. Competencies for providing modulated human touch are identified and linked to the supporting literature.

NEUROMOTOR CONSIDERATIONS

A mother's womb provides 9 months of an ideal environment of safety and support for optimal neuromotor development of the fetus. The fetus enjoys circumferential boundaries, which encourage flexed, midline-oriented, and symmetrical resting postures of the neck, thoracolumbar spine, and extremities (Altimier & Phillips, 2016; Ferrari et al., 2007;

Madlinger-Lewis et al., 2014). The flexed, symmetrical posture afforded by the mother's uterus supports the fetus in developing body awareness when the hands touch the chest or face area and when the legs or feet touch each other. The semi-flexed posture allows the fetus to practice movements of the hand to mouth and thumb or fingers in mouth, which later provide a mechanism for assisting in self-calming (Jarus et al., 2011) and emotional regulation (Altimier & Phillips, 2016; King & Norton, 2017; Madlinger-Lewis et al., 2014).

The flexible nature of the uterine wall offers dynamic resistance and varying sensory feedback as the fetus experiences spontaneous movements. With fetal growth throughout gestation, the dynamic resistance to movement and intensity of sensory feedback increase proportionally to the fetus's changes in body size, muscle properties, strength, and movement patterns. After birth, the infant is then prepared for movement, progressive motor development, and functional skills, all in the presence of gravity. These neonatal movement competencies result in self-calming (hands to mouth, face or body), self-movement of the body toward comfort, and exploration of the environment (King & Norton, 2017; Madlinger-Lewis et al., 2014). Neurologically intact infants born at term gestation benefit from the match of endogenous neuromuscular development with the exogenous, extrauterine environment.

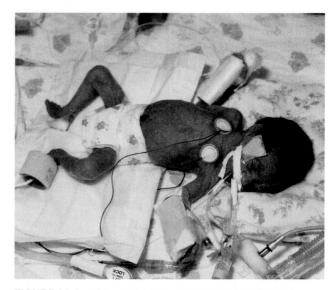

FIGURE 14-1. Without therapeutic positioning, the "W" configuration of shoulders and arms, "frogged" posture of legs and asymmetric head position may promote positional deformities and developmental gaps or delays. [Reprinted with permission from Hunter, J. G. (2010). The neonatal intensive care unit. In Case-Smith, J. (Ed.), *Occupational therapy for children* (6th ed.). Mosby.]

Extrauterine Motor Challenges

Many strategies have been designed by NICU teams to modify environmental sound, light, and day/night cycling, thereby addressing stressful and disruptive environmental input to the immature visual, auditory, and sleep systems of the infants (Altimier & Phillips, 2016; Casavant et al., 2017; Coughlin et al., 2009; Griffiths et al., 2019; Lipner & Huron, 2018; Wiley et al., 2020). Care procedures are often grouped to allow uninterrupted periods of rest (Altimier & Phillips, 2016; Coughlin et al., 2009; Griffiths et al., 2019). The often complex medical needs of infants born preterm may limit the extent the NICU environment can be modified to resemble or recreate the supportive, intrauterine environment.

An infant born preterm is equipped with neuromuscular properties (i.e., muscle fiber ratios) and abilities appropriate for the infant's gestational age and designed only for the intrauterine environment (Pineda et al., 2013; Sweeney & Gutierrez, 2002). After preterm birth, the infant is faced with a mismatch between neuromuscular properties, corresponding motor abilities, and the challenges of moving against gravity in the extrauterine environment (Altimier & Phillips, 2016). Lacking the strength and motor control of a full-term infant, the infant born preterm is dominated by gravity (Gomes et al., 2019; Picheansathian et al., 2009). In the supine position infants demonstrate neck extension, head rotated to one side, and upper extremities resting flat against the supporting surface with shoulder external rotation (Sweeney & Gutierrez, 2002). Lower extremities are abducted, externally rotated ("frog" posture) and also resting against the supporting surface (Sweeney & Gutierrez, 2002; Figure 14-1).

Combined with hypotonia and ligamentous laxity corresponding to gestational age, time spent in this position creates a muscle and soft tissue bias that favors neck and trunk extension, shoulder external rotation, and hip abduction/external rotation (Sweeney & Gutierrez, 2002; Teledevara et al., 2019). Infants born full term enter the antigravity developmental sequence with a flexion bias. Compared with the flexion postures of term infants, the extension predisposition of many preterm infants creates a postural set inadequately supporting extremity movement choices (Picheansathian et al., 2009; Pineda et al., 2013). Potential developmental sequelae of atypical positioning are summarized in Table 14-1. Musculoskeletal malalignment and functional limitations in infants are also described in Table 11-2 in Chapter 11.

Consequences of a static resting position are compounded by the movement difficulties often experienced by infants born preterm. It is difficult for the infant to develop the midline orientation, symmetry, strength, and coordination needed for effective function against gravity (Eskandari et al., 2020; Sweeney & Gutierrez, 2002). Limited strength for anti-gravity movement combined with a high energy cost may decrease the frequency of movement in infants born prematurely (Picheansathian et al., 2009). The infant's spontaneous movements may lack controlled variability, particularly at the elbow and knee, making small, independent position changes for comfort difficult to attain. For example, movement excursions may be large and abrupt sometimes creating stressful rather than self-comforting strategies (Ferrari et al., 2007). Without the maternal uterine wall to dampen movements, provide kinesthetic feedback, and guide

TABLE 14-1 Potential Consequences of Postural Malalignment in the NICU

Neonatal Posture	Potential Consequences in Infancy
Head turned to side 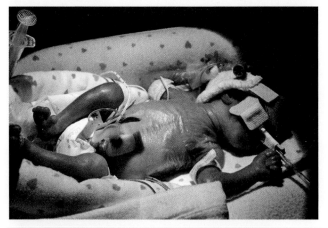	• Contributes to dolichocephaly [narrow head shape] • Generates potential head turn preference and plagiocephaly risk [asymmetrical skull flattening] • Creates risk for torticollis if prolonged asymmetrical head turn preference occurs • May contribute to challenges in eye coordination or tracking and binocular vision development if asymmetrical head position is prolonged • Creates challenges in developing midline head control • Contributes to potential interference with later eye–hand play activities in midline
Neck hyperextension 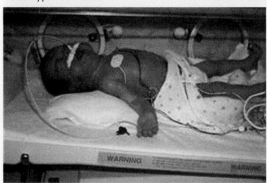	• Creates breathing patterns linked to extended neck position • Contributes to delayed development of head and shoulder postural control • Interferes with chin tuck for downward gaze during eye–hand play activities • Generates difficulty with latch and sucking pattern related to open mouth position with neck hyperextension posture • May produce inefficient swallowing with increased risk of aspiration
Elevated, retracted shoulders 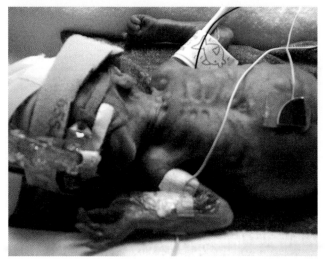["W" shoulder-elbow posture]	• Interferes with shoulder stability for upper extremity function like reaching and grasping • Contributes to delayed head and shoulder postural control • Generates difficulty with hands to midline for play, hands to mouth for self-calming, and body exploration • Interferes with development of rolling skills

(Continued)

TABLE 14-1 Potential Consequences of Postural Malalignment in the NICU (Continued)

Neonatal Posture	Potential Consequences in Infancy
Asymmetrical trunk with trunk 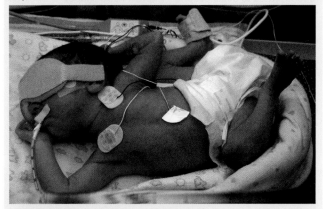 Extension	• Generates need for careful surveillance of potential risk for scoliosis if trunk asymmetry pattern persists • Creates potential consequences in rib cage development and respiratory support for breathing, voice production, and volume • Contributes to decreased postural control of the trunk affecting balance and gross motor skills (transitioning in and out of positions)
Hip abduction and external rotation 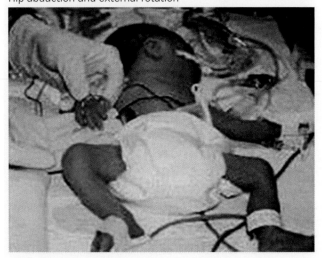	• Creates challenges in learning to roll and move into and out of sitting • Contributes to a wide base of support for gait, which may interfere with walking patterns and running • Develops tendency for abnormal leg position, which may interfere with learning coordination skills for participation in group motor activities

Sources for possible consequences of inadequate neonatal positioning consist of the following references as well as clinical observation in follow-up settings that are linked to NICU environment and postures (Georgieff & Bernbaum, 1986; Gorga et al., 1988; Katz et al., 1991; Klimo et al., 2016; McCarty et al., 2017; Monterosso et al., 2003; Riegger-Krugh, 1993; Sweeney & Gutierrez, 2002; Vaivre-Douret et al., 2004).

movement back toward a more flexed, midline-oriented and symmetrical posture, the preterm infant is disadvantaged in accessing and practicing movements that could enhance comfort and behavioral control (Altimier & Phillips, 2016; Picheansathian et al., 2009). The infant's new (extrauterine) environment no longer provides dynamic resistance for developing changes in muscle architecture, strength, and movement control that support flexion-biased function.

Therapeutic Positioning

Historically, therapeutic positioning was viewed within the context of re-creating the transient phase of physiologic extremity flexion demonstrated by healthy infants born full term. Most infants born preterm do not have, and will never develop, the extremity tissue tightness and flexion recoil that comprise physiological flexion (Dubowitz et al., 1999; Pineda

et al., 2013; Ricci et al., 2008; Sweeney & Gutierrez, 2002). An important role of therapeutic positioning is to provide support for comfortable, safe resting postures that offer the preterm infant the same positional support for the flexed position provided for the fetus and full-term infant (Altimier & Phillips, 2016; King & Norton, 2017; Madlinger-Lewis et al., 2014; Picheansathian et al., 2009; Santos et al., 2017). Varied body positions can decrease occurrence of atypical muscle and soft tissue tightness in medically fragile preterm infants, potentially associated with reduced mobility from long-term use of respiratory equipment, tubes, and lines (Sweeney & Gutierrez, 2002). Equally important, a dynamic, supportive environment can be created that allows the infant to rest or to move in extremity ranges other than full flexion or full extension. Midrange extremity positions are often inaccessible to the infant, given the motor limitations of prematurity (Altimier & Phillips, 2016; Ferrari et al., 2007;

Zahed et al., 2015). Muscles can change and grow when dynamic resistance from flexible containment nests and swaddling materials support rather than restrict spontaneous infant movements (Sweeney & Gutierrez, 2002). Therapeutic positioning enables the infant to perform self-initiated functional and developmental activities such as body exploration with hand to hand, hand to mouth, foot to foot, or foot to leg (Altimier & Phillips, 2016; Byrne & Garber, 2013; Sweeney & Gutierrez, 2002; Zahed et al., 2015). The neuromotor system "learns" from the repetition of self-initiated movements that have function and "meaning" performed at times chosen by the infant. Even very ill, low-birth-weight, and medically unstable infants initiate movement to attempt to meet needs for comfort, physiological and behavioral regulation, and short-duration interaction.

SKIN CONSIDERATIONS

Infants born preterm and hospitalized in the NICU are at substantial risk of skin injury related to medical care (Albahrani & Hunt, 2019; August et al., 2018; Behr et al., 2020; Liversedge et al., 2018). Preterm infants demonstrate increased susceptibility to skin injury related to gestational age, birthweight, and medical device application (i.e., monitors, catheters, and mechanical ventilation (Afsar, 2009; August et al., 2018; de Faria et al., 2019; Liversedge et al., 2018). Skin injuries further jeopardize the health of hospitalized preterm infants by increasing pain, lengthening hospitalization, and creating long-term scarring (Sardesai et al., 2011; Visscher & Taylor, 2014). Four mechanical forces responsible for skin injury in infants born preterm are stripping, pressure, friction, and shear (August et al., 2018). Skin injuries are grouped below into two categories: epidermal stripping injuries and pressure injuries.

Epidermal Stripping Injuries

Epidermal stripping injuries are usually caused by adhesive removal (August et al., 2018; de Faria et al., 2019). The immature skin of infants born preterm has a weak dermal–epidermal junction until 34 weeks' gestation (Ness et al., 2013). Stripping injuries of fragile, thin preterm skin occur due to the stronger bond of the adhesive with the epidermis compared with the bond between the epidermis and dermis (Afsar, 2009; Behr et al., 2020; Lund, 2014; Ness et al., 2013). In addition to using adhesive remover products, diligent body positioning can protect stripping injuries after they occur by decreasing direct pressure to support circulation and healing (Behr et al., 2020).

Pressure Injuries

The National Pressure Ulcer Advisory Panel defined a pressure injury as "localized damage to the skin and underlying soft tissue usually over a bony prominence or related to a medical or other device" (August et al., 2018; Edsberg et al., 2016).

Pressure, friction, and sheer are primary causes of pressure injuries, but interactions among the three forces are poorly understood (August et al., 2018). Preterm infants are predisposed to pressure-based injuries from the presence of thin, fragile skin combined with decreased frequency of movement resulting in extended periods of pressure from bed surfaces and medical equipment (Behr et al., 2020; Hutchinson & Wayne, 2016; Ness et al., 2013; Razmus et al., 2008). Friction and sheer-based skin injury are common in infants with Neonatal Opiate Withdrawal or extreme agitation (Ness et al., 2013). Pressure injuries occur frequently in the NICU setting with reported incidences of 9.25% to 43.1% (August et al., 2018; Behr et al., 2020; Liversedge et al., 2018; Ness et al., 2013). Most frequent sites for pressure injuries are the occiput, nose, ears, neck, foot, and heel (Behr et al., 2020; Hutchinson & Wayne, 2016; Liversedge et al., 2018; Ness et al., 2013).

August et al. (2018) and de Faria et al. (2019) concluded that, in addition to treatment of existing skin injuries, prevention of skin injury for neonates is an essential part of neonatal care (August et al., 2018; de Faria et al., 2019). Consistent repositioning of the infant's body and medical equipment (such as noninvasive respiratory devices) paired with application of skin barriers is essential for prevention of pressure injuries (Behr et al., 2020; Ness et al., 2013). The 2014 International Pressure Ulcer Guidelines, supported by other NICU research, recommended change of body and mechanical device position every 2 hours for optimal pressure injury prevention (Behr et al., 2020; de Faria et al., 2019; Haesler et al., 2017; Ness et al., 2013; Yilmazer & Tuzer, 2019).

RESPIRATORY CONSIDERATIONS

Positioning is an important component in the care of infants born preterm with respiratory complications. Frequent and extended intermittent hypoxemic events correlate with later bronchopulmonary dysplasia and possible pulmonary dysfunction in adulthood (Fairchild et al., 2019; Poets et al., 2015; Raffay et al., 2019). Neonatal positioning should be individualized to accommodate the essential medical support equipment while adhering as closely as possible to body alignment and positioning principles. Infants with respiratory complications often seek positions of neck and trunk extension. Caregivers must respect the infant's respiratory needs by individualizing optimal neck and trunk flexion postures within the respiratory comfort and capabilities of each infant. Tolerance for optimal, neutral neck alignment and mild trunk flexion postures will increase as the infant's respiratory status begins to improve.

Historically, the prone position has been credited with short-term increase in oxygen saturation and thoracoabdominal synchrony as well as decreased hypoxemic episodes in infants born preterm (Oishi et al., 2018; Picheansathian et al., 2009). Recent systematic reviews and a meta-analysis show that evidence is insufficient to support any single position for prolonged respiratory benefits (Ballout et al., 2017; Rivas-Fernandez et al., 2016). Compared with supine position effects, short-term benefits for improved oxygenation and respiratory rate in the prone position were found for infants on noninvasive mechanical ventilation and also for infants diagnosed with respiratory distress syndrome (Ghorbani et al., 2013; Hough et al., 2012; Rivas-Fernandez et al., 2016). Examination of a group of infants born with very low birth weight (VLBW) and on noninvasive mechanical support also revealed increased oxygenation and stability in the prone position (Miller-Barmak et al., 2020). The quarter prone position has shown respiratory benefits similar to the prone position and superior to the supine position (Hough et al., 2012; Montgomery et al., 2014; Tane et al., 2019; Utario et al., 2017). Sufficient evidence was not found in a recent review for improved oxygenation during prone positioning of spontaneously breathing infants with significant apnea (Ballout et al., 2017). Conclusions for insufficiency of evidence in current reviews were based on small cohorts, participant heterogeneity, study design, and conflicting results among qualifying studies. Although positioning has not decreased apnea in spontaneously breathing infants, Oishi et al. (2018) found that near-term infants demonstrated fewer episodes of desaturation when positioned prone compared with supine and lateral positions.

A variety of positions (prone, quarter prone, right lateral, supine, and left lateral) may be used to assist infants with respiratory difficulties. Hough et al. (2016) found an effect of time on respiratory efficiency. Respiratory function improved with a change of position for infants on respiratory support following the common lung function peak at 2 hours (Hough et al., 2016). The prone position provided benefits of improved oxygenation and stability for all NICU infants on noninvasive mechanical respiratory support, particularly VLBW infants (Ghorbani et al., 2013; Miller-Barmak et al., 2020; Oishi et al., 2018; Rivas-Fernandez et al., 2016). Use of the prone position should be limited to NICU infants on cardiorespiratory monitoring unless the infant is awake and under direct supervision of a caregiver or NICU team member (Gillies et al., 2012; Picheansathian et al., 2009; Rivas-Fernandez et al., 2016).

GASTROINTESTINAL CONSIDERATIONS

Nutrition is essential for growth and development of infants in the NICU. Feeding intolerance can result in feeding schedule disruptions, low weight gain, abdominal discomfort, and prolonged hospitalization (Elser, 2012; Jadcherla et al., 2013). Due to immature anatomical and neurological development, difficulties resulting in gastrointestinal reflux and gastric residual are common in infants born preterm (Khatony et al., 2019). Therapeutic positioning is an accepted nonpharmacological approach to assist in the management of gastrointestinal symptoms and feeding intolerance.

Gastroesophageal Reflux

It is essential that healthcare providers consider the possible cause(s) of feeding intolerance in each infant and individualize positioning accordingly. Gastroesophageal reflux is defined as movement of gastric content into the esophagus, with or without vomiting (Imam et al., 2018). It is commonly diagnosed on the basis of clinical or behavioral signs. Some proposed causes of reflux and possible resulting aspiration include displacement of the lower esophageal sphincter to a position above the diaphragm, immature motor responses of the upper esophageal sphincter prior to 33 weeks' gestation, gastric distention, mechanical ventilation, immature swallow mechanism, and immature airway protective reflexes (Jadcherla et al., 2003; Omari et al., 2004; Schurr & Findlater, 2012).

Prone and left side positions after feeding are used to decrease the frequency and duration of gastroesophageal reflux episodes (Ewer et al., 1999). Although both the prone and left side positions are more effective than supine and right lateral positions in reducing reflux, supervised prone positioning remains the optimal antireflux position (Ewer et al., 1999). Infants no longer on continuous cardiorespiratory and oxygen saturation monitoring and not under immediate supervision by a parent or healthcare provider should not be left in a prone position according to Back to Sleep recommendations (Eichenwald, 2018; Picheansathian et al., 2009; Task force on Sudden Infant Death Syndrome, 2016).

Gastric Residual and Gastric Emptying

In contrast to the beneficial effects of left lateral positioning in infants with gastroesophageal reflux, left lateral positioning is the least advantageous position for gastric emptying (Khatony et al., 2019). Instead, significant gastric emptying documented in the right lateral body position makes it the recommended position post-feeding to reduce gastric residual (Khatony et al., 2019). Infants demonstrating both gastroesophageal reflux and gastric residual can be managed with either prone or right-side positioning with repositioning based on behavioral cues (Chen et al., 2013; Elser, 2012; Khatony et al., 2019; Yayan et al., 2018). The majority of gastric emptying has been shown to occur in the first half hour post-feeding (Chen et al., 2013). Chen et al. (2013) recommended placing infants prone for 30 minutes immediately after feeding then transitioning to another position according to the infant's behavioral cues.

Aspiration

Aspiration is a particular concern for ventilated infants with gastroesophageal reflux and a contributing factor to ventilator-associated pneumonia (Garland et al., 2014). Using pepsin levels found in tracheal aspirate as a marker for aspiration, researchers found reduced tracheal aspiration (pepsin levels) in supine, ventilated, low-birth-weight infants when positioned with 14 or greater degrees of head of bed elevation rather than flat (Garland et al., 2014). Head elevation for infants positioned in supine was considered effective in the early days of ventilation (Garland et al., 2014). The right lateral position was a preferred position for decreased tracheal aspirate over the supine position when compared in a flatbed position (Imam et al., 2018). Comparisons between head elevated prone and supine tracheal aspirate levels were not reported.

Supine Positioning With Elevation

Elevation of the head of the crib or supporting surface is often the initial approach recommended for infants in management of reflux and aspiration. The position taken by authors of current research, with policy support from the American Academy of Pediatrics (AAP), head elevation of cribs is *not* effective in decreasing reflux (American Academy of Pediatrics, 2008; Eichenwald, 2018; Moon, 2016; Task force on Sudden Infant Death Syndrome, 2016; Tobin et al., 1997). Other concerns included infants scooting or rolling to the bottom of the crib and ending in a position that accidentally compromised the airway (Eichenwald, 2018; Moon, 2016; Task force on Sudden Infant Death Syndrome, 2016; Tobin et al., 1997).

Further increased supine elevation by placing the infant in a car seat or infant seat is a favored position caregivers may use after feeding medically stable infants. Placement in a car seat or infant seat has been repeatedly shown to greatly increase symptoms of gastroesophageal reflux and is *not* recommended for infants in general (Eichenwald, 2018; Orenstein, 1990; Orenstein et al., 1983).

Research on the impact of head of bed elevation and supine semi-reclined positions exists only for older infants. General consensus affirms that results would be similar for infants born preterm (Eichenwald, 2018). Exceptions to effectiveness of head elevation have been demonstrated within the first few days of ventilation in VLBW infants for whom head elevation greater than 14° is promising for reduction of tracheal aspirate in any body position (Garland et al., 2014).

SLEEP AND COMFORT

The preservation of infant sleep is critical in NICU care (van den Hoogen et al., 2017). Immaturity of the central nervous system and discomfort result in difficulty with sleep–wake organization for infants born preterm (Bennet et al., 2018; Çakıcı & Mutlu, 2020). Development of sensory systems, brain plasticity, learning, long-term memory, growth hormone secretion, energy storage, feeding progression, and recovery from illness are all dependent on quality sleep–wake cycles for infants during NICU hospitalization (Bonan et al., 2015; Calciolari & Montirosso, 2011; Graven & Browne, 2008; Park et al., 2020). Although the literature is generally heterogenous in methodology and design, numerous authors concluded that prematurity was linked to later "sleep-related" disorders and neurodevelopmental differences (Bennet et al., 2018; Gogou et al., 2019; Stangenes et al., 2017). Bundled care, light restriction, and noise reduction are essential environmental interventions for improving the NICU sleep environment (Orsi et al., 2017; van den Hoogen et al., 2017). Skin-to-skin parental holding has also shown positive effects on the sleep–wake cycles of NICU infants (Bastani et al., 2017; Feldman & Eidelman, 2003; Ludington-Hoe et al., 2006). However, even in the most advantageous situations, infants in the NICU spend a substantial percentage of time (Gaultier, 1995) not being held by a parent or caregiver, and medical care often necessitates increased environmental stresses. Therapeutic positioning must be prioritized as a critical element of care to support the infant through periods of stress in lieu of and in addition to other supports in bundled care protocols (Lan et al., 2018; Valizadeh et al., 2016).

Sleep positioning of NICU infants is complex. Sleep–wake cycles are influenced by environmental factors, gestational age, illness, and medical equipment use (Collins et al., 2015; Park, 2020; van den Hoogen et al., 2017). Individualization and prioritization of medical and comfort needs must inform sleep positioning strategies for each infant (Çakıcı & Mutlu, 2020). Sleep position should support and modulate the body system(s) causing behavioral instability and discomfort. Careful observation of the frequency of arousals from sleep can help guide caregivers in individualizing selection of sleep comfort positions within the constraints of medical priorities (Modesto et al., 2016; Park, 2020).

Comfort

Body positioning was found to have a positive influence on the duration of sleep (Valizadeh et al., 2016). Compared with the "free body" position, facilitated tucking increased sleep time in both lateral and supine positions for hospitalized preterm infants. Furthermore, authors compared lateral with supine facilitated tuck positions and found that the mean duration of sleep was greater in the lateral tucked position than in the supine tucked position (Valizadeh et al., 2016). Similar results were found for more rapid acquisition of sleep state and increased sleep duration with better outcomes in the tucked prone position compared with tucked lateral and supine positions (Jarus et al., 2011; Peng et al., 2014; Tane et al., 2019; Çakıcı & Mutlu, 2020).

Factors contributing to increased comfort and sleep duration in a tucked body position vary. Reduced movement, increased energy efficiency, and strategic support for self-calming and self-regulation provided by a tucked body position may support improved sleep in preterm infants. The tucked position in prone was found to be most effective in enhanced sleep comfort and duration compared with lateral and supine tucked positions (Bhat et al., 2006; Cândia et al., 2014; Jarus et al., 2011; Lan et al., 2018; Peng et al., 2018; Tane et al., 2019; Valizadeh et al., 2016; Çakıcı & Mutlu, 2020).

Cardiorespiratory and Sleep

The effect of body position on body systems may vary between wake and sleep states. Oishi et al. (2018) examined this relationship for the respiratory and cardiac systems in near-term infants. Body position effects on oxygen saturation and stability were found to be similar between sleep and wake states; desaturations were less frequent in the prone position than in the lateral or supine position.

Differences between wake and sleep responses to body position were determined for the cardiac system (Oishi et al., 2018). In the awake state, bradycardia was observed more frequently when the infants were placed in a lateral position. During sleep, infants demonstrated bradycardia more frequently when positioned in supine. The prone position was concluded to be the most advantageous for decreasing bradycardia in both wake and sleep states (Oishi et al., 2018).

BACK TO SLEEP CONSIDERATIONS

The Back to Sleep campaign was adopted in the United States by the AAP in 1994 in an effort to reduce the incidence of sudden infant death (SIDs). Healthy infants were to be placed on the back or side position for sleep. The guidelines in 2000 indicated that the supine position was preferred over side lying and expanded the recommendations to include sleep on a flat, firm surface with no soft objects or loose bedding (American Academy of Pediatrics, 2000). By 2005, the recommendation indicated supine positioning as the only position that should be used for sleep. In the 2016 guideline, exemptions to supine sleeping were noted. Although infants diagnosed with gastroesophageal reflux disease (GERD) are generally included in supine sleep guidelines, sleep in positions other than supine may be considered if their risk of death from GERD exceeds the risk of death from SIDs (Task force on Sudden Infant Death Syndrome, 2016). Authors provided the following examples: "upper airway disorders in which airway-protective mechanisms are impaired, including infants with anatomic abnormalities, such as type 3 or 4 laryngeal clefts, who have not undergone anti-reflux surgery" (Task force on Sudden Infant Death Syndrome, 2016).

Initially the guidelines addressed infants in general with no specific directions for infants in the NICU. The guideline update of 2016 specifically addressed prematurely born infants as follows:

> Preterm infants should be placed supine as soon as possible. Preterm infants are at increased risk of SIDS, and the association between prone sleep position and SIDS among low birth weight and preterm infants is equal to, or perhaps even stronger than, the association among those born at term. The task force concurs with the AAP Committee on Fetus and Newborn that "preterm infants should be placed supine for sleeping, just as term infants should, and the parents of preterm infants should be counseled about the importance of supine sleeping in preventing SIDS. Hospitalized preterm infants should be kept predominantly in the supine position, at least from the postmenstrual age of 32 weeks onward, so that they become acclimated to supine sleeping before discharge.
>
> (American Academy of Pediatrics, 2008; Task force on Sudden Infant Death Syndrome, 2016, p. 3)

Healthcare providers are responsible for making individualized positioning decisions for young medically fragile infants in the NICU, balancing the infants' needs for supportive medical care, and positioning benefits with safety. Considerations for supine sleep positioning should be given to any medically stable, nonmonitored NICU infant, especially those of 32 weeks' postmenstrual age and onward. Emphasis on supine sleep practices and family education is essential in preparation for discharge home (American Academy of Pediatrics, 2008; Bredemeyer & Foster, 2012; Task force on Sudden Infant Death Syndrome,

2016). Please see Chapter 13 related to infant sleep for more details on how to support sleep in the high-risk infant.

SHORT- AND LONG-TERM NEUROBEHAVIORAL EFFECTS

Beyond immediate detrimental physiologic responses (Pados, 2019) to stress and pain experienced by infants while in the NICU, significant short-and long-term difficulties are documented in the literature for infants, children, and adults born preterm (Allin et al., 2011; Arpi & Ferrari, 2013; Barrero-Castillero et al., 2019; Casavant et al., 2019; Everts et al., 2019; Haraldsdottir et al., 2018; Johnson et al, 2010a, 2010b; Karvonen et al., 2019; Linsell et al., 2019; Moreira et al., 2014; Spittle & Orton, 2014; Sullivan et al., 2012; van Veen et al., 2017; Vollmer & Stalnacke, 2019; Winchester et al., 2018). Outcomes include altered brain development (Als et al., 2004; Brummelte et al., 2012; Lammertink et al., 2021; Rogers et al., 2017; Smith et al., 2011) and epigenetic changes (Barrero-Castillero et al., 2019; Casavant et al., 2019; Provenzi et al., 2015). Neurobehavioral outcomes in individuals born preterm include, but are not limited to, difficulties with self-regulation, attention, autism spectrum disorder, anxiety, and depression (Arpi & Ferrari, 2013; D'Agata et al., 2017; Johnson & Marlow, 2011; Rogers et al., 2017).

Positioning and Toxic Stress

Guided by the 2011 technical report of the AAP, a new understanding was established and emphasis placed on the important link between high levels of infant stress and potentially compromised child/adult health outcomes (Shonkoff et al., 2012). Authors of the AAP report described three levels of stress: positive stress, tolerable stress, and toxic stress (Shonkoff et al., 2012). The three stress levels differ in frequency, intensity, and duration of stress (Shonkoff et al., 2012; Weber & Harrison, 2019). Positive stress, and sometimes tolerable stress, can be beneficial when facing common life adversities (Shonkoff et al., 2012; Weber & Harrison, 2019). Toxic stress is characterized by frequent, often intense stress occurring over an extended period of time (Shonkoff et al., 2012). Increased risk of long-term harm is linked to toxic stress due to dysregulation across body systems (Casavant et al., 2019; Sanders & Hall, 2018; Shonkoff et al., 2012; Weber & Harrison, 2019). The NICU hospitalization and medical treatment needed to support infants born preterm are often associated with frequent, intense, and chronic stress (Cong et al., 2017). Common NICU-associated stressors include extended separation from parents, altered infant–parent bonding, light, noise, and stressful or painful procedures (Barrero-Castillero et al., 2019; Bergman et al., 2015; Casavant et al., 2019; Cruz et al., 2016; Shah et al., 2016; Weber & Harrison, 2019). Gomes et al. (2019) stated that inadequate positioning stresses the infant's immature autonomic nervous system (Gomes et al., 2019). Consequently, body malalignment and inadequate postural support must now be recognized as a factor contributing to toxic stress in the NICU. The complexity and multifaceted nature of stressors associated with NICU hospitalization have been the basis for toxic stress identified as medical trauma or IMTN (Infant Medical Trauma in the Neonatal Intensive Care Unit) (D'Agata et al., 2016; D'Agata et al., 2017).

Toxic stress must be addressed using a combination of reducing and buffering approaches in neonatal practice. Buffering of toxic stress is attributed to the presence of strong supportive relationships (Shonkoff et al., 2012), primarily between the infants and parents (Sanders & Hall, 2018). In the absence of continuous parental presence, nurses and other healthcare professionals may be the closest supportive relationships available to infants in the NICU (Weber & Harrison, 2019). The needs for consistent caregiving staff, gentle human touch, four-handed care, and individualized positioning are essential (Altimier & Phillips, 2016; Weber & Harrison, 2019; Wiley et al., 2020). Within the void between parent or caregiver interactions and after painful or stressful procedures, the infants must rely on their own resiliency. Inherent resiliency varies among infants and depends on factors such as the infant's genetic profile, gestational age at birth, and degree of illness (D'Agata et al., 2016). Diligent, individualized, and appropriate positioning supports the infant for self-regulation and self-calming (Altimier & Phillips, 2016; Eskandari et al., 2020; Grenier et al., 2003; Santos et al., 2017), thus improving opportunities for the infant to practice activities that may build resiliency. Gomes et al. (2019) observed reduced stress behaviors during appropriate positioning and with increased parasympathetic activity and heart rate variability indicating improved function of the infant's autonomic nervous system (Gomes et al., 2019). Reduced stress during painful procedures (heel stick) was also documented when infants were positioned in a nested prone position (Kahraman et al., 2018).

Less stress related to consistent, individualized positioning appears to reduce the overall toxic stress load allowing preterm infants the opportunity to build resiliency over time. The large number of studies showing a positive impact of positioning on body systems, comfort, and self-regulation in infants born preterm clearly demonstrates the essential role of consistent positioning in NICU care and stress reduction for preterm infants.

HUMAN TOUCH

The sense of touch reportedly develops as early as 8 to 14 weeks in fetal development (Anand et al., 2007). In addition to touch from the walls of the uterus, the fetus was observed (ultrasound imaging) to self-touch the face by 13 weeks' gestation (de Vries et al., 1985). This earliest sensory perception capability is a key path for evolving infant–caregiver communication of discomfort and calming.

Touch is an integral part of all caregiving and medical procedures. In addition to communication with the infant, the dosage of touch (duration, intensity, location) has varied effects on physiological and behavioral stability. Individualized combinations of touch to the head and chest, head and under feet, or hand and mouth (pacifier) areas are advised when infants are awake or in a distressed state, not when sleeping (Harrison et al., 2000; Harrison & Brown, 2017; Modrcin-Talbott et al., 2003; Smith, 2012). Gentle touch without stroking helps stabilize infant behavior and prevents tactile overstimulation and state disorganization. A form of gentle touch known as "facilitated tucking" provides a swaddling effect from the caregiver's hands around the infant's body. Hartley et al. (2015) presented a facilitated tucking protocol and reviewed emerging evidence of positive nonpharmacological pain management through gentle touch and facilitated tucking during aversive procedures. In addition, four-handed care (two providers) offers stabilizing gentle touch for fragile infants during medical procedures (Cone et al., 2013) and with repositioning fragile infants on mechanical ventilation.

The steady touch of skin-to-skin contact of infants held at parent's chests can create an optimal experience for communication, calming, infant sleep cycling, and attachment for both infant and parent (Feldman & Eidelman, 2003; Feldman et al., 2002; Ludington-Hoe et al., 2006). When parents are available, this skin-to-skin holding is emerging as a preferred touch and positioning approach for stabilizing infants during heel lances, gavage feeding, and procedural pain (Johnston et al., 2017). Individualized holding, positioning, and handling methods can modulate inadvertent tactile and kinesthetic overstimulation of vulnerable infants. A traditional care procedure in many cultures, infant swaddling is also used effectively in assisting behavioral regulation of infants with opiate withdrawal and procedural pain (Zeller & Giebe, 2014). Body overheating and inadvertent extremity malalignment may occur during swaddling from excessive tightness of the wrap causing restricted leg movement and decreased hand to mouth engagement (Fletcher et al., 2018). Attention to providing space for leg movement (hip flexion and abduction) is critical for decreasing hip dysplasia risk and for modeling "hip-healthy swaddling" for parents (Shaw et al., 2016). Elasticity in wrapping and positioning materials may provide dynamic resistance for limb movement or inadvertently contribute to limitation of spontaneous movement and hip abduction when fastened or secured with excessive stretch. Strategies for varied infant positioning procedures are detailed with photos, body alignment analyses, and instruction in a manual by Fern (2011) and described in the neonatal nursing literature (Drake, 2017; Gardner & Goldson, 2021; Sweeney & Gutierrez, 2002). The key to success in implementing effective body positioning is collaboration among the NICU interdisciplinary team and parents and guided by each infant's alignment and comfort. Neonatal positioning resources are outlined in Table 14-4. Clinical competencies for neonatal touch are described with evidence-based practice recommendations in Table 14-3.

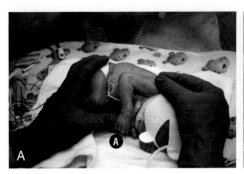
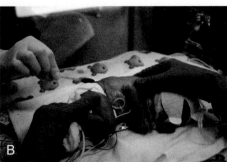

FIGURE 14-2. A and B. Tucked position for lumbar puncture **A.** Containment is provided by facilitated tuck procedure for midline alignment of extremities and head. Eyes are protected with phototherapy mask. Infant's relaxed hand is wrapped about caregiver's thumb. **B.** Four-handed care during lumbar puncture.

TOUCH AND POSITIONAL SUPPORT DURING MEDICAL PROCEDURES

Postural alignment and behavioral support for medical procedures require strategic actions before, during, and after the procedure. Parent(s) should be given the option to participate in positional and calming support with medical procedures if they are comfortable and medical complexity allows. Before the procedure, plans may include documenting baseline physiological and behavioral status, gathering positional support materials, and determining nonpharmacologic (pacifier, swaddling, sucrose, facilitated tucking, skin-to-skin holding) and pharmacologic needs. During the procedure, moving and stabilizing the infant into a supported position may be optimized by two team members (four-handed care) with one handling the positional, behavioral, and physiological stability management (Figure 14-2). After the procedure, the priority is the transition into a calm, comfortable recovery position and environment with return to the physiological baseline.

Medical procedures are critical in neonatal intensive care and may be urgent. They can be stressful, painful, and physiologically destabilizing. Postural alignment and behavioral support may play an important role in contributing to the effectiveness of the medical procedure by modulating infant stress, decreasing pharmacologic support, and promoting caregiver efficiency for a shorter procedure time. Continual developmental awareness and individualized care practices balance the often invasive medical support.

NEONATAL POSITIONING STANDARDS AND COMPETENCIES

Neonatal positioning standards and competencies are based on a practice framework of infant and family-centered developmental care. This framework, implementation process, evaluation models, and NICU system organizational complexity are presented in the following sections.

Framework

Practice frameworks of standards and competencies provide guidance for teaching, guiding, and evaluating professional practice. Developmental care standards and competencies for NICU settings were designed and recently reported by an interdisciplinary panel on Infant and Family-Centered Developmental Care (Consensus Committee of the Standards, 2019). The panel members were selected by their respective national professional organizations in the United States and represented the multiple disciplines on neonatal care teams. An interdisciplinary consensus process was used among the expert panel and nationally recognized content experts from each discipline and international consultants provided external review. The evidence-based neonatal touch and positioning standards and competencies were developed and reviewed by neonatal physical therapists (Sweeney & McElroy, 2019). Refer to Tables 14-2 and 14-3 for summarized neonatal positioning competencies or neonatal touch competencies.

Implementation

The positioning and touch standards and competencies are intended for implementation in varied NICU practice procedures. They may guide orientation and skills training of trainees and new professionals to the NICU team in the areas of evidence-based postural alignment for infants with respiratory or gastrointestinal conditions. Prevention of extremity malalignment, torticollis, or positional skull deformity can be targeted and guided by the practice recommendations. Performance assessment of NICU team members should include interval competency evaluations of positioning and touch procedures with follow-up teaching to maintain consistency in clinical practice.

Family teaching may be enhanced by the care principles embedded in the positioning and touch competencies. Learning to interpret behavioral signs of comfort or stress and to adjust infant body alignment for calming enhances parent confidence and communication with the baby. Parent satisfaction surveys can indicate if they were taught and guided to

TABLE 14-2 Neonatal Positioning Competencies, Practice Recommendations, and Level of Evidence

Clinical Competency	Practice Recommendations	Evidence Level	References
Administer and monitor duration of infant position	***General*** • Change infant position every 3–4 hours rotating	Level II	Vaivre-Douret et al. (2004)
	Skin Injuries • Change infant position and medical equipment every 2 hours	Level I Level III Level VII Level I	Behr et al. (2020) de Faria et al. (2019) Haesler et al. (2017) Ness et al. (2013)
	IVH Precaution • Use minimal handling and maintain head in midline and elevated 15°–30° during position changes within the first 72 hours • Clinically, many NICUs limit routine care episodes to every 6 hours during this time period	Level I Level I	Romantsik et al. (2017) Wilson et al. (2020)
Positioning Competency 1			
Individualize body position with monitoring of head, trunk, and extremity alignment and spontaneous movement	***Supine*** • Align head and trunk in neutral (not flexed or extended) position with semiflexed extremity posture and use of nested containment with positioning materials	Level III Level III Level II Level II Level II Level II	Eskandari et al. (2020) Ferrari et al. (2007) Madlinger-Lewis et al. (2014) Vaivre-Douret et al. (2004) Valizadeh et al. (2016) Zahed et al. (2015)
	• Place head in midline position in supine and side lying to minimize potential risk of germinal matrix-intraventricular hemorrhage during the first 3 days after birth in babies born at or less than 32 weeks of gestation • Provide space within the positional support materials or aids to promote and not restrict spontaneous extremity movement	Level I Level I	Romantsik et al. (2017) Romantsik et al. (2020)
	• Prior to discharge, transition medically stable babies previously positioned therapeutically in varied sleep positions to the supine position on a flat, firm bed surface without positioning aids or loose bedding materials	Level I Level VII Level I	Brodomoyor and Foster (2012) Picheansathian et al. (2009) Task force on Sudden Infant Death Syndrome (2016)
	Prone • Use continuous cardiorespiratory and oxygen saturation monitoring for preterm babies positioned in prone	Level I Level I Level III	Gillies et al. (2012) Gomes et al. (2019) Picheansathian et al. (2009)
	• Place a vertical positioning roll (from clavicle to pubis) to facilitate extremity flexion in the prone position	Level IV Level I	Monterosso et al. (2003) Picheansathian et al. (2009)
	• Move mechanically ventilated preterm babies with judicious handling to prone to improve oxygenation	Level I	Rivas-Fernandez et al. (2016)
	Side • Use side-lying position on an individualized basis for spontaneously breathing preterm babies	Level I	Ballout et al. (2017)

(Continued)

TABLE 14-2 Neonatal Positioning Competencies, Practice Recommendations, and Level of Evidence (Continued)

Clinical Competency	Practice Recommendations	Evidence Level	References
	Swaddling • Provide optimal body alignment within a swaddling blanket by placing hands toward the mouth or face, moving legs into a semiflexed, abducted position, and keeping neck and trunk alignment neutral without flexion or extension	Level I	van Sleuwen et al. (2007)
	• Create space for spontaneous kicking inside the swaddled containment to reduce the risk of hip dysplasia from excessive hip adduction and extension posture	Level VII	Shaw et al. (2016)
	• Apply swaddling during weighing, bathing, and heel lance to modulate physiological and behavioral stress during routine care	Level III Level II Level I Level III	Bembich et al. (2017) Edraki et al. (2014) Freitas et al. (2014) Neu and Browne (1997)
	• Use swaddling as a nonpharmaco-logical comfort strategy for babies with behavioral irritability or opiate withdrawal symptoms	Level I Level II Level V	Huang et al. (2004) Ryan et al. (2019) van Sleuwen et al. (2007)
Positioning Competency 2 Assess, implement, document, and monitor cranial shape and neck alignment to prevent positional skull deformity and muscular torticollis	• Promote cranial shaping and prevent muscular torticollis by frequent variation of head positions (lateral and midline) and repositioning the crib for head turn variation within the assigned bed space	Level IV Level IV Level III Level IV	Ifflaender et al. (2013) McCarty et al. (2016) McCarty et al. (2018) Nuysink et al. (2013)
	• Refer to Neonatal Physical Therapy inpatient examination for infants demonstrating asymmetrical head position preference and skull deformation	Level IV	Nuysink et al. (2013)
	• Coordinate outpatient infant physical therapy referral during discharge planning for infant reassessment and family teaching if skull asymmetry or neck asymmetry remains at discharge	Level I Level II	Klimo et al. (2016) van Vlimmeren et al. (2008)
Positioning Competency 3 Individualize positioning for infants with gastroesophageal reflux or gastric residual	• After feeding, place babies with gastroesophageal reflux in *prone* (optimal) or on the *left* side	Level II	Ewer et al. (1999)
	• After feeding, position babies with gastric residual in *prone* or on the *right* side	Level III Level II	Chen et al. (2013) Sangers et al. (2013)
	• Right side lying position to decrease aspiration of gastric residual	Level II	Imam et al. (2018)
	• Provide bed elevation (14°–15°) to reduce tracheal aspirate in ventilated babies	Level IV Level VII Level II	Chen et al., 2013 Elser, 2012 Garland et al., 2014

TABLE 14-3 Neonatal Touch Competencies, Practice Recommendations, and Level of Evidence

Competency	Practice Recommendations	Evidence Level	References
Competency 1 Implement parent participation in supporting infants during selected stressful caregiving procedures	• Invite and guide parents to participate with the primary caregiver and provide infant support during potentially stressful caregiving and medical procedures	Level I Level III	Balice-Bourgois et al. (2020) Hartley et al. (2015)
Competency 2 Organize personnel staffing for intermittent procedural assistance in providing touch and comfort during complex procedures	• When parents are unavailable, a second caregiver should provide touch and positional support during stressful procedures	Level III	Cone et al. (2013)
	• Advocate for and organize staffing options to support infant behavioral stability and comfort during medical procedures or stressful caregiving activities	Level I Level I Level III Level III Level III	Alinejad-Naeini et al. (2014) Cone et al. (2013) Hartley et al. (2015) Herrington and Chiodo. (2014) Pillai Riddell et al. (2011)
Competency 3 Apply individualized gentle touch to support behavioral stability and prevent sensory overstimulation	• Provide individualized gentle touch when the baby is in an awakened or distressed state, rather than during quiet sleeping • Create a steady touch without stroking on the head, chest, back, or under the feet	Level I Level VII	Byrne and Garber (2013) Smith (2012)
Competency 4 Evaluate the baby's responses to the touch interaction	• Determine the timing and amount of gentle touch by evaluating the baby's behavioral and physiological parameters before, during, and after the touch interaction • Avoid overstimulation by diligent observation of behavioral cues of stress and fatigue	Level I	Smith (2012)
Competency 5 Assess and monitor physiological and behavioral tolerance and modify or stop during touch interventions for babies with low gestational age and high acuity	• Use supplemental gentle touch judiciously with diligent monitoring for babies with low gestational age and high acuity to ensure stability and avoid behavioral agitation, oxygen desaturation, and bradycardia	Level II	Harrison et al. (2000)
Competency 6 Apply stabilizing hand support and slow movement transitions for infants with fragile bones or respiratory equipment	• Demonstrate stabilizing hand support and slow movement transitions during routine caregiving tasks for infants with fragile bones, infusion lines and tubes, and ventilator or respiratory equipment	Level VII	Altimier and Phillips (2016)

effectively increase infant comfort and thereby help the babies manage stress.

NICU Organizational System

The NICU is a complex organizational system in continual adaptation to changes in patient care, staffing, technology, and environment factors and stressors. The effectiveness of programs for individualized touch, body alignment, and postural care depends on NICU culture and system support for focused teaching, positioning equipment access, staffing adequacy, team dynamics and communication, and family inclusion. The dynamic nature of the NICU system can either create opportunities for clinical problem solving or provide organizational obstacles to implementing therapeutic positioning and touch interventions. To minimize variability and promote consistency in neonatal positioning among practitioners, the need emerged to create and implement body positioning evaluation processes within the NICU system.

Neonatal Positioning Evaluation Models

Coughlin designed a clinical model, the Infant Positioning Assessment Tool (IPAT), to guide neonatal team members in learning and evaluating appropriate supine position alignment of six specific body regions. A scoring system for each body region distinguished between ideal, acceptable, or unacceptable alignment (Coughlin, 2017b; Infant Positioning Assessment Tool (IPAT), 2018). Coughlin et al. (2010) later reported reliability and effectiveness of applying

the IPAT during neonatal nursing care practices (Coughlin et al., 2010). Coughlin's IPAT model has been implemented internationally to guide infant alignment and postural care in NICUs in Lebanon, India, Netherlands, and Egypt (Abusaad et al., 2017; Charafeddine et al., 2018; Diertens & Wielenga, 2018; Upadhyay et al., 2021).

The Neonatal Postural Assessment Worksheet (neoPAW) (Coughlin, 2017a) is a corollary to the IPAT and was expanded by neonatal researchers in the Netherlands. This postural assessment tool offered two additional items on scapular and trunk alignment, included prone and side positions, and displayed infant photos for eight body regions. A similar scoring system was maintained in the IPAT and neoPAW assessments. Feasibility for use of the neoPAW with infants in incubators on respiratory equipment was demonstrated in 30 infants (median age 34 weeks post conception at testing) in the Netherlands with head alignment and hand position showing lower scores (less optimal alignment) than other body regions (Diertens & Wielenga, 2018).

A mobile application was designed to support learning of neonatal postural alignment in NICU settings. The neoPAL BASIC (Caring Essentials Collaborative, LLC) (Coughlin, 2017a; Table 14-4) application was created as a contemporary teaching tool for competency-based positioning practices and quality improvement initiatives. Neonatal nurses and therapists may find this mobile application to be a useful resource for enhancing learning in neonatal positioning and also in addressing other care priorities (e.g., discharge teaching topics) in the future.

TABLE 14-4 Positioning Equipment Resources

Category	Product	Corporate Address
Body containment	Snuggle Up Dandle Wrap Dandle Roo	www.philips.com/mothersandchild.com www.dandlelionmedical.com
Positioning roll	Fluidized rolls (Z flo) Bendy Bumper Cozy Cub	www.molnlycke.us/products-solutions-z-flo-fluidized-positioner-neonatal www.philips.com/othersandchild.com www.dandlelionmedical.com
Cushion, mattress, pillow	Fluidized mats (Z flo) Gel pillow (Gel-E-Donut) Prone Plus Squishon Mattress	www.molnlycke.us/products-solutions-z-flo-fluidized-positioner-neonatal www.philips.com/mothersandchild.com www.philips.com/mothersandchild.com www.philips.com/mothersandchild.com
Head alignment device	Crown Cradle Tortle Midliner Head Positioner	www.dandlelionmedical.com www.tortle.com/medical/cranial-asymmetry
Swaddling garment	Dandle Wrap Stretch Baby Sleep Sacks Cotton Muslin Swaddle Blankets	www.dandlelionmedical.com www.halosleep.com www.swaddledesigns.com
Tub bathing system	Turtle Tub Dandle LION Bathing System	www.catapult-products.com www.dandlelionmedical.com
Positioning assessment and training tools	neoPAL–Neonatal basic training app Triangle Factory neoPAL BASIC by Caring Essentials Collaborative, LLC	https://www.triangle-factory.be/portfolio/neopal https://appadvice.com/app/neopal-basic/ 1029603403

CONCLUSION

Body positioning and touch are therapeutic for neonates only when they are applied within a synchronous communication with the baby and adapted in each care episode to meet physiological and behavioral needs. The NICU setting and medical equipment provide many challenges to creating optimal neonatal biomechanical alignment and comfort, but they also offer numerous opportunities for modeling varied strategies for parents to communicate with their infant by individualized position and touch. These positive caregiving interactions contribute to stress reduction in both infants and parents in the NICU and can influence communication and behavioral dynamics throughout infancy and beyond.

Using current research evidence to update clinical competencies and practice is an ongoing, essential process. Our future practice decisions and innovations must be guided by continued investigation on effectiveness of current and future neonatal positioning procedures and equipment and by focused quality improvement studies on positioning practices.

Potential Research Questions

1. What are the psychometric properties of reliability and validity in neonatal positioning assessment tools?
2. What critical gestational age periods present the highest risk for development of positional skull deformity by infants in the NICU?
3. What are the parents' view of (1) most effective techniques learned for calming and comforting their infants and (2) caregiving procedures involving moving the baby's body they found most difficult?
4. What differences occur in preterm infant skin integrity, behavioral stability, sleep cycles, and physiological effects among "containment nesting" positioning systems?
5. What spontaneous movements occur in infants positioned in containment nests at varied gestational periods?

ACKNOWLEDGMENT

We appreciate the support of Jan Hunter MA, OTR and Dana Fern OTR/L for contribution of infant photos.

REFERENCES

Abusaad, F., El Aziz, R., & Nasef, N. (2017). The effectiveness of developmentally supportive positioning on preterm infants' pain response at neonatal intensive care units. *American Journal of Nursing Science, 6*(1), 63–71. https://doi.org/10.11648/j.ajns.20170601.18

Afsar, F. S. (2009). Skin care for preterm and term neonates. *Clinical and Experimental Dermatology, 34*(8), 855–858. https://doi.org/10.1111/j.1365-2230.2009.03424.x

Albahrani, Y., & Hunt, R. (2019). Newborn skin care. *Pediatric Annals, 48*(1), e11–e15. https://doi.org/10.3928/19382359-20181211-01

Alinejad-Naeini, M., Mohagheghi, P., Peyrovi, H., & Mehran, A. (2014). The effect of facilitated tucking during endotracheal suctioning on procedural pain in preterm neonates: A randomized controlled crossover study. *Global Journal of Health Science, 6*(4), 278–284. https://doi.org/10.5539/gjhs.v6n4p278

Allin, M. P., Kontis, D., Walshe, M., Wyatt, J., Barker, G. J., Kanaan, R. A., McGuire, P., Rifkin, L., Murray, R. M., & Nosarti, C. (2011). White matter and cognition in adults who were born preterm [Research Support, Non-U.S. Gov't]. *PLoS One, 6*(10), e24525. https://doi.org/10.1371/journal.pone.0024525

Als, H., Duffy, F. H., McAnulty, G. B., Rivkin, M. J., Vajapeyam, S., Mulkern, R. V., Warfield, S. K., Huppi, P. S., Butler, S. C., Conneman, N., Fischer, C., & Eichenwald, E. C. (2004). Early experience alters brain function and structure. *Pediatrics, 113*(4), 846–857. http://www.ncbi.nlm.nih.gov/entrez/query.fcgi?cmd=Retrieve&db=PubMed&dopt=Citation&list_uids=15060237; https://pediatrics.aappublications.org/content/113/4/846

Altimier, L., & Phillips, R. (2016). The neonatal integrative developmental care model: Advanced clinical applications of the seven core measures for neuroprotective family-centered developmental care. *Newborn and Infant Nursing Reviews, 16*(4), 230–244. https://doi.org/10.1053/j.nainr.2016.09.030

American Academy of Pediatrics. (2000) Changing Concepts of sudden infant death syndrome: Implications for infant sleeping environment and sleep position. *Pediatrics, 105*(3), 650–656. https://doi.org/10.1542/peds.105.3.650

American Academy of Pediatrics. (2008). Hospital discharge of the high-risk neonate. *Pediatrics, 122*(5), 1119–1126. https://doi.org/10.1542/peds.2008-2174

Anand, K., Stevens, B., & McGrath, P. (2007). *Pain in neonates and infants* (3rd ed.). Elsevier.

Arpi, E., & Ferrari, F. (2013). Preterm birth and behaviour problems in infants and preschool-age children: A review of the recent literature. *Developmental Medicine & Child Neurology, 55*(9), 788–796. https://doi.org/10.1111/dmcn.12142

August, D., New, K., Ray, R., & Kandasamy, Y. (2018). Frequency, location and risk factors of neonatal skin injuries from mechanical forces of pressure, friction, shear, and stripping: A systematic literature review. *Journal of Neonatal Nursing, 24*, 173–180. http://dx.doi.org/10.1016/j.jnn.2017.08.003

Balice-Bourgois, C., Zumstein-Shaha, M., Simonetti, G. D., & Newman, C. J. (2020). Interprofessional collaboration and involvement of parents in the management of painful procedures in newborns. *Frontiers in Pediatrics, 8*, 394. https://doi.org/10.3389/fped.2020.00394

Ballout, R. A., Foster, J. P., Kahale, L. A., & Badr, L. (2017). Body positioning for spontaneously breathing preterm infants with apnoea. *Cochrane Database Systematic Reviews, 1*, Cd004951. https://doi.org/10.1002/14651858.CD004951.pub3

Barrero-Castillero, A., Morton, S. U., Nelson, C. A., III, & Smith, V. C. (2019). Psychosocial stress and adversity: Effects from the perinatal period to adulthood. *NeoReviews, 20*(12), e686–e696. https://doi.org/10.1542/neo.20-12-e686

Bastani, F., Rajai, N., Farsi, Z., & Als, H. (2017). The effects of kangaroo care on the sleep and wake states of preterm infants. *Journal of Nursing Research, 25*(3), 231–239. https://doi.org/10.1097/jnr.0000000000000194

Behr, J. H., Wardell, D., Rozmus, C. L., & Casarez, R. L. (2020). Prevention strategies for neonatal skin injury in the NICU. *Neonatal Network, 39*(6), 321–329. https://doi.org/10.1891/0730-0832/11-t-623

Bembich, S., Fiani, G., Strajn, T., Sanesi, C., Demarini, S., & Sanson, G. (2017). Longitudinal responses to weighing and bathing procedures in preterm infants. *Journal of Perinatal & Neonatal Nursing, 31*(1), 67–74. https://doi.org/10.1097/JPN.0000000000000228

Bennet, L., Walker, D. W., & Horne, R. S. C. (2018). Waking up too early- the consequences of preterm birth on sleep development. *Journal of Physiology, 596*(23), 5687–5708. https://doi.org/10.1113/JP274950

Bergman, K. S., Beekmans, V., & Stromswold, J. (2015). Considerations for neuroprotection in the traumatic brain injury population. *Critical Care Nursing Clinics of North America, 27*(2), 225–233. https://doi.org/10.1016/j.cnc.2015.02.009

Bhat, R. Y., Hannam, S., Pressler, R., Rafferty, G. F., Peacock, J. L., & Greenough, A. (2006). Effect of prone and supine position on sleep, apneas, and arousal in preterm infants. *Pediatrics, 118*(1), 101–107. https://doi.org/10.1542/peds.2005-1873

Bonan, K. C., Pimentel Filho Jda, C., Tristao, R. M., Jesus, J. A., & Campos Junior, D. (2015). Sleep deprivation, pain and prematurity: A review study. *Arquivos de Neuro-Psiquiatria, 73*(2), 147–154. https://doi.org/10.1590/0004-282X20140214

Bredemeyer, S. L., & Foster, J. P. (2012). Body positioning for spontaneously breathing preterm infants with apnoea [Meta-Analysis Research Support, N.I.H., Extramural Research Support, Non-U.S. Gov't Review]. *Cochrane Database Systematic Reviews, 6*, CD004951. https://doi.org/10.1002/14651858.CD004951.pub2

Brummelte, S., Grunau, R. E., Chau, V., Poskitt, K. J., Brant, R., Vinall, J., Gover, A., Synnes, A. R., & Miller, S. P. (2012). Procedural pain and brain development in premature newborns. *Annals of Neurology, 71*(3), 385–396. https://doi.org/10.1002/ana.22267

Byrne, E., & Garber, J. (2013). Physical therapy intervention in the neonatal intensive care unit. *Physical & Occupational Therapy in Pediatrics, 33*(1), 75–110. https://doi.org/10.3109/01942638.2012.750870

Çakıcı, M., & Mutlu, B. (2020). Effect of body position on cardiorespiratory stabilization and comfort in preterm infants on continuous positive airway pressure. *Journal of Pediatric Nursing, 54*, e1–e8. https://doi.org/10.1016/j.pedn.2020.06.015

Calciolari, G., & Montirosso, R. (2011). The sleep protection in the preterm infants. *The Journal of Maternal-Fetal & Neonatal Medicine, 24*(Suppl. 1), 12–14. https://doi.org/10.3109/14767058.2011.607563

Cândia, M. F., Osaku, E. F., Leite, M. A., Toccolini, B., Costa, N. L., Teixeira, S. N., Costa, C. R., Piana, P. A., Cristovam, M. A., & Osaku, N. O. (2014). Influence of prone positioning on premature newborn infant stress assessed by means of salivary cortisol measurement: Pilot study. *Revista Brasileira de Terapia Intensiva, 26*(2), 169–175. https://doi.org/10.5935/0103-507x.20140025

Casavant, S. G., Bernier, K., Andrews, S., & Bourgoin, A. (2017). Noise in the neonatal intensive care unit: What does the evidence tell us? *Advances in Neonatal Care, 17*(4), 265–273. https://doi.org/10.1097/ANC.0000000000000402

Casavant, S. G., Cong, X., Moore, J., & Starkweather, A. (2019). Associations between preterm infant stress, epigenetic alteration, telomere length and neurodevelopmental outcomes: A systematic review. *Early Human Development, 131*, 63–74. https://doi.org/10.1016/j.earlhumdev.2019.03.003

Charafeddine, L., Masri, S., Ibrahim, P., Badin, D., Cheayto, S., & Tamim, H. (2018). Targeted educational program improves infant positioning practice in the NICU. *International Journal for Quality in Health Care, 30*(8), 642–648. https://doi.org/10.1093/intqhc/mzy123

Chen, S. S., Tzeng, Y. L., Gau, B. S., Kuo, P. C., & Chen, J. Y. (2013). Effects of prone and supine positioning on gastric residuals in preterm infants: A

time series with cross-over study. *International Journal of Nursing Studies, 50*(11), 1459–1467. https://doi.org/10.1016/j.ijnurstu.2013.02.009

Collins, C. L., Barfield, C., Davis, P. G., & Horne, R. S. (2015). Randomized controlled trial to compare sleep and wake in preterm infants less than 32 weeks of gestation receiving two different modes of non-invasive respiratory support. *Early Human Development, 91*(12), 701–704. https://doi.org/10.1016/j.earlhumdev.2015.09.011

Cone, S., Pickler, R. H., Grap, M. J., McGrath, J., & Wiley, P. M. (2013). Endotracheal suctioning in preterm infants using four-handed versus routine care. *Journal of Obstetric, Gynecologic & Neonatal Nursing, 42*(1), 92–104. https://doi.org/10.1111/1552-6909.12004

Cong, X., Wu, J., Vittner, D., Xu, W., Hussain, N., Galvin, S., Fitzsimons, M., McGrath, J. M., & Henderson, W. A. (2017). The impact of cumulative pain/stress on neurobehavioral development of preterm infants in the NICU. *Early Human Development, 108*, 9–16. https://doi.org/10.1016/j.earlhumdev.2017.03.003

Consensus Committee of the Standards, Competencies, and Best Practices for Infant and Family-Centered Developmental Care in the Intensive Care Unit. (2019). *Developmental care standards for infants in intensive care* https://nicudesign.nd.edu/nicu-care-standards/

Coughlin, M., Gibbins, S., & Hoath, S. (2009). Core measures for developmentally supportive care in neonatal intensive care units: Theory, precedence and practice. *Journal of Advances in Nursing, 65*(10), 2239–2248. https://doi.org/10.1111/j.1365-2648.2009.05052.x

Coughlin, M., Lohman, M., & Gibbons, S. (2010). Reliability and effectiveness of an Infant Positioning Assessment Tool to standardize developmentally supportive positioning practices in the neonatal intensive care unit. *Newborn and Infant Nursing Reviews, 10*, 104–106.

Coughlin, M. (2017a). *Trauma-Informed Care in the NICU: Evidence-based practice guidelines for neonatal clinicians.* Springer Publishing.

Coughlin, M. (2017b). *Transformative nursing in the NICU: Evidence-based practice guidelines for neonatal clinicians.* Springer Publishing.

Cruz, M. D., Fernandes, A. M., & Oliveira, C. R. (2016). Epidemiology of painful procedures performed in neonates: A systematic review of observational studies. *European Journal of Pain, 20*(4), 489–498. https://doi.org/10.1002/ejp.757

D'Agata, A., Young, E, Cong, X, Grasso, D, McGrath, J. (2016). Infant medical trauma in the neonatal intensive care unit (IMTN): A proposed concept for science and practice. *Advance in Neonatal Care, 16*(4), 289–297. https://doi.org/10.1097/ANC.0000000000000309

D'Agata, A. L., Sanders, M. R., Grasso, D. J., Young, E. E., Cong, X., & McGrath, J. M. (2017). Unpacking the burden of care for infants in the NICU. *Infant Mental Health Journal, 38*(2), 306–317. https://doi.org/10.1002/imhj.21636

de Faria, M. F., Ferreira, M. B. G., Felix, M., Calegari, I. B., & Barbosa, M. H. (2019). Factors associated with skin and mucosal lesions caused by medical devices in newborns: Observational study. *Journal of Clinical Nursing, 28*(21–22), 3807–3816. https://doi.org/10.1111/jocn.14998

de Vries, J. I. P., Visser, G. H. A., & Prechtl, H. F. R. (1985). The emergence of fetal behaviour. II. Quantitative aspects. *Early Human Development, 12*(2), 99–120. https://doi.org/10.1016/0378-3782(85)90174-4

Diertens, D., & Wielenga, J. (2018). Developmentally accurate body posture of newborn infants: A quality assessment using the neoPAW score. *Infant, 14*, 32–35.

Drake, E. (2017). *Positioning the neonate for best outcomes.* National Association of Neonatal Nurses. https://www.pampersprofessional.com/sfsites/c/resource/PositioningtheNeonate

Dubowitz, L., Dubowitz, V., & Mercuri, E. (1999). *The neurological assessment of the preterm and full-term newborn infant* (2nd ed., Vol. 79). MacKeith Press.

Edraki, M., Paran, M., Montaseri, S., Razavi Nejad, M., & Montaseri, Z. (2014). Comparing the effects of swaddled and conventional bathing methods on body temperature and crying duration in premature infants: A randomized clinical trial. *Journal of Caring Sciences, 3*(2), 83–91. https://doi.org/10.5681/jcs.2014.009

Edsberg, L. E., Black, J. M., Goldberg, M., McNichol, L., Moore, L., & Sieggreen, M. (2016). Revised national pressure ulcer advisory panel pressure injury staging system: Revised pressure injury staging system. *Journal of Wound, Ostomy, and Continence Nursing, 43*(6), 585–597. https://doi.org/10.1097/WON.0000000000000281

Eichenwald, E. C. (2018). Diagnosis and management of gastroesophageal reflux in preterm infants. *Pediatrics, 142*(1), e20181061. https://doi.org/10.1542/peds.2018-1061

Elser, H. E. (2012). Positioning after feedings: What is the evidence to reduce feeding intolerances? *Advances in Neonatal Care, 12*(3), 172–175. https://doi.org/10.1097/ANC.0b013e318256b7c1

Eskandari, Z., Seyedfatemi, N., Haghani, H., Almasi-Hashiani, A., & Mohagheghi, P. (2020). Effect of nesting on extensor motor behaviors in preterm infants: A randomized clinical trial. *Iranian Journal of Neonatology, 11*(3), 65–70.

Everts, R., Schone, C. G., Murner-Lavanchy, I., & Steinlin, M. (2019). Development of executive functions from childhood to adolescence in very preterm-born individuals-A longitudinal study. *Early Human Development, 129*, 45–51. https://doi.org/10.1016/j.earlhumdev.2018.12.012

Ewer, A. K., James, M. E., & Tobin, J. M. (1999). Prone and left lateral positioning reduce gastro-oesophageal reflux in preterm infants. *Archives of Disease in Childhood Fetal & Neonatal Edition, 81*(3), F201–F205. https://www.ncbi.nlm.nih.gov/pubmed/10525024

Fairchild, K. D., Nagraj, V. P., Sullivan, B. A., Moorman, J. R., & Lake, D. E. (2019). Oxygen desaturations in the early neonatal period predict development of bronchopulmonary dysplasia. *Pediatric Research, 85*(7), 987–993. https://doi.org/10.1038/s41390-018-0223-5

Feldman, R., & Eidelman, A. I. (2003). Skin-to-skin contact (Kangaroo Care) accelerates autonomic and neurobehavioural maturation in preterm infants. *Developmental Medicine & Child Neurology, 45*(4), 274–281. https://doi.org/10.1111/j.1469-8749.2003.tb00343.x

Feldman, R., Eidelman, A. I., Sirota, L., & Weller, A. (2002). Comparison of skin-to-skin (kangaroo) and traditional care: Parenting outcomes and preterm infant development. *Pediatrics, 110*(1 Pt. 1), 16–26. https://doi.org/10.1542/peds.110.1.16

Ferrari, F., Bertoncelli, N., Gallo, C., Roversi, M. F., Guerra, M. P., Ranzi, A., & Hadders-Algra, M. (2007). Posture and movement in healthy preterm infants in supine position in and outside the nest. *Archives Disease in Childhood Fetal & Neonatal Edition, 92*(5), F386–F390. https://doi.org/10.1136/adc.2006.101154

Fletcher, L., Pham, T., Bar, S., Li, D., Spinazzola, R., Papaioannou, H., & Milanaik, R. (2018). Variation in neonate swaddling techniques. *Advances in Neonatal Care, 18*(4), 302–306. https://doi.org/10.1097/ANC.0000000000000506

Freitas, P. D., Marques, S. R., Alves, T. B., Takahashi, J., & Kimura, A. F. (2014). Changes in physiological and behavioral parameters of preterm infants undergoing body hygiene: A systematic review. *Revista da Escola de Enfermagem da USP, 48*(Spec No:178–183), 178–183. https://doi.org/10.1590/S0080-623420140000600025

Gardner, S., & Goldson, E. (2021). *The neonate and the environment impact* (9th ed.). Elsevier.

Garland, J. S., Alex, C. P., Johnston, N., Yan, J. C., & Werlin, S. L. (2014). Association between tracheal pepsin, a reliable marker of gastric aspiration, and head of bed elevation among ventilated neonates. *Journal of Neonatal-Perinatal Medicine, 7*(3), 185–192. https://doi.org/10.3233/npm-14814020

Gaultier, C. (1995). Cardiorespiratory adaptation during sleep in infants and children. *Pediatric Pulmonology, 19*(2), 105–117. https://doi.org/10.1002/ppul.1950190206

Georgieff, M. K., & Bernbaum, J. C. (1986). Abnormal shoulder girdle muscle tone in premature infants during their first 18 months of life. *Pediatrics, 77*(5), 664–669.

Ghorbani, F., Asadollahi, M., & Valizadeh, S. (2013). Comparison the effect of sleep positioning on cardiorespiratory rate in noninvasive ventilated premature infants. *Nursing and Midwifery Studies, 2*(2), 182–187.

Gillies, D., Wells, D., & Bhandari, A. P. (2012). Positioning for acute respiratory distress in hospitalised infants and children. *Cochrane Database of Systematic Reviews, *(7), Cd003645. https://doi.org/10.1002/14651858.CD003645.pub3

Gogou, M., Haidopoulou, K., & Pavlou, E. (2019). Sleep and prematurity: Sleep outcomes in preterm children and influencing factors. *World Journal of Pediatrics, 15*(3), 209–218. https://doi.org/10.1007/s12519-019-00240-8

Gomes, E., Santos, C. M. D., Santos, A., Silva, A. G. D., França, M. A. M., Romanini, D. S., Mattos, M. C. V., Leal, A. F., & Costa, D. (2019). Autonomic responses of premature newborns to body position and environmental noise in the neonatal intensive care unit. (Respostas autonômicas de recém-nascidos prematuros ao posicionamento do corpo e ruídos ambientais na unidade de terapia intensiva neonatal). *Revista Brasileira de Terapia Intensiva, 31*(3), 296–302. https://doi.org/10.5935/0103-507x.20190054

Gorga, D., Stern, F. M., Ross, G., & Nagler, W. (1988). Neuromotor development of preterm and full-term infants. *Early Human Development, 18*(2–3), 137–149. http://www.ncbi.nlm.nih.gov/entrez/query.fcgi?cmd=Retrieve&db=PubMed&dopt=Citation&list_uids=3224576 http://www.sciencedirect.com/science?_ob=ArticleURL&_udi=B6T65-4C3C7PK-4C&_user=10&_rdoc=1&_fmt=&_orig=search&_sort=d&_docanchor=&view=c&_acct=C000050221&_version=1&_urlVersion=0&_userid=10&md5=26ce03c6912fef767b8f4d8b841eb27c

Graven, S., & Browne, J. (2008). Sleep and brain development. *Clinics in Perinatology, 33*(3), 693–706, vii. https://doi.org/10.1016/j.clp.2006.06.009

Grenier, I. R., Bigsby, R., Vergara, E. R., & Lester, B. M. (2003). Comparison of motor self-regulatory and stress behaviors of preterm infants across body positions. *American Journal of Occupational Therapy, 57*(3), 289–297. http://www.ncbi.nlm.nih.gov/entrez/query.fcgi?cmd=Retrieve&db=PubMed&dopt=Citation&list_uids=12785667

Griffiths, N., Spence, K., Loughran-Fowlds, A., & Westrup, B. (2019). Individualised developmental care for babies and parents in the NICU: Evidence-based best practice guideline recommendations. *Early Human Development, 139*, 104840. https://doi.org/10.1016/j.earlhumdev.2019.104840

Haesler, E., Kottner, J., Cuddigan, J., & International Guideline Development Group, . (2017). The 2014 international pressure ulcer guideline: Methods and development. *Journal of Advanced Nursing, 73*(6), 1515–1530. https://doi.org/10.1111/jan.13241

Haraldsdottir, K., Watson, A. M., Goss, K. N., Beshish, A. G., Pegelow, D. F., Palta, M., Tetri, L. H., Barton, G. P., Brix, M. D., Centanni, R. M., & Eldridge, M. W. (2018). Impaired autonomic function in adolescents born preterm. *Physiological Reports, 6*(6), e13620. https://doi.org/10.14814/phy2.13620

Harrison, T., & Brown, R. (2017). Autonomic nervous system function under a skin-to-skin intervention in infants with congenital heart disease. *Journal of Cardiovascular Nursing, 32*(5), E1–E13.

Harrison, L. L., Williams, A. K., Berbaum, M. L., Stem, J. T., & Leeper, J. (2000). Physiologic and behavioral effects of gentle human touch on preterm infants. *Research in Nursing & Health, 23*(6), 435–446. https://doi.org/10.1002/1098-240X(200012)23:6<435::AID-NUR3>3.0.CO;2-P

Hartley, K. A., Miller, C. S., & Gephart, S. M. (2015). Facilitated tucking to reduce pain in neonates: Evidence for best practice. *Advances in Neonatal Care, 15*(3), 201–208. https://doi.org/10.1097/anc.0000000000000193

Herrington, C. J., & Chiodo, L. M. (2014). Human touch effectively and safely reduces pain in the newborn intensive care unit. *Pain Management Nursing, 15*(1), 107–115. https://doi.org/10.1016/j.pmn.2012.06.007

Hough, J. L., Johnston, L., Brauer, S. G., Woodgate, P. G., Pham, T. M., & Schibler, A. (2012). Effect of body position on ventilation distribution in preterm infants on continuous positive airway pressure. *Pediatric Critical Care Medicine, 13*(4), 446–451. https://doi.org/10.1097/PCC.0b013e31822f18d9

Hough, J., Trojman, A., & Schibler, A. (2016). Effect of time and body position on ventilation in premature infants. *Pediatric Research, 80*(4), 499–504. https://doi.org/10.1038/pr.2016.116

Huang, C. M., Tung, W. S., Kuo, L. L., & Ying-Ju, C. (2004). Comparison of pain responses of premature infants to the heelstick between containment and swaddling. *Journal of Nursing Research, 12*(1), 31–40.

Hutchinson, G., & Wayne, R. (2016). From surviving to thriving: The impact of cranial deformation and pressure ulcers in the hospitalized infant. *Neonatal Intensive Care, 29*(2), 44–47.

Ifflaender, S., Rudiger, M., Konstantelos, D., Wahls, K., & Burkhardt, W. (2013). Prevalence of head deformities in preterm infants at term equivalent age. *Early Human Development, 89*(12), 1041–1047.

Imam, S. S., Shinkar, D. M., Mohamed, N. A., & Mansour, H. E. (2018). Effect of right lateral position with head elevation on tracheal aspirate pepsin in ventilated preterm neonates: Randomized controlled trial. *Journal of Maternal-Fetal & Neonatal Medicine, 32*(22), 3741–3746. https://doi.org/10.1080/14767058.2018.1471674

Infant Positioning Assessment Tool (IPAT). (2018). *Koninklijke Phillips.* http://images.philips.com/is/content/PhilipsConsumer/Campaigns/HC20140401_DG/Documents/ipat_sheet.pdf

Jadcherla, S. R., Duong, H. Q., Hoffmann, R. G., & Shaker, R. (2003). Esophageal body and upper esophageal sphincter motor responses to esophageal provocation during maturation in preterm newborns. *Journal of Pediatrics, 143*(1), 31–38. https://doi.org/10.1016/S0022-3476(03)00242-7

Jadcherla, S. R., Slaughter, J. L., Stenger, M. R., Klebanoff, M., Kelleher, K., & Gardner, W. (2013). Practice variance, prevalence, and economic burden of premature infants diagnosed with GERD. *Hospital Pediatrics, 3*(4), 335–341. https://doi.org/10.1542/hpeds.2013-0036

Jarus, T., Bart, O., Rabinovich, G., Sadeh, A., Bloch, L., Dolfin, T., & Litmanovitz, I. (2011). Effects of prone and supine positions on sleep state and stress responses in preterm infants. *Infant Behavior and Development, 34*(2), 257–263. https://doi.org/10.1016/j.infbeh.2010.12.014

Johnson, S., & Marlow, N. (2011). Preterm birth and childhood psychiatric disorders. *Pediatric Research, 69*(5 Pt. 2), 11R–18R. https://doi.org/10.1203/PDR.0b013e318212faa0

Johnson, S., Hollis, C., Kochhar, P., Hennessy, E., Wolke, D., & Marlow, N. (2010a). Autism spectrum disorders in extremely preterm children. *Journal of Pediatrics, 156*(4), 525–531.e2. https://doi.org/10.1016/j.jpeds.2009.10.041

Johnson, S., Hollis, C., Kochhar, P., Hennessy, E., Wolke, D., & Marlow, N. (2010b). Psychiatric disorders in extremely preterm children: Longitudinal finding at age 11 years in the EPICure study. *Journal of the American Academy of Child and Adolescent Psychiatry, 49*(5), 453–463.e1. https://www.ncbi.nlm.nih.gov/pubmed/20431465

Johnston, C., Campbell-Yeo, M., Disher, T., Benoit, B., Fernandes, A., Streiner, D., Inglis, D., & Zee, R. (2017). Skin-to-skin care for procedural pain in neonates. *Cochrane Database of Systematic Reviews, 2*, CD008435. https://doi.org/10.1002/14651858.CD008435.pub3

Kahraman, A., Başbakkal, Z., Yalaz, M., & Sözmen, E. Y. (2018). The effect of nesting positions on pain, stress and comfort during heel lance in premature infants. *Pediatrics and Neonatology, 59*(4), 352–359. https://doi.org/10.1016/j.pedneo.2017.11.010

Karvonen, R., Sipola, M., Kiviniemi, A., Tikanmaki, M., Jarvelin, M. R., Eriksson, J. G., Tulppo, M., Vaarasmaki, M., & Kajantie, E. (2019). Cardiac autonomic function in adults born preterm. *Journal of Pediatrics, 208*, 96–103.e4. https://doi.org/10.1016/j.jpeds.2018.12.061

Katz, K., Krikler, R., Wielunsky, E., & Merlob, P. (1991). Effect of neonatal posture on later lower limb rotation and gait in premature infants. *Journal of Pediatric Orthopedics, 11*(4), 520–522. https://doi.org/10.1097/01241398-199107000-00019

Khatony, A., Abdi, A., Karimi, B., Aghaei, A., & Brojeni, H. S. (2019). The effects of position on gastric residual volume of premature infants in NICU. *Italian Journal of Pediatrics, 45*(1), 6. https://doi.org/10.1186/s13052-018-0591-9

King, C., & Norton, D. (2017). Does therapeutic positioning of preterm infants impact upon optimal health outcomes? A literature review. *Journal of Neonatal Nursing, 23*(5), 218–222. https://doi.org/https://doi.org/10.1016/j.jnn.2017.03.004

Klimo, P. J., Lingo, P. R., Baird, L. C., Bauer, D. F., Beier, A., Durham, S., Lin, A. Y., McClung-Smith, C., Mitchell, L., Nikas, D., Tamber, M. S., Tyagi, R., Mazzola, C., & Flannery, A. M. (2016). Congress of neurological surgeons systematic review and evidence-based guideline on the management of patients with positional plagiocephaly: The role of repositioning. *Neurosurgery, 79*(5), E627–E629. https://doi.org/10.1227/neu.0000000000001428

Lammertink, F., Vinkers, C. H., Tataranno, M. L., & Benders, M. J. N. L. (2021). Premature birth and developmental programming: Mechanisms of resilience and vulnerability [review]. *Frontiers in Psychiatry, 11*(1515). https://doi.org/10.3389/fpsyt.2020.531571

Lan, H. Y., Yang, L., Hsieh, K. H., Yin, T., Chang, Y. C., & Liaw, J. J. (2018). Effects of a supportive care bundle on sleep variables of preterm infants during hospitalization. *Research in Nursing & Health, 41*(3), 281–291. https://doi.org/10.1002/nur.21865

Linsell, L., Johnson, S., Wolke, D., Morris, J., Kurinczuk, J. J., & Marlow, N. (2019). Trajectories of behavior, attention, social and emotional problems from childhood to early adulthood following extremely preterm birth: A prospective cohort study. *European Child & Adolescent Psychiatry, 28*(4), 531–542. https://doi.org/10.1007/s00787-018-1219-8

Lipner, H. S., & Huron, R. F. (2018). Developmental and interprofessional care of the preterm infant: Neonatal intensive care unit through high-risk infant follow-up. *Pediatric Clinics of North America, 65*(1), 135–141. https://doi.org/10.1016/j.pcl.2017.08.026

Liversedge, H., Bader, D., Schoonhoven, L., & Worsley, P. (2018). Survey of neonatal nurses' practices and beliefs in relation to skin health. *Journal of Neonatal Nursing, 24*, 86–93. https://doi.org/10.16/j.jnn.2017.07.007

Ludington-Hoe, S. M., Johnson, M. W., Morgan, K., Lewis, T., Gutman, J., Wilson, P. D., & Scher, M. S. (2006). Neurophysiologic assessment of neonatal sleep organization: Preliminary results of a randomized, controlled trial of skin contact with preterm infants. *Pediatrics, 117*(5), e909–e923. https://doi.org/10.1542/peds.2004-1422

Lund, C. (2014). Medical adhesives in the NICU. *Newborn and Infant Nursing Reviews, 14*(4), 160–165. https://doi.org/10.1053/j.nainr.2014.10.001

Madlinger-Lewis, L., Reynolds, L., Zarem, C., Crapnell, T., Inder, T., & Pineda, R. (2014). The effects of alternative positioning on preterm infants in the neonatal intensive care unit: A randomized clinical trial. *Research in Developmental Disabilities, 35*(2), 490–497. https://doi.org/10.1016/j.ridd.2013.11.019

McCarty, D. B., Peat, J. R., Malcolm, W. F., Smith, P. B., Fisher, K., & Goldstein, R. F. (2016). Dolichocephaly in preterm infants: Prevalence, risk factors, and early motor outcomes. *American Journal of Perinatology, 34*(4), 372–378. https://doi.org/10.1055/s-0036-1592128

McCarty, D. B., Peat, J. R., Malcolm, W. F., Smith, P. B., Fisher, K., & Goldstein, R. F. (2017). Dolichocephaly in preterm infants: Prevalence, risk factors, and early motor outcomes. *American Journal of Perinatology, 34*(4), 372–378. https://doi.org/10.1055/s-0036-1592128

McCarty, D. B., O'Donnell, S., Goldstein, R. F., Smith, P. B., Fisher, K., & Malcolm, W. F. (2018). Use of a midliner positioning system for prevention of dolichocephaly in preterm infants. *Pediatric Physical Therapy, 30*(2), 126–134. https://doi.org/10.1097/PEP.0000000000000487

Miller-Barmak, A., Riskin, A., Hochwald, O., Haddad, J., Dinur, G., Vortman, R., Kugelman, A., & Borenstein-Levin, L. (2020). Oxygenation instability assessed by oxygen saturation histograms during supine vs prone position in very low birthweight infants receiving noninvasive respiratory support. *Journal of Pediatrics, 226*, 123–128. https://doi.org/10.1016/j.jpeds.2020.06.066

Modesto, I. F., Avelar, A. F., Pedreira Mda, L., Pradella-Hallinan, M., Avena, M. J., & Pinheiro, E. M. (2016). Effect of sleeping position on arousals from sleep in preterm infants. *Journal for Specialists in Pediatric Nursing, 21*(3), 131–138. https://doi.org/10.1111/jspn.12147

Modrcin-Talbott, M. A., Harrison, L. L., Groer, M. W., & Younger, M. S. (2003). The biobehavioral effects of gentle human touch on preterm infants. *Nursing Science Quarterly, 16*(1), 60–67. http://www.ncbi.nlm.nih.gov/entrez/query.fcgi?cmd=Retrieve&db=PubMed&dopt=Citation&list_uids=12593316

Monterosso, L., Kristjanson, L. J., Cole, J., & Evans, S. F. (2003). Effect of postural supports on neuromotor function in very preterm infants to term equivalent age. *Journal of Paediatrics and Child Health, 39*(3), 197–205. https://www.ncbi.nlm.nih.gov/pubmed/12654143

Montgomery, K., Choy, N. L., Steele, M., & Hough, J. (2014). The effectiveness of quarter turn from prone in maintaining respiratory function in premature infants. *Journal of Paediatrics and Child Health, 50*(12), 972–977. https://doi.org/10.1111/jpc.12689

Moon, R. Y. (2016). SIDS and other sleep-related infant deaths: Evidence base for 2016 updated recommendations for a safe infant sleeping environment. *Pediatrics, 138*(5). https://doi.org/10.1542/peds.2016-2940

Moreira, R. S., Magalhaes, L. C., & Alves, C. R. (2014). Effect of preterm birth on motor development, behavior, and school performance of school-age children: A systematic review. *Jornal de Pediatria (Rio J), 90*(2), 119–134. https://doi.org/10.1016/j.jped.2013.05.010

Ness, M. J., Davis, D. M. R., & Carey, W. A. (2013). Neonatal skin care: A concise review. *International Journal of Dermatology, 52*(1), 14–22. https://doi.org/10.1111/j.1365-4632.2012.05687.x

Neu, M., & Browne, J. V. (1997). Infant physiologic and behavioral organization during swaddled versus unswaddled weighing. *Journal of Perinatology, 17*(3), 193–198. https://www.ncbi.nlm.nih.gov/pubmed/9210073

Nuysink, J., Eijsermans, M. J., van Haastert, I. C., Koopman-Esseboom, C., Helders, P. J., de Vries, L. S., & van der Net, J. (2013). Clinical course of asymmetric motor performance and deformational plagiocephaly in very preterm infants. *Journal of Pediatrics, 163*(3), 658–665.e1.

Oishi, Y., Ohta, H., Hirose, T., Nakaya, S., Tsuchiya, K., Nakagawa, M., Kusakawa, I., Sato, T., Obonai, T., Nishida, H., & Yoda, H. (2018). Combined effects of body position and sleep status on the cardiorespiratory stability of near-term infants. *Scientific Reports, 8*(1), 8845. https://doi.org/10.1038/s41598-018-27212-8

Omari, T. I., Rommel, N., Staunton, E., Lontis, R., Goodchild, L., Haslam, R. R., Dent, J., & Davidson, G. P. (2004). Paradoxical impact of body positioning on gastroesophageal reflux and gastric emptying in the premature neonate. *Journal of Pediatrics, 145*(2), 194–200. https://doi.org/10.1016/j.jpeds.2004.05.026

Orenstein, S. R., Whitington, P. F., & Orenstein, D. M. (1983). The infant seat as treatment for gastroesophageal reflux. *The New England Journal of Medicine, 309*(13), 760–763. https://doi.org/10.1056/nejm198309293091304

Orenstein, S. R. (1990). Effects on behavior state of prone versus seated positioning for infants with gastroesophageal reflux. *Pediatrics, 85*(5), 765–767.

Orsi, K. C., Avena, M. J., Lurdes de Cacia Pradella-Hallinan, M., da Luz Goncalves Pedreira, M., Tsunemi, M. H., Machado Avelar, A. F., & Pinheiro, E. M. (2017). Effects of handling and environment on preterm newborns sleeping in incubators. *Journal of Obstetric, Gynecologic & Neonatal Nursing, 46*(2), 238–247. https://doi.org/10.1016/j.jogn.2016.09.005

Pados, B. F. (2019). Physiology of stress and use of skin-to-skin care as a stress-reducing intervention in the NICU. *Nursing for Womens Health, 23*(1), 59–70. https://doi.org/10.1016/j.nwh.2018.11.002

Park, J., Silva, S. G., Thoyre, S. M., & Brandon, D. H. (2020). Sleep-wake states and feeding progression in preterm infants. *Nursing Research, 69*(1), 22–30. https://doi.org/10.1097/nnr.0000000000000395

Park, J. (2020). Sleep promotion for preterm infants in the NICU. *Nursing for Womens Health, 24*(1), 24–35. https://doi.org/10.1016/j.nwh.2019.11.004

Peng, N. H., Chen, L. L., Li, T. C., Smith, M., Chang, Y. S., & Huang, L. C. (2014). The effect of positioning on preterm infants' sleep-wake states and stress behaviours during exposure to environmental stressors. *Journal of Child Health Care, 18*(4), 314–325. https://doi.org/10.1177/1367493513496665

Peng, H. F., Yin, T., Yang, L., Wang, C., Chang, Y. C., Jeng, M. J., & Liaw, J. J. (2018). Non-nutritive sucking, oral breast milk, and facilitated tucking relieve preterm infant pain during heel-stick procedures: A prospective, randomized controlled trial. *International Journal of Nursing Studies, 77*, 162–170. https://doi.org/10.1016/j.ijnurstu.2017.10.001

Picheansathian, W., Woragidpoonpol, P., & Baosoung, C. (2009). Positioning of preterm infants for optimal physiological development: A systematic review. *JBI Library of Systematic Reviews, 7*(7), 224–259. https://www.ncbi.nlm.nih.gov/pubmed/27820087

Pillai Riddell, R., Racine, N., Turcotte, K., Uman, L., Horton, R., Din Osmun, L., Ahola Kohut, S., Hillgrove-Stuart, J., Stevens, B., & Lisi, D. (2011). Nonpharmacological management of procedural pain in infants and young children: An abridged cochrane review. *Pain Research & Management, 16*(5), 321–330.

Pineda, R. G., Tjoeng, T. H., Vavasseur, C., Kidokoro, H., Neil, J. J., & Inder, T. (2013). Patterns of altered neurobehavior in preterm infants within the neonatal intensive care unit. *Journal of Pediatrics, 162*(3), 470–476.e1. https://doi.org/10.1016/j.jpeds.2012.08.011

Poets, C. F., Roberts, R. S., Schmidt, B., Whyte, R. K., Asztalos, E. V., Bader, D., Bairam, A., Moddemann, D., Peliowski, A., Rabi, Y., Solimano, A., Nelson, H., & for the Canadian Oxygen Trial Investigators. (2015). Association between intermittent hypoxemia or bradycardia and late death or disability in extremely preterm infants. *Journal of American Medical Association, 314*(6), 595–603. https://doi.org/10.1001/jama.2015.8841

Provenzi, L., Fumagalli, M., Sirgiovanni, I., Giorda, R., Pozzoli, U., Morandi, F., Beri, S., Menozzi, G., Mosca, F., Borgatti, R., & Montirosso, R. (2015). Pain-related stress during the Neonatal Intensive Care Unit stay and SLC6A4 methylation in very preterm infants. *Frontiers in Behavioral Neuroscience, 9*, 99. https://doi.org/10.3389/fnbeh.2015.00099

Raffay, T. M., Dylag, A. M., Sattar, A., Abu Jawdeh, E. G., Cao, S., Pax, B. M., Loparo, K. A., Martin, R. J., & Di Fiore, J. M. (2019). Neonatal intermittent hypoxemia events are associated with diagnosis of bronchopulmonary dysplasia at 36 weeks postmenstrual age. *Pediatric Research, 85*(3), 318–323. https://doi.org/10.1038/s41390-018-0253-z

Razmus, I., Lewis, L., & Wilson, D. (2008). Pressure ulcer development in infants: State of the science. *Journal of Healthcare Quality, 30*(5), 36–42. https://doi.org/10.1111/j.1945-1474.2008.tb01160.x

Ricci, D., Romeo, D. M., Haataja, L., van Haastert, I. C., Cesarini, L., Maunu, J., Pane, M., Gallini, F., Luciano, R., Romagnoli, C., de Vries, L. S., Cowan, F. M., & Mercuri, E. (2008). Neurological examination of preterm infants at term equivalent age. *Early Human Development, 84*(11), 751–761. https://doi.org/10.1016/j.earlhumdev.2008.05.007

Riegger-Krugh, C. (1993). Relationship of mechanical and movement factors to prenatal musculoskeletal development. *Physical & Occupational Therapy in Pediatrics, 4*, 19–37.

Rivas-Fernandez, M., Roque, I. F. M., Diez-Izquierdo, A., Escribano, J., & Balaguer, A. (2016). Infant position in neonates receiving mechanical ventilation. *Cochrane Database of Systematic Reviews, 11*, Cd003668. https://doi.org/10.1002/14651858.CD003668.pub4

Rogers, C. E., Sylvester, C. M., Mintz, C., Kenley, J. K., Shimony, J. S., Barch, D. M., & Smyser, C. D. (2017). Neonatal amygdala functional connectivity at rest in healthy and preterm infants and early internalizing symptoms. *Journal of the American Academy of Child & Adolescent Psychiatry, 56*(2), 157–166. https://doi.org/10.1016/j.jaac.2016.11.005

Romantsik, O., Calevo, M. G., & Bruschettini, M. (2017). Head midline position for preventing the occurrence or extension of germinal matrix-intraventricular hemorrhage in preterm infants. *Cochrane Database of Systematic Reviews, 7*, CD012362. https://doi.org/10.1002/14651858.CD012362.pub2

Romantsik, O., Calevo, M. G., & Bruschettini, M. (2020). Head midline position for preventing the occurrence or extension of germinal matrix-intraventricular haemorrhage in preterm infants. *Cochrane Database of Systematic Reviews, 7*(7), Cd012362. https://doi.org/10.1002/14651858.CD012362.pub3

Ryan, G., Dooley, J., Gerber Finn, L., & Kelly, L. (2019). Nonpharmacological management of neonatal abstinence syndrome: A review of the literature. *Journal of Maternal-Fetal & Neonatal Medicine, 32*(10), 1735–1740. https://doi.org/10.1080/14767058.2017.1414180

Sanders, M. R., & Hall, S. L. (2018). Trauma-informed care in the newborn intensive care unit: Promoting safety, security and connectedness. *Journal of Perinatology, 38*(1), 3–10. https://doi.org/10.1038/jp.2017.124

Sangers, H., de Jong, P. M., Mulder, S. E., Stigter, G. D., van den Berg, C. M., te Pas, A. B., & Walther, F. J. (2013). Outcomes of gastric residuals whilst feeding preterm infants in various body positions. *Journal of Neonatal Nursing, 19*(6), 337–341. https://doi.org/10.1016/j.jnn.2012.12.003

Santos, A., Viera, C., Bertolini, G., Osaku, E., Costa, C. d. M., & Grebinski, A. (2017). Physiological and behavioural effects of preterm infant positioning in a neonatal intensive care unit. *British Journal of Midwifery, 25*(10), 647–654. https://doi.org/10.12968/bjom.2017.25.10.647

Sardesai, S. R., Kornacka, M. K., Walas, W., & Ramanathan, R. (2011). Iatrogenic skin injury in the neonatal intensive care unit. *Journal of Maternal-Fetal & Neonatal Medicine, 24*(2), 197–203. https://doi.org/10.3109/14767051003728245

Schurr, P., & Findlater, C. K. (2012). Neonatal myth busters: Evaluating the evidence for and against pharmacologic and nonpharmacologic management of gastroesophageal reflux. *Neonatal Network, 31*(4), 229–241. https://www.ncbi.nlm.nih.gov/pubmed/22763250

Shah, A. N., Jerardi, K. E., Auger, K. A., & Beck, A. F. (2016). Can hospitalization precipitate toxic stress? *Pediatrics, 137*(5). https://doi.org/10.1542/peds.2016-0204

Shaw, B. A., Segal, L. S., & Section on Orthopedics. (2016). Evaluation and referral for developmental dysplasia of the hip in infants. *Pediatrics, 138*(6). https://doi.org/10.1542/peds.2016-3107

Shonkoff, J. P., Garner, A. S., Committee on Psychosocial Aspects of Child and Family Health, Committee on Early Childhood, Adoption, and Dependent Care, Section on Developmental, & Behavioral Pediatrics. (2012). The lifelong effects of early childhood adversity and toxic stress. *Pediatrics, 129*(1), e232–e246. https://doi.org/10.1542/peds.2011-2663

Smith, G. C., Gutovich, J., Smyser, C., Pineda, R., Newnham, C., Tjoeng, T. H., Vavasseur, C., Wallendorf, M., Neil, J., & Inder, T. (2011). Neonatal intensive care unit stress is associated with brain development in preterm infants. *Annals of Neurology, 70*(4), 541–549. https://doi.org/10.1002/ana.22545

Smith, J. (2012). Comforting touch in the very preterm hospitalized infant: An integrative review. *Advances in Neonatal Care, 12,* 349–365. https://doi.org/10.1097/ANC.0b013e31826093ee

Spittle, A. J., & Orton, J. (2014). Cerebral palsy and developmental coordination disorder in children born preterm. *Seminars in Fetal & Neonatal Medicine, 19*(2), 84–89. https://doi.org/10.1016/j.siny.2013.11.005

Stangenes, K. M., Fevang, S. K., Grundt, J., Donkor, H. M., Markestad, T., Hysing, M., Elgen, I. B., & Bjorvatn, B. (2017). Children born extremely preterm had different sleeping habits at 11 years of age and more childhood sleep problems than term-born children. *Acta Paediatrica, 106*(12), 1966–1972. https://doi.org/10.1111/apa.13991

Sullivan, M. C., Msall, M. E., & Miller, R. J. (2012). 17-year outcome of preterm infants with diverse neonatal morbidities: Part 1—Impact on physical, neurological, and psychological health status. *Journal of Specialists in Pediatric Nursing, 17*(3), 226–241. https://doi.org/10.1111/j.1744-6155.2012.00337.x

Sweeney, J. K., & Gutierrez, T. (2002). Musculoskeletal implications of preterm infant positioning in the NICU. *Journal of Perinatal and Neonatal Nursing, 16*(1), 58–70. http://www.ncbi.nlm.nih.gov/entrez/query.fcgi?cmd=Retrieve&db=PubMed&dopt=Citation&list_uids=12083295

Sweeney, J., & McElroy, J. (2019). *IFCDC-recommendations for best practice for positioning and touch.* https://nicudesign.nd.edu/nicu-care-standards/ifcdc--recommendations-for-best-practice-for-positioning-and-touch/

Tane, R., Rustina, Y., & Waluyanti, F. T. (2019). Nesting with fixation and position to facilitate quiet sleep and oxygen saturation on low-birth weight infants. *Comprehensive Child and Adolescent Nursing, 42*(Suppl. 1), 29–37. https://doi.org/10.1080/24694193.2019.1577923

Task Force on Sudden Infant Death Syndrome. (2016). SIDS and other sleep-related infant deaths: Updated 2016 recommendations for a safe infant sleeping environment. *Pediatrics, 138*(5). https://doi.org/10.1542/peds.2016-2938

Teledevara, S., Rajeswari, M., Kumar, R. S., & Udayakumar, N. (2019). Factors associated with low muscle tone and impact of common musculoskeletal problems on motor development in preterm infants at one year of corrected age [article]. *Journal of Clinical & Diagnostic Research, 13*(3), 12–16. https://doi.org/10.7860/JCDR/2019/39551.12675

Tobin, J. M., McCloud, P., & Cameron, D. J. (1997). Posture and gastrooesophageal reflux: A case for left lateral positioning. *Archives of Disease in Childhood, 76*(3), 254–258. https://doi.org/10.1136/adc.76.3.254

Upadhyay, J., Singh, P., Digal, K. C., Shubham, S., Grover, R., & Basu, S. (2021). Developmentally supportive positioning policy for preterm low birth weight infants in a tertiary care neonatal unit: A quality improvement initiative. *Indian Pediatrics.* Advance online publication. https://www.ncbi.nlm.nih.gov/pubmed/33408277

Utario, Y., Rustina, Y., & Waluyanti, F. T. (2017). The quarter prone position increases oxygen saturation in premature infants using continuous positive airway pressure. *Comprehensive Child and Adolescent Nursing, 40*(Suppl. 1), 95–101. https://doi.org/10.1080/24694193.2017.1386976

Vaivre-Douret, L., Ennouri, K., Jrad, I., Garrec, C., & Papiernik, E. (2004). Effect of positioning on the incidence of abnormalities of muscle tone in low-risk, preterm infants. *European Journal of Paediatric Neurology, 8*(1), 21–34. https://doi.org/10.1016/j.ejpn.2003.10.001. pii: S1090379803001521.

Valizadeh, L., Ghahremani, G., Gharehbaghi, M. M., & Jafarabadi, M. A. (2016). The effects of flexed (fetal tucking) and extended (free body) postures on the daily sleep quantity of hospitalized premature infants: A randomized clinical trial. *Journal of Research in Medical Sciences, 21,* 124. https://doi.org/10.4103/1735-1995.196606

van den Hoogen, A., Teunis, C. J., Shellhaas, R. A., Pillen, S., Benders, M., & Dudink, J. (2017). How to improve sleep in a neonatal intensive care unit: A systematic review. *Early Human Development, 113,* 78–86. https://doi.org/10.1016/j.earlhumdev.2017.07.002

van Sleuwen, B. E., Engelberts, A. C., Boere-Boonekamp, M. M., Kuis, W., Schulpen, T. W., & L'Hoir, M. P. (2007). Swaddling: A systematic review. *Pediatrics, 120*(4), e1097–e1106. https://doi.org/10.1542/peds.2006-2083

van Veen, S., Aarnoudse-Moens, C. S. H., Oosterlaan, J., van Sonderen, L., de Haan, T. R., van Kaam, A. H., & van Wassenaer-Leemhuis, A. G. (2017). Very preterm born children at early school age: Healthcare therapies and educational provisions. *Early Human Development, 117,* 39–43. https://doi.org/10.1016/j.earlhumdev.2017.12.010

van Vlimmeren, L. A., van der Graaf, Y., Boere-Boonekamp, M. M., L'Hoir, M. P., Helders, P. J., & Engelbert, R. H. (2008). Effect of pediatric physical therapy on deformational plagiocephaly in children with positional preference: A randomized controlled trial. *Archives of Pediatrics & Adolescent Medicine, 162*(8), 712–718. https://doi.org/10.1001/archpedi.162.8.712

Visscher, M., & Taylor, T. (2014). Pressure ulcers in the hospitalized neonate: Rates and risk factors. *Scientific Reports, 4,* 7429. https://doi.org/10.1038/srep07429

Vollmer, B., & Stalnacke, J. (2019). Young adult motor, sensory, and cognitive outcomes and longitudinal development after very and extremely preterm birth. *Neuropediatrics, 50*(4), 219–227. https://doi.org/10.1055/s-0039-1688955

Weber, A., & Harrison, T. M. (2019). Reducing toxic stress in the neonatal intensive care unit to improve infant outcomes. *Nursing Outlook, 67*(2), 169–189. https://doi.org/10.1016/j.outlook.2018.11.002

Wiley, F., Raphael, R., & Ghanouni, P. (2020). NICU positioning strategies to reduce stress in preterm infants: A scoping review. *Early Child Development and Care,* 1–18. https://doi.org/10.1080/03004430.2019.1707815

Wilson, D., Kim, D., & Breibart, S. (2020). Intraventricular hemorrhage and posthemorrhagic ventricular dilation: Current approaches to improve outcomes. *Neonatal Network,* (3), 158–169. https://doi.org/10.1891/0730-0832.39.3.158

Winchester, S. B., Sullivan, M. C., Roberts, M. B., Bryce, C. I., & Granger, D. A. (2018). Long-term effects of prematurity, cumulative medical risk, and proximal and distal social forces on individual differences in diurnal cortisol at young adulthood. *Biological Research for Nursing, 20*(1), 5–15. https://doi.org/10.1177/1099800417718955

Yayan, E. H., Kucukoglu, S., Dag, Y. S., & Karsavuran Boyraz, N. (2018). Does the post-feeding position affect gastric residue in preterm infants? *Breastfeeding Medicine, 13*(6), 438–443. https://doi.org/10.1089/bfm.2018.0028

Yilmazer, T., & Tuzer, H. (2019). Pressure ulcer prevention care bundle: A cross-sectional, content validation study. *Wound Management & Prevention, 65*(5), 33–39.

Zahed, M., Berbis, J., Brevaut-Malaty, V., Busuttil, M., Tosello, B., & Gire, C. (2015). Posture and movement in very preterm infants at term age in and outside the nest. *Childs Nervous System, 31*(12), 2333–2340.

Zeller, B., & Giebe, J. (2014). Pain in the neonate: Focus on nonpharmacologic interventions. *Neonatal Network, 33*(6), 336–340. https://doi.org/10.1891/0730-0832.33.6.336

CHAPTER 15

Oral Feeding and the High-Risk Infant

Jacqueline M. McGrath, Barbara Medoff-Cooper, Ashley Darcy-Mahoney, Kelly Sharmane McGlothen-Bell, and Annalyn Velasquez

---

IFCDC Standards in Collaborative Practice

Standard 1: Systems Thinking
- The intensive care unit (ICU) shall exhibit an infrastructure of leadership, mission, and a governance framework to guide the performance of the collaborative practice of Infant- and Family-Centered Developmental Care (IFCDC).

Standard 2: Systems Thinking
- The intensive care unit shall provide a professionally competent interprofessional collaborative practice team to support the baby, parent, and family's holistic physical, developmental, and psychosocial needs from birth through the transition of hospital discharge to home and assure continuity to follow-up care.

Standard 3: Feeding
- Nutrition shall be optimized during the ICU period.

Standard 4: Feeding
- M/others shall be supported to be the primary feeders of their baby.

Standard 5: Feeding
- Caregiving activities shall consider baby's response to input, especially around face/mouth, and aversive noncritical care oral experiences shall be minimized.

Standard 6: Feeding
- Professional staff shall consider smell and taste experiences that are biologically expected.

Standard 7: Feeding
- Support of baby's self-regulation shall be encouraged, especially as it relates to sucking for comfort.

Standard 8: Feeding
- Environments shall be supportive of an attuned feeding for both the feeder and the baby.

Standard 9: Feeding
- Feeding management shall focus on establishing safe oral feedings that are comfortable and enjoyable.

Standard 10: Feeding
- ICUs shall include interprofessional perspectives to provide best feeding management.

Standard 11: Feeding
- Feeding management shall consider short- and long-term growth and feeding outcomes.

INTRODUCTION

Many times the importance of feeding interventions and techniques are lost or forgotten in the high-tech environment of the NICU.

Conway (1994, p. 71)

Although the above quote may seem outdated, for the most part the environment of the neonatal intensive care unit (NICU) continues to be mostly noxious to infants and families. Many improvements have occurred over time, and the NICU has become more supportive with increasing understanding of the developmental needs of the high-risk infant. Yet, it is still not the best environment to support the maturation and acquisition of oral feeding skills. As previous sections of this text have indicated, the environment plays a significant role in the infant's and family's development. Research in the area of "environmental neonatology" continues to grow; however, evidence of the long-term consequences remains largely abstract and not very predictable. Given this situation, avoidance of prolonged hospitalization in the NICU is an appropriate goal. Most low-birth-weight (LBW), preterm infants are discharged from the NICU sometime between 36 and 40 weeks postmenstrual age (PMA). The criteria used to determine the stability of the preterm infant often include cardiorespiratory stability, consistent weight gain, and successful bottle-feeding (even when the mother intends to breastfeed)

Suggested Criteria for Early Discharge

- Cardiorespiratory stability
- No apnea or bradycardia for 3–5 days
- Consistent weight gain
- Thermal regulation
- Successful bottle-feeding [even if the mother intends to breastfeed]

- Parents actively participating in caregiving
- Parents confident in caregiving and feeding skills
- Home environment prepared for care of infant

Data from Boykova et al., 2020; Edwards et al., 2019; Lean et al., 2018.

(Boykova et al., 2020; Edwards et al., 2019; Lean et al., 2018) (Box "Suggested Criteria for Early Discharge"). These criteria continue to be the "gold standard" for integrity and stability in the preterm infant before discharge. Thus, implementation of interventions that support successful gastric and, later, oral breastfeeding or bottle-feeding in the NICU is a critical developmental milestone for infants leaving the NICU.

In this chapter, oral feeding is reviewed, both as a physiologic and developmental milestone. Recommendations and interventions to successfully support this process are reviewed with examination of the evidence to support these practices. Focus is on best practices related to supporting the infant and their family during the transition to oral feeding and the transition to home. Feeding directly at the breast given that breastmilk is the optimal nutrition for high-risk infants is the optimal goal. Yet, many preterm infants may not fully achieve this goal prior to discharge so we will discuss both oral feeding at the breast and from a bottle as important milestones for both the NICU infant and parent.

Generally, bottle-feeding a preterm or high-risk infant has not been recognized as an intervention requiring expertise. Bottle-feeding a newborn infant is commonly thought to be instinctual for both the infant and the caregiver; therefore, it is believed that *anyone can feed a baby*. The skills for both partners are believed to develop naturally with time and patience. Yet, research has demonstrated this is not true for development of oral feeding for the high-risk preterm infant; both maturation and experience often play a part in the development of these skills (Edwards et al., 2019). When oral feeding is unsuccessful, the caregiver is just as likely to be found at fault as the infant making feeding an important aspect of confidence and competence for mothering.

Feeding success has implications for fostering parent–child bonding (Korja et al., 2009). Often times, the first task a new mother judges herself on is the ability to feed her infant; feeding her child often becomes a lifelong benchmark she uses to evaluate her parenting success (McGrath, 2007b). For families, mealtime is a social event involving interaction and interchange as well as nourishment. It is usually a time of family bonding, sharing, and togetherness. Many cultural celebrations (e.g., holidays, birthdays, weddings, birth, and death ceremonies) involve meals. Thus, when a family has a child who is a difficult eater, the entire family is affected.

Feeding issues are even more significant for preterm infants because of the relative uncertainty of their growth

and development. Once the preterm infant has attained cardiorespiratory stability, successful gastric feeding and breast or bottle-feeding is the next major objective of NICU care. PMA along with consistent weight gain continues to be used to assess oral bottle-feeding readiness; however, some practitioners are beginning to use behavioral competencies as useful criteria (Edwards et al., 2019). However, nursing practices and protocols in the NICU generally are based more on routines ("the way we've always done it") than on research findings. As Conway (1994; p. 71) stated, "Few other routine tasks of neonatal nursing require as much expertise and offer as few objective measurements of the outcome as bottle-feeding the premature infant." Although this quote is dated, in reality it could be said today because oral feeding is not an area of great interest for caregivers and researchers. There are only a handful of nurse researchers who are examining oral feeding and strategies to best support infant and family success in this crucial area of NICU caregiving.

Families of preterm infants might not be well prepared to feed their high-risk infants. The NICU's emphasis on technology and numbers rather than on infant behaviors as well as the standardized way in which care is delivered leads to what has been termed as the "medicalization" of families in the NICU (McGrath, 2000). The importance of feeding can get lost amid the chaos and routines, and thus, families might not be well prepared to feed their infants after discharge. Families of preterm infants are already at greater risk for difficulties with bonding, attachment, and parenting that can only be compounded by problems with breast or bottle-feeding (Cannella, 2005; D'Agata et al., 2016). Therefore, oral feeding is an area of neonatal care that cannot be overlooked. It might even need to be assigned a higher priority, given our greater understanding of the need to positively affect the bond between the mother and infant to support long-term development. It is also concerning that preterm infants might continue to be discharged more immature and at earlier PMAs with breastfeeding or bottle-feeding interventions occurring more and more in the home environment.

GASTROINTESTINAL TRACT: ANATOMIC AND PHYSIOLOGIC LIMITATIONS

At birth, the neonate's gastrointestinal (GI) system must be able to provide a multitude of functions, including nutrient digestion and absorption, fluid and electrolyte maintenance, and immunologic protection against various toxins and bacteria. To support the neonate's energy requirements for basal metabolism and growth, the GI tract must have the functional capacity for efficient digestion and absorption of carbohydrates, fats, and proteins.

In utero, the placenta provides for the nutritional needs of the fetus and facilitates function of the fetal gastrointestinal tract while it is maturing. Although the anatomic development of the fetal gut is essentially complete by 20 weeks' gestation, maturation of physiologic function does not occur until later in gestation and extends throughout the early postnatal period (Ngo & Shah, 2020). Thus, at full-term birth, although structurally mature, the functional ability of the GI tract of the neonate is continuing to develop and is somewhat inefficient in its capabilities for digestion, fluid and electrolyte maintenance, and immunologic protection. These concerns are even more apparent for the preterm infant (see Box "Postconceptual Age and Associated Feeding Behaviors").

The fetal intestine is derived from the endoderm germ layer, and by 12 weeks all anatomic divisions of the intestinal tract are present. The development of the fetal intestine is divided into four processes that occur during gestation: cytodifferentiation, digestion, absorption, and motility (Ngo & Shah, 2020). Many of the complications of the preterm infant are dependent on the timing of delivery and the corresponding fetal GI development.

At approximately 4 weeks' gestation, the stomach develops from the ectoderm. The length of the intestine at 21 weeks is approximately 50 cm, and by 40 weeks the length has exponentially grown to 200 cm (Sato & Chang, 2016). The mesoderm is believed to be responsible for expression of the first digestive enzymes. Functionality of the gastrointestinal tract begins with the development of these enzymes. Intestinal villi begin to develop at 7 weeks and develop throughout the entire intestine by 14 weeks (Kenner, 2020).

By week eight, enzymes including aminopeptidase, sucrase, and lactase begin to emerge. These enzymes are most abundant in the jejunum. Lactase activity does not reach the maximum until 40 weeks of gestation (Sato & Chang, 2016). This low level of lactase is thought to be a contributing factor to preterm infant's intolerance and malabsorption of growth factors and nutrients. For this reason, lactose comprises only 40% of total carbohydrates in preterm formula. The process of absorption is also highly dependent on lactase (Sato & Chang, 2016). This enzyme is crucial for the digestion of carbohydrates in breast milk. The ability to absorb glucose from lactose digestion develops near birth. This insufficient activity of the lactase enzyme in the preterm infant is what often leads to malabsorption and feeding intolerance.

The GI tract has a muscular structure that consists of two layers—an inner circular sheath overlaid by an outer longitudinal coating of muscle tissues. The circular layer begins to develop at 5 weeks' gestation, whereas the outer layer is not appreciated until approximately 8 weeks' gestation. The layers thicken with increasing gestational age and are responsible for motility within the GI tract. Intestinal motility in four stages with increasing gestational age: disorganized motility from 25 to 40 weeks, the fetal complex from 30 to 33 weeks, propagation of the migrating motor complex from 33 to 36 weeks, and mature interdigestive motility from 36 weeks to term (Ngo & Shah, 2020). Thus, an infant born at 25 weeks' gestation has gastric motility that is approximately 60% of that of a term infant (Ngo & Shah, 2020).

Intestinal motility has been described and identified by the PMA at which motility dramatically improves (Kenner, 2020) Considerable improvement has been noted at 32 weeks' gestation, and with infants whose mothers had received prenatal steroids it demonstrated a more mature pattern than that of infants of comparable gestations. Motility appears to be a function of gestation, postnatal maturation, and disease state, with a link to central nervous system (CNS) maturation. There is a 4-fold increase noted in gastric motility between 28 and 38 weeks PMA. If intestinal motility is

---

Postconceptual Age and Associated Feeding Behaviors

Postconceptional Age (weeks)	Behavior
9.5	Perioral stimulation produces mouth opening and movement
12–17	Active swallowing and sucking routinely noted
14	Basic taste bud morphology and nerve supply develops
16–17	Swallowing regulates the amount of amniotic fluid
24	Ganglion cells have innervated the gastrointestinal system
28	Rooting, swallowing, and sucking reflex are present but slow/imperfect
32	Gag reflex present
	Nonnutritive sucking present
34	Functional suck/swallow/breath pattern but poor endurance
36	Coordinated suck/swallow/breath pattern

Data from Ngo, K. D., & Shah, M. (2020). Gastrointestinal system. In Kenner, C., Altimier, L. B., & Boykova, M. V. (Eds.], *Comprehensive neonatal nursing care: A physiologic perspective* (6th ed., pp. 179–210). Springer.

the limiting factor in the progression of enteral feedings, it should be identified as such before several formula changes are tried. It is essential to identify the specific source of the enteral feeding characteristics so that a plan can be devised to eliminate the causative factor.

In the premature and critically ill child, the provision of adequate nutritional support for growth and development is an ongoing challenge. Limitations of gastrointestinal function cause the infants to be at risk for dehydration, reflux, malabsorption, electrolyte imbalance, and necrotizing enterocolitis (NEC). Because the development of motility and peristalsis occurs during the third trimester, premature infants have higher risks. Infants who have cardiorespiratory disease require assisted ventilation, and those who are physiologically unstable will also have a delay in oral motor coordination as well as GI function, as the gut might be compromised secondary to these other medical conditions (Ngo & Shah, 2020).

Gastrointestinal function that is immature at birth increases the risk of malabsorption and malnutrition. Functional and anatomic maturation includes the suck–swallow reflexes, esophageal motility, function of the lower esophageal sphincter, gastric emptying, intestinal motility, and development of the absorptive surface area. Esophageal motility is decreased in the newborn during the first 12 hours. The lower esophageal sphincter is primarily above the diaphragm and subject to intrathoracic pressures, which results in esophageal reflux. Esophageal reflux is common and can be seen on a radiographic film in 38% of normal term infants in the first week of life; more than 70% of preterm infants have reflux; however, most are asymptomatic. The sphincter remains small and inadequate in these high-risk infants for the first 6 to 12 months. Gastric emptying takes a minimum of 2 to 6 hours.

When determining the preterm infant's physiologic capacity for safe and effective oral feeding, the infant's gestational age (GA) and PMA are important factors to consider. This means that the infant's ability to establish and maintain successful oral feeding by breast or bottle will primarily depend on the degree of structural and functional development of the preterm infant's GI tract and oral cavity (Table 15-1). There are several developmental handicaps that might disrupt or delay the successful transition to oral feeds: (1) immature suck–swallow–breathe coordination, (2) absent or weak cough and gag reflexes, (3) incompetent gastroesophageal sphincter, (4) delayed gastric emptying, (5) decreased intestinal motility, (6) incompetent ileocecal valve, and (7) impaired rectosphincteric reflex. Each of these needs to be considered and evaluated within a careful nutritional assessment to best understand what exactly is delaying the successful transition to oral feeding.

ENTERAL FEEDING

Gavage Feedings

Gavage feedings are provided for premature infants before the maturation of suck, swallow, and breathing. Box "Postconceptual Age and Associated Feeding Behaviors" shows the progression of sucking and swallowing development. The gavage tube can be placed either orally or nasally and is usually a semisoft catheter of 3.5 to 8 Fr, depending on the size of the infant. Feedings can then be delivered via gravity or over a pump to control the duration of the feeding.

Tube Placement

For placement, the tube is first measured by extending it from the xiphoid process to the ear of the infant and then to the mouth or nares and adding 1 cm. The tube can be inserted quickly and smoothly into the nares or mouth while the infant is offered a pacifier. Insertion orally can be slightly more difficult; however, the same technique can be utilized to decrease the stress of insertion. The tube is secured to the side of the mouth or nares with tape or other clear adhesive dressing. Many of the clear adhesive dressings are kinder and gentler to the delicate skin of the preterm infant. The tube can be

TABLE 15-1 Anatomical Differences Between the Full-Term Infant and Preterm Infant Mouth and Pharynx		
Structure	Full-Term Infant	Preterm Infant
Oral cavity	"Potential space"	Large space
Buccal pads	Large	Small or absent
Lips	Large, inactive	Small, inactive
Tongue	Relative size	Small
Soft palate	Full closure	Weak, incomplete
Jaw	Stable	Hypermobile
Hyoid	Stable	Unstable
Larynx	Muscular closure	Weak closure
Arytenoids	Large	Smaller bulk
Nasal passage	Nose breathers	Often O_2 dependent

removed after each feeding or left indwelling for 1 to 3 days. However, some of the softer Silastic tubes might be left in place for a month or more. In the past, checking for placement was done by inserting air into the tube and listening for a gastric bubble; recently this technique has been found to be somewhat inaccurate, and checking the aspirate from the tube for gastric pH might be a more reliable technique for assessing tube placement into the stomach of infants (Farrington et al., 2009; de Souza Barbosa Dias et al., 2017).

Trophic Feedings

Trophic gavage feedings provided within the first few days of life to preterm infants are the standard of care in many NICUs. These early subnutritional feedings are usually small (a few milliliters), dilute (often 50%-strength formula or expressed breast milk), and frequent (approximately every 2 hours). These feedings are most often provided by gravity via a gavage tube (Ehrenkranz, 2007). Results from research are varied; however, there seems to be greater evidence from both retrospective analysis and controlled trials of increased feeding tolerance, fewer residuals, and fewer numbers of days to full feeding with a decreased incidence of NEC (Gephart et al., 2012). Infants who received early feedings experience less time to full enteral feedings and regained any weight loss experienced and decreased days on the ventilator and on aminophylline than those infants who received later supplementation. However, in a recent Cochrane review conducted by Morgan et al. (2013) the evidence remains mixed and no recommendations could be made, because the important benefits could not be said to outweigh potential risks; more research is needed. In addition, it is important to note that how fast these early feedings are progressed is important as well as the number of calories and osmolarity of the feedings in relationship to the development of NEC (Gephart et al., 2012; Gregory, 2008). Thinking about these feedings as "gut priming" rather than truly providing nutrition in the early weeks of care may be important in our management of early feeding of very-low-birth-weight (VLBW) infants.

Orogastric Feedings Versus Nasogastric Feedings

Enteral tube feedings minimize the premature infant's energy expenditure during feeding; however, which method is best, nasogastric (NG) or orogastric (OG)? This issue has been debated throughout the literature, and practice differs from nursery to nursery as well as from individual caregiver to caregiver. With proper tube placement into the stomach and not into the lower end of the esophagus, Hawes et al. (2004) found no difference in weight gain, apnea, or bradycardia between preterm infants who received either indwelling NG or intermittent OG feedings. However, it has been hypothesized that the nasal feeding tube might be less optimal because of the increased airway resistance in the nares and the continuous inhibition of the esophageal sphincter, increasing the risk of reflux. Even the placement of the tube

can cause irritability in the infant and adversely affect breathing. Indwelling tubes might be more economical (changed less often), and this may be cited as the only clinically significant difference in the two methods of enteral feedings. Irrespective of which method the caregiver chooses, insertion might be what causes the greatest distress for the infant and should be done skillfully with a pacifier in a fluid process. Once the tube is placed, the feeding should be administered by gravity for 15 to 30 minutes; if too large a feeding tube is used, the feeding could flow in too fast and increase the risk for reflux. In addition, it is best if the tube feeding is attended; that is, that the nurse remain at the bedside and be available should the infant have difficulty with the feeding. Some of the newest research actually suggest that holding the infant during the gastric feeding may have better long-term outcomes; however, the findings are mixed and more research is needed (Peters et al., 2008; Pickler et al., 2020).

Continuous Versus Bolus Feedings

Other research has focused on the use of continuous feedings versus intermittent gavage feedings rather than just the question of an indwelling catheter or not. In a systematic review conducted by Premji and Chessell (2011), infants across the studies were all premature and weighed less than 1,500 g. They found that it was difficult to make comparisons across groups because consistent variables and outcomes were not examined and most studies had very small sample sizes. Although no recommendation as to which feeding method to use could be made, they did find that continuous feedings resulted in a longer period of time to reach full enteral feedings. There were no differences in days to maximal growth or discharge or in the incidence of NEC. Dsilna et al. (2005) found that continuously fed VLBW infants achieved full gavage feeding faster and gained more efficiently; however, no long-term effects were examined in this randomized controlled trial (RCT). In a more recent RCT, Dsilna et al. (2008) examined the stress response of preterm infants with intermittent orogastric or nasogastric gavage feedings compared with those with continuous nasogastric gavage feeding. Those in the intermittent groups demonstrated a statistically significant higher need for behavioral and physiologic stabilization during the feeding. The stress was not significantly different between the two intermittent groups. Given these results continuous gastric feedings might be more appropriate for the easily stressed, extremely low-birth-weight infant during the first weeks of life with transition to intermittent feedings at a later time. More research in this area is needed if we are to better understand ways to best feed the high-risk preterm infant.

Nursing Interventions During Gavage Feedings

Routine nursing care during gavage feedings should include abdominal assessments consisting of palpation, auscultation, and abdominal girths at least every 4 hours, with more close assessment when any one parameter has changed in the previous 4 hours. It has been suggested that aspirates/residuals should not be checked routinely and that checking for residuals could actually cause more harm than good (Parker et al., 2015; Parker et al., 2019b). However, if the infant is demonstrating other signs of feeding intolerance, then possibly checking a residual seems appropriate, but not routinely checking for residuals. The infant's behavioral cues also need to be a part of this routine assessment. Always consider what has been happening to and around the infant when examining the infant; their behaviors tell you much about how they are feeling. The duration of tube feedings is also related to the duration of the hospital stay. Those with a longer duration of tube feedings generally have longer hospitalizations (Griffith et al., 2018).Transition to bottle-feeding can be facilitated during gavage feeding in a number of ways. Several strategies are listed in Box "Interventions to Facilitate Transition to Oral Feeding," with supporting rationale and evidence from the literature. Transition to oral feeding also has implications for mother–infant interaction. Infants who have little difficulty with the transition to oral feeding also seem more available for mother–infant interactions while those that have more difficulties are often perceived to be more difficult (Silberstein et al., 2009). In general, mothers of infants who have difficult transitions have poorer interactions with their infants.

BREASTFEEDING

Decreasing the length of stay of infants in the NICU continues to be a focus of care with an important emphasis on discharging functional, mature infants (Lean et al., 2018). General standards exist to guide the preparation of families for NICU discharge and includes content related to technical baby skills (Smith et al., 2013). Such readiness skills include physiological stability, consistent weight gain, and successful oral feeding from a bottle or breast (Kish, 2014; Smith et al., 2013). Successful oral feeding is an exceptionally complex task of infancy (Briere et al., 2014b). Moreover, the mastery of bottle-feeding is often perceived to be a marker of feeding success (Collins et al., 2016; Kanhadilok & McGrath, 2015; McGrath & Braescu, 2004) and is required before discharge even if the mother intends to breastfeed (Collins et al., 2016).

More understanding and research are needed to support breastfeeding as the standard of care for this vulnerable population. It is highly recommended that all infants

Interventions to Facilitate Transition to Oral Feeding

Nursing Intervention	Supportive Rationale	Level of Evidence	References
Oral stimulation prior to feeding and support of chin and cheeks during feeding	Has been shown to positively affect feeding success. The facial muscles of the preterm infant are underdeveloped, and the infant has no buccal pads to support the intensity of sucking needed to generate milk flow	III IV	Boiron et al. [2007] Hwang et al. [2010] Fucile et al. [2012] Kish [2014]
Nonnutritive sucking	Accelerates maturation of the sucking reflex Improves weight gain Decreases oxygen consumption Facilitates earlier advancement to full oral feeding and earlier discharge	I II II III IV	Foster et al. [2016] Pineda et al. [2019] Yildiz and Arikan [2012] Bingham et al. [2010] Rocha et al. [2007] Hanzer et al. [2009]
Tactile and kinesthetic interventions prior to feeding	Behavioral calming of infant provided infant with increased alertness for feeding	II	Fucile et al. [2012]
Prone or side-lying position during and after feeding	Improves gastric emptying Decreases regurgitation and aspiration	III	Ramirez et al. [2006]
Reduction of noxious environmental stimulation	Reduces hypoxia Decreases fluctuations in oxygenation that could affect the GI tract Promotes behavioral state that is conducive to social interaction [alertness]	IV II III	Silberstein et al. [2009]
Skin-to-skin contact [Kangaroo care]	Decreases stress and increases sleep Increases social interaction	II III	Briere et al. [2014a] Conde-Agudelo et al. [2016] Demirci et al. [2015]

exclusively breastfeed for the first 6 months of life with continued breastfeeding until 1 year (Kleinman & Greer, 2020). Recent recommendations also suggest the extension of complimentary breastfeeding until 2 years (Dietary Guidelines Advisory Committee, 2020). Implementation of this guideline for the high-risk preterm infant is even more critical (Boquien, 2018). Research has demonstrated many benefits of breast milk and breastfeeding for this population, including a protective effect on infant mortality (Jeeva et al., 2015), protection against infection and NEC (Gephart et al., 2012; Victora et al., 2016), and improved neurodevelopmental outcomes (Boquien, 2018; Rozé et al., 2012). Furthermore, immunologic enhancement, GI growth, and fewer morbidities are associated with breastfeeding (Gregory & Walker, 2013; Jakaitis & Denning, 2014).

Findings from a Centers for Disease Control and Prevention (CDC) report (2019) revealed the prevalence of infants receiving any breast milk varied by gestational age, with 71.3% of extremely preterm infants, 76.0% of early preterm infants, 77.3% of late preterm infants (LPIs), and 84.6% of term infants receiving any breast milk (Chiang et al., 2019). Several factors are associated with disparities in receipt of breast milk across gestational age groups, which largely include sociodemographic factors (Brownell et al., 2014; Casavant et al., 2015; Chiang et al., 2019). As such, many infants who would greatly benefit from the receipt of breast milk do not receive it. Therefore, a review of strategies to support breastfeeding for preterm infants is warranted.

Nursing Interventions to Support Breastfeeding

Research from several studies suggests the need for additional efforts to support breastfeeding in the NICU setting (Cricco-Lizza, 2016; Spatz, 2018). Findings from a study conducted by Hallowell et al. (2014) revealed that only 51% of NICUs in the United States reported having lactation consultants on staff in the NICU (Hallowell et al., 2014; Spatz, 2018). Furthermore, only 13% of NICU infants in the national sample received nurse-reported breastfeeding assistance (Hallowell et al., 2014; Spatz, 2018).

Yet, even equipped with this evidence, changing caregiving practices to best support mothers in breastfeeding and the provision of human milk to preterm infants appear to be highly influenced by the attitudes and beliefs of health professionals in the NICU. It has been found that nurses' attitudes and beliefs about their level of competency and ability to offer evidenced-based care influences the level of support that they provide to mothers in the face of breastfeeding challenges (Cricco-Lizza, 2016; Tuthill et al., 2014; Tuthill et al., 2016).

Several programmatic initiatives are available as models of care for the provision of breastfeeding in the NICU, including Meier et al. (1993) five-phase temporal model to support lactation in the NICU (Meier et al., 1993), Spatz 10-step model for human milk and breastfeeding (Spatz, 2004), the Breastfeeding Resource Model (Spatz et al., 2015), and the Ten Steps to Successful Breastfeeding into Neonatal Intensive Care (Neo-BFHI) (Nyqvist et al., 2013, 2015).

The Spatz (2021) five-phase temporal model for supporting lactation in the NICU is still in use today. This model is based on research in the area of breastfeeding support. The five phases are (1) assisting the mother with milk collection and storage, (2) gavage feeding of expressed mother's milk, (3) managing in-hospital breastfeeding, (4) breastfeeding support following the infant's discharge, and (5) consultation with the family or NICU staff/lactation consultant or both (Lucas & McGrath, 2016; Meier & Mangurten, 1993). This model incorporates use of nonpharmacologic supports to increase milk volume and ease of breastfeeding. Supports consistent across all breastfeeding models in the NICU include use of breast pumps at the infant's bedside, kangaroo care or skin-to-skin contact, and nonnutritive sucking (NNS) (Briere et al., 2014a; Foster et al., 2016).

Mothers face many challenges when providing human milk to preterm infants. Some challenges to breastfeeding in the NICU include (1) initiating and maintaining a milk supply; (2) transition from gavage to feeding at the breast; (3) infant coordination of the sucking, swallowing, and breathing necessary to both stimulate the breast and transfer milk; (4) mother–infant separation (D'Agata et al., 2016); and (5) quantifying milk transfer (how much milk is the baby getting?) (Casey et al., 2018; Hallowell et al., 2016). As such, models to support breastfeeding should tackle each of these issues holistically.

For most women, the decision to breastfeed most often occurs before birth and many times is based on family cultural norms that can be influenced by education and support antenatally (Pitts et al., 2015); however, for mothers of preterm infants, this decision is often made very quickly following the premature birth of their infant (Esquerra-Zwiers et al., 2016). Furthermore, the needs of the preterm infant for breast milk are somewhat unique and information about the importance of breast milk may not have been provided even if breastfeeding information was received in prenatal classes. In addition, preterm mothers may not have attended prenatal classes given the preterm birth. Whether or not a decision to breastfeed was made prior to birth, mothers should be approached and provided information about the benefits of breast milk and breastfeeding for the preterm infant so they can make an informed decision related to the individual needs of their infant. Mothers will often make the effort to provide breast milk once they understand the implications for their infant (Esquerra-Zwiers et al., 2016). On the other hand, if the mother ultimately chooses not to initiate lactation, care for the mother and infant should be equally as supportive to the mother's needs and choice.

Optimally, lactation is initiated in the first hour of life and is supported by a hospital-grade electric pump (Khan et al., 2015; Parker et al., 2015). Mothers will require information about pump use and human milk storage. Use of a milk production log during those first few days can be useful in helping mothers to pump regularly and build a good milk supply (Meier et al., 2013, 2017). Although there is evidence that a good maternal milk supply is correlated with more sustained lactation, milk supply in the NICU has not been correlated with increased duration of breastfeeding after discharge (Briere et al., 2014a; Hoban et al., 2018). More research needs to occur to better understand the breastfeeding needs of preterm mothers and infants after discharge.

The available evidence suggests that transitioning from gavage feedings directly to breastfeeding is optimal; however, additional research in this area is warranted (Briere et al., 2014a; Briere et al., 2015; Collins et al., 2016; Kliethermes et al., 1999). Nonetheless, use of a bottle during the first oral feeding is not necessary. Supporting mothers and infants so the first oral feeding is at the breast should be the goal. Subsequent oral feedings can be at the breast when the mother is present and by bottle when she cannot be available in the NICU. Lactation support during this transition is very important (Briere et al., 2014a; Briere et al., 2016; Ikonen et al., 2015; Mercado, Vittner, Drabant, & McGrath, 2019; Mercado, Vittner, & McGrath, 2019). Preterm infants often have weak sucks, and irregular sucking rhythms, which can be disheartening to a new mother. Mothers will require coaching and extra support to be successful with milk transfer particularly if they are young or first-time mothers (Casey et al., 2018; Kanhadilok & McGrath, 2015; Meier et al., 2010, 2017; Nyqvist et al., 2013). Nipple shields have been found to enhance milk transfer for some preterm infants and should be considered if infants are struggling with latching on to the breast. In addition, test weights before and after breastfeeding can be used to easily calculate milk transfer (Meier et al., 2013, 2017). Cup-feeding or using supplemental feeding devices may also be considered, but the research on each is mixed and both have been used more successfully in developing countries (Penny, Brownell, et al., 2018; Penny, Judge, et al., 2018). More evidence is needed to understand how best to support the mother and infant during the transition to fully directly breastfeeding particularly if the mother prefers the infant not be bottle-fed.

Supporting breastfeeding in the NICU can be time intensive for the nurse at the bedside. Many patterns of caregiving in the NICU decrease the likelihood that mothers will be encouraged or supported to provide breast milk or to breastfeed their preterm infants (Briere et al., 2014a; Cricco-Lizza, 2016). Nurses are at the crux of the institutional culture in the NICU, which is regulated through policies and procedures—both written and unwritten. Furthermore, the culture of the NICU often rewards technical proficiency and adherence to the guidelines, policies, and procedures that may encourage less than optimal engagement with the family; however, such engagement often is necessary to promote and support successful initiation of maternal milk supply and maintain breastfeeding (Briere et al., 2014a; Cricco-Lizza, 2016).

There is no shortage of reasons for why breastfeeding disparities exist in the NICU (Cartagena et al., 2021). Funding for breastfeeding research remains inadequate.

Thus, research findings are growing but are still not sufficient to fully guide caregiving in this area. Knowledge about the properties of breast milk (Wu et al., 2018) and the implementation of breastfeeding in the NICU (Esquerra-Zwiers et al., 2016) remain limited for both nursing and medicine. These topics are often brief in basic educational programs and may not be considered essential material for orientation to the NICU. In addition, if there is didactic content, clinical experience related directly to implementation is seldom a requirement. Breastfeeding remains marginalized in the quantitative world of medicine. Since parental nutrition and formulas designed specifically to meet the needs of the preterm infants are easily available, they are often used as the first line of care. In contrast, provision of mother's own milk or donor human milk and ultimately breastfeeding are often seen as adjunct but not central to the nutritional support of the preterm infant. Furthermore, the industrial influence of formula companies and the lack of support for breastfeeding mothers in the workplace add to implementation barriers. Finally, nursing attitudes and social pressure within the NICU culture also have a significant impact on the intention to perform interventions (Cricco-Lizza, 2016). With the advent of evidence-based practice thinking and protocols, the relative importance and prioritization of breastfeeding interventions has the potential to change if time, resources, and support are provided to mothers/infants, bedside nurses, and all NICU health professionals.

Several strategies have been utilized to support mothers in breastfeeding their preterm infants, including (1) provision of information about benefits as well as the anatomy and physiology of breastfeeding; (2) provision of support such as peer mentors, family support, and nursing support; and (3) provision of resources such as breast pumps, milk storage supplies, and use of equipment to support lactoengineering (Lucas et al., 2014; Merewood et al., 2006; Spatz, 2004, 2005, 2006). Ultimately, implementation of these strategies requires nurses to have expert knowledge in this area. Spatz (2005) has successfully implemented a comprehensive program to support nurses who are providing breastfeeding care to mothers/infants at the bedside in the NICU. This comprehensive program addresses all areas of caregiving and includes 16 hours of didactic classes. Several topics are integrated into the content outline, such as benefits of breast milk, role of culture and support, resources in the institution to support breastfeeding, anatomy and physiology of breastfeeding, composition of breast milk, maternal nutritional requirements, breast pumping issues, lactoengineering, transition to the breast, care of the breast, work and breastfeeding, human milk banking, and sexuality issues. In addition, the participants have the opportunity to evaluate a breastfeeding session, including latching-on, positioning, and interventions to support the mother as well as test weights for estimating consumption. The classes are interactive and have received excellent reviews. The classes are not required for the staff nurse to work in the NICU; however, paid time to attend is provided. More than half of the staff has participated and found the information to be beneficial and meaningful to their caregiving (Spatz, 2005). Similar programs must be implemented with all NICU professionals to best support the initiation of milk expression and breastfeeding, so these practices become routine in the care of preterm infants.

BREASTFEEDING IN OTHER HIGH-RISK NICU POPULATIONS

Breastfeeding the Late Preterm Infant

Like the other premature infant literature, much of the neonatal breastfeeding literature is focused on infants less than 33 weeks' gestation. According to the National Institute of Child Health and Human Development (NICHD), infants born between 34 0/7 and 36 6/7 weeks of gestation are considered as late preterm (Engle, 2006). This designation establishes a standard terminology and underscores the fact that these infants' characteristics align closer with those of preterm infants as opposed to term infants (Boies & Vaucher, 2016; Engle, 2006). Evidence suggests the importance of feeding considerations for LPIs and emphasizes the feeding-related morbidities experienced by LPIs compared with term infants (Boies & Vaucher, 2016; Ray & Lorch, 2013; Young et al., 2013). Feeding the LPI presents a challenge to care providers, as the infant may not be able to fully coordinate the suck–swallow–breathe pattern and can result in fatigue (Cartwright et al., 2017). In addition, neurodevelopmental immaturity may inhibit these infants to give feeding readiness cues and thus make oral feeding difficult (Pike et al., 2017).

Breastfeeding provides an even greater challenge with greater risk for inadequate nutrition particularly if discharge occurs prior to the mother's milk coming in and successful feeding establishment. These infants had fewer awake periods and less stamina and generally did a poorer job of stimulating and emptying the breast, often resulting in poor milk production (Briere, Lucas, et al., 2015; Cartwright et al., 2017). Many times, milk supply is not established prior to discharge of infants in well-baby nurseries, and when coupled with the LPI's inability to stimulate supply, these infants are at high risk for readmission (Boies & Vaucher, 2016; Ray & Lorch, 2013; Young et al., 2013).

The Academy of Breastfeeding Medicine (ABM, 2016) provides guidelines regarding breastfeeding the LPI (Boies & Vaucher, 2016). Parents must be educated on what cues their infants will give and when to wake their infant up to feed them if the infant is sleepy. Furthermore, establishing how much intake their infant will require and what kind of assistance a breastfeeding mother may need should be determined prior to discharge. Close interaction with the lactation team to help determine milk supply and transfer will ensure better hydration and weight gain for these infants. This guideline states that breastfed infants should be seen by their healthcare provider 48 hours after discharge and visiting nursing services should be offered as a resource to assist in proper hydration

and weight gain for the LPI (Boies & Vaucher, 2016). There are many aspects of breastfeeding that are beyond the scope of this book; however, the Academy of Breastfeeding Medicine guidelines provides several principles of care for the LPI available for review (Boies & Vaucher, 2016).

Breastfeeding Infants With Prenatal Opioid Exposure

The resulting impact of the "opioid epidemic" in the United States has immensely affected pregnant and parenting women and their infants (Grossman et al., 2017). Prenatal exposure to opioids (POE) is associated with opioid withdrawal causing severe CNS and gastrointestinal irritability in infants (Klaman et al., 2017). If symptoms persist, an infant with POE may be subsequently diagnosed with neonatal abstinence syndrome (NAS), sometimes called neonatal opioid withdrawal symptom (Klaman et al., 2017). Symptoms of withdrawal may influence their feeding behaviors and subsequently the mother–infant relationship (Maguire et al., 2015). Moreover, several studies suggest that breastfeeding is a nonpharmacologic intervention that has the capacity to reduce NAS symptom severity and, thus, pharmacological treatment and length of hospital stay (LOS) (Cirillo & Francis, 2016; Dryden et al., 2012; Favara et al., 2019). Several professional organizations subscribe to the safety of breastfeeding for mothers receiving medication-assisted treatment (MAT) for opioid use disorder (OUD) and recommend it for infants with POE (Clark, 2019). Despite the evidence regarding the importance of feeding as a growth-fostering process, breastfeeding rates for mother–infant dyads affected by POE are disparate, with breastfeeding cessation most often occurring in the first week post birth (Demirci et al., 2015).

Several barriers to breastfeeding in this population exist, including misinformation regarding the safety of breastfeeding and MAT for OUD, stigma laden care, and mother–infant separation, which often excludes the mother from care participating in the care of her infant (D'Agata et al., 2016; Demirci et al., 2015; McGlothen et al., 2018). Furthermore, findings from a recent integrative review highlights the inconsistency in evidence regarding feeding behaviors specific to infants with prenatal opioid exposure or the subsequent diagnosis of NAS; however, the literature suggests that the sucking and behavioral states may be different in infants with prenatal opioid exposure when compared with those without exposure (McGlothen-Bell et al., 2020). Nurses may support mothers of infants with POE to breastfeed by offering support and education regarding the safety of breastfeeding (Demirci et al., 2015; Groer et al., 2018; McGlothen & Cleveland, 2018; McGlothen et al., 2018). Furthermore, nurses can support the mother to engage in the care of her infant, offering nonjudgmental care, encouraging the use of kangaroo care or skin-to-skin care, and teaching the mother to read infant feeding cues to support breastfeeding (Demirci et al., 2015; McGlothen et al., 2018; McGlothen-Bell et al., 2021).

MYTHS ABOUT BREASTFEEDING IN THE NICU

In addition, there are several myths about breastfeeding and the high-risk infant that need to be addressed and disqualified so they do not continue to influence nursing caregiving practices.

1. *Myth—Successful bottle-feeding is necessary prior to initiating breastfeeding for the preterm infant.* In fact, breastfeeding increases physiologic stability in the preterm infant and is NOT more difficult than bottle-feeding (Davanzo et al., 2014; Lubbe, 2018; Park et al., 2015). Greater physiologic stability and less physical distress have been demonstrated with breastfeeding compared with bottle-feeding in preterm infants (Lin et al., 2013; Lubbe, 2018; Campbell & Miranda, 2018). There is no evidence to support the need to bottle-feed preterm infants prior to placing them at the breast (Davanzo et al., 2014; Lubbe, 2018; Park et al., 2015). This medicalization of preterm infant feeding is often a professional need to control the feeding related to amount, flow speed, and timing, and the necessity needs to be reconsidered on an individual basis.

2. *Myth—Racial and ethnic minority mothers are less likely to desire to breastfeed their preterm infants.* Moreover, breastfeeding rates in the United States are often the highest among Asian and Hispanic mothers (Beauregard et al., 2019). Although racial and ethnic disparities in breastfeeding do exist for some mother–infant dyads in the NICU, often these mothers do desire and intend to breastfeed. Evidence is growing that these disparities are more driven by the social determinants of health than other factors (DeVane-Johnson et al., 2017). For example, Parker, Weaver, et al. (2019) found that disparities in mother's milk feedings among black mothers of VLBW infants were not seen early in the NICU stay; in fact, the mothers participated in early breastfeeding initiation. However, the disparities began emerging after 3 weeks. This suggests that factors both inside and outside the hospital play a key role. As such, multilevel approaches to address social determinants of health are warranted (Cartagena et al., 2021; Howell & Ahmed, 2019).

3. *Myth—Bottle-feeding is easier, and infants are bigger and healthier with formula feeding.* There is no evidence to support this myth, and the research findings that link bottle-feeding with increased risk for diabetes and obesity indicate the conflicting findings (Section on Breastfeeding, 2012). Yet, this message is sent to mothers in many ways including pictures of smiling babies with bottles and gifts of free formula, as well as even more subliminal messages such as breastfeeding bans in public places, no place to breastfeed or use a breast pump in the workplace, and a sense that breastfeeding is somehow sexual in nature and thus needs to occur out of sight (Jones, 2012).

Myths are barriers to full integration of breastfeeding practices into routine caregiving and must be overcome with appropriate education and support for all who interact with vulnerable infants and mothers. It is important to remember that the crisis of preterm birth is a process of physiologic and psychological change for both the infant and the mother in which the need for professional support is great. Nurses in the NICU play a unique role in launching these special families. It is often the support of the nurse at the bedside that will be the deciding factor in the initiation and continued provision of breast milk and breastfeeding. Finding ways to best support nurses in the provision of role requires increased education, vigilance, and a belief that breastfeeding is as essential and important to the long-term outcomes for the infant and families as other caregiving tasks.

PHYSIOLOGY AND DEVELOPMENT OF SUCKING AND SWALLOWING

Sucking and swallowing develop in utero and mature in the fetus during the third trimester (McGrath & Braescu, 2004). Physiologic maturation appears to have a greater influence on the development of nutritive sucking (NS) abilities and swallowing than "experience" with bottle-feeding, although there is some evidence to support experience playing a complimentary role in the development of NS. This area needs to be further explored. Coordination of suck, swallow, and breathing has been considered the most complex task of infancy. At 9.5 weeks, the fetus will open its mouth following perioral stimulation, but the actual sucking response is not present until 13 to 18 weeks. Swallowing has been observed at 18 weeks, and between 28 and 30 weeks, rooting, sucking, and swallowing reflexes have all been established; however, they are not at all mature.

The swallowing reflex is well developed by 28 to 30 weeks but is easily exhausted. The swallowing reflex is completely functional by 34 weeks PMA. NS can be demonstrated in infants by 26 weeks, but a rhythmic pattern is not developed until 32 to 34 weeks. The gag reflex is complete at 34 weeks. Coordination of breath, suck, and swallow occurs beginning at 32 to 34 weeks for short periods; however, these mechanisms are not yet coordinated enough to sustain the infant's nutritional needs (see Box "Postconceptual Age and Associated Feeding Behaviors"). True synchrony of suck, swallow, and breath in a 1:1:1 pattern does not occur until 36 to 38 weeks PMA. Infants with a physiologic disability in which the absence or the weakness of the gag and cough reflexes exist should be monitored for an increased risk of aspiration. The assessment for the presence of a gag reflex can be performed by direct observation during the passing of a feeding tube. However, the adequacy of the gag reflex can be more difficult to assess and the risk of aspiration should be a consideration in all infants receiving nasal or orogastric tube feeding.

The development of competent oral feeding skills is a requisite for physiologic adaptation and survival during infancy. Oral feeding is a highly organized and intricate behavior that encompasses the activities of food seeking/obtaining, ingestion, and swallowing (McGrath & Braescu, 2004). Physiologically, oral feeding involves complex interaction of the brain and

CNS, oral motor reflexes, and multiple muscles of the mouth, pharynx, esophagus, and face (Barlow, 2009; Delaney & Arvedson, 2008). Infant oral feeding requires the rhythmic coordination of sucking and swallowing a bolus of fluid while at the same time balancing the demands for breathing (Barlow, 2009; Stumm et al., 2008). Oral feeding has been regarded as the most highly organized behavioral activity of early infancy.

For term infants, oral feeding is a "natural physiologic process" that proceeds with minimal difficulty during the first days of life. However, the transition to oral or bottle-feedings in preterm infants might be significantly delayed as a result of anatomic and functional immaturity of the gastrointestinal system, PMA, acute and/or chronic illness, neurobehavioral maturation, oral motor dysfunction, and behavioral aversion (Box "Physiologic Influences on the Efficacy of Sucking in the Preterm Infant").

The development and physiologic process of infant oral feeding has been extensively discussed in numerous clinical and research-based publications. Conceptually, oral feeding is defined as a multifaceted series of events involving the activities of food seeking, ingestion, and deglutition (swallowing) (Lau, 2007). In addition, oral feeding is described as a highly integrated neurobehavioral process whereby the evolution of oral motor skills parallels the general sequence of fine and gross motor skill acquisition during infancy (de Costa et al., 2008; Delaney & Arvedson, 2008; Lau, 2007). Developmentally, it is suggested that the early primitive and reflex patterns of infant oral feeding are sequentially extinguished and replaced by mature feeding patterns as a result of maturational changes within the brain and CNS (Delaney & Arvedson, 2008; Lau, 2007). Research has documented a positive correlation between brain maturation and the emergence of higher-level behavioral skills (Rossier, 2009; Turk-Browne et al., 2008). Oral feeding is commonly portrayed as a three-stage process (Box "Oral Feeding: A Three-Stage Process").

Although neonates and young infants rely on parents and other caregivers to provide the nutrients needed for adequate growth and development, the establishment of competent oral feeding skills requires an intact and functioning brain and CNS, as well as the ability to rhythmically coordinate the neuromotor activities of sucking, swallowing, and breathing. During infancy, sucking, swallowing, and breathing are the essential motor components of the oral feeding process. The following sections will discuss each of these components in greater detail.

ANATOMY OF ORAL FEEDING

Sucking

Investigations of the development of oral feeding during infancy have primarily focused on bottle-feeding. Research has primarily focused on describing the neonatal sucking response, a major component of oral feeding. Sucking is a rhythmic action of the tongue and jaw that causes fluid to flow out of a nipple or maternal teat due to changes in intraoral pressure. Sucking includes both negative (suction) and positive (compression) pressure components. Sucking has been described as a push–pulling action, whereby the positive pressure changes created by the rhythmic compression of the nipple between the tongue and palate acts to push fluid out of a nipple into the oral cavity and negative pressure

---

Physiologic Influences on the Efficacy of Sucking in the Preterm Infant

- Immature sucking response
- Decreased muscle tone
- Poor state regulation
- Autonomic instability
- Disorganized sucking, swallowing, and breathing patterning

- Inability to effectively switch from nonnutritive to nutritive sucking.

Data from Case-Smith, J., Cooper, P., & Scala, V. (1989). Feeding efficiency of premature neonates. *American Journal of Occupational Therapy, 43*(4), 245–250.

Oral Feeding: A Three-Stage Process

Stage I   Entails the recognition of hunger by the infant or caregiver; acknowledgment of infant hunger cues; the process of obtaining food substances; and ingestion

Stage II   Involves the complex motor activities of deglutition (swallowing); deglutition is a complex series of neuromotor activities functioning to transport food and fluids from the mouth to the stomach while preventing the aspiration of food substances into the trachea and lungs

Stage III Entails the activities of esophageal swallowing and gastrointestinal absorption

Modified from Tuchman, D. N., & Walter, R. S. (Eds.). (1994). *Disorders of feeding and swallowing in infants and children: Pathophysiology, diagnosis, and treatment.* Singular.

changes function to draw fluid from the nipple (Lau, 2007). Negative or suction pressure is generated through rhythmic contractions of jaw muscles and tongue movements working in concert to pull fluid out of the nipple into the mouth. In bottle-feeding, the tongue appears to move in a piston-like fashion; whereas in breastfeeding, there is more of a rolling movement of the tongue.

The anatomic configuration of the mouth and pharynx support the act of suckling. Infants have a mandible that is disproportionately small compared with the skull and a tongue that fills the oral cavity leaving little space for much variation in tongue movements. The fat pads in the cheeks narrow the oral cavity further facilitating sucking action (Arvedson & Brodsky, 2002; Crapnell et al., 2013). Term infants have the capability to both organize their sucking and regulate the amount of pressure that is generated during sucking (Lau, 2007), whereas the preterm infant may not be able to achieve a similar level of sucking organization until 34 to 35 weeks PMA (Medoff-Cooper et al., 2009). In contrast, LPIs, those born between 34 1/7 and 36 6/7 weeks, are typically total oral feeders, although many show evidence of disorganized sucking patterns (Delaney & Arvedson, 2008).

A systematic review of early sucking and swallowing problems considered predictors of long-term neurodevelopmental outcomes in children with neonatal brain injury. Slattery et al. (2012) found that, in infants with hypoxic ischemic encephalopathy (HIE) and strokes in the perinatal and/or neonatal period, there is a greater than 40% incidence of difficulties with coordination necessary for successful sucking and swallowing and a 35% incidence for those with mixed brain injury diagnoses. Infants diagnosed with severe sucking difficulties during the neonatal period were reported to have severe disability on the Bayley Scales of Infant Development (BSID) at follow-up (Slattery et al., 2012). Specific sucking elements at 44 to 46 weeks PMA were found to be associated with neurodevelopmental outcomes in preterm infants at 24 months corrected age. This period might be a sensitive time of infant development in which sucking behavior is an early marker of abnormal developmental outcomes. These findings may provide opportunities for individualizing early intervention (Wolthuis-Stigter et al., 2015). In comparison with controls, infants with HIE may display significant hypertonicity of skeletal muscle components, impairment of pharyngeal provocation-induced reflexes, and smooth muscle contractile vigor, reflecting poor propagation with maturation. These mechanisms may be responsible for inadequate clearance of secretions, ascending refluxate, and oropharyngeal bolus in HIE infants (Jensen et al., 2017).

Nonnutritive Sucking

There are two types of sucking that have been described in the literature since the late 1960s—nonnutritive (NNS) and nutritive sucking (NS). NNS is defined as a repetitive pattern of mouthing activity on a pacifier and is a precursor to

NS behavior. From a developmental perspective, NNS and spontaneous mouthing movements have been observed in utero as early as 15 to 18 weeks' gestation, with maturational changes in patterns of NNS noted over time. NNS is described as alternating periods of short sucking bursts and pauses. The rate of sucking is approximately two sucks per second, with a suck-to-swallow ratio of six to eight sucks per swallow. NS occurs spontaneously or might be initiated by the presence of a pacifier in the infant's mouth. Furthermore, NS only takes place during oral feeding, whereas NNS has been observed during all sleep–wake cycles (Hanzer et al., 2009) (see Fig. 15-1), might occur at the end of a feeding, or might be interspersed between bursts of NS. NNS has been recommended for full-term infants as preventive of sudden infant death syndrome because of the way infants breathe during active NNS and how NNS activity appears to regulate breathing in the neonate (Hanzer et al., 2010; Hauck et al., 2005). It has been recommended that NNS be encouraged during sleep especially during the first 6 months of life and then weaned over the next 6 months to prevent otitis media.

Measures of NNS organization has been studied as a predictor for NS in preterm infants (Bingham et al., 2010; Psaila & Patterson, 2016). Bingham et al. (2010) found that infants with a more organized NNS sucking pattern transitioned from first oral feeding to full oral feedings faster. However, GA and PMA of the infants were also highly linked with transition times. More recently, the findings of Pineda et al. (2019) concur with these previous results. They also found that NNS integrity increased with PMA and maybe correlated with medical complications; however, the sample size for this study was small (Pineda et al., 2019). A Cochrane review found that NNS is associated with decreased length of stay (LOS) and earlier and faster transitions to full oral feeding such that NNS should be offered with all gavage feedings (Foster et al., 2016). Rocha et al. (2007) examined the use of NNS with sensory stimulation prior to the introduction of oral feedings in

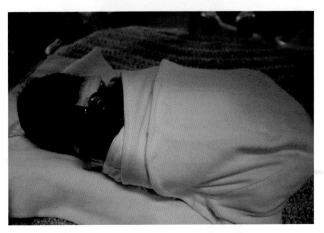

FIGURE 15-1. Infant swaddled with pacifier and hands free near face. [Photo courtesy of Joan Smith, RN, MNS, NNP-BC and Mary Raney, RN, MSN, NNP-BC, St. Louis Children's Hospital, NICU.]

preterm infants and found that infants initiated oral feeding sooner and progressed to full feedings more quickly with a decreased LOS (see Figs. 15-2 and 15-3). Because of the association between NNS and better oral feeding progression Neiva and associates (2008) created a scoring system to use as a means to evaluate when oral feeding in preterm infants might begin. More research needs to be done with this tool before predictive validity can be established. NNS just before bottle-feeding has been found to be associated with improved oxygen saturations. However, in a more recent study, Pickler and Reyna (2004) did not find that prefeeding NNS affected NS, breathing during feeding, or other behavioral characteristics. The relationship between NNS and NS remains an area where more understanding is needed.

Another aspect of NNS that is under investigation is long-term effects on dental formation (Warren & Bishara, 2002). In an epidemiologic study of children aged 1 to 3 years (Jorge et al., 2009) prevalence of dental trauma and NNS habits were not statistically related. However, Ferrini et al. (2008) found an increased prevalence of enamel defects in very-low- and extremely low-birth-weight infants that was highly correlated with NNS sucking habits. Benefits and risks of interventions always need to be weighed in caregiving decisions. The long-term effects must be part of our considerations when it comes to all aspects of feeding.

Nutritive Sucking

In contrast, NS is defined as the pattern of sucking that occurs when a bolus of fluid is introduced into the infant's mouth (Conway, 1994). NS is organized as a continuous sequence of long and slow bursts of sucking at pressures sufficient to deliver fluid from a nipple. Research has described the developmental progression and maturation of NS following birth.

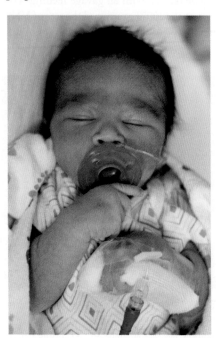

FIGURE 15-2. Infant alert with pacifier for self-regulation. [Used with parental permission. Photo courtesy of family.]

Infants born before 32 weeks GA demonstrate mouthing movements not associated with effective sucking. Between 32 and 36 weeks' gestation, preterm infants display an immature pattern of sucking that consists of short sucking bursts occurring at a rate of 1 to 1.5 sucks per second. In this stage of development, swallowing either precedes or follows each sucking burst. A more mature pattern of NS usually emerges by 35 to 36 weeks' gestation and is characterized by prolonged bursts of 10 to 30 sucks per second with a suck-to-swallow ratio of 1:1 (da Costa et al., 2010; McGrath et al., 2021).

In addition, physiologic studies of neonatal sucking during bottle-feeding have found that NS comprises two distinct phases: a continuous sucking phase and an intermittent sucking phase. Continuous sucking patterns occur during the first 2 minutes of oral feeding and are depicted by long, uninterrupted sucking bursts accompanied by brief pauses in sucking. As sucking continues, an intermittent pattern of NS emerges, which is characterized by shorter bursts of sucking alternating with three to five periods of sucking pauses. It also appears that sucking patterns change during the course of breastfeeding. Research suggests that sucking frequency, patterning of bursts and sucking pauses, and ratio of sucks to swallows are significantly influenced by changes in rate of milk flow during maternal "let down."

da Costa et al. (2010) showed that small for gestation age (SGA) infants demonstrated lack of coordination more often than their age appropriate (AGA) peers. The SGA infants took a median of 6 weeks longer to reach "normal sucking patterns" when compared with AGA infants, thus leading to gavage-assisted feeds for a longer period of time. Gestational age and birth weight were two factors that explained 35% of the variance between normal and abnormal sucking patterns. This study connected impaired sucking patterns with neurologic dysfunction (da Costa et al., 2010).

Milk Volume Intake During Nutritive Sucking

Research suggests that the volume of fluid expressed per suck is regulated by a combination of factors including nipple flow rates, sucking efficiency, sucking patterns, taste, and characteristics of containers used for bottle-feeding (Pados et al., 2019; Pados et al., 2016). In studies investigating the effects of various types of nipple units upon milk flow during bottle-feeding for term and preterm infants, Pados et al. (2016, 2019) found wide variability in milk flow within and among the various types of nipples that are used for bottle-feeding term and preterm infants. The firmness or pliability of the nipple and size of the nipple hole are important determinants of milk flow during bottle-feeding. High-flow nipple units, such as those used for preterm infants, are generally softer in consistency and have larger feeding holes (Pados et al., 2019; Scheel et al., 2005). Nipples used for term or older preterm infants might be stiffer in consistency, with a wide range of feeding hole sizes. All nipple-unit types have similar flow patterns—the bigger the hole, the larger the flow of milk (Chang et al., 2007; Pados et al., 2019).

The use of high-flow nipple units for bottle-feeding preterm infants has been based on the assumption that

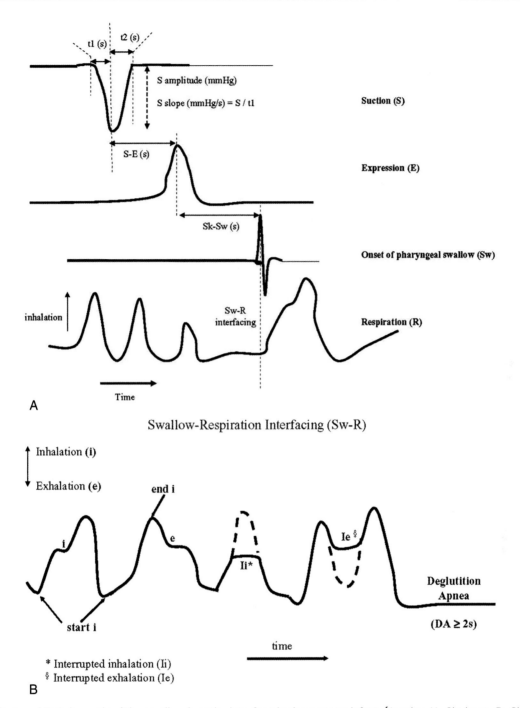

FIGURE 15-3. A and **B.** Schematic of the swallow breathe interface in the preterm infant. [Amaizu, N., Shulman, R., Shanler, R., & Lau, C. [2008]. Maturation of oral feeding skills in preterm infants. *Acta Pediatrica, 97*[1], 61–67.]

faster milk flow compensates for the preterm infant's limited ability to generate sufficient pressures requisite for oral feeding (Scheel et al., 2005). However, there are limited empiric data to support this premise (Pados et al., 2019). Stable respiratory patterns and better oxygenation and less drooling and choking have been associated with use of orally supportive nipples with low flow (Pados et al., 2019). Research also suggests that the rate of milk flow might be affected by the characteristics of the containers used during bottle-feeding and the osmolality of the milk. Collapsible feeding bags were associated with faster

feeding rates compared with the slower feeding demonstrated with the use of glass containers. It is thought that the vacuum created during sucking from a glass container limits the amount of milk expression from the bottle. Most standard nipples used today have vent holes to overcome the vacuum effect created during sucking from glass containers. Milk (formula) that is thickened can decrease the flow and make it more difficult for the infant to suck (Pados & Mellon, 2020). The size of the nipple hole must be considered so the infant does not struggle to take in thickened feedings.

Sucking efficiency is another determinant of milk volume expression during oral feeding. The presence of congenital and/or acquired defects of the lip and/or palate and abnormalities in oral motor muscle tone (paralysis, weakness, hypertonia) can limit both the infant's ability to form an adequate lip seal and the ability to generate sufficient pressure changes required for effective sucking. Sucking efficiency can also be influenced by characteristics associated with prematurity, including an immature sucking response, low muscle tone, poor state regulation, autonomic instability, disorganized sucking–swallowing and breathing patterning, and the inability to effectively switch from NNS to NS. Given the existing evidence, some neonatal care providers choose not to routinely use preemie nipples because of the increased milk flow they provide. They use standard nipples right from the initiation of oral feeding because they will not provide increased flow during a time when the infant is just learning to coordinate the highly organized process of bottle-feeding. However, what might be best of all is choosing a particular nipple for a particular baby and not having any standard process for nipple selection during initiation of bottle-feeding. Individualizing the process requires accurate assessment and a team of professionals working together to facilitate infant success during the process.

Swallowing

Swallowing, or deglutition, is also an integral component of infant oral feeding and includes the entire act from fluid placement in the mouth until the fluid enters the stomach (Dodds, 1989). Swallowing is a complex and coordinated motor activity that functions to transport food and fluids from the mouth to the stomach while preventing the aspiration of food substances into the trachea and lungs. Swallowing undergoes developmental maturation during the fetal period, which continues after birth. The control of swallowing occurs in multiple levels of the nervous system. There are both sensory and motor systems relevant to swallowing and thus oral feeding. There are three distinct phases of swallowing—oral, pharyngeal, and esophageal. During early infancy, the oral phase of deglutition is a reflex activity that initiates with NS.

The second phase of deglutition, known as the pharyngeal phase, comprises a sequential series of semiautomatic movements that are triggered by the presence of liquid or solid food in the oral cavity. Pharyngeal deglutition involves the preparation of the oral–nasal cavity, airway, and esophagus for the movement of fluid or food bolus into the pharynx and ultimately into the esophagus. As the infant swallows, breathing is "reflexively" suppressed, and the upward movement of the epiglottis closes the airway and laryngohyoid complex, thereby preventing the aspiration of food contents into the tracheobronchial tree.

Phase III, or esophageal deglutition, entails the delivery of food or liquids into the stomach by the peristaltic contractions of the esophagus and the concurrent automatic inhibition of the upper esophageal sphincter. Esophageal deglutition is activated by the presence of food in the esophagus and is thought to be a continuation of pharyngeal deglutition. Developmental patterns of swallowing in preterm infants have been described. Preterm infants establish a swallow rhythm as early as 32 weeks PMA, which remains unchanged through 40 weeks PMA. Beyond term, the maturation of swallowing rates is characterized by increased frequency and coordination with sucking behaviors (Lau et al., 2003).

Breathing

Breathing is an autonomic process that we seldom acknowledge except when we have a cold or increased work of breathing, such as during exercise. In the full-term infant, the process is much the same. However, the immaturity of the preterm respiratory system impairs the mechanics of breathing. Preterm infants are at increased risk for aspiration, apnea, and periodic breathing, which is increasingly apparent during feeding (Barlow, 2009; Thoyre & Carlson, 2003) especially for infants who already have respiratory compromise such as those with bronchopulmonary dysplasia (Howe, Sheu, et al., 2007; Mizuno et al., 2007; Vice & Gewolb, 2008). The issue of coordination of sucking, swallowing, and breathing is of concern for these infants.

Sucking, Swallowing, and Breathing

Safe and successful oral feeding in neonates requires well-coordinated sucking, swallowing, and breathing sequencing (Delaney & Arvedson, 2008; Kelly et al., 2007). Coordination of sucking, swallowing, and breathing is related to the type of sucking (NNS or NS), the flow of the milk (a little to swallow or a lot), and the neuromaturation of the infant. The rhythms of suck, swallow, and breathe appear to follow a quantifiable maturational pattern that correlates with increasing PMA suggesting that these patterns are innately programmed (Amaizu et al., 2008; Barlow, 2009; Barlow & Estep, 2006). See Figure 15-3 for a drawing of the relationship between suck, swallow, and breathe in the preterm infant. Understanding the multifaceted relationship of these parameters is ongoing; however, it is safe to note that the complexity is still beyond our understanding and more research is needed to understand how each affects the other and how interventions can support the integration of all three parameters. Sex-related differences have been reported across the second and third trimesters for sucking and swallowing behaviors as measured by sonographic images (Miller et al., 2006). The male and female pace of physical growth was similar. However, there were significant differences in the development of pharyngeal structures and oral–lingual movements. Overall females attained oral motor skills at an earlier stage of prenatal development, which has implications for defining sex-specific indices of maturation during the introduction of oral feeding in the preterm infant.

A great deal of organization is required for this process; thus, the infant's energy resources, developmental maturation, and the environment will have an impact on the infant's ability to be successful (McGrath et al., 2021). Evidence to support earlier introduction of oral feedings, requiring coordination of suck, swallow, and breathing in synchronization with improvement of the transition from tube to oral feeding, is growing (Barlow, 2009; Gewolb & Vice, 2008; Lau & Smith, 2012a; Simpson et al., 2002). Given these findings, it is important to be able to assess feeding readiness accurately.

ASSESSMENT OF FEEDING READINESS

The questions of when and how to introduce oral feeds to hospitalized preterm infants are controversial issues for which there are still no clear answers. Although the literature and anecdotal reports indicate that several criteria have been used by NICU staff to determine preterm infant readiness for initiating oral feedings, numerous publications report that, for the most part, feeding-related decisions are typically not research based (Gennattasio et al., 2015). For example, it is customary practice for oral feedings to be delayed until the infant reaches a weight of 1,500 grams and/or is 32 to 35 weeks PMA (Mason-Wyckoff et al., 2003). There is no evidence to support the maturation of suck–swallow coordination with weight; however, this parameter traditionally has been used to assess feeding readiness. Indeed, recent research suggests that young preterm infants might be able to initiate and sustain breastfeeding activities as early as 32 weeks PMA (Nye, 2008; Pickler, Best, et al., 2006; Pickler, Chiaranai, et al., 2006). However, for preterm infants with bronchopulmonary dysplasia, the impact of increased respiratory effort on breathing patterning during oral feeding should be considered in feeding-related decisions (Howe, Sheu, et al., 2007; Mizuno, et al., 2007; Vice & Gewolb, 2008). For these infants, the transition to oral feedings may be significantly delayed.

Generally, the literature suggests that decisions of when and how to introduce oral feedings are primarily guided by established nursery routines or customs, caregiver preference, or what is most convenient for the staff. It is also common practice for clinicians to utilize what Merenstein calls a "trial-and-error" approach, whereby specific interventions are introduced, continued, or deleted based on infant response or tolerance. Consequently, feeding practices are likely to vary from nursery to nursery and might even vary from caregiver to caregiver within the same unit, often based on subjective assumptions of the caregiving team.

Once respiratory stability is established in the preterm infant, successful oral feeding is a major priority for discharge decision-making. Yet, no objective measures for oral feeding readiness or progression exists. The Feeding Readiness and Progression in Preterms Scale (FRAPPS) is a 10-item pen-and-paper instrument designed to easily assess a variety of physiologic and behavioral parameters that appear to influence oral feeding readiness/progression. Content and face validity have been established (McGrath,

2006). In nonexperimental design feeding readiness was examined using the FRAPPS (McGrath et al., 2008). Within the FRAPPS tool, hunger, control of tone, and the ability to manage the environment variables changed significantly over time and other variables did change over time but the change was not significant. Hunger was also significantly correlated with the number of sucks and number of sucks per burst. The variables to be included in the FRAPPS were refined based upon this analysis. The psychometric properties of the now 8-item tool are reliable and valid. Cronbach's alpha was 0.784 for the 8-item tool. These results led us to believe that the refined FRAPPS is a reliable and valid measure sensitive to feeding readiness and progression during the transition to oral feeding. Decision-making during this process seldom takes into account a full picture of the interwoven physiologic and behavioral variables. Use of the FRAPPS in the clinical setting and research should enhance this process. More research that tests the predictive validity of the FRAPPS is needed for further validation of its use to initiate and advance feedings in the clinical setting. See Box "Indications of Neurobehavioral Readiness for Feeding" for parameters to be included in an assessment of feeding readiness.

Research that examines interventions to increase readiness for oral feeding has also become more predominate in the literature. Increasing behavioral organization and alert states has been studied and found to positively impact feeding readiness and performance (Giannì et al., 2017; White-Traut et al., 2005). Oral stimulation is another strategy that has been examined and found to be somewhat effective. In a small RCT, Fucile et al. (2005) provided an oral stimulation program for 15 minutes each day for 10 days prior to the initiation of oral feeding and found that the infants in the intervention group achieved full oral feedings 7 days sooner than those in the control group. Intervention infants also demonstrated a more efficient sucking pattern as more milk transfer and greater amplitude of sucking were noted.

SETTING THE STAGE FOR FIRST AND SUBSEQUENT FEEDING SUCCESS

Oral feeding of the high-risk infant takes careful decision-making. Once the decision to provide bottle-feeding has been made, there are many subsequent decisions that must be made by the caregiver. If left to chance, as is often the case in the NICU, these choices can ultimately determine the successful attainment of bottle-feeding by the preterm infant. These decisions focus on how and when caregivers should intervene and support the infant through the process. From a macro- to microperspective, the environment of the NICU and, specifically, that of the infant must first be addressed; both are important in supporting the infant during this process (Garber, 2013; Lau & Smith, 2012a; Lau & Smith, 2012b; Pickler et al., 2013) (Box "Steps to Consider When Preparing for Bottle-Feeding").

A difficult or immature feeder might display more incoordination of sucking, swallowing, and breathing, requiring more intensive intervention and attention. These infants

Indications of Neurobehavioral Readiness for Feeding

Neurobehavioral maturation–Conceptualized through Als' Synactive Theory of Development (Als, 1982)

- Gestation age versus postconceptual age (PCA)
- Older than 32 weeks PCA

Physiologic/behavioral stability

- Respirations fairly regular, rate of 40–60 breaths per minute
- Physiologic and behavioral cues–signs of stress
- Approach versus avoidance cues
- Can the baby manage their environment?

Hunger cues such as mouthing, rooting, and waking for feedings
Behavioral state–ability to be available, attentiveness

- Smooth behavioral state transitions with a wide variety of states available
- Ability to reach and maintain an alert state

Motor development–ability to hold themselves together

- Low versus high tone

Limp vs. flexed and tucked

- Oral motor development

Good facial tone
Energy resources

Data from McGrath, J. M., & Braescu, A. V. B. (2004). State of the science: Feeding readiness in the preterm infant. *Journal of Perinatal and Neonatal Nursing, 18*(4), 353–368. https://doi.org/10.1097/00005237-200410000-00006

Steps to Consider When Preparing for Bottle-Feeding

Assess the infant's neurobehavioral readiness for feeding

- Use Als' Synactive Theory of Development as a framework for intervention
- Respiratory stability

Is there a time of day when this infant is more awake?
Consider the environment

- Light, noise, activity, space: How do these affect *this* infant?
- What else has happened in this infant's day or the past 24 hours that could affect feeding success?
- What in the environment facilitates state transition for *this* infant?

Preparation of the care provider

- Does this care provider know *this* baby?
- Commitment of this care provider to the infant's success: Do they have the time to provide the support *this* infant will need?

Data from Als, H. (1982). Toward a synactive theory of development: Promise for the assessment of infant individuality. *Infant Mental Health Journal, 3,* 229–243.

are often easily overstimulated and tire quickly with bottle-feeding. Careful attention to their individualized needs is required for these infants to become successful with bottle-feeding (Lau & Smith, 2012a; Torola et al., 2012).

Infant–caregiver interaction, coregulation, and caregiver commitment to feeding must be considered. Feeding success for the infant is largely dependent on the care providers' attention to the individualized needs of the infant (Premji et al., 2004; Thoyre et al., 2012). Reciprocity must exist between the infant and the caregiver for successful oral feeding to occur. This reciprocity might be difficult to achieve if there is no consistency in care providers; thus, consistency of care is an issue of concern when promoting feeding

success. Documentation of feeding readiness cues and stress behaviors during the feeding, as well as interventions used to support the infant, can promote feeding success when several care providers feed the preterm infant. It is also important to note that not every intervention is necessary for every infant; feeding should be individualized to the infant. When providing intervention, we should never do for the infant what they can do for themselves. Box "Interventions That Facilitate Breast and/or Bottle-Feeding Success" contains interventions to promote feeding success, and Box "Caregiver Actions That Can Detract From Feeding Success" contains nursing actions that have been found to detract from the infant's ability to achieve success (Shaker, 2013).

Interventions That Facilitate Breast and/or Bottle-Feeding Success

Intervention	Rationale	Level of Evidence	References
Decreasing environmental stimulation during feeding	Allows the infant to be focused on the feeding. This can include dimming bright lights, choosing a place that is quiet and away from activity. This might be difficult in the environment of the NICU but should be a priority in preparation	III V	Gennattasio et al. [2015] Shaker [2013]
Facilitating alertness—prior to and during the feeding	Facilitating alertness has been found to be correlated to more efficient feeding Alertness can be facilitated through cue-based feeding strategies	II	Giannì et al. [2017] Gennattasio et al. [2015] Griffith et al. [2017] Park et al. [2016] Park et al. [2020]
Held in caregiver arms in a folded and flexed and semiupright position during feeding	Promotes flexed posture Encourages social interaction Decreases regurgitation and aspiration	II	Peters et al. [2008] Pickler et al. [2020]
Type of nipple	Must be individualized to the infant. The care provider must continuously assess sucking, milk flow, and seal for determination of appropriateness of nipple type. There should be no set routine for what nipple to use first or when, but it should be individualized based on the infant's behaviors and cues	I III	Pados et al. [2016] Pados et al. [2019] Scheel et al. [2005]
Coregulatory approach to feeding that provides a patterned approach to the feeding event	Protocol approach to feeding that provides consistent feeding approach for infant Promotes behavioral state that is conducive to social interaction [alertness]	II II II IV	Thoyre et al., 2013, 2016 Pickler et al. [2015] Reyna et al. [2012] Thoyre et al. [2012] Kish [2014]
Auditory, Tactile, Visual, Vestibular [ATVV]	Increased sucking maturation and progression to full oral feedings as well as time to discharge	II	Medoff-Cooper et al. [2015]
Swaddling the infant	Supports flexion with hands up and into body; supports development of flexion as well as decreases disorganized behaviors that could detract from feeding success. Positioning the infant so that the head is higher than the torso and holding the infant close to your body, supporting flexion and organization	VI	Shaker [2013]
Burping	Can be very stressful for most preterm infants; however, there are strategies to make this intervention less stressful. When possible, infants should be placed on the shoulder for support, and rubbing of the back is less stressful than patting. If a shoulder position is not tolerated, holding the infant upright on your lap with their head curled forward over your hand and rubbing the back should facilitate burping	VII	Expert opinion

[Continued]

Interventions That Facilitate Breast and/or Bottle-Feeding Success (Continued)

Intervention	Rationale	Level of Evidence	References
Side-lying feeding	Increases stability during oral bottle-feeding for some preterm infants	I II	Park et al. [2018] Park, Thoyre, and Knafl [2015]
Infant-paced feeding	Allow the infant to decide when to suck and when to pause. Pausing allows the infant who has difficulty coordinating sucking, swallowing, and breathing to reorganize and continue with the feeding. Pausing is not the time for intervention; allow the infant to pace the feeding	II III	Pineda Law-Morstatt et al. [2003]
Cue-based feeding approaches	Using a cue-based approach is less stressful and facilitates alertness as well as transition to full oral feedings	I VI I IV	Settle and Francis [2019] Fry et al. [2018] Watson and McGuire [2016] Ludwig & Waitzman [2007]
Skin-to-skin contact Kangaroo care	Kangaroo care before bottle-feeding might facilitate alertness and transition to quieter states, which could promote feeding success. Kangaroo care does not tire the infant and should not be avoided because the infant needs to rest for bottle-feeding	I II	Conde-Agudelo, & Díaz-Rossello, [2016] Pike et al. [2017]

Caregiver Actions That Can Detract From Feeding Success

- Twisting and turning the nipple in the infant's mouth
- Pushing/pulling the bottle in and out of the infant's mouth
- Using a nipple with too large a hole or one that is too soft
- Pushing infants to suck when they tire or are pausing, taking a break

- Putting vitamins or medications into the feeding, which might alter the taste. Preterm infants have been found to have a keener sense of taste than previously thought.

Data from Shaker, C. S. [2013]. Cue-based feeding in the NICU: using the infant's communication as a guide. *Neonatal Network*, *32*[6], 404–408. https://doi.org/10.1891/0730-0832.32.6.404

Many preterm infants have trouble with reflux related to oral feeding. GI reflux is abnormal frequent passage of gastric contents into the esophagus. Reflux can detract from feeding success as well as delay growth and development. Remember that more than 70% of preterm infants have reflux, although only a few are symptomatic enough to require intervention. Interventions should be only provided as needed and should be related to the symptoms (Box "Interventions to Support Infant With Symptomatic Reflux or Feeding Intolerance"). Slocum et al. (2009) examined the incidence of apnea, bradycardia, and desaturations related to gastroesophageal reflux and did not find a relationship. Most of the infants did demonstrate GER, but there was no increase in the prevalence of other symptoms.

Pharmacologic interventions should be reserved for when all other interventions have failed and should be monitored closely; these medications are not without their own issues and concerns. Adding a thickening agent to the formula such as *Simply Thick* or rice cereal is a nonpharmacologic intervention that has been used with some success for some infants but again the strategy needs to be individualized to the needs of the infant (Pados & Mellon, 2020).

A difficult or immature feeder might display more incoordination of sucking, swallowing, and breathing, requiring more intensive intervention and attention. These infants are often easily overstimulated and tire quickly with bottle-feeding (Hwang et al., 2012). Careful attention to their individualized needs is required for

---

Interventions to Support Infant With Symptomatic Reflux or Feeding Intolerance

- Elevating the head of the bed at least 30°.
- Positioning the infant in prone or side-lying position.
- Providing frequent feedings of small volumes to decrease gastric distention.
- Many care providers choose to thicken feedings with cereal; however, this practice must be done with consistency to be successful. The research that suggests thickening of feedings found that prethickened infant formulas (by the manufacturer) seemed to be tolerated best. However, because these are seldom available, a consistent approach that guarantees uniformity is required.
- Do not add cereal to formula until just before that feeding; cereal left in formula for extended periods becomes very thick and chunky in nature, diminishing the infant's ability to extract it from the nipple.
- Cross-cut nipples or large, single-hole nipples are suggested. Nipples that are cut by nursing staff at each feeding are inappropriate because the inconsistent size of the cut detracts from the infant's ability to regulate their own feeding. Sometimes the flow is too fast (large cuts in nipples increases chances for reflux), sometimes too slow (small cuts in nipple hole tire the infant quickly).
- Pharmacologic interventions should be reserved for when all other interventions have failed and should be monitored closely; they are not without their own issues and concerns.
- Gastrointestinal reflux is abnormal frequent passage of gastric contents into the esophagus. Reflux is experienced by many preterm infants and might detract from feeding success as well as delay growth and development.

---

these infants to become successful with bottle-feeding (Pineda et al., 2020).

Lastly, infant-caregiver interaction, co-regulation, and caregiver commitment to feeding must be considered. Feeding success for the infant is largely dependent on the care providers' attention to the individualized needs of the infant (Shaker, 2013). Reciprocity must exist between the infant and the caregiver for successful oral feeding to occur. This reciprocity might be difficult to achieve if there is no consistency in care providers; thus, consistency of care is an issue of concern when promoting feeding success. Documentation of feeding readiness cues and stress behaviors during the feeding, as well as interventions used to support the infant, can promote feeding success when several care providers feed the preterm infant. It is also important to note that not every intervention is necessary for every infant; feeding should be individualized to the infant. When providing intervention, we should never do for the infant what they can do for themselves. Box "Interventions That Facilitate Breast and/or Bottle-Feeding Success" contains interventions to promote feeding success, and Box "Caregiver Actions That Can Detract From Feeding Success" contains nursing actions that can detract from the infant's ability to achieve success. Assessment during the feeding itself is important and could provide important predictors for long-term development; research in this area is ongoing (Kwon et al., 2020).

Cue-Based Feeding

There are now several published studies and quality improvement projects to support the feeding of preterm infants on a cue-based or within a demand schedule. This approach focuses on behavioral and hunger cues from the infant that demonstrate feeding readiness rather than a predetermined feeding schedule. Researchers have found that the staff must be trained to recognize these subtle signs in the preterm infant and must respond quickly with a feeding opportunity. If this does not occur, the infant may move from a state of alertness and feeding readiness to one of disorganization rather quickly, which would negatively impact the feeding opportunity (Park et al., 2020). In addition, coordination and support of the caregiving team is important to the successful implementation of demand feeding in the NICU. Demand feeding provides better support for the preterm infant in reaching alert states that have been repeated, correlated with increased feeding success (Medoff-Cooper et al., 2000; Park et al., 2020). For best success a "demand feeding protocol" with a decision-tree for implementation of demand feeding is needed to increase success of the NICU caregiving team. For example, NICUs where demand feeding has been successful found they needed a cutoff time for when to wake a sleeping infant who has not fed for a long period of time and parameters for acceptable weight loss after the infant is initially placed on a demand schedule. A recent Cochrane review recommends that additional research is necessary to develop specific recommendations to support the implementation of demand feedings (McCormick et al., 2010).

Neonatal nurses have tremendous observation skills regarding feeding readiness. Too often these skills are overshadowed by the pressure to "get" the infant to eat at the scheduled feeding time as a means to facilitate the transition to full feedings and discharge (Ludwig & Waitzman, 2007). Cue-based feeding requires the bedside nurse to identify infant feeding readiness signs to establish when an infant is ready to attempt oral nipple feedings. Cues include alertness and signs of hunger (see Fig. 15-4). When this approach is applied correctly, the oral feeding is infant driven not caregiver driven; a successful feeding is no longer that of an empty bottle and/or what strategies the caregiver used

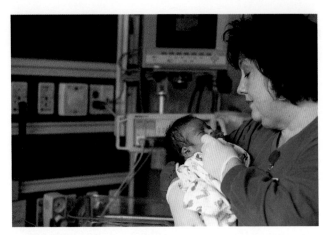

FIGURE 15-4. Infant alert with pacifier prior to feeding. [Used with parental permission. Photo courtesy of family.]

to achieve the task. According to Ludwig and Waitzman (2007), a successful feeding in an infant-driven model of care includes the achievement of several goals: the feeding is (1) safe, (2) functional, (3) nurturing, and (4) individualized and (5) developmentally appropriate. Two different systematic reviews (Settle & Francis, 2019; Watson & McGuire, 2016) identified how feeding preterm infants according to their behavioral cues might enhance the infants' and parents' satisfaction; however, the level of evidence was low and more research is needed to validate this intervention strategy. Since that time several quality improvement initiatives have been successfully implemented demonstrating that weight gain, time to full oral feedings, and decreased length of stay maybe positive outcomes to cue-based feeding protocols (Fry et al., 2018). More quality improvement and research in this area is needed with sicker, less stable preterm infants. To support the implementation of cue-based feeding, Ludwig and Waitzman (2007) developed a documentation flowsheet to provide information about how an infant behaved during the feeding and what activities of the nurse supported the oral feeding as a means to communicate this information to the caregiving team facilitating more positive outcomes for the preterm infant.

Coregulatory Feeding

Coregulatory feeding is similar to cue-based feeding; however, the nurse caregiver needs to be even more in tune with the behaviors and cues of the infant before, during, and after the feeding event so they can guide the mother in providing the feeding to her high-risk preterm infant. The whole dynamics of the event need to be evaluated including the effects of the macro environment of the NICU, the skills of the caregiver (mother), as well as the behaviors of the infant. The nurse needs to reflect about what competencies the infant brings to the feeding so that interventions can be targeted specifically to that infant (Thoyre et al., 2013).

The nurse uses reflection from previous feeding experiences with that infant and mother while supporting guided participation during the feeding event and thus increasing their chances for an optimal feeding experience. Coregulatory interventions might include reinforcing the mother's ability to read her infants cues, supporting the infant during the feeding through pacing to coregulating breathing, providing motoric stability, regulating milk flow, and providing rest periods (Thoyre et al., 2016). Mothers can easily be distressed when their infant is not progressing with feeding or experiences feeding intolerance. This type of approach provides support so they become increasingly knowledgeable about their infant and more involved in the infant's care. Providing a means of understanding and growing sense of competency can increase confidence and decrease distress for mothers (Park et al., 2016).

Postural support is often one of the individualized interventions used during coregulatory feeding. For example, semielevated side-lying position is a strategy used to support breathing during feeding (Park et al., 2014). Park et al. (2014) found that this position appears to increase stability for the infant because it decreases heart-rate and breathing variability; however, more study of this intervention is needed. In a systematic review conducted by Park and associates in 2018, only four studies were identified with conflicting results demonstrating the need for greater understanding of how this intervention works and for which infants it is best suited (Park et al., 2018). A large trial with a diverse group of high-risk preterm infants is needed to determine the overall effects of the side-lying position for supporting the optimal feeding experience.

Pacing of Feeding

Building on the framework of cue-based feeding is facilitating the infant to pace the feeding. In the past neonatal caregivers were noted to manipulate the bottle or nipple in the infant's mouth to try to increase the flow ("to get the feeding done more quickly") or when the infant appeared to take a break and stopped sucking ("to get them to keep going and finish the feeding"). In addition, sometimes a preterm infant will continue to suck even when their oxygen saturation is declining, with pacing, the bottle may be tipped back briefly (3 to 5 seconds) to give the infant a break and recover before continuing with the feeding (see Fig. 15-5). In a nonrandomized experimental design Law-Morstatt et al. (2003) examined a paced feeding protocol with 36 preterm infants. Although there was no significant difference in weight gain or length of stay with this protocol, infants did demonstrate significantly less bradycardia during feeding and appeared to have a more developmentally mature sucking pattern at discharge. Transitioning preterm infants to full feedings is often times stressful for the infant, and finding ways to best support the infant and decrease stress must continue to be a focus in facilitating oral feeding success. During transition too much milk flow can also be an issue for the preterm infants that

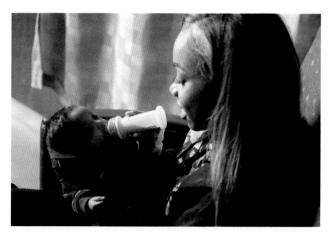

FIGURE 15-5. Infant alert during feeding. (Used with parental permission. Photo courtesy of family.)

may be influenced by pacing. Traditional bottles will provide milk even if the infant is not sucking. Lau et al. (2015) have studied a bottle system that only delivered the milk when the infant is sucking and found that this self-pacing unit was effective in facilitating the transition to full oral feedings in preterm infants born at less than 30 weeks' gestation who may have more difficulty handling increased flow during the transition to full oral feeding. Flow of milk has implications for breathing and swallowing as well as safety during the oral feeding. More research is needed to understand whether development of new and different bottles and nipples would best support the oral feeding transition of preterm infants.

Effects of Experience on Feeding

Pickler et al. (2006a, 2006b, 2008, 2010, 2015) found that experience at nipple feeding had the greatest effect on suck–swallow–breathing performance, which also impacted overall consumptions and success rates. This trajectory of research demonstrates the interaction between maturation, oral feeding skill development, and neurobehavioral organization in the preterm infant. It must be noted, however, that the preterm infants in this study were not "forced" to complete the oral feeding. They were provided the "opportunity" for oral feeding. No interventions that would push or force the feeding were provided during the feeding where data was collected and the remainder of the feeding was provided by gavage tube if the infant did not finish the ordered amount. The rooting reflex was initiated and the nipple was offered; what the infant did was up to that infant at that feeding. Infants are learning while they are in the NICU, and just as with any learning activity both good and bad patterns/habits can be initiated. Providing more opportunities for oral feeding may be important in facilitating the transition to full oral feeding in the preterm infant. Cunha et al. (2009) compared the NS patterns of VLBW preterm infants with that of full-term newborns and found that experience was an influencing factor in the change of the NS pattern in the

preterm infants, further validating the effect of experience on preterm infant feeding performance.

Feeding Issues of the Late Preterm Infant

The LPI, born at 34 1/6 to 36 6/7 weeks, has been reported to have feeding problems (Wight, 2003) that is understandable in that the development of synchrony between sucking and swallowing reflexes is typically not completed until 36 to 38 weeks' gestation. Immature muscle tone and neurologic processes necessary to maintain an airway and effective sucking behaviors are often not present putting these infants at risk for poor intake. Feeding problems are most often related to immature suck and swallowing reflexes that may make proper latch-on necessary for successful breastfeeding difficult. Failure to coordinate breathing, sucking, and swallowing predisposes the most immature LPI to apneic events, bradycardia and oxygen desaturation, and fatigue during feeding (Lau et al., 2003; McGrath & Medoff-Cooper, 2001). Complicating feeding progression is the inability of the LPI to maintain an active or quiet alert state, a necessary component of feeding success (Park et al., 2020).

Medoff-Cooper et al. (2001) reported differences in feeding behaviors in LPIs as compared with those infants with a gestational age of >38 weeks PMA. Infants with a PMA of 35 to 36 weeks produced fewer sucks, fewer sucks per burst, and lower mean maximum pressure during a 5-minute sucking assessment as compared with full-term infants, providing further evidence that the LPI is at risk for feeding problems. The LPI has a higher risk of discharge delay due to additional nutritional support (defined as intravenous fluids, total parenteral nutrition, or gavage feeds)—after correcting for comorbidities (respiratory distress syndrome, surgical). The preterm infant's need for longer hospitalization periods compared with term counterparts accounts mainly for the time needed to mature suck/swallow coordination in this GA (Giannì et al., 2015). Furthermore, researchers have reviewed sucking behavior in infants born preterm and their developmental outcomes in school. They found. That persistent abnormal sucking behavior between 42 weeks and 50 weeks PMA was associated with developmental outcomes at primary school age. Wolthuis et al. (2017) argue that, rather than representing a maturational process, these persistent sucking difficulties may be an early sign of brain dysfunction that may indicate an increased risk of developmental difficulties, not only at preschool but at school age as well (Wolthuis et al., 2017).

PSYCHOSOCIAL AND FAMILY ISSUES: PREPARING FOR DISCHARGE

Parents are essential to caregiving in the NICU and need to be included in every aspect of the care of their infant (McGrath & Vittner, 2020). Successful oral feeding of the preterm infant is often one of the greatest priorities for families prior to NICU discharge. This goal is unchanged whether the infant is breast or bottle-feeding. However, it must be noted that the route (breast or bottle) is the mother's choice not the health professional's. As soon as possible, parents must be facilitated to provide as much of the routine caregiving as they are available and willing to do. Participating in feeding increases the parents' feelings of involvement and contribution to their infant's well-being (Buchan & Bennett, 2020). During gavage feeding, parents should be encouraged to hold the infant, provide skin-to-skin contact, or support the infant who is learning to integrate NNS (supporting the pacifier). Social interaction during gavage feeding should be based on the infant's availability and behavioral cues.

Mothers often judge their parenting ability by how well their infant is growing. Statements such as, "My baby weighs almost 10 pounds," are statements of pride (McGrath, 2007b). Providing a nurturing environment in which their infant can grow and thrive is important to mothers. Nursing is in an optimal position to support mothers (and families) in their transition to caring for their infant in the NICU. Family participation in caregiving begins optimally at birth even when the infant is born preterm and/or very ill. Family participation in feeding can begin with participation in the delivery of gavage feedings and the transition to oral feedings in the NICU. Dennis and McQueen (2009) conducted a systematic review and found that women with depressive symptomatology in the early postpartum period may be at increased risk for negative infant feeding outcomes. These findings support the need to facilitate family competence with feeding the preterm infant.

The implications of feeding for families of preterm infants are great given the critical care ambience of the NICU. The technology, attention to numbers, rather than infant behaviors, and, the nonindividualized way in which care is often delivered leads to what has been termed the "medicalization" of families (McGrath, 2007a). The importance of feeding may get lost in all the chaos and routines, and thus, families may not be as well prepared to feed their infants after discharge. Parents may be too stressed to really concentrate on the issues related to care of their infant after discharge (Estrem et al., 2017). In addition, preterm families are already at greater risk for having difficulties with attachment and parenting that can only be further diminished by problematic oral feeding (Estrem et al., 2020; Reyna et al., 2006; Thoyre et al., 2005). Thus, the importance of successful oral feeding is an area of neonatal nursing care that cannot be overlooked and may even need to be given higher priority (Thomas, 2007).

A priority in supporting families in the feeding of their preterm infant in the NICU includes altering schedules so that families (mothers) are supported to provide the *FIRST* oral feeding. There is **NO** documented evidence that the provision of the first oral feeding by a health professional is warranted. Mothers will, however, require more education and encouragement to successfully support their infant during the first oral feeding. Issues to address include positioning the infant for support, providing a quiet environment with few distractions for the infant and choices of feeding supplies to best support the infant (nipple shields, nipples, etc.) (Thomas et al., 2021). Few preterm infants are excellent feeders during the first oral feeding, and thus, mothers need information about what to expect of their infant's performance. Preterm infants are messy, often have a poor seal, and usually take very little volume during the first feeding. Sharing this information will help to increase the mother's confidence about her feeding ability. In addition, offering to finish the first feeding because the infant does not complete the prescribed amount, will only serve to diminish the mother's confidence, and does it really matter? Sometimes the infant is unable to complete the volume offered during an early feeding, so giving the remainder by gavage is a better solution for both the mother and the infant. Feeding schedules can also be adjusted to coincide with parental availability in the NICU. If parents are truly considered partners in the caregiving of their infant, then their schedule is important and takes precedence for providing oral feedings.

Whenever possible, the parents should provide the feeding, be it bottle and of course breast. This might mean the feeding schedule is adjusted to the visiting schedule of the parent. Initially, the nurse may need to be present for the entire oral feeding to offer advice, provide demonstrations, and answer questions or address specific concerns. As the parent and infant become more comfortable and successful, the nurse may only need to check on the progress of the infant periodically during the oral feeding session. Parents should not be denied the opportunity to feed even the most difficult infant; remember, this is their baby! Helping the mother and infant to establish synchrony during feeding is important as it will help increase maternal confidence (Reyna et al., 2012). Consider ways to reinforce maternal reading of infant feeding cues and behaviors as a means of increasing synchrony within the dyad.

Parents are often provided with lots of information about how their infant should be fed at home. Although anticipatory guidance is important in supporting families' on their own, decision-making is also an important consideration. Families should be asked what their plans are for feeding their infant. Mothers often make decisions about how they plan to feed their infant before birth, even when the child is born preterm (Brown, 2007; Thoyre, 2007). This can include choice of route or choice of bottle and nipple type. The mother who is bottle-feeding may encounter several unanticipated problems as she prepares for the discharge from the hospital setting of her preterm infant (Brown et al., 2009). Many of the nipples and bottles used in the NICU are not available commercially outside the hospital environment. Some nurseries provide supplies for the transition to home and some do not. The number of different types of nipples and bottles available is staggering. Making the best choice for the preterm is difficult without good information about the needs of the preterm infant. Mothers are often confused about the issues of high-flow versus low-flow nipples. Some commercially available high-flow nipples still state on the label they are best for preterm infants. In addition, mothers may already have a supply of bottles or nipples at home that they are anticipating using after discharge that may not be appropriate for supporting their preterm infant. Asking mothers about their plans or asking them to bring in their nipples and bottles can be helpful in providing support for preterm infants and families for the transition to home. The care provider must have the knowledge to be able to continuously assess sucking, milk flow, and seal for determination of appropriateness of nipple type (Scheel et al., 2005). Nipple and bottle choice is, thus, individualized based on the infant's behaviors (Chang et al., 2007).

Parents also need information about infant behaviors and hunger cues related to oral feeding. Reyna et al. (2006) found that parents seldom were able to describe cues that told them when their infant was ready for a feeding. They also were unable to identify cues about satiation. In the NICU infants are often fed on a schedule and hunger cues are often considered a nonissue, so importance of these behaviors may not have been role modeled for families or addressed in discussions about how and when to best feed the preterm infant after discharge. Mothers in this study were reluctant to move to an ad libitum schedule after discharge because the scheduled feedings seemed so important in the hospital setting. Remember what we do sometimes speaks volumes, whereas what we say sometimes gets lost in the translation. Parents are always watching; they have trusted the nursing staff with a very precious possession, so of course what they see is often what they do after discharge.

Many parents also need more direction about advancement of feeding volume after discharge; they may be reluctant to advance feedings on their own (Reyna et al., 2006). Helping them to anticipate this need and set up networks of support within their extended family and community prior to discharge can be helpful (McGrath, 2007a; Pridham et al., 2007; Stevens et al., 2014; Thoyre, 2007; Thoyre et al., 2005). Admitting they need help after the infant is already home may be difficult for some mothers. Mothers have a great need to feel competent in the care of their infant, and knowing that the need for help is normal will increase their sense of competence in caring for their infant. Phone calls from the NICU about the adjustment to home can be helpful as well as the ability for parents to call back to the NICU with questions as they develop. Visits to the pediatrician or pediatric nurse practitioner should be scheduled before discharge and occur within 1 to 2 weeks of discharge. The needs of the preterm infant and family do not end with the transition to home; in some ways they are just beginning and we need to continue to find ways to better support these families in successful oral feeding while increasing parent competence during this transition (Brown, 2007; Brown et al., 2009; Pickler et al., 2012).

Novel Coronavirus-19 and Feeding Practices

The COVID-19 pandemic challenged maternal–child healthcare providers and best practices in dyadic care in the early part of the pandemic when there were few guidelines and little evidence on the transmission of SARS-CoV-2, the virus that causes COVID-19, with respect to neonates. Initially, there were limited reports on intrauterine, intrapartum, or peripartum transmission, but as the pandemic continued, the extent of vertical transmission from mother to infant remained rare. The CDC and American Academy of Pediatrics offered rapid cycle clinical guidelines based on the best available evidence for neonatal care, including feeding (AAP, 2021; CDC, 2020).

As noted earlier in the chapter, maternal milk supply is established during the first weeks postpartum, which is a critical time for lactation. To date, no study has found the live severe acute respiratory syndrome coronavirus-2 (SARS-CoV-2) that causes COVID-19 in breast milk (Chen et al., 2020; Pereira et al., 2020). The CDC offers guidance and considerations for breastfeeding that can be used to council breastfeeding dyads that are in isolation and quarantine as well as precautions to take while feeding at the breast, expressing milk, or feeding from a bottle when one or both members of the dyad has suspected or confirmed COVID-19. In particular, hand washing, mask wearing, and cleansing and sanitizing breast pumps are among the most important precautions (Amatya et al., 2020; CDC, 2020).

As we consider the implications of COVID-19 on future public health disasters, it is important to consider that the maternal child health community used evidence-based policy decisions to the best extent possible and deployed recommendations as quickly as possible to reduce any unnecessary separation between mothers and babies. Although some may have viewed these as too fast or too slow, the guidance was made with the best available data. As important, the barriers to accessing NICUs and labor and delivery units and the impact of restrictions on parental presence were profound. They caused distress to families and from a feeding perspective (Erdei & Liu, 2020) also decreased the availability of lactation and oral feeding support (Darcy Mahoney et al., 2020). Lessons learned from this pandemic with respect to harm reduction and trauma informed care practices related to maternal–child health must be considered in future disasters and in disaster preparedness for the nursing workforce.

FUTURE RESEARCH IMPLICATIONS

The interaction between the preterm infant, the care provider, and the environment during bottle-feeding has been studied systematically in parts, but the dynamics of the entire holistic process still needs more attention so that infants and mothers feel supported (Park et al., 2016). Hill (2002) systematically explained the literature to design a theory of feeding efficiency for preterm infants; however, as yet this theory is untested. For example, coordination of sucking, swallowing, and breathing has been systematically studied, yet all the factors that contribute or diminish feeding success appear ambiguous (Case-Smith et al., 1989).

The debate over the role of feeding experience versus neurologic maturation as the major driver of sucking organization continues. Although there is no doubt that feeding experience adds to overall feeding efficiency, increasing sensory and motor CNS maturation is critical (da Costa et al., 2008). There is an urgent need for reliable and noninvasive tools that objectively measure sucking and swallowing movements and to assess the coordination between sucking, swallowing, and breathing (da Costa et al., 2008). Few interventions to improve feeding organization have been systematically studied, but chin and cheek support appears to be effective; still, more research with other interventions is needed. Assessment of bottle-feeding success before discharge from the NICU is essential, so that infants and, thus, families are not at risk for feelings of failure, poor attachment, and/or rehospitalization related to failure to thrive. More research is needed on aspects of breastfeeding, including use of an interdisciplinary, family-centered approach; factors that enhance breastfeeding success; and physiologic aspects on infant outcomes. Another important area of research is the impact on methods of feeding during the initiation of oral feeding on long-term consequences of development beyond the NICU and infancy periods. Finally, understand the dynamics of ways to best support families not only during the transition to oral feeding but after discharge are important to long-term outcomes.

CONCLUSION

Feeding preterm infants is often considered a routine task, rather than a critical element in the care of the preterm infant. The ambiance of the NICU places increased emphasis on maintaining physiologic stability in the acute period after the birth of a preterm infant rather than on a skill that is often considered to be a simple reflex. However, it is the delay in obtaining feeding skills that is the most frequent cause of prolonged hospitalization (Bakewell-Sachs et al., 2009). Research that holistically examines the dynamic process of oral feeding initiation will enhance the maturation of feeding behaviors and transition of these infants from hospital to home. More importantly, it must be noted that bottle-feeding/breast feeding is an interactive process that requires reciprocity between the caregiver and infant; both members of the feeding dyad must be competent. Yet, no definition or set of objective components could be found in the literature that clearly delineated all the criteria that care providers use to describe "successful bottle-feeding." Furthermore, given the recognized importance of successful bottle-feeding of preterm infants before discharge from the NICU, the lack of identified guidelines and criteria in regard to successful bottle-feeding and the need for more research in this area are serious concerns. Although the number of studies is growing, the sample sizes remain small and the generalizability of the results are limited. Continued research that examines all the aspects of the NICU that impact this process will provide a better understanding of what is needed to further facilitate the transition

from hospital to home for these high-risk infants and families. Feeding practices and their promotion in the NICU environment constitute a benchmark that is now a part of many parent-satisfaction surveys as well as a method of benchmarking for quality improvement regarding individualized, family-centered, developmental care (IFDC) (Saunders et al., 2003). Feeding is one aspect of IFDC that requires a commitment to using infant and family cues to set up a plan of care. Feeding is a critical element in determining morbidity and mortality of infants, and we must recognize that use of individualized developmental family-centered care is as well.

The interaction between preterm infant, the care provider, and the environment during bottle-feeding has been studied systematically in parts, but the dynamics of the entire holistic process remains basically untouched. Hill (2002) systematically explained the literature to design a theory of feeding efficiency for preterm infants; however, as yet this theory is untested. For example, coordination of sucking, swallowing, and breathing has been systematically studied, yet all the factors that contribute or diminish feeding success appear ambiguous (Case-Smith et al., 1989). Few interventions have been systematically studied, but chin and cheek support appears to be effective; still, more research with other interventions is needed. Coregulatory interventions are beginning to show promise, but the time investment of the staff is high for this intervention to be successful. Assessment of bottle-feeding success before discharge from the NICU is essential, so that infants and, thus, families are not at risk for feelings of failure, poor attachment, and/or rehospitalization related to failure to thrive. More research is needed on aspects of breastfeeding, including use of an interdisciplinary, family-centered approach; factors that enhance breastfeeding success; and physiologic aspects on infant outcomes. Another important area of research is the impact on methods of feeding on long-term consequences of development beyond the NICU and infancy periods.

REFERENCES

Als, H. (1982). Toward a synactive theory of development: Promise for the assessment of infant individuality. *Infant Mental Health Journal, 3,* 229–243.

Amaizu, N., Shulman, R., Shanler, R., & Lau, C. (2008). Maturation of oral feeding skills in preterm infants. *Acta Paediatrica, 97*(1), 61–67.

Amatya, S., Corr, T., Gandhi, C., Glass, K., Kresch, M., Mujsce, D., Oji-Mmuo, C., Mola, S., Murray, Y., Palmer, T., Singh, M., Fricchione, A., Arnold, J., Prentice, D., Bridgeman, C., Smith, B., Gavigan, P., Ericson, J., Miller, J., … Kaiser, J. (2020). Management of newborns exposed to mothers with confirmed or suspected COVID-19. *Journal of Perinatology, 40*(7), 987–996. https://doi.org/10.1038/s41372-020-0695-0

American Academy of Pediatrics. (2021). *Breastfeeding guidance post hospital discharge for mothers or infants with suspected or confirmed SARS-Co V-2 infection.* https://services.aap.org/en/pages/2019-novel-coronavirus-covid-19-infections/clinical-guidance/breastfeeding-guidance-post-hospital-discharge/

Arvedson, J. C., & Brodsky, L. (2002). *Pediatric swallowing and feeding: Assessment and management.* Singular Publishing.

Bakewell-Sachs, S., Medoff-Cooper, B., Escobar, G. J., Silber, J. H., & Lorch, S. A. (2009). Infant functional status: The timing of physiologic maturation of premature infants. *Pediatrics, 123*(5), e878–e886.

Barlow, S. M., & Estep, M. (2006). Central pattern generation and the motor infrastructure for suck, respiration and speech. *Journal of Communication Disorders, 39*(5), 366–380.

Barlow, S. M. (2009). Oral and respiratory control for preterm feeding. *Current Opinion in Otolaryngology & Head and Neck Surgery, 17*(3), 179–186.

Beauregard, J. L., Hamner, H. C., Chen, J., Avila-Rodriguez, W., Elam-Evans, L. D., & Perrine, C. G. (2019). Racial disparities in breastfeeding initiation and duration among U.S. Infants born in 2015. *MMWR Morbidity Mortality Weekly Report, 68*, 745–748. http://dx.doi.org/10.15585/mmwr.mm6834a3

Bingham, P. M., Ashikaga, T., & Abbasi, S. (2010). Prospecitve study of non-nutritive sucking and feeding skills in premature infants. *Archives of Diseases in Childhood Fetal and Neonatal Edition, 95*(3), F194–F200. https://doi.org/10.1136/adc.2009.164186

Boies, E. G., Vaucher, Y. E., & Academy of Breastfeeding Medicine. (2016). ABM clinical protocol #10: Breastfeeding the late preterm (34–36 6/7 weeks of gestation) and early term infants (37–38 6/7 weeks of gestation), second revision 2016. *Breastfeeding Medicine, 11*, 494–500. https://doi.org/10.1089/bfm.2016.29031.egb

Boiron, M., Da Nobrega, L., Roux, S., Henrot, A., & Saliba, E., (2007). Effects of oral stimulation and oral support on non-nutritive sucking and feeding performance in preterm infants. *Developmental Medicine and Child Neurology, 49*(6), 439–444.

Boquien, C. (2018). Human milk: An ideal food for nutrition of preterm newborn. *Frontiers in Pediatrics, 6*, 295. https://doi.org/10.3389/fped.2018.00295

Boykova, M. V., Kenner, C., Walker, K., & Discenza, D. A. (2020). Postdischarge care of the newborn, infant, and families. In Kenner, C., Altimier, L. B., & Boykova, M. V. (Eds.), *Comprehensive neonatal nursing care: A physiologic perspective* (6th ed., pp. 795–822). Springer.

Briere, C., McGrath, J., Cong, X., & Cusson, R. (2014a). An integrative review of factors that influence breastfeeding duration for premature infants after NICU hospitalization. *Journal of Obstetric, Gynecologic, and Neonatal Nursing: JOGNN, 43*(3), 272–281. https://doi.org/10.1111/1552-6909.12297

Briere, C., McGrath, J., Cong, X., & Cusson, R. (2014b). State of the science: A contemporary review of feeding readiness in the preterm infant. *The Journal of Perinatal & Neonatal Nursing, 28*(1), 51–E54. https://doi.org/10.1097/JPN.0000000000000011

Briere, C. E., Lucas, R., McGrath, J. M., Lussier, M., & Brownell, E. (2015a). Establishing breastfeeding with late preterm infants in the NICU. *JOGNN: Journal of Obstetrical, Gynecological and Neonatal Nursing, 44*(1), 102–113. https://doi.org/10.1111/1552-6909.12536

Briere, C. E., McGrath, J. M., Cong, X., Brownell, E., & Cusson, R. (2015b). Direct-breastfeeding premature infants in the neonatal intensive care unit, *Journal of Human Lactation, 31*(3), 386–392. https://doi.org/10.1177/0890334415581798

Briere, C. E., Cusson, R., Cong, X., & McGrath, J. M. (2016). Preterm infant breastfeeding trajectories. *Applied Nursing Research, 32*, 47–51. http://dx.doi.org/10.1016/j.apnr.2016.04.004

Brown, L. F., Thoyre, S., Pridham, K., & Schubert, C. (2009). The mother-infant feeding tool. *JOGNN: Journal of Obstetrical, Gynecologic,and Neonatal Nursing, 38*(4), 491–503.

Brown, L. (2007). Heart rate variability in premature infants during feeding. *Biological Research for Nursing, 8*(4), 283–293.

Brownell, M. A., Lussier, M. M., Hagadorn, J. I., McGrath, J. M., Marinelli, K. A., & Herson, V. C. (2014). Independent predictors of human milk receipt at NICU discharge. *American Journal of Perinatology, 31*(10), 891–898. https://doi.org/10.1055/s-0033-1363500

Buchan, J. L., & Bennett, C. T. (2020). Promoting infant mental health through evidence-informed interventions to support infant feeding and the transition to parenthood: A clinical practice example. *Canadian Journal of Nursing Research, 52*(2), 100–107. https://doi.org/10.1177/0844562120908755

Campbell, A. G., & Miranda, P. Y. (2018). Breastfeeding trends among very low birth weight, and normal birth weight infants. *Journal of Pediatrics, 200*, 71–78. https://doi.org/10.1016/j.jpeds.2018.04.039

Cannella, B. L. (2005). Maternal-fetal attachment an integrative review. *Journal of Advanced Nursing, 50*(1), 60–68.

Cartagena, D., Renya, B., McGrath, J. M., & Parker, L. (2021). Strategies to improve mother's own milk expression in Black and Hispanic mothers of premature infants, *Advances in Neonatal Care.* https://doi.org/10.1097/ANC.0000000000000866

Cartwright, J., Atz, T., Newman, S., Mueller, M., & Demirci, J. (2017). Integrative review of interventions to promote breastfeeding in the late preterm infant. *Journal of Obstetric, Gynecologic, and Neonatal Nursing: JOGNN, 46*(3), 347–356. https://doi.org/10.1016/j.jogn.2017.01.006

Casavant, S. G., McGrath, J. M., Burke, G., & Briere, C. E. (2015). Caregiving factors affecting breastfeeding duration within a neonatal intensive care unit. *Advances in Neonatal Care, 15*(6), 421–428.

Case-Smith, J., Cooper, P., & Scala, V. (1989). Feeding efficiency of premature neonates. *American Journal of Occupational Therapy, 43*(4), 245–250.

Casey, L., Fucile, S., & Dow, K. (2018). Determinants of successful direct breastfeeding at hospital discharge in high-risk premature infants. *Breastfeeding Medicine, 13*(5), 346–351. https://doi.org/10.1089/bfm.2017.0209

Centers for Disease Control. (2020). *Care for breastfeeding people interim guidance on breastfeeding and breast milk feeds in the context of COVID-19.* https://www.cdc.gov/coronavirus/2019-ncov/hcp/care-for-breastfeeding-women.html

Chang, Y. J., Lin, C. P., Lin, Y. J., & Lin, C. H. (2007). Effects of single-holed and cross-cut nipple units on feeding efficiency and physiologic parameters in premature infants. *Journal of Nursing Research, 15*(3), 215–223.

Chen, H., Guo, J., Wang, C., Luo, F., Yu, X., Zhang, W., Li, J., Zhao, D., Xu, D., Gong, Q., Liao, J., Yang, H., Hou, W., & Zhang, Y. (2020). Clinical characteristics and intrauterine vertical transmission potential of COVID-19 infection in nine pregnant women: A retrospective review of medical records. *Lancet, 395*(10226), 809–815.

Chiang, K., Sharma, A., Nelson, J., Olson, C., & Perrine, C. (2019). Receipt of breast milk by gestational age - United States, 2017. *MMWR Morbidity Mortality Weekly Report, 68*, 489–493. https://doi.org/10.15585/mmwr.mm6822a1

Cirillo, C., & Francis, K. (2016). Does breast milk affect neonatal abstinence syndrome severity, the need for pharmacologic therapy, and length of stay for infants of mothers on opioid maintenance therapy during pregnancy? *Advances in Neonatal Care, 16*(5), 369–378. https://doi.org/10.1097/anc.0000000000000330

Clark, R. R. S. (2019). Breastfeeding in women on opioid maintenance therapy: A review of policy and practice. *Journal of Midwifery & Women's Health, 64*(5), 545–558. https://doi.org/10.1111/jmwh.12982

Collins, C., Gillis, J., McPhee, A., Suganuma, H., & Makrides, M. (2016). Avoidance of bottles during the establishment of breast feeds in preterm infants. *Cochrane Database of Systematic Reviews,* (10). https://doi.org/10.1002/14651858.CD005252.pub4

Conde-Agudelo, A., Díaz-Rossello, J. L., & Conde-Agudelo, A. (2016). Kangaroo mother care to reduce morbidity and mortality in low birth-weight infants. *Cochrane Library, 2017*(2), CD002771. https://doi.org/10.1002/14651858.CD002771.pub4

Conway, A. (1994). Instruments in neonatal research: Measuring preterm infant feeding ability, Part 1. Bottle-feeding. *Neonatal Network, 13*(4), 71–73.

Crapnell, T. L., Rogers, C.E., Neil, J. J., Inders, T. E., Woodward, L. J., & Pineda, R. G. (2013). Factors associated with feeding difficulties in very preterm infants. *Acta Paediatrica, 102*, e539–e545. https://doi.org/10.1111/apa.12393

Cricco-Lizza, R. (2016). Infant feeding beliefs and day-to-day feeding practices of NICU nurses. *Journal of Pediatric Nursing, 31*(2), e91–e98. https://doi.org/10.1016/j.pedn.2015.10.012

Cunha, M., Barreiros, J., Goncalves, I., & Figueiredo, H. (2009). Nutritive sucking pattern—from very low birth weight preterm to term newborn. *Early Human Development, 85*(2), 125–130.

da Costa, S. P., van den Engel-Hoek, L., & Bos, A. F. (2008). Sucking and swallowing in infants and diagnostic tools. *Journal of Perinatology, 28*(4), 247–257.

da Costa, S. P., van der Schans, C. P., Zweens, M. J., Boelema, S. R., van der Meij, E., Boerman, M. A., & Bos, A. F. (2010). Development of sucking patterns in preterm infants with BPD. *Neonatology, 98,* 268–277. https://doi.org/10.1159/000281106

D'Agata, A., Young, E., Cong, X., Grasso, D. J., & McGrath, J. M. (2016). Infant medical trauma in the neonatal intensive care unit (IMTN): A proposed concept for science and practice. *Advances in Neonatal Care, 16*(4), 289–297. https://doi.org/10.1097/ANC.0000000000000309

Darcy Mahoney, A., White, R., Velasquez, A., Barrett, T., Clark, R., & Ahmad, K. (2020). Impact of restrictions on parental presence in neonatal intensive care units related to coronavirus disease 2019. *Journal of Perinatology, 40*(Suppl. 1), 36–46. https://doi.org/10.1038/s41372-020-0753-7

Davanzo, R., Strajn, T., Kennedy, J., Crocetta, A., & De Cunto, A. (2014). From tube to breast: The bridging role of semi-demand breastfeeding. *Journal of Human Lactation, 30*(4):405–409. https://doi.org/10.1177/0890334414548697

de Souza Barbosa Dias, F., Emidio, S. C. D., de Moraes Lopes, M. H. B., Shimo, A. K. K., Beck, A. R. M., & Carmona, E. V. (2017). Procedures for measuring and verifying gastric tube placement in newborns: An integrative review. *Reviews Latino-Americana de Enfermagem, 25,* e2908. https://doi.org/10.1590/1518-8345.1841.2908

Delaney, A. L., & Arvedson, J. C. (2008). Development of swallowing and feeding: Prenatal through first year of life. *Developmental Disability Research Review, 14*(2), 105–117.

Demirci, J., Bogen, D., & Klionsky, Y. (2015). Breastfeeding and methadone therapy: The maternal experience. *Substance Abuse, 36*(2), 203–208.

Dennis, C. L., & McQueen, K. (2009). The relationship between feeding outcomes and postpartum depression: A qualitative systematic review. *Pediatrics, 123*(4), e736–e751.

DeVane-Johnson, S., Woods-Giscombé, C., Thoyre, S., Fogel, C., & Williams, R. (2017). Integrative literature review of factors related to breastfeeding in African American women: Evidence for a potential paradigm shift. *Journal of Human Lactation, 36*(6), 359–367. https://doi.org/10.1891/0730-0832.36.6.359

Dietary Guidelines Advisory Committee. 2020. *Scientific report of the 2020 dietary guidelines advisory committee: Advisory report to the secretary of agriculture and the secretary of health and human services.* U.S. Department of Agriculture, Agricultural Research Service.

Dodds, W. (1989). The physiology of swallowing. *Dysphagia, 3,* 171–179.

Dryden, C., Young, D., Campbell, N., & Mactier, H. (2012). Postnatal weight loss in substitute methadone-exposed infants: Implications for the management of breast feeding. *Archives of Disease in Childhood: Fetal & Neonatal, 97*(3), F214–F216. https://doi.org/10.1136/adc.2009.178723

Dsilna, A., Christensson, K., Alfredsson, , Lagercrantz, H., & Blennow, M. (2005). Continuous feeding promotes gastrointestinal tolerance and growth in very low birth weight infants. *Journal of Pediatrics, 147*(1), 43–49.

Dsilna, A., Christensson, K., Gustafsson, A.-S., Lagercrantz, H., & Alfredsson, L. (2008). Behavioral stress is affected by the mode of tube feeding in very low birth weight infants. *Clinical Journal of Pain, 24,* 447–455.

Edwards, L., Cotton, C. M., Smith, P. B., Goldberg, R., Saha, S., Das, A., Laptook, A. R., Stoll, B. J., Bell, E. F., Carlo, W. A., D'Angio, CT., DeMauro, S. B., Sanchez, PJ., Shankaran, S., van Meurs, K. P., Vohr, B. R., Walsh, M. C., Malcolm, W. F., & Eunice Kennedy Shriver National Institute of Child Health and Human Development. (2019). Inadequate oral feeding as a barrier to discharge in moderately preterm infants. *Journal of Perinatology, 39*(9), 1219–1228. https://doi.org/10.1038/s41372-019-0422-x

Ehrenkranz, R. A. (2007). Early aggressive nutritional management for very low birth weight infants: What is the evidence? *Seminars in Perinatology, 31*(2), 48–55.

Engle, W. A. (2006). A recommendation for the definition of "late preterm" (near-term) and the birth weight-gestational age classification system. *Seminars in Perinatology, 30*(1), 2–7. https://doi.org/10.1053/j.semperi.2006.01.007

Erdei, C., & Liu, C. (2020). The downstream effects of COVID-19: A call for supporting family wellbeing in the NICU. *Journal of Perinatology, 40*(9), 1283–1285. https://doi.org/10.1038/s41372-020-0745-7

Esquerra-Zwiers, A., Rossman, B., Meier, P., Engstrom, J., Janes, J., & Patel, A. (2016). "It's somebody else's milk": Unraveling the tension in mothers of preterm infants who provide consent for pasteurized donor human milk. *Journal of Human Lactation, 32*(1), 95–102. https://doi.org/10.1177/0890334415617939

Estrem, H. H., Pados, B. F., Park, J., Knafl, K. A., & Thoyre, S. M. (2017). Feeding problems in infancy and early childhood: Evolutionary concept analysis. *Journal of Advanced Nursing, 73*(1):56–70. https://doi.org/10.1111/jan.13140

Estrem, H. H., Pados, B. F., Park, J., Thoyre, S. M., McComish, C., & Ngyuen, T. (2020). The impact of feeding on the parent and family Scales (feeding impact Scales): Development and psychometric testing. *Journal of Nursing Measurement.* https://doi.org/10.1891/JNM-D-20-00008

Farrington, M., Cullen, L., Lang, S., & Stewart, S. (2009). Nasogastric tube placement verification in pediatric and neonatal patients. *Pediatric Nursing, 35*(1), 17–24.

Favara, M. T., Carola, D., Jensen, E., Cook, A., Genen, L., Dysart, K., Greenspan, J. S., & Aghai, Z. H. (2019). Maternal breast milk feeding and length of treatment in infants with neonatal abstinence syndrome. *Journal of Perinatology, 39*(6), 876–882. https://doi.org/10.1038/s41372-019-0374-1

Ferrini, F. R., Marba, S. T., & Gaviao, M. B. (2008). Oral conditions in very low birth and extremely low birth weight children. *Journal of Dentistry for Children, 75*(3), 235–242.

Foster, J. P., Psaila, K., & Patterson, T. (2016). Non-nutritive sucking for increasing physiologic stability and nutrition in preterm infants. *Cochrane Database of Systematic Reviews, 10*(10), CD001071. https://doi.org/10.1002/14651858.CD001071.pub3

Fry, T. J., Marfurt, S., & Wengier, S. (2018). Systematic review of quality improvement initiatives related to cue-based feeding in preterm infants. *Nursing for Womens Health, 22*(5):401–410. https://doi.org/10.1016/j.nwh.2018.07.006

Fucile, S., Gisel, E. G., & Lau, C. (2005). Effect of an oral stimulation program on sucking skill maturation of preterm infants. *Developmental Medicine and Child Neurology, 47*(3), 158–162.

Fucile, S., McFarland, D. H., Gisel, E. G., & Lau, C. (2012). Oral and nonoral sensorimotor interventions facilitate suck-swallow-respiration functions and their coordination in preterm infants. *Early Human Development, 88*(6), 345–350. https://doi.org/10.1016/j.earlhumdev.2011.09.007

Garber, J. (2013). Oral-motor function and feeding intervention. *Physical and Occupational Therapy in Pediatrics, 33*(1), 111–138. https://doi.org/10.3109/01942638.2012.750864

Gennattasio, A., Perri, E. A., Baranek, D., & Rohan, A. (2015). Oral feeding readiness assessment in premature infants. *MCN: American Journal of Maternal Child Nursing, 40*(2), 96–104. https://doi.org/10.1097/NMC.0000000000000115

Gephart, S., McGrath, J., Effken, J., & Halpern, M. (2012). Necrotizing enterocolitis risk: State of the science. *Advances in Neonatal Care, 12*(2), 77–87. https://doi.org/10.1097/ANC.0b013e31824cee94

Gewolb, I. H., & Vice, F. L. (2008). Maturational changes in the rhythms, patterning, and coordination of respiration and swallow during feeding in preterm and term infants. *Developmental Medicine and Child Neurology, 48*(7), 589–594.

Gianni, M., Roggero, P., Piemontese, P., Liotto, N., Orsi, A., Amato, O., Taroni, F., Morlacchi, L., Consonni, D., & Mosca, F. (2015). Is nutritional support needed in late preterm infants? *BMC Pediatrics, 15*(1), 194. https://doi.org/10.1186/s12887-015-0511-8

Gianni, M. L., Sannino, P., Bezze, E., Plevani, L., Esposito, C., Muscolo, S., Roggero, P., & Mosca, F. (2017). Usefulness of the Infant Driven Scale in the early identification of preterm infants at risk for delayed oral feeding independency. *Early Human Development, 115,* 18–22. https://doi.org/10.1016/j.earlhumdev.2017.08.008

Gregory, K. E., & Walker, W. A. (2013). Immunologic factors in human milk and disease prevention in the preterm infant. *Current Pediatrics Reports, 1*(4). https://doi.org/10.1007/s40124-013-0028-2

Gregory, K. E. (2008). Clinical predictors of necrotizing enterocolitis in premature infants. *Nursing Research, 57*(4), 260–270.

Griffith, T., Rankin, K., & White-Traut, R. (2017). The relationship between behavioral states and oral feeding efficiency in preterm infants.

Advances in Neonatal Care, 17(1), E12–E19. https://doi.org/10.1097/ANC.0000000000000318

Griffith, T. T., Bell, A. F., White-Traut, R., Medoff-Cooper, B., & Rankin, K. (2018). Relationship between duration of tube feeding and success of oral feeding in preterm infants. *Journal of Obstetrical Gynecological and Neonatal Nursing, 47*(5), 620–631. https://doi.org/10.1016/j.jogn.2018.06.002

Groer, M., Panel, B. E., Maguire, D., Panel, B. E., & Taylor, K. (2018). Supporting breastfeeding for infants born to opioid dependent mothers. *Nursing Outlook, 66*(5), 496–498. https://doi.org/10.1016/j.outlook.2018.07.003

Grossman, M. R., Berkwitt, A. K., Osborn, R. R., Xu, Y., Esserman, D. A., Shapiro, E. D., & Bizzarro, M. J. (2017). An initiative to improve the quality of care of infants with neonatal abstinence syndrome. *Pediatrics, 139*(6), e20163360. https://doi.org/10.1542/peds.2016-3360

Hallowell, S., Spatz, D., Hanlon, A., Rogowski, J., & Lake, E. (2014). Characteristics of the NICU work environment associated with breastfeeding support. *Advances in Neonatal Care, 14*(4), 290–300. https://doi.org/10.1097/ANC.0000000000000102

Hallowell, S., Rogowski, J., Spatz, D., Hanlon, A., Kenny, M., & Lake, E. (2016). Factors associated with infant feeding of human milk at discharge from neonatal intensive care: Cross-sectional analysis of nurse survey and infant outcomes data. *International Journal of Nursing Studies, 53*, 190–203. https://doi-org.libproxy.uthscsa.edu/10.1016/j.ijnurstu.2015.09.016

Hanzer, M., Zotter, H., Sauseng, W., Pichler, G., Müller, W., & Kerbl, R. (2009). Non-nutritive sucking habits in sleeping infants. *Neonatology (Basel, Switzerland), 97*(1), 61–66. https://doi.org/10.1159/000231518

Hanzer, M., Zotter, H., Sauseng, W., Pichler, G., Muller, W., & Kerbl, R. (2010). Non-nutritive sucking habits in sleeping infants. *Neonatology, 97*(1) 61–66.

Hauck, F. R., Omojokun, O. O., & Siadatay, M. S. (2005). Do pacifiers reduce the risk of sudden infant death syndrome? A meta-anlysis. *Pediatrics, 116*(5), e716–e723.

Hawes, J., McEwan, P., & McGuire, W. (2004). Nasal versus oral route for placing feeding tubes in preterm or low birth weight infants. *Cochrane Database of Systematic Reviews, (3)*, CD003952.

Hill, A. S. (2002). Toward a theory of feeding efficiency for bottle-fed preterm infants. *The Journal of Theory Construction & Testing, 6*(1), 75–81.

Hoban, R., Bigger, H., Schoeny, M., Engstrom, J., Meier, P., & Patel, A. (2018). Milk volume at 2 weeks predicts mother's own milk feeding at neonatal intensive care unit discharge for very low birthweight infants. *Breastfeeding Medicine, 13*(2), 135–141. https://doi.org/10.1089/bfm.2017.0159

Howe, T. S., Sheu, C. F., & Holzman, I. R. (2007). Bottle-feeding behaviors in preterm infants with and without bronchopulmonary dysplasia. *American Journal of Occupational Therapy, 61*(4), 378–383.

Howell, E. A., & Ahmed, Z. N. (2019). Eight steps for narrowing the maternal health disparity gap: Step-by-step plan to reduce racial and ethnic disparities in care. *Contemporary Obstetrics and Gynecology, 64*(1), 30–36.

Hwang, Y.-S., Vergara, E., Lin, C.-H., Coster, W. J., Bigsby, R., & Tsai, W.-H. (2010) Effects of prefeeding oral stimulation on feeding performance of preterm infants. *Indian Journal of Pediatrics, 77*(8), 869–873.

Hwang, Y.-S., Ma, M.-C., Chen-Sea, M.-J., Kao, H.-M., Tsai, W.-H. (2012). Factors affecting early feeding performance in preterm infants below 32 weeks gestation. *Journal of Tropical Pediatrics, 58*(1), 77–78. https://doi.org/10.1093/tropej/fmr008

Ikonen, R., Paavilainen, E., & Kaunonen, M. (2015). Preterm infant's mothers' experiences with milk expression and breastfeeding: An integrative review. *Advances in Neonatal Care, 15*(6), 394–406. https://doi.org/10.1097/ANC.0000000000000232

Jakaitis, B. M., & Denning, P. W. (2014). Human breast milk and the gastrointestinal innate immune system. *Clinics in Perinatology, 41*(2), 423–435. https://doi.org/10.1016/j.clp.2014.02.011

Jeeva, S., Bireshwar, S., Ranadip, C., Nita, B., Sunita, T., Jose, M., & Bahl, R. (2015). Optimal breastfeeding practices and infant and child mortality: A systematic review and meta-analysis. *Acta Paediatrica, 104*, 3–13. https://doi.org/10.1111/apa.13147

Jensen, P., Gulati, I., Shubert, T., Sitaram, S., Sivalingam, M., Hasenstab, K., El-Mahdy, M., & Jadcherla, S. (2017). Pharyngeal stimulus-induced reflexes are impaired in infants with perinatal asphyxia: Does maturation modify? *Neurogastroenterology and Motility, 29*(7), e13039. https://doi.org/10.1111/nmo.13039

Jones, L. (2012). Oral feeding readiness in the neonatal intensive care unit. *Neonatal Network, 31*(3), 148–155.

Jorge, K. O., Moyses, S. J., Ferreira e Fefferra, E., Ramos-Jorge, M. L., & de Araujo Zara, P. M. (2009). Prevalence and factors associated to dental trauma in infants 1 to 3 years of age. *Dental Traumatology, 25*(2), 185–189.

Kanhadilok, S., & McGrath, J. M. (2015). An integrative review of breastfeeding influencing factors in adolescent mothers. *Journal of Perinatal Education, 24*(2), 119–127. https://doi.org/10.1891/1946-6560.24.2.119

Kelly, B. N., Huckabee, M. L., Jones, R. D., & Frampton, C. M. (2007). The early impact of feeding infant breathing-swallowing coordination. *Respiratory Physiologic Neurobiology, 156*(2), 147–153.

Kenner, C. (2020). Fetal development: Environmental influences and critical periods. In Kenner, C., Altimier, L. B., & Boykova, M. V. (Eds.), *Comprehensive neonatal nursing care: A physiologic perspective* (6th ed., pp. 1–20). Springer.

Khan, J., Vesel, L., Bahl, R., & Martines, J. (2015). Timing of breastfeeding initiation and exclusivity of breastfeeding during the first month of life: Effects on neonatal mortality and morbidity—A systematic review and meta-analysis. *Maternal & Child Health Journal, 19*(3), 468–479. https://doi.org/10.1007/s10995-014-1526-8

Kish, M. (2014). Improving preterm infant outcomes: Implementing an evidence-based oral feeding advancement protocol in the neonatal intensive care unit. *Advances in Neonatal Care, 14*(5), 346–353. https://doi.org/10.1097/ANC.0000000000000099

Klaman, S. L., Isaacs, K., Leopold, A., Perpich, J., Hayashi, S., Vender, J., Campopiano, M., & Jones, H. E. (2017). Treating women who are pregnant and parenting for opioid use disorder and the concurrent care of their infants and children: Literature review to support national guidance. *Journal of Addiction Medicine, 11*(3), 178–190. https://doi.org/10.1097/ADM.0000000000000308

Kleinman, R. E., & Greer, F. R. (2020). *Pediatric nutrition: Policy of the American academy of pediatrics* (8th ed.). American Academy of Pediatrics.

Kliethermes, P., Cross, M., Lanese, M., Johnson, K., & Simon, S. (1999). Transitioning preterm infants with nasogastric tube supplementation: Increased likelihood of breastfeeding. *Journal of Obstetric, Gynecologic, and Neonatal Nursing: JOGNN, 28*(3), 264–273. https://doi.org/10.1111/j.1552-6909.1999.tb01991.x

Korja, R., Savonlahti, E., Haataja, L., Lapinleimu, H., Manninen, H., Piha, J., Lehtonen, L., & PIPARI Study Group, . (2009). Attachment representations in mothers of preterm infants. *Infant Behavior and Development, 32*(3), 305–311.

Kwon, J., Kellner, P., Wallendorf, M., Smith, J., & Pineda, R. (2020). Neonatal feeding performance is related to feeding outcomes in childhood. *Early Human Development, 151*, 105202. https://doi.org/10.1016/j.earlhumdev.2020.105202

Lau, C., & Smith, E. (2012a). Interventions to improve oral feeding performance of preterm infants. *Acta Pediatrica, 101*, e269–e274.

Lau, C., & Smith, E. O. (2012b) A novel approach to assess oral feeding skills of preterm infants. *Neonatology, 100*, 64–70.

Lau, C., Smith, E., & Schandler, R. O. (2003). Coordination of suck-swallow and swallow respiration in preterm infants. *Acta Paediatrica, 92*(6), 721–727.

Lau, C., Fucile, S., & Schanler, R. J., (2015). A self-paced oral feeding system that enhances preterm infants' oral feeding skills *Journal of Neonatal Nursing, 21*(3), 121–126. https://doi.org/10.1016/j.jnn.2014.08.004

Lau, C. (2007). Development of oral feeding skills in the preterm infant. *Archives of Pediatrics, 1*, S35–S41.

Law-Morstatt, L., Judd, D. M., Snyder, P., Baier, R. J., & Dhaniereddy, R. (2003). Pacing as a treatment technique for transitional sucking patterns. *Journal of Perinatology, 23*, 483–488.

Lean, R. E., Rogers, C. E., Paul, R. A., & Gerstein, E. D. (2018). NICU hospitalization: Long-term implications on parenting and child behaviors. *Current Treatment Options in Pediatrics, 4*(1), 49–69.

Lin, S. C., Lin, C. H., Zhang, J. W., Chen, S. M., Chen, C. L., & Huang, M. C. (2013). Breast- and bottle-feeding in preterm infants: A comparison of behavioral cues. *Hu Li Za Zhi, 60*(6), 27–34. https://doi.org/10.6224/JN.60.6.27

Lubbe, W. (2018). Clinicians guide for cue-based transition to oral feeding in preterm infants: An easy-to-use clinical guide. *Journal of Evaluation in Clinical Practice, 24*(1), 80–88. https://doi.org/10.1111/jep.12721

Lucas, R., & McGrath, J. M. (2016). Managing pain related to breastfeeding. *Topics in Pain Management: Current Concepts and Treatment Strategies, 32*(3), 1–12.

Lucas, R., Paquette, R. J., Briere, C. E., & McGrath, J. M. (2014). Furthering our understanding of the needs of mothers who are pumping breast milk for infants in the NICU: An integrative review. *Advances in Neonatal Care, 14*(4), 241–252.

Ludwig, S. M., & Waitzman, K. A. (2007). Changing feeding documentation to reflect infant-driven feeding practice. *Newborn and Infants Nursing Reviews, 7*(3), 155–160.

Maguire, D. J., Rowe, M. A., Spring, H., & Elliott, A. F. (2015). Patterns of disruptive feeding behaviors in infants with neonatal abstinence syndrome. *Advances in Neonatal Care, 15*(6), 429–439. https://doi.org/10.1097/ANC.0000000000000204

Mason-Wyckoff, M., McGrath, J. M., Griffin, T., Malan, J., & White-Traut, R. C. (2003). Nutrition: physiologic basis of metabolism and management of enteral and parenteral nutrition. In Kenner, C., & Wright, L. J., (Eds.), *Comprehensive neonatal nursing: a physiologic persepective* (3rd ed., pp. 425–447). Saunders.

McCormick, F. M., Tosh, K. & McGuire, W. (2010). Ad libitum or demand/semi-demand feeding versus scheduled interval feeding for pretem infants. *Cochrane Database of Systematic Reviews*, (2), CD005255. https://doi.org/10.1002/14651858.CD005255.pub3

McGlothen, K. S., & Cleveland, L. M. (2018). The right to mother's milk: A call for social justice that encourages breastfeeding for women receiving medication-assisted treatment for opioid use disorder. *Journal of Human Lactation, 34*(4), 799–803. https://doi.org/10.1177/0890334418789401

McGlothen, K., Cleveland, L., & Gill, S. (2018). "I'm Doing the Best that I Can for Her": Infant-Feeding decisions of mothers receiving medication-assisted treatment for an opioid use disorder. *Journal of Human Lactation, 34*(3), 535–542.

McGlothen-Bell, K., Cleveland, L., Recto, P., Brownell, E., & McGrath, J. (2020). Feeding behaviors in infants with prenatal opioid exposure: An integrative review. *Advances in Neonatal Care, 20*(5), 374–383. https://doi.org/10.1097/ANC.0000000000000762

McGlothen-Bell, K., Recto, P., McGrath, J. M., Brownell, E., & Cleveland, L. (2021). Recovering together: Mothers' experiences providing skin-to-skin care for their infants with NAS. *Advances in Neonatal Care, 21*(1), 16–22. https://doi.org/10.1097/ANC.0000000000000819

McGrath, J. M., & Braescu, A. V. B. (2004). State of the science: Feeding readiness in the preterm infant. *Journal of Perinatal and Neonatal Nursing, 18*(4), 353–368. https://doi.org/10.1097/00005237-200410000-00006

McGrath, J. M., & Medoff-Cooper, B. (2001). Apnea and periodic breathing during bottle feeding of premature infants. *Communicating Nursing Research, 34*(9), 220.

McGrath, J. M., & Vittner, D. (2020). Family: Essential partner in care. In Kenner, C., Altimier, L. B., & Boykova, M. V. (Eds.), *Comprehensive neonatal nursing care: A physiologic perspective* (6th ed., pp. 753–783). Springer.

McGrath, J. M., Lewis, M., & Pickler, R. (October, 2008). Psychometric testing of the feeding readiness and progression in preterms Scale. Conference proceedings: 2008 National State of the Science Congress in Nursing Research. Washington, DC.

McGrath, J. M., Bromiker, R., Hanlon, A., McGlothen-Bell, K., & Medoff-Cooper, B. (2021). Correlates and trajectories of preterm infant sucking patterns and sucking organization at term age. *Advances in Neonatal Care, 21*(2), 152–159. https://doi.org/10.1097/ANC.0000000000000810

McGrath, J. M. (2000). Developmentally supportive caregiving and technology in the NICU: Isolation or merger of intervention strategies? *Journal of Perinatal and Neonatal Nursing, 14*(3), 78–91.

McGrath, J. M. (2006, March). *Factors related to feeding readiness in early born preterm infants.* Conference proceedings: Inaugural NANN Research Summit. Scottsdale, AZ.

McGrath, J. M. (2007a). Breastfeeding success for the high-risk infant and family: Nursing attitudes and beliefs. *Journal of Perinatal and Neonatal Nursing, 21*(3), 183–185.

McGrath, J. M. (2007b). "My Baby weighs almost 10 pounds" Families and feeding the preterm infant. *Newborn and Infant Nursing Reviews, 7*(3), 173–174.

Medoff-Cooper, B., McGrath, J. M., & Bilker, W. (2000). Nutritive sucking and neurobehavioral development in preterm infants from 34 weeks PCA to term. *MCN: American Journal of Maternal Child Nursing, 25*(2), 64–70.

Medoff-Cooper, B., Bilker, W., & Kaplan, J. (2001). Suckling behavior as a function of gestational age: A cross-sectional study. *Infant Behavior and Development, 24*, 83–94.

Medoff-Cooper, B., Shults, J., & Kaplan, J. (2009). Sucking behavior of preterm neonates as a predictor of developmental outcomes. *Journal of Developmental and Behavioral Pediatrics, 30*(1), 16–22.

Medoff-Cooper, B., Rankin, K., Li, Z., Liu, L., & White-Traut, R. (2015). Multisensory intervention for preterm infants improves sucking organization. *Advances in Neonatal Care, 15*(2), 142–149.

Meier, P., Engstrom, J., Mangurten, H., Estrada, E., Zimmerman, B., & Kopparthi, R. (1993). Breastfeeding support services in the neonatal intensive-care unit. *Journal of Obstetric, Gynecologic, and Neonatal Nursing: JOGNN, 22*(4), 338–347. https://doi.org/10.1111/j.1552-6909.1993.tb01814.x

Meier, P. P., Engstrom, J. L., Patel, A. L., Jegier, B. J., & Bruns, N. E. (2010). Improving the use of human milk during and after the NICU stay. *Clinics in Perinatology, 37*(1), 217–245. https://doi.org/10.1016/j.clp.2010.01.013

Meier, P., Patel, A., Bigger, H., Rossman, B., & Engstrom, J. (2013). Supporting breastfeeding in the neonatal intensive care unit: Rush Mother's Milk Club as a case study of evidence-based care. *Pediatric Clinics of North America, 60*(1), 209–226. https://doi.org/10.1016/j.pcl.2012.10.007

Meier, P., Johnson, T., Patel, A., & Rossman, B. (2017). Evidence-based methods that promote human milk feeding of preterm infants: An expert review. *Clinics in Perinatology, 44*(1), 1–22. https://doi.org/10.1016/j.clp.2016.11.005

Mercado, K., Vittner, D., Drabant, B., & McGrath, J. M. (2019a). Neonatal intensive care unit-specific lactation support and maternal breast milk availability for very low birthweight infants. *Advances in Neonatal Care, 19*(6), 474–481. https://doi.org/10.1097/ANC.0000000000000684

Mercado, K., Vittner, D., & McGrath, J. M. (2019b). What is the impact of NICU dedicated lactation consultants? An evidence-based brief. *Advances in Neonatal Care, 19*(5), 383–393. https://doi.org/10.1097/ANC.0000000000000602

Merewood, A., Chamberlain, L. B., Cook, J. T., Philipp, B. L., Malone, K., & Bauchner, H. (2006). The effect of peer counselors on breastfeeding rates in the neonatal intensive care unit. *Archives of Pediatric and Adolescent Medicine, 160*, 681–685.

Miller, J. L., Macedonia, C., & Sonies, B. C. (2006). Sex differences in prenatal oral-motor function and development. *Developmental Medicine and Child Neurology, 48*(6), 465–470.

Mizuno, K., Nishida, Y., Taki, M., Hibino, S., Murase, M., Sakurai, M., & Itabashi, K. (2007). Infants with bronchopulmonary dysplasia suckle with weak pressures to maintain breathing during feeding. *Pediatrics, 120*(4), e1035–e1042.

Morgan, J., Bombell, S., & McGuire, W. (2013). Early trophic feeding for very low birth weight infants. *Cochrane Database of Systematic Reviews*, (3), CD000504. https://doi.org/10.1002/14651858.CD000504.pub4

Neiva, F., Leone, C., & Leone, C. (2008). Non-nutritive sucking scoring system for preterm newborns. *Acta Pædiatrica, 97*(10), 1370–1375. https://doi.org/10.1111/j.1651-2227.2008.00943.x

Ngo, K. D., & Shah, M. (2020). Gastrointestinal system. In Kenner, C., Altimier, L. B., & Boykova, M. V. (Eds.), *Comprehensive neonatal nursing care: A physiologic perspective* (6th ed., pp. 179–210). Springer.

Nye, C. (2008). Transitioning premature infants from gavage to breast. *Neonatal Network, 27*(1), 7–13.

Nyqvist, K., Haggkvist, A., Hansen, M., Kylberg, E., Frandsen, A., Maastrup, R., Ezeonodo, A., Hannula, L., Haiek, L., & Baby-Friendly Hospital Initiative Expert Group. (2013). Expansion of the Baby-Friendly Hospital Initiative ten steps to successful breastfeeding into neonatal intensive care: Expert group recommendations. *Journal of Human Lactation, 29*(3), 300–309.

Nyqvist, K. H., Maastrup, R., Hansen, M. N., Haggkvist, A. P., Hannula, L., Ezeonodo, A., Kylberg, E., Frandsen, A. L., & Haiek, L. N. (2015). *Neo-BFHI: The Baby-friendly Hospital Initiative for Neonatal Wards.* Core document with recommended standards and criteria. Nordic and Quebec Working Group; 2015. This document can be found at the International Lactation Consultant Association (ILCA) website:http://www.ilca.org/i4a/pages/index.cfm?pageid=4214

Pados, B. F., & Mellon, M, (2020). Effect of thickening on flow rates through bottle nipples. *JOGNN: Journal of Obstetrical, Gynecological and Neonatal Nursing, 50*(1), P78–P87. https://doi.org/10.1016/j.jogn.2020.09.153

Pados, B. F., Park, J., Thoyre, S. M., Estrem, H., & Nix, W. B. (2016). Milk Flow Rates from bottle nipples used after hospital discharge. *MCN: American Journal of Maternal Child Nursing, 41*(4)–237–243. https://doi.org/10.1097/NMC.0000000000000244

Pados, B. F., Park, J., & Dodrill, P. (2019). Know the flow: Milk flow rates from bottle nipples used in the hospital and after discharge. *Advances in Neonatal Care, 19*(1), 32–41. https://doi.org/10.1097/ANC.0000000000000538

Park, J., Thoyre, S., Knafl, G. J., Hodges, E. A., & Nix, W. B. (2014). Efficacy of semielevated side-lying positioning during bottle-feeding of very preterm infants: A pilot study. *Journal of Perinatal and Neonatal Nursing, 28*(1), 69–79. https://doi.org/10.1097/JPN.0000000000000004

Park, J., Knafl, G., Thoyre, S., & Brandon, D. (2015). Factors associated with feeding progression in extremely preterm infants. *Nursing Research, 64*(3), 159–167. https://doi.org/10.1097/NNR.0000000000000093

Park, J., Thoyre, S., & Knafl, G. (2015). Four measures of change in physiologic state during the feeding period of very premature infants. *Biological Research for Nursing, 17*(5), 503–509.

Park, J., Thoyre, S., Estrem, H., Pados, B. F., Knafl, G. J., & Brandon, D. (2016) Mothers' psychological distress and feeding of their preterm infants. *MCN: American Journal of Maternal Child Nursing, 41*(4), 221–229. https://doi.org/10.1097/NMC.0000000000000248

Park, J., Pados, B. F., & Thoyre, S. M. (2018). Systematic review: What is the evidence for the side-lying position for feeding preterm infants? *Advances in Neonatal Care, 18*(4):285–294. https://doi.org/10.1097/ANC.0000000000000529

Park, J., Silva, S. G., Thoyre, S. M., & Brandon, D. H. (2020). Sleep-wake states and feeding progression in preterm infants. *Nursing Research, 69*(1), 22–30. https://doi.org/10.1097/NNR.0000000000000395

Parker, L. A., Torrazza, R. J. M., Yuefeng, L. Talaga, E. Shuster, J., & Neu, J. (2015). Aspiration and evaluation of gastric residuals in the NICU: State of the science. *Journal of Perinatal and Neonatal Nursing, 29*(1), 51–59. https://doi.org/10.1097/JPN.0000000000000080

Parker, L. A., Weaver, M., Torrazza, R. J. M., Shuster, J., Krueger, C., & Neu, J. (2019a). Effect of gastric residual evaluation on enteral intake in extremely preterm infants. *JAMA Pediatrics, 173*(6), 534–543. https://doi.org/10.1001/jamapediatrics.2019.0800

Parker, M. G., Greenberg, L. T., Edwards, E. M., Ehret, D., Belfort, M. B., & Horbar, J. D. (2019). National trends in the provision of human milk at hospital discharge among very low-birth-weight infants. *JAMA Pediatrics, 173*(10), 961–968. https://doi.org/10.1001/jamapediatrics.2019.2645

Penny, F., Brownell, E., Judge, M., & McGrath, J. M. (2018a). Cup feeding as a supplemental, alternative feeding method for preterm breastfed infants: An integrative review. *Maternal and Child Health Journal, 22*(11), 1568–1579. https://doi.org/10.1007/s10995-018-2632-9

Penny, F., Judge, M., Brownell, E., & McGrath, J. M. (2018b). What is the evidence for use of the supplemental feeding tube device as an alternative supplemental feeding method for breastfed infants? *Advances in Neonatal Care, 18*(1), 31–37. https://doi.org/10.1097/ANC.0000000000000446

Pereira, A., Cruz-Melguizo, S., Adrien, M., Fuentes, L., Marin, E., Forti, A., & Perez-Medina, T. (2020). Breastfeeding mothers with COVID-19 infection: A case series. *International Breastfeeding Journal, 15*(1), 1–8. https://doi.org/10.1186/s13006-020-00314-8

Peters, A., McGrath, J. M., Doggett, M., Langley, K., & Weller, M. (2008). *Outcomes of holding premature infants during gavage feedings. Conference proceedings: 2008 National State of the Science Congress in Nursing Research.* Washington, DC.

Pickler, R. H., & Reyna, B. A. (2004). Effects of non-nutritive sucking on nutritive sucking, breathing, and behavior during bottle feedings of preterm infants. *Advances in Neonatal Care, 4*(4), 226–234.

Pickler, R. H., Best, A. M., Reyna, B. A., Gutcher, G., & Wetzel, P. A. (2006a). Predictors of nutritive sucking in preterm infants. *Journal of Perinatology, 26*(11), 693–699.

Pickler, R. H., Chiaranai, C., & Reyna, B. A. (2006b). Relationship of the first suck to feeding outcomes in preterm infants. *Journal of Perinatal and Neonatal Nursing, 20*(2), 157–162.

Pickler, R. H., Best, A., & Crosson, D. (2008). The effect of feeding experience on clinical outcomes in preterm infants. *Journal of Perinatology, 29*(2), 124–129.

Pickler, R. H., McGrath, J. M., Reyna, B. A., McCain, N., Lewis, M., Cone, S., Best, A., & Wetzel, P. (2010). A Model of neurodevelopmental risk and protection for preterm infants. *Journal of Perinatal and Neonatal Nursing, 24*(4), 356–365.

Pickler, R. H., Reyna, B. A, Griffin, J. B., Lewis, M., & Thompson, A. M. (2012). Changes in oral feeding in preterm infants two weeks after hospital discharge. *Newborn and Infant Nursing Reviews, 12*(4), 202–206. https://doi.org/10.1053/j.nainr.2012.09.012

Pickler, R. H., McGrath, J. M., Reyna, B., Cooley, H. T., Best, A., Lewis, M., Cone, S., & Wetzel, P. (2013). Effects of the neonatal intensive care unit environment on preterm-infant oral feeding. *Research and Reports in Neonatology, 2013*(3), 15–20.

Pickler, R. H., Wetzel, P. A., Meinzen-Derr, J, Tubs-Cooley, H. L., & Moore, M. (2015). Patterned feeding experience for preterm infants: Study protocol for a randomized controlled trial. *BMC Trials, 16*, 255. https://doi.org/10.1186/s13063-015-0781-3

Pickler, R. H., Meinzen-Derr, J, Moore, M., Sealscott, S., Tepe, K. (2020). Effect of tactile experience during preterm infant feeding on clinical outcomes. *Nursing Research, 69*(5 Suppl. 1), S21–S28. https://doi.org/10.1097/NNR.0000000000000453

Pike, M., Kritzinger, A., & Krüger, E. (2017). Breastfeeding characteristics of late-preterm infants in a kangaroo mother care unit. *Breastfeeding Medicine, 12*(10), 637–644. https://doi.org/10.1089/bfm.2017.0055

Pineda, R., Dewey, K., Jacobsen, A., & Smith, J. (2019). Non-nutritive ducking in the preterm infant. *American Journal of Perinatology, 36*(3), 268–276. https://doi.org/10.1055/s-0038-1667289

Pineda, R., Prince, D., Reynolds, J., Grabill, M., & Smith, J. (2020). Preterm infant feeding performance at term equivalent age differs from that of full-term infants. *Journal of Perinatology, 40*(4), 646–654. https://doi.org/10.1038/s41372-020-0616-2

Pitts, A., Faucher, M. A., & Spencer, R. (2015). Incorporating breastfeeding education into prenatal care. *Breastfeeding Medicine, 10*(2), 118–123. https://doi.org/10.1089/bfm.2014.0034

Premji, S. S., & Chessell, L. L. (2011). Continuous nasogastric milk feeding versus intermittent bolus milk feeding for premature infants less than 1500 grams. *Cochrane Database of Systematic Reviews, 2011*(11), CD001819. https://doi.org/10.1002/14651858.CD001819.pub2

Premji, S. S., McNeil, D. A., & Scotland, J. (2004). Regional neonatal oral feeding protocol: The ethos of feeding preterm infants. *Journal of Perinatal and Neonatal Nursing, 18*(4), 371–384.

Pridham, K., Steward, D., Thoyre, S., Brown, R., & Brown, L. (2007). Feeding skill performance in premature infants during the first year of life. *Early Human Development, 83*(5), 293-305.

Psaila, K., & Patterson, T. (2016). Non-nutritive sucking for increasing physiologic stability and nutrition in preterm infants. *Cochrane Database of Systematic Reviews, 10*(10), CD001071. https://doi.org/10.1002/14651858.CD001071.pub3

Ramirez, A., Wong, W. W., & Shulman, R. J. (2006). Factors regulating gastric emptying in preterm infants. *Journal of Pediatrics, 149*(4), 475–479.

Ray, K. N., & Lorch, S. A. (2013). Hospitalization of early preterm, late preterm, and term infants during the first year of life by gestational age. *Hospital Pediatrics, 3*(3), 194–203. https://doi.org/10.1542/hpeds.2012-0063

Reyna, B. A., Pickler, R. H., & Thompson, A. (2006). A descriptive study of mothers' experiences feeding their preterm infants after discharge. *Advances in Neonatal Care, 6*(6), 333–340.

Reyna, B. A., Brown, L. F., Pickler, R. H., Myers, B. J., & Younger, J. B. (2012). Mother-infant synchrony during infant feeding. *Infant Behavior and Development, 35*(4), 669–677. https://doi.org/10.1016/j.infbeh.2012.06.003

Rocha, A. D., Moreira, M. E., Pimenta, H. P., Ramos, J. R., & Lucena, S. L. (2007). A randomized study of the efficacy of sensory-motor-oral stimulation and non-nutritive sucking in very low birth weight infants. *Early Human Development, 83*(6), 385–388.

Rossier, J. (2009). Wiring and plumbing in the brain. *Frontiers in Human Neuroscience, 3*(2),1–2.

Rozé, J., Darmaun, D., Boquien, C., Flamant, C., Picaud, J., Savagner, C., Claris, O., Lapillonne, A., Mitanchez, D., Branger, B., Simeoni, U., Kaminski, M., & Ancel, P. Y. (2012). The apparent breastfeeding paradox in very preterm infants: Relationship between breast feeding, early weight gain and neurodevelopment based on results from two cohorts, EPIPAGE and LIFT. *BMJ Open, 2*(2), e000834. https://doi.org/10.1016/j.peds.2012.11.090

Sato, T. T., & Chang, H. L. (2016). Abnormal rotation of the and the fixation of the intestines. In Wyllie, R., Hyams, H. S., & Kay, M. (Eds.), *Pediatric gastric and liver and liver disease* (5th ed., pp. 640–647), Elsevier.

Saunders, R. P., Abraham, M. R., Crosby, M. J., Thomas, K., & Edwards, W. H. (2003). Evaluation and development of potentially better practices for improving family-centered care in neonatal intensive care units. *Pediatrics, 111*(4 Pt. 2), e437–e449.

Scheel, C. E., Schanler, R. J., & Lau, C. (2005). Does the choice of bottle nipple affect the oral feeding performance of very-low-birthweight (VLBW) infants? *Acta Paediatrica, 94*(9), 1266–1272.

Section on Breastfeeding. (2012). Breastfeeding and the use of human milk. *Pediatrics, 129*(3), e827–e841. https://doi.org/10.1542/peds.2011-3552

Settle, M., & Francis, K. (2019). Does the infant-driven feeding method positively impact preterm infant feeding outcomes? *Advances in Neonatal Care, 19*(1), 51–55. https://doi.org/10.1097/ANC.0000000000000577

Shaker, C. S. (2013). Cue-based feeding in the NICU: Using the infant's communication as a guide. *Neonatal Network, 32*(6), 404–408. https://doi.org/10.1891/0730-0832.32.6.404

Silberstein, D., Geva, R., Feldman, R., Gardner, J. M., Karmel, B. Z., Rozen, H., & Kuint, J. (2009). The transition to oral feeding in low-risk premature infants: Relation to infant neurobehavioral functioning and mother–infant feeding interaction. *Early Human Development, 85*(3),157–162.

Simpson, C., Schanler, R. J., & Lau, C. (2002). Early introduction of oral feeding in preterm infants. *Pediatrics, 110*(3), 517–522.

Slattery, J., Morgan, A., & Douglas, J. (2012). Early sucking and swallowing problems as predictors of neurodevelopmental outcome in children with neonatal brain injury: A systematic review. *Developmental Medicine and Child Neurology, 54*(9), 796–806. https://doi.org/10.1111/j.1469-8749.2012.04318.x

Slocum, C., Arko, M., Di Fiore, J., Martin, R. J., & Hibbs, A. M. (2009). Apnea, bradycardia and desaturation in preterm infants before and after feeding. *Journal of Perinatology, 29*(3), 209–212. https://doi.org/10.1038/jp.2008.226

Smith, V., Hwang, S., Dukhovny, D., Young, S., & Pursley, D. (2013). Neonatal intensive care unit discharge preparation, family readiness and infant outcomes: Connecting the dots. *Journal of Perinatology, 33*(6), 415–421.

Spatz, D., Froh, E., Flynn-Roth, R., & Barton, S. (2015). Improving practice at the point of care through the optimization of the breastfeeding resource nurse model. *Journal of Obstetric, Gynecologic, and Neonatal Nursing: JOGNN, 44*(3), 412–418. https://doi.org/10.1111/1552-6909.12570

Spatz, D. L. (2004). Ten steps to promoting and protecting breastfeeding for vulnerable infants. *Journal of Perinatal and Neonatal Nursing, 18*, 385–396.

Spatz, D. L. (2005). Report of a staff program to promote and support breastfeeding in the care of vulnerable infants at a Children's Hospital. *The Journal of Perinatal Education, 14*(1), 30–38. https://doi.org/10.1624/105812405X23630

Spatz, D. L. (2006). State of the science: use of human milk and breast-feeding for vulnerable infants. *The Journal of Perinatal & Neonatal Nursing, 20*(1), 51–55. https://doi.org/10.1097/00005237-200601000-00017

Spatz, D. (2018). Beyond BFHI: The Spatz 10-step and breastfeeding resource nurse model to improve human milk and breastfeeding outcomes. *Journal of Perinatal & Neonatal Nursing, 32*, 164–174. https://doi.org/10.1097/JPN.0000000000000339

Spatz, D. L. (2021). The use of human milk and breastfeeding in the neonatal intensive care unit. In Wamback, K., & Spencer, B. (Eds.), *Breastfeeding and human lactation.* Jones & Bartlett Publishers, Inc.

Stevens, E. E., Gazza, E., & Pickler, R. (2014). Parental experience learning to feed their preterm infants. *Advances in Neonatal Care, 14*(5), 354–361. https://doi.org/10.1097/ANC.0000000000000105

Stumm, S. L., Barlow, S. M., Estep, M., Lee, J., Cannon, S., Carlson, J., & Finan, D. (2008). Respiratory distress syndrome degrades the fine structure of the non-nutritive suck in preterm infants. *Journal of Neonatal Nursing, 14*(1), 9–16.

Thomas, T., Goodman, R., Jacob, A., & Grabher, D. (2021). Implementation of cue-based feeding to improve preterm infant feeding outcomes and promote parents' involvement. *Journal of Obstetrical Gynecological and Neonatal Nursing, 50*(3), 328–339. https://doi.org/10.1016/j.jogn.2021.02.002

Thomas, A. (2007). Guidelines for bottle feeding your premature infant. *Advances in Neonatal Care, 7*(6), 311–318.

Thoyre, S. M., & Carlson, J. R. (2003). Preterm infants' behavioural indicators of oxygen decline during bottle feeding. *Journal of Advanced Nursing, 43*(6), 631–641. https://doi.org/10.1046/j.1365-2648.2003.02762.x

Thoyre, S. M., Shaker, C. S., Pridham, K. F. (2005). The early feeding skills assessment for preterm infants. *Neonatal Network, 24*(3), 7–16.

Thoyre, S., Holditch-Davis, D., Schwartz, T. A., Melendez Roman, C. R., & Nix, W. (2012). Coregulated approach to feeding preterm infants with lung disease, effects during feeding. *Nursing Research, 61*(4), 242–251.

Thoyre, S., Park, J., Pados, B., & Hubbard, C. (2013). Developing a Coregulated, cue-based feeding practice: The critical role of assessment and reflection. *Journal of Neonatal Nursing, 19*(4), 139–148. https://doi.org/10.1016/j.jnn.2013.01.002

Thoyre, S. M., Hubbard, C., Park, J., Pridham, K., & McKechnie, A. (2016). Implementing Co-regulated feeding with mothers of preterm infants. *MCN: American Journal of Maternal Child Nursing, 41*(4), 204–211. https://doi.org/10.1097/NMC.0000000000000245

Thoyre, S. M. (2007). Feeding outcomes of extremely premature infants after neonatal care. *JOGNN: Journal of Obstetric, Gynaecologic and Neonatal Nursing, 36*(4), 366–375.

Torola, H., Lehtihalmes, M., Yloherva, A., & Olsen, P. (2012). Feeding skill milestones of preterm infants born extremely low birth weight. *Infant Behavior and Development, 35*(2), 187–194. https://doi.org/10.1016/j.infbeh.2012.01.005

Turk-Browne, N. B., Scholl, B. J., & Chun, M. M. (2008). Babies and brains: Habituation in infant cognition and functional neuroimaging, *Frontiers in Human Neuroscience, 2*, 1–11.

Tuthill, E. L., Butler, L., McGrath, J. M., Cusson, R., Makiwani, N. G., Gable, R. K., & Fisher, J. D. (2014). Cross-cultural adaptation of instruments assessing breastfeeding determinants: A multi-step approach. *International Breastfeeding Journal, 9*(16), 9–16. https://doi.org/10.1186/1746-4358-9-16. http://www.internationalbreastfeeding-journal.com/content/9/1/16

Tuthill, E. L., McGrath, J. M., Graber, M. Cusson, R. M., & Young, S. L. (2016). Breastfeeding self-efficacy: A critical review of available instruments. *Journal of Human Lactation, 32*(1), 35–45. https://doi.org/10.1177/0890334415599533

Vice, F. L., & Gewolb, I. H. (2008). Respiratory patterns and strategies during feeding in preterm infants. *Developmental Medicine and Child Neurology, 50*(6), 467–372.

Victora, C., Bahl, R., Barros, A., Franca, G., Horton, S., Krasevec, J., Murch, S., Sankar, M. J., Walker, N., Rollins, N. C., & Lancet Breastfeeding Series Group. (2016). Breastfeeding in the 21st century: Epidemiology, mechanisms, and lifelong effect. *Lancet, 387*, 475–490). https://doi.org/10.1016/S0140-6736(15)01024-7

Warren, J. J., & Bishara, S. E. (2002). Duration of nutritive and non-nutritive sucking behaviors and their effects on the dental arches in the primary dentition. *American Journal of Orthodontics & Dentofacial Orthopedics, 121*(4), 347–356.

Watson, J., & McGuire, W. (2016). Responsive versus scheduled feeding for preterm infants. *Cochrane Database of Systemic Reviews, (8)*, CD005255. https://doi.org/10.1002/14651858.CD005255.pub5

White-Traut, R. C., Berbaum, M. L., Lessen, B., McFarlin, B., & Cardenas, L. (2005). Feeding readiness in preterm infants: The relationship between preterm behavioral state and feeding readiness behaviors and efficiency during transition from gavage to oral feeding. *MCN: American Journal of Maternal Child Nursing, 30*(1), 52–59.

Wight, N. (2003). Breastfeeding the borderline (near-term) preterm infant. *Pediatric Annals, 32*(5), 329–336.

Wolthuis, M., da Costa, S., Bos, A., Krijnen, W., van der Schans, C., & Luinge, M. (2017). Sucking behaviour in infants born preterm and developmental outcomes at primary school age. *Developmental Medicine and Child Neurology, 59*(8), 871–877. https://doi.org/10.1111/dmcn.13438

Wolthuis-Stigter, M., Luinge, M., da Costa, S., Krijnen, W., van der Schans, C., & Bos, A. (2015). The association between sucking behavior in preterm infants and neurodevelopmental outcomes at 2 years of age. *The Journal of Pediatrics, 166*(1), 26–30.e1. https://doi.org/10.1016/j.jpeds.2014.09.007

Wu, X., Jackson, R. T., Khan, S. A., Ahuja, J., & Pehrsson, P. R. (2018). Human milk nutrient composition in the United States: Current knowledge, challenges, and research needs. *Current Developments in Nutrition, 2*(7), nzy025. https://doi.org/10.1093/cdn/nzy025

Yildiz, A., & Arikan, D. (2012) The effects of giving a pacifier to premature infants and making them listen to lullabies on their transition period to total oral feeding and sucking success. *Journal of Clinical Nursing, 5*(3), 644–656. https://doi.org/10.1111/j.1365-2702.2010.03634.x

Young, P. C., Korgenski, K., & Buchi, K. F. (2013). Early readmission of newborns in a large health care system. *Pediatrics, 131*(5), e1538–e1544. https://doi.org/10.1542/peds.2012-2634

CHAPTER 16

Skin-to-Skin Contact Optimizes Outcomes for Infants and Families

Dorothy Vittner and Jacqueline M. McGrath

> **Standard 3, Systems Thinking:** The practice of Infant and Family-Centered Developmental Care (IFCDC) in the intensive care unit (ICU) shall be based on evidence that is ethical, collaborative, safe, timely, quality driven, efficient, equitable, and cost-effective.
>
> **Standard 6, Systems Thinking:** The interprofessional collaborative team should provide IFCDC through transition to home and continuing care for the baby and family to support the optimal physiologic and psychosocial health needs of the baby and family.
>
> **Standard 1, Skin-to-Skin Contact:** Parents shall be encouraged and supported in early, frequent, and prolonged skin-to-skin contact (SSC) with their babies.
>
> **Standard 2, Skin-to-Skin Contact:** Education and policies in support of skin-to-skin contact between parents and their baby shall be developed, implemented, monitored, and evaluated by an interprofessional collaborative team.
>
> **Standard 3, Skin-to-Skin Contact:** Babies shall be evaluated to (a) determine their readiness for transfer to KC, (b) assess stability during transfer from bed to parent's chest, (c) assess baby's response to SSC, and (d) assess their stability during and after transfer back to the bed.
>
> **Standard 4, Skin-to-Skin Contact:** Parents shall be provided information about the benefits of SSC that continue for babies and parents after discharge.
>
> **Standard 1, Pain and Stress, Families:** The interprofessional team shall document increased parental/caregiver well-being and decreased emotional distress during the intensive care hospital (ICU) stay. Distress levels of baby's siblings and extended family should also be considered.
>
> **Standard 2, Pain and Stress, Babies:** The interprofessional collaborative team shall develop care practices that prioritize multiple methods to optimize baby outcomes by minimizing the impact of stressful and painful stimuli.

INTRODUCTION

Individualized developmental care in the neonatal intensive care unit (NICU) aims to support the infant's physiologic stabilization, neurobehavioral functioning, and emotional and social well-being, which ultimately facilitates the infant's short- and long-term growth and development. Yet, it is well known that infant cannot be stable if separated from their mothers/caregivers and the needs of mothers/caregivers must also be addressed as inseparable from providing care to the high-risk infant. The impact of infant separation has been well documented within the Infant Medical Trauma in the NICU (IMTN) model by D'Agata et al. (2016, 2017). The critical components of the model define the traumatic experience of the infant, which includes the complex relationships between

stress and allostasis, parental separation and pain (D'Agata et al., 2016). The unique feature of IMTN, as opposed to pediatric medical trauma is that, this framework, hinges on increasing one's understanding of the influence of early life traumatic events within the NICU. The traumatic events, individually and cumulatively have both short and long-term effects on neurodevelopmental and genetic vulnerability for infants receiving care in the NICU (D'Agata et al., 2016). The IMTN model provides language to articulate the infant's lived experience in the NICU where the importance of family can often be lost among the other medical priorities. We begin by discussing this issue because mother–infant separation cannot be minimized for this already medically traumatized population.

Based on each infant's individual maturity, competencies, vulnerabilities, and status of subsystem functioning, developmental care integrates a mutually supportive physical and social environment, individualized assessment and interventions, infant and family-centered care, and a collaborative clinical practice model to provide personalized and consistent infant care activities that supports and encourages parent engagement and participation in caregiving. Thus, it is essential that all NICU care is provided with awareness and integration of infant's current developmental functioning and neurobehavioral competence to consider opportunities to diffuse stress and support the infant and family to benefit from the unique competencies they each bring into interactions. Appropriate care encompasses awareness of sensory experiences within the overall physical environment, sometimes referred to as the macroenvironment, as well as provision of the environment immediately around the infant, which can also be referred to as the microenvironment, to support appropriate and responsiveness to the infant's neurobehavioral cues.

Fundamental to the infant's developmental trajectory is early parent–infant contact. Parent–infant contact through touch, especially during skin-to-skin contact (SSC), has the potential to reduce the adverse consequences of prematurity. SSC is defined as a diaper-clad infant on a parent's bare chest. SSC is also referred to as Kangaroo Care given its historical underpinning. Kangaroo Mother Care (KMC) is considered a model of care that includes interventions such as nonseparation of infant and mother, extensive SSC, opportunities for exclusive breastfeeding, potential earlier hospital discharge, and follow-up care (Chan et al., 2016; Kostandy & Ludington-Hoe, 2019). Benefits of SSC are thought to occur though physiological changes in the infant and parents that facilitate increased feelings of comfort, attachment, and physiologic stability (Mori et al., 2010; Vittner et al., 2019). SSC is an evidence-based holding strategy that increases the opportunity for parental proximity and provides a continuous interactive environment known to enhance infant physiologic stability and affective closeness within the parent–infant dyad (Chan et al., 2016; Ludington-Hoe, 2011; Moore et al., 2016).

There is a plethora of evidence to support routine integration of SSC practices with hospitalized infants (healthy newborns, critically ill newborns, premature infants, infants with complex heart disease, etc.). However, the purpose of this chapter is to provide the evidence documenting responses of high-risk infants and families to SSC within the context of the NICU environment. Evidence for use of SSC with other populations can be found elsewhere in the literature; SSC is an intervention strategy to foster mother/caregiver attachment and engagement, autonomic and physiologic, cognitive and motor, as well as state development with facilitation of prolonged periods of restorative sleep. SSC is also an effective care practice to enhance positive feeding experiences, infection control, thermoregulation, and comfort dimensions for provision of individualized developmental care model. This chapter will also discuss implementation strategies as well as barriers to SSC implementation in the NICU with recommendations for overcoming these barriers.

BENEFITS TO FAMILY (MATERNAL AND PATERNAL)

Fundamental to the infant's developmental trajectory is early parent–infant contact, which benefits infant, mother, father, and family caregivers. Overall, the effects of parent–child separation are consistently negative on children's social-emotional development, well-being, and mental health (Bentley Waddoups et al., 2019). Parental touch, especially during SSC can reduce the adverse consequences of prematurity. As stated above, SSC is an evidence-based holding strategy that increases parental proximity and provides a continuous interactive environment known to enhance infant physiologic stability and affective closeness within the parent–infant dyad (Feldman, 2015b; Uvnäs Moberg, Gross, et al., 2020). Holding is a powerful strategy to enhance the developing infant–parent relationship (Vittner et al., 2016). Recently published long-term outcomes documented with high-risk infants held SSC during early infancy have shown improved physiology, improved executive functioning, and increased mother–child reciprocity at 10 years post NICU (Feldman, 2015b). SSC also improves mother–infant interaction and maternal bonding during early infancy (Bigelow et al., 2012). Father–infant SSC had positive impacts on infants' outcomes, including temperature and pain, biophysiological markers, and behavioral response (Shorey et al., 2016). SSC also enhances father's parental role attainment and paternal interaction behavior and decreases paternal stress and anxiety (Shorey et al., 2016; Vittner et al., 2018).

Underlying Mechanism of SSC—Oxytocin. So, why is implementation of SSC important? Evidence suggests that SSC activates oxytocin release for mother, father, and infant (Carter, 2014; Carter et al., 2020, Cong et al., 2015; Vittner et al., 2018). Oxytocin was originally identified as a female hormone because of its important roles in birth and lactation (Erlandsson et al., 2007; Lee et al., 2009; Ross & Young, 2009). However, in the lay literature, oxytocin is often referred to as the love hormone. Oxytocin is a vital and integrative component of a comprehensive neurochemical system that regulates positive interaction and exerts powerful antistress and restorative effects on all developing relationships (Uvnäs Moberg, Gross, et al., 2020). Another key role that the oxytocinergic system plays is in bond formation and parenting (Feldman, 2015a). Oxytocin stimulates various kinds of social interactive behaviors including maternal behavior and bonding (Feldman, 2015a; Uvnäs Moberg, Ekström, et al., 2020). It decreases fear and the sensation of pain, and it may promote trust and well-being. In addition, oxytocin induces powerful anti-inflammatory and antistress effects including lowering of blood pressure, heart rate, and cortisol levels (Uvnäs Moberg, Gross, et al., 2020). Oxytocin is produced primarily in the supraoptic nucleus and paraventricular nucleus of the hypothalamus (Gordon et al., 2017).

In limited human studies, parental plasma oxytocin concentrations were positively related to mother–infant affectionate contact and father–infant stimulatory contact at 6 months postpartum (Ross & Young, 2009). Oxytocin is reported to be involved in the control of stress, anxiety, and autonomic functions, such as heart rate; high oxytocinergic activity is stress relieving and anxiolytic in animals and humans (Uvnäs Moberg, Gross, et al., 2020). Mothers of preterm infants are more likely to have difficulty with attachment than mothers of full-term infants (Lee et al., 2009). This can be attributed to decreased synchrony or responsiveness with parent–infant interactions as well as the subtle behavioral cues among premature infants that are difficult to interpret (Vittner et al., 2018, 2019). Evidence suggests that early dysfunctional contacts due to the infant's disorganized behavioral patterns between the infant and parent lead to poorer attachment and behavioral problems in childhood (Feldman et al., 2014). Conversely, early responsive and synchronous contact may positively influence cognitive and developmental outcomes for the child (Feldman, 2015b). Feldman defines sensitive periods of development as opportunities to identify essential biobehavioral experiences that trigger specific neurological or endocrine systems that influence gene expression, brain development, and social fitness that exist in early infant–parent environments (Feldman, 2015b).

Increases in oxytocin levels in infants have been associated with increased reciprocity and responsiveness within parent–infant interactions (Vittner et al., 2018). Evidence suggests that fathers with higher oxytocin and lower testosterone levels engaged in more affectionate touch during observed interactions with their infants (Gordon et al., 2017). Higher oxytocin can help focus attention toward socially salient contexts, regardless of whether they have positive or negative valence (Crespi, 2016). Recent evidence suggests that the mechanisms for oxytocin release may be different for fathers as compared with mothers, indicating minimal oxytocin responses for fathers during the first episode of SSC, but increasing with successive episodes (Gettler et al., 2021). Interestingly, infants held within SSC by their fathers later displayed significantly more play between fathers and infants if their oxytocin levels increased indicating support for implementing SSC influencing long-term development (Gettler et al., 2021).

Effects on Depression and Well-being. The birth of preterm or critically ill infants can be a highly emotional and distressing period for families. Parents of these infants face unique challenges, including coping with the complex health conditions of their infants, disruption of family routines due to hospital stay, and prolonged physical separation from their infant. Mothers of hospitalized infants have an increased risk of postpartum depression (PPD) compared with mothers of full-term infants, with prevalence as high as 40% in the first year after birth versus 15% to 20% of all new mothers. A recent systematic review and meta-analysis identified that SSC has a small protective effect on maternal depressive scores (Scime et al., 2019). SSC may affect maternal PPD through various mechanisms such as activation of the oxytocinergic system as evidenced by increases

in salivary oxytocin (Cong et al., 2015; Vittner et al., 2018). SSC may protect mothers from psychological vulnerabilities linked with PPD and possibly from other areas of mental distress like anxiety that are disproportionately high in the NICU population (Bigelow et al., 2012; Roque et al., 2017). More confidence and competence in caring for their infant (Scime et al., 2019) and enhanced maternal behaviors with the infant (Baley, 2015) and improved maternal–infant interactions at 1 year of life due to SSC right after birth have been reported. Now SSC is emerging as a therapy for maternal depression, decreasing maternal anxiety (Athanasopoulou & Fox, 2014), decreasing the number of preterm birth mothers with clinically manifested depression (Kirca & Adibelli, 2021), decreasing the severity of depression in preterm birth mothers (Athanasopoulou & Fox, 2014), and showing promise in prevention of depression (Kirca & Adibelli, 2021). Minimization of maternal stress also occurs with SSC (Handlin et al., 2009), and maternal and neonatal stress levels synchronously decrease during SSC (Vittner et al., 2018). Maternal satisfaction with SSC is high (Cong et al., 2015; Vittner et al., 2018). Physical improvement in the mother's postpartum condition (higher hematocrit, less lochia, faster involution, and shorter length of postpartum stay) has been attributable to SSC (Conde-Agudelo & Díaz-Rossello, 2016).

SSC has many benefits for fathers in context of more responsive attachment (Chen et al., 2017), increased confidence (Scime et al., 2019), more active caregiving, and more responsive interactions (Vittner et al., 2018) with their preterm infants. Paternal SSC also increases depth of respirations in the newly born term infant (Shorey et al., 2016). Thus, SSC has been considered the optimal family-centered approach for newborn care and is leading institutions to find ways to better support the continuation of SSC 24/7 throughout the mother's postpartum stay (Kostandy & Ludington-Hoe, 2019).

The evidence supporting integration of SSC for high-risk infants and families has been appraised using the system in which the following levels have specific meaning: level I, evidence identified from a systematic review or meta-analysis of all relevant randomized controlled trials (RCTs) or evidence-based clinical guidelines based on systematic reviews of RCTs; level II, evidence obtained from well-designed RCT; level III, evidence obtained from well-designed controlled trials without randomization; level IV, evidence from well-designed case-controlled and cohort studies; level V, evidence from systematic reviews of descriptive and qualitative studies; level VI, evidence from a single descriptive or qualitative study; level VII, evidence from opinion of authorities and/or reports of expert committees. Tables in this chapter summarize the recommendation for practice, level of evidence, and key references. Table 16-1 provides the evidence for benefits to parents and caregivers as a result of participating in SSC with their high-risk infant.

References are not inclusive of all studies because of the plethora of evidence to support SSC, which has been studied since 1972. Earlier findings are well represented

TABLE 16-1 Evidence to Support Maternal, Paternal, and Family Benefits of SSC

Benefits for:	Rationale for SSC Implementation	Level of Evidence	References
Mothers	Decreased separation; increased bonding and attachment	I, II, III, IV	Kostandy and Ludington-Hoe [2019] Groer and Morgan [2007] Ross and Young [2009] Cong et al. [2015] Vittner et al. [2018] Baley [2015]
	Strategy to decrease postpartum depression and increase overall well-being	II, III	Roque et al. [2017] Athanasopoulou and Fox [2014], de Alencar et al. [2009]
	Increased physical improvement and recovery from birth	III	Conde-Agudelo and Díaz-Rossello [2016]
Fathers	Increases sense of attachment with infant	II, III	Cong et al. [2015] Shorey et al. [2016] Vittner et al. [2018] Gettler et al. [2021]
Both	Decreased separation; increased bonding and attachment	I, II, III	Uvnäs Moberg, Ekström, et al. [2020] Uvnäs Moberg, Gross, et al. [2020] Cong et al. [2015] Vittner et al. [2018] Feldman [2015a, 2015b]
	Increased competence, confidence, and satisfaction with parenting and NICU experience	I, II	Scime et al. [2019] Cong et al. [2015] Vittner et al. [2018]
Infants in relationship to parent-attachment	More positive long-term relationships with the child and better developmental outcomes for child	I, II	Kostandy and Ludington-Hoe [2019] Shorey et al. [2016] Bystrova et al. [2009] Bracht et al. [2013]

*Whenever possible, references were limited to last 10 years to demonstrate the most recent evidence to support SSC integration with high-risk infants and families in the NICU.

within a recent systematic review of SSC effects in preterm infants (Chan et al., 2016) as well as within a comprehensive review of SSC in full-term infants (Karimi et al., 2019). Please find more about strategies for enhancing and facilitating the benefits for families later in the chapter within the sections on SSC education, safety, and implementation.

BENEFITS FOR INFANTS

SSC may be used as an intervention to help stabilize the critically ill infant's physiologic stability and autonomic organization. A wealth of evidence exists demonstrating effects of SSC on several physiologic parameters. Ludington-Hoe clearly articulates that the autonomically organized infant maintains physiologic stability in the presence of environmental disturbances (Ludington-Hoe, 2011). Stability in physiologic levels is demonstrated by decreased variation in the rates and smaller standard deviations in each parameter during and/or following SSC (Boundy et al., 2016). Table 16-2 provides the level of evidence for physiologic benefits to infants as a result of participating in SSC.

Physiologic Stability. Current evidence continues to validate the positive effect of SSC on heart rate stability (Linner et al., 2020). Several RCTs included in a meta-analysis and Cochrane Review demonstrates that increases in heart rate (HR) during SSC are minimal, HR remains within normal limits, and greater stability in HR is present during SSC than during incubator care, crib care, and swaddled holding in preterm infants Boundy et al., 2016; Conde-Agudelo & Díaz-Rosello, 2016). Increased physiologic stability with lasting effects through the first 10 years after SSC during infancy has also been documented (Feldman et al., 2014). Better stability of cardiorespiratory status was also observed when preterm and full-term infants were transported to and from the NICU in SSC rather than in incubators. Thus, SSC transport is believed to offer advantages over incubator transport. The evidence strongly suggests that SSC enhances physiologic stability, which includes an absence of bradycardia during SSC with high-risk infants (Chi Luong et al., 2016; Linner et al., 2020; Lorenz et al., 2017).

Heart rate variability. Heart rate variability (HRV) is a measure of the variation from one heartbeat to the next; this physiological phenomenon of HRV can provide additional

TABLE 16-2 Practice Recommendations for Physiologic Outcomes for High-Risk Infants Experiencing Skin-to-Skin Contact With a Parent

Physiologic Variable	Rationale for SSC Implementation	Level of Evidence	References
Heart rate	• Heart rate stability is increased during standing transfer for SSC • Heart rate stability is increased during SSC that lasts greater than 1 hour • Increased stability during SSC with decreased episodes of bradycardia	I, II, III	Linner et al. (2020) Boundy et al. (2016) Conde-Agudelo & Díaz-Rosello (2016) Mori et al. (2010) Ludington-Hoe (2011) Feldman et al. (2014)
Heart rate variability	• Expect no difference in HRV during SSC • Increase in sympathetic tone with parasympathetic predominance during SSC • Increased coregulation between infant and parent	III, IV, V	Kommers et al. (2018) Joshi et al. (2019) Schrod and Walter (2002)
Respiratory patterns	• Increased stability • Decreased episodes of irregular breathing/apnea • Respiratory rate might rise up to 10 breaths/min with transfer • RR might decrease slightly for a short time (3 minutes) after SSC implementation	I, II, III, IV	Vogl et al. (2021) Moore et al. (2016) Chi Luong et al. (2016) Lee et al. (2021) Linnér et al. (2020), Lorenz et al. (2017) Boundy et al. (2016)
Oxygenation	• SaO_2 fluctuations should be within normal ranges during implementation of SSC • SaO_2 may drop during transfer but quickly recovers • Cerebral oxygenation improves during SSC • SaO_2 changes during breastfeeding in SSC are rare	I, II, III, IV	Mori et al. (2010) Conde-Agudelo & Díaz-Rossello (2016) Mori et al. (2010) Boundy et al. (2016) Begum et al. (2009) Conde-Agudelo & Díaz-Rossello (2016) Shattnawi and Al-Ali (2019)
Temperature	• Infants ≥ 28 weeks postmenstrual age are warmer in SSC than anywhere else • Infants < 28 weeks PMA do not warm up in SSC alone • Infants < 28 weeks PMA may need heat lamp during SSC to maintain body temperature • Maternal breasts/Paternal chest warm up and conduct heat to regulate infant temperature in SSC (however, paternal chests may not regulate as well so please monitor infant temperature with fathers) • SSC prevents hypothermia, beginning at birth, and SSC is superior to swaddling for prevention of hypothermia • SSC is recommended for rewarming of infants	I, II, III, IV	Kostandy and Ludington-Hoe (2019) Srivastava et al. (2014) Boundy et al. (2016) Oras et al. (2016) Abdulghani et al. (2018) and Feldman-Winters et al. (2016) AAP and American Heart Association, 2016 Kristoffersen et al. (2016)

*Whenever possible, references were limited to last 10 years to demonstrate the most recent evidence to support SSC integration with high-risk infants and families in the NICU.

physiological insight into regulatory changes that occur for high-risk infants. HRV reflects the dynamic, rapidly occurring changes in autonomic regulation caused by the primary systems controlling the infant's heart rate (Kommers et al., 2018). In addition to humoral factors, the sympathetic nervous system and the parasympathetic nervous system (PSNS) can influence HRV quickly (Rajendra Acharya et al., 2006). HRV provides an opportunity to noninvasively track the regulatory activity of the infant's autonomic nervous system.

This autonomic regulation in preterm infants is distinctly affected by intra- versus extrauterine maturation (Joshi et al., 2019). Thus, HRV adequately measures the effect of the environment on autonomic functioning. SSC and associated parental coregulation seem to trigger an immediate transition toward the more stable HRV regulation offered by the myelinated vagus (Kommers et al., 2017). The regulation offered by this branch of the PSNS encourages efficient usage of energy and rapid regulation of cardiac output. The parasympathetic activation that occurs during SSC was probably due to the calming, soothing, nature of SSC, but other factors inherent in SSC may also come into play. For example, SSC usually occurs in an inclined position; infants are more horizontal when laying on incubator or crib mattress. Being inclined activates parasympathetic nerves; returning to a horizontal position incites sympathetic activation indicating horizontal positioning is more stressful than inclined positioning.

Respiratory Patterns: Apnea/Periodic Breathing/ Irregular Breathing. Respiratory rate changes might be expected during SSC either because infants fall asleep (respiratory rate decreases) or because infants are warmed by their mothers (respiratory rates increase). Yet, evidence indicates that SSC has stabilizing effects on respiratory rates and infants show greater stability than seen in an incubator (Moore et al., 2016; Vogl et al., 2021). Knowing the impact of SSC on apnea frequency is important (Mallet et al., 2007), especially because apnea and bradycardia can trigger changes in cerebral autoregulation of blood flow, intracranial pressure, cerebral oxygenation, and carbon dioxide tension, putting infants at greater risk of postnatal intraventricular hemorrhage. Thus, many investigations have measured apnea and irregular breathing as an outcome (Table 16-2). The predominant finding in randomized controlled clinical trials is that apnea decreases during SSC as compared with incubator (Lee & Bang, 2011) SSC brings about fewer and shorter episodes of apnea and periodic breathing because apneas and unsteady breathing occur during indeterminate sleep. Across subgroup analysis, SSC is associated with lower respiratory rates and higher oxygen saturations (Boundy et al., 2016). Indeterminate sleep does not seem to occur during SSC, and the number of arousals from sleep is decreased during SSC.

Oxygenation. Oxygenation usually changes during SSC, but the direction and magnitude of change vary across the studies (Table 16-2). Levels of oxygen saturation during SSC have been found to increase over incubator-based values (Conde-Agudelo & Díaz-Rossello, 2016), have decreased by 0.5% to 1.0% over 1 to 3 hours of SSC (Mori et al., 2010), and have remained the same in SSC as in the incubator before or after SSC or remained the same as in control infants who never received SSC (Boundy et al., 2016). Better stability in oxygen saturation values during SSC has also been found (Boundy et al., 2016; Conde-Agudelo & Díaz-Rossello, 2016). A meta-analysis of case controlled (pre-SSC—SSC—post-SSC) studies showed that oxygen saturation drops by 0.6% during SSC (Mori et al., 2010). Nonetheless, oxygen saturation changes during SSC are predominantly within normal limits for variability and accompanied by increased stability, with values commonly remaining within clinically

acceptable range. Thus, **desaturation** events are rare, either not occurring at all, occurring less frequently with SSC, or occurring slightly more frequently (Boundy et al., 2016) during SSC than during incubator care. In one study, **cerebral oxygenation** of the left and right hemispheres increased slightly (from 46.8% to 47.3% in the left and from 48.6% to 49.1% in the right) over incubator values during 1 hour of SSC (Begum et al., 2009). Regardless of changes in oxygen saturation levels, several studies have reported that an increase in oxygen consumption does not occur during SSC (Conde-Agudelo & Díaz-Rossello, 2016), suggesting that changes in peripheral oxygen saturation are not accompanied by systemic changes in the infant. Nonetheless, SSC predominantly has positive effects on infant cardiorespiratory status and has been shown to facilitate recovery from respiratory distress (Conde-Agudelo & Díaz-Rossello, 2016). Given that the decision to practice SSC is often based on the infant's existing HR, respiratory rate (RR), and arterial oxygen saturation (SaO_2) rather than weight and infant postmenstrual age (PMA) (Shattnawi & Al-Ali, 2019), the data on cardiorespiratory outcomes improving during SSC support SSC as adjunctive to routine respiratory care seems expected and appropriate.

Temperature Stability with SSC. The majority of preterm, full-term, ventilated, twin, and triplet infants are found to be warmer in SSC than anywhere else, and SSC is more effective in preventing hypothermia and rewarming infants than any other technique, including swaddled holding (Srivastava et al., 2014). A recent meta-analysis provided strong evidence that revealed compared with conventional care, SSC was associated with 78% lower risk of hypothermia (Boundy et al., 2016). This effect was similar across different types of KMC and infant characteristics (Table 16-2). Interestingly, researchers have found that infants are warmer when breastfeeding in SSC than when being bottle fed held SSC (Oras et al., 2016). Because of the overwhelmingly consistent results among all types of studies and particularly among the RCTs and meta-analyses, SSC immediately after vaginal or cesarean birth (Akbari et al., 2018; Boundy et al., 2016) has become one of the five components of essential care for all newborns around the world (Abdulghani et al., 2018; Feldman-Winters et al., 2016). Further recognition of the strength of the data showing SSC warms infants is the inclusion of SSC as a strategy for thermoregulation in the guidelines for neonatal resuscitation (AAP & American Heart Association, 2016). The phenomenon that mothers are able to thermoregulate (instantaneously and spontaneously without conscious effort increase or decrease the breast temperature in response to the infant's temperature) (Kostandy & Ludington-Hoe, 2019) is a caregiving strategy to which healthcare professionals need to become more accustomed to and trust more than they currently do. It is well documented that mothers make many more temperature adjustments and are more effective than incubators (Conde-Agudelo & Díaz-Rossello, 2016; Kostandy & Ludington-Hoe et al., 2019). Nevertheless, three nuances of SSC's temperature effects need to be considered. First, infants under 28 weeks gestational and postmenstrual age do not gain body warmth in SSC and may lose up to 1.0°C temperature, although this rarely occurs (Kristoffersen et al., 2016). SSC with extremely low-birth-weight infants improves thermal control during the golden hours transition with decreased oxygen needs (Linner et al., 2020). Second, during paternal SSC infant temperatures may continue to rise resulting in hyperthermia, especially in tropical environments, thus requiring the need for close observation by the healthcare professional (Kostandy & Ludington-Hoe, 2019). Paternal chests do not make the multiple adjustments to prevent hypo- and hyperthermia in the infant that women's chests do, yet they are effective in keeping their infant warm (Boundy et al., 2016). Third, immediately after birth the infant should be well dried and may need a head cap to prevent hypothermia while held in SSC. The maintenance of the infant's temperature during SSC has been a concern for preterm and full-term infants given the plethora of existing studies examining this issue.

Often times infants requiring phototherapy for **hyperbilirubinemia** are denied SSC so phototherapy treatment can continue. However, the evidence does not support denying infants and parents this opportunity (Kostandy & Ludington-Hoe, 2019) Infants can experience SSC with a fiberoptic bili-light blanket being used up against the infant's back beneath the blankets used to insulate and contain the preterm infant in SSC. Infants can then be cared for under bank lights when not being held in SSC.

SSC Effects on Infection. Currently, conflicting data exist about the effect of SSC on infections in preterm and full-term infants, even though a Cochrane meta-analysis in 2016 (Conde-Agudelo & Díaz-Rossello, 2016) revealed that SSC was associated with reduction of nosocomial infections. Several studies have shown that preterm infants who received SSC during hospitalization had fewer infections (or none at all) than infants who did not receive SSC (Kostandy & Ludington-Hoe, 2019). However, the exact mechanism of SSC's role in reducing infections is still unknown.

In summary, the **goal** of care for hospitalized infants in the autonomic and physiologic dimension is promotion of physiologic stability in the face of environmental disturbances and continued development of the autonomic nervous system so homeostasis is sustained such that growth and development can occur. The effects of SSC on all physiologic systems are predominantly positive and the benefits outweigh the few risks that have been identified, especially when vigilant monitoring is available to each parent and infant. Autonomic and physiologic organization (stability, vital signs remaining within normal limits, breathing patterns more regular, hormonal secretion, and developmental normal) characterize the infant's condition during maternal and paternal SSC of preterm and full-term infants (Vogl et al., 2021). The infant's brainstem itself needs maternal touch to normally function (normal functioning is manifested by homeostasis in all cardiorespiratory and state systems), and when brainstem-related physiologic regulation occurs, such

as happens under SSC, emotion, attention, and higher-level processing such as self-regulation, inhibitory control, and cognitive development foster experience-dependent plasticity of neurobiological systems that support social functioning (Feldman, 2015a).

SHORT- AND LONG-TERM EFFECTS ON FEEDING, GROWTH, DEVELOPMENT, AND MATERNAL–INFANT INTERACTION OUTCOMES

SSC Effects on Feeding. In preterm and term infants SSC clearly promotes initiation of prefeeding behaviors (Oras et al., 2016), initiation of breastfeeding (Mekonnen et al., 2019; Wang et al., 2020), exclusivity of breastfeeding (Elhalik & El-Atawi, 2016; Sharma, 2016), longer duration of breastfeeding (Quigley & McGuire, 2014; Tully et al., 2016), better recognition of mother's milk, and higher milk production. Meta-analysis and systematic review (Elhalik & EL-Atawi, 2016; Sharma, 2016) have shown that even short periods of SSC increase the duration of breastfeeding for 4 to 6 weeks post discharge and that SSC offers greater advantage for the preterm infant in terms of breastfeeding outcome than expressing milk, galactogogues, support, peer counseling, test weighing, nipple shields, and finger and cup feedings (Quigley & McGuire, 2014). In addition, the oxytocin released during SSC positively affects vagal nerve activity linked to increased gastrointestinal functioning and enhances anabolic metabolism (Uvnäs Moberg, Ekström, et al., 2020). More SSC infants breastfeed at discharge than infants who did not receive SSC (Moore et al., 2016; Quigley & McGuire, 2014; Tully et al., 2016), and given that exclusive breast milk feedings at discharge was made an evaluation criterion of the Joint Commission for Accreditation of Healthcare Organizations (JCAHO) as of April 1, 2010 (Feldman-Winter et al., 2013), SSC's role as an independent predictor of breastfeeding (Moore et al., 2016) supports routine use of SSC starting at birth and continuing throughout hospitalization so all infants are receiving exclusive breast milk feedings in the neonatal period. A priority is to educate NICU healthcare professionals about daily SSC, and SSC as a prefeeding intervention has shown evidence of increasing the breast milk feeding rate at discharge in preterm infants (Agudelo et al., 2020). The evidence base for SSC effects on breastfeeding is robust and has been subjected to meta-analyses that confirm more preterm and full-term infants who receive SSC will breastfeed than infants who do not receive SSC (Moore et al., 2016) and is included in breastfeeding clinical guidelines for safe sleep and Baby Friendly implementation in the neonatal period (Moon, 2016; Sampaio et al., 2016).

Growth. To determine if SSC promotes infant growth and development, several biomarkers have been examined, such as effects of SSC on blood glucose, metabolic hormones such as thyroxin, gastrin, cholecystokinin, and somatostatin. None of these parameters demonstrated negative effects, and in fact positive effects were often noted. For example, a Cochrane meta-analysis has confirmed that full-term infants who have SSC will have higher blood glucose levels at the end of SSC than infants who did not have SSC (Conde-Agudelo & Díaz-Rossello, 2016). The ultimate end point of metabolism is **somatic growth**. Growth in infants is most commonly measured by weight gain. Weight changes in response to SSC have been extensively studied, and the majority of the reports identify increased daily weight gain in SSC in comparison with no-SSC, regardless of duration (Table 16-3). However, several RCTs have shown no effect of SSC on weight change, yet meta-analyses (Conde-Agudelo &

Díaz-Rossello, 2016) confirm that across all studies preterm infants experiencing SSC demonstrated greater weight gain than infants not experiencing SSC.

Cognitive and Motor Development Effects. Evidence suggests that SSC positively effects cognitive development. When receiving SSC during NICU hospitalization preterm infants have exhibited more alertness and less gaze aversion, more rapid maturation of vagal tone and state organization, more quiet sleep, more alert wakefulness, less active sleep, better habituation and orientation skills on the Neonatal Behavioral Assessment Scale (NBAS), and higher mental and motor scores on the Bayley Scales of Infant and Toddler

TABLE 16-3 Practice Recommendations for Growth, Development, and Maternal–Infant Interaction Outcomes Related to Skin-to-Skin Contact With a Parent

Variable	Rationale for SSC Implementation	Level of Evidence	References
Weight gain	• SSC infants generally gain 15–30 g/d after 30 weeks PMA with implementation of SSC • Expect swifter birth weight recovery with SSC	I, II,	Conde-Agudelo and Díaz-Rossello (2016)
Feeding	• Enhances prefeeding activities • For mothers SSC enhances milk production • Enhances breastfeeding with longer durations of breastfeeding • Enhances exclusive breastfeeding • Enhances increased oxytocin release • Enhances the chances that the high-risk infant will continue breastfeeding to and after discharge from NICU		Oras et al. (2016) Wang et al. (2020) Sharma et al. (2016), Tully et al. (2016) Quigley and McGuire (2014) Elhalik and El-Atawi (2016) Uvnäs-Moberg et al. (2020a, 2020b) Agudelo et al. (2020) Moore et al. (2016) Moon (2016)
Mental development	• Brain maturation and mental development (higher Bayley scores) is enhanced when SSC is provided for at least 60 minutes daily • Fewer and less severe IVH with implementation of SSC		Akbari et al. (2018) Kaffashi et al. (2013) Feldman (2015a, 2015b)
Motor development	• Motor development is enhanced with daily SSC implementation	I, II,III, VI	Akbari et al. (2018) Kaffashi et al. (2013)
State: alert, sleep, and regulation	• SSC implementation enhances alert period duration and better orientation in infants after 38 weeks PMA • SSC implementation reduces crying • SSC implementation enhances duration and quality (fewer arousals) of quiet sleep	III II III, V IV	Kaffashi et al. (2013) Campbell-Yeo et al. (2015) Scher et al. (2009) Moore et al. (2016), van Sleuwen et al. (2007) Cong et al. (2015)
Maternal–infant interaction	• SSC implementation improves interactions due to proximity and release of oxytocin • Implementation of regular (daily) SSC leads to more positive maternal behaviors and better quality of maternal–infant interaction in the first year of life • Mothers believe SSC promotes better relationship with infants, and SSC moms are satisfied with their interactions with their babies regardless of severity of illness	I, II, III	Uvnäs Moberg, Ekström, et al. (2020) Uvnäs Moberg, Gross, et al. (2020) Cong et al. (2015) Vittner et al. (2019) Feldman (2015a, 2015b) Bracht et al. (2013) Carter (2014) Carter et al. (2020), Vittner et al. (2018) Scatliffe et al. (2019)

*Whenever possible, references were limited to last 10 years to demonstrate the most recent evidence to support SSC integration with high-risk infants and families in the NICU.
IVH, intra-ventricular hemorrhage.

Development. Preterm infants >32 weeks PMA who received 24/7 SSC in the hospital and at home demonstrated similar developmental outcomes as infants who did not receive SSC, with no difference in development as measured by the Griffiths Mental Development Scales at 6 and 12 months corrected age, and no differences in the incidence of cerebral palsy, visual deficits, and hearing impairments at 12 months of age (Kostandy & Ludington-Hoe, 2019). Geva and Feldman (2008) ho reported that maternal touch provides a set of biobehavioral regulators for the infant's brainstem development. Vittner and colleagues reported similar results with improved neurobehavioral competencies for healthy preterm infants who were held SSC (Vittner et al. under review). Maternal touch affects the secretion of brainstem-related biochemical substances and brainstem coordination of the developing circadian rhythms of the infant (Geva & Feldman, 2008). Feldman and colleagues reported enhanced child cognitive development and executive functions for participants from 6 months to 10 years (Feldman et al., 2014). Furthermore by 10 years of age, children receiving SSC showed attenuated stress responses, improved autonomic functioning, more organized sleep, and better cognitive control. Improved autonomic functioning and maternal behavior were dynamically interrelated over time, which leads to better physiology, executive functions, and mother–child reciprocity at 10 years (Feldman et al., 2014).

Several studies of SSC effects on motor development have been conducted (Table 16-3). Akbari et al. (2018) conducted a meta-analysis of studies pertaining to biopsychosocial outcomes within the first year. SSC was compared with incubator care, among low-birth-weight premature infants; SSC compared with conventional care was associated with improved infant self-regulation. Moderated effects were identified for cognitive and motor development correcting for duration of SSC, country-level mortality ratio, and infant gender (Akbari et al., 2018). Previous systematic review of studies of many different types of early intervention, some beginning in the NICU, concluded that SSC enhanced motor development and that preterm infants benefitted most from intervention programs that acknowledge the need for a multifaceted sensory environment (Als & McAnulty, 2011). SSC provides a sensory rich environment for infants with opportunities to hear parental heart rate and body sounds; opportunities to feel maternal respiratory movements and nurturing touch; opportunities for the unique parental scent, warmth, and contained flexed positioning; and opportunities to see the parents' facial expressions. Evidence suggests that the use of SSC influences infant self-regulation that has lasting effects (Akbari et al., 2018). SSC is widely regarded as a developmentally appropriate intervention to improve both mental and motor development outcomes (Akbari et al., 2018).

In addition, the **motor** system is definitely affected by SSC as the infant's position changes from being supine or prone and mostly horizontal in an incubator (or under a radiant warmer) to being more upright, prone, and confined between breasts or constrained on the chest. The more upright position of SSC fosters outward recoil of the chest. Interestingly, outward recoil of an infant's chest is limited when the infant lies supine. Once the infant is more upright, the contents of the abdominal cavity can shift away from the upper abdomen, creating an increase in negative subdiaphragmatic pressure, a change that favors outward recoil of the chest wall, enhancing the efficiency of the diaphragm and pulmonary functions. While in SSC, the infant's head should be kept at a 30° to 60° upright angle, allowing for better pulmonary functional residual capacity and easier breathing.

Effects of SSC on State Organization. Infant state organization refers to appropriate and smooth transitions from one state to another on the continuum of deep sleep through wakefulness to robust crying. Smooth transitions mean that changes in state occur with physiologic compromise and behavioral agitation. When infants are held SSC, they often are in a deep restorative sleep and seldom arouse and are thus able to maintain healthy durations of quiet sleep (Campbell-Yeo et al., 2015), durations that maximize memory and brain development (Kaffashi et al., 2013). SSC also has some behavioral effects on the infant, which include better sleep cycles, decreased crying, and an analgesic effect on the infant during painful procedures (Disher et al., 2017; Johnston et al., 2017; Mörelius et al., 2015).

The sleep/wake cycle for infants defines each state as quiet/deep sleep, active sleep, drowsy, quiet alert, awake and active, and fussy (Brazelton, 1978). Electroencephalographic studies have confirmed that infants fall more quickly into quiet sleep, have longer periods of quiet sleep, have more clearly defined sleep states, have fewer arousals from sleep, and have better cyclicity of sleep in SSC than when in an incubator (Kaffashi et al., 2013). In fact, sleep in the incubator is generally chaotic and fragmented and riddled with long-duration arousals (Scher et al., 2009). Crying is also reduced when an infant, both preterm and full term, is held SSC (Moore et al., 2016) or swaddled in maternal arms (Moore et al., 2016). Preterm and full-term infant crying are clearly reduced by SSC according to meta-analyses (Moore et al., 2016).

SSC Effects on Comfort and Pain. Evidence suggests that SSC appears to be an effective intervention to decrease composite pain indicators with both physiological and behavioral indicators and, independently, using heart rate and crying time, and safe for a single painful procedure (Johnston et al., 2017). Reducing agitation is one method for enhancing comfort. In premature infants, environmental disturbances can cause physiologic and behavioral (motoric and state) agitation. Heart rate, respiratory rate, and oxygen indices will fluctuate widely with any disturbance at low gestational ages, but as the infant matures, maintenance of homeostatic values ensues. Behavioral disorganization also occurs with environmental disruptions, resulting in arms flailing, legs extending, trunk lifting and arching, head turning side to side, and facial grimacing. A priority of developmental care is to minimize agitated, energy-depleting movements and reduce the infant's overreaction to changes in the environment. SSC efficiently relaxes infants, dampens infant's responses to environmental events, and induces sleep, permitting the infant a short reprieve from the stimulation onslaught characterizing neonatal intensive care (Moore et al., 2016). The containment provided by secure placement in SSC between breasts and up against the parental chest clearly evokes quiescence and relaxation in preterm and full-term infants (Oras et al., 2016; Vittner et al., 2018). Feldman has defined a sensitive period of development that is essential for infant experiences that trigger specific neurobiological processes with the neurological and endocrine system that influence gene expression, brain development, and social connectedness that has life-long effects (Feldman, 2015a). When skin-to-skin, evidence suggests that the neuropeptide oxytocin is activated and plays a pivotal role as a neuromodulator and contributes to social sensitivity and attunement developing relationships (Carter, 2014; Carter et al., 2020; Scatliffe et al., 2019; Vittner et al., 2018).

In addition to behavioral quiescence, SSC also minimizes hormonal signs of **stress**. Salivary and serum cortisol have been measured extensively in preterm infants (Table 16-4). The preterm infant who is at rest and undisturbed in an incubator has levels of circulating cortisol that markedly exceed the 150 nmol/L that is associated with eustress. High cortisol levels signal stress, even when the infant appears to be resting and calm. Stress in the neonatal period has been clearly identified as a precursor to adult-age cardiovascular disease and dementia (Champagne & Curley, 2009; Nuyt, 2008). Infant stress is significantly reduced by SSC (Vittner et al., 2018). Evidence continues to suggest that as little as 20 minutes of SSC reduces cortisol levels by 60% in infants 25 weeks PMA and older (Mörelius et al., 2015). Preterm infant and mother cortisol levels tend to be synchronous; with infant–mother SSC, they mutually and simultaneously reduce their cortisol levels (Hardin et al., 2020; Mörelius et al., 2015; Vittner et al., 2018). So, with stressful experiences such as invasive procedures, intubation, medical handling, diapering, weaning from a ventilator, medical and neurobehavioral assessments

gavage, and tube feedings, SSC should be given to calm and comfort the infants because SSC is a very effective simple form of tactile stimulation that is as close to natural maternal care giving as can be and is more customary than keeping a hand on the thigh or head or stroking and massaging an infant.

Pain is a pernicious developmental event, and premature infants are commonly subjected to repeated and prolonged painful and stress procedures throughout their hospital stay (D'Agata et al., 2017). Unrelieved pain due to invasive procedures has been associated with increased heart rate, increased blood pressure, increased oxygen consumption, stress hormone secretion, and fluctuations in intracranial pressure (Johnston et al., 2017). The preterm infant's reactivity to pain is a marker of neuromotor development (Young et al., 2017) and overrepeated unrelieved pain experiences, diminished behavioral reactivity, and diminished cortisol secretion occur (Young et al., 2017), indicating significant influence on infant development (Abdulkader et al., 2008; D'Agata et al., 2017). In fact, the more the invasive procedures and infant experiences during hospitalization, the poorer the infant's cognitive and motor function will be at 8 and 18 months corrected age (O'Reilly et al., 2020). So, many pharmacologic and nonpharmacologic interventions to alleviate pain have been scientifically tested to assist in the management of physiologically destabilizing and developmentally challenging pain experiences. Incorporation of the mother to touch and soothe her infant during painful procedures has been encouraged. SSC is an evidence-based approach to the pain interventionist's armamentarium and works well for procedural pain in preterm and full-term infants even when morphine and other opioids do not (Anand, 2008; Lago et al., 2009) (Table 16-4). SSC reduces infant pain responses (Cong et al., 2011). SSC is effective in reducing pain due to heel sticks in premature infants (Johnston et al., 2017). Because nurses have positive attitudes about relieving procedural pain with nonpharmacologic interventions, and because SSC has been found to be more effective than sucrose in reducing pain, the use of SSC to minimize heel stick and injection pain

TABLE 16-4 Practice Recommendations for Comfort and Pain Outcomes

Variable	Rationale for SSC Implementation	Level of Evidence	References
Relaxation and stress reduction	• SSC induces calm/relaxation in both infants and parents • Infant stress is decreased rapidly during SSC • Parent stress is decreased during SSC • SSC assists in palliative care	I, II, III,	Johnston et al. [2017] Moore et al. [2016] Oras et al. [2016] Vittner et al. [2018] Feldman [2015a, 2015b]
Pain reduction	• SSC minimizes pain responses to minor procedural pain [i.e., heel lance, venipuncture, shots] • SSC is more effective than swaddling in reducing infant pain • SSC may also reduce maternal pain	I, II, III	Cong et al. [2011] Disher et al. [2017] Johnston et al. [2017] Moore et al. [2016]

*Whenever possible, references were limited to last 10 years to demonstrate the most recent evidence to support SSC integration with high-risk infants and families in the NICU.

should be implemented as an evidence-based developmental intervention. Maternal holding, whether by SSC or facilitated tucking, generally is more effective than oral glucose and opioids in reducing pain (Johnston et al., 2017).

SSC minimizes pain through several pathways. One pathway is by causing release of oxytocin in the infant; oxytocin raises the pain threshold (Carter, 2014). SSC also promotes the release of opioid peptides and cholecystokinin, both of which reduce pain sensitivity. Another pathway is by blocking passage of pain pathways to the brain, and another is by maternal presence alone. Also, during SSC the infant often falls into a restful asleep, and the level of arousal at the time of the pain stimulus independently and strongly predicts pain response. SSC has also been identified as a palliative treatment to promote relaxation and pain relief in infants with life-limiting conditions. Thus, published recommendations to use SSC for minor procedural infant pain are now available (Disher et al., 2017; Feldman-Winters et al., 2016).

RECOMMENDATIONS FOR PRACTICE

Mentorship education for SSC. There continues to be a knowledge–practice gap surrounding SSC despite the array of education efforts over the past 20 years related to various aspects of SSC implementation. Perinatal/neonatal nurses continue to have educational gaps related to the positive physiologic effects of SSC on infants, safe and effective transfer techniques, and best strategies to support the parent–infant dyad with appropriate use of SSC (Vittner et al., 2016). Nurses need continued education across perinatal settings with accurate information regarding the benefits and importance of SSC to augment nonseparation of the infant–mother dyad to enhance the infants' developmental trajectory. For increased integration of SSC into routine caregiving, nurses must design strategies to ensure that each infant is supported to participate in daily SSC.

Safety during SSC. To increase safety during implementation, SSC needs to be considered a process rather than a task. For best implementation, provision of SSC demands a modified sensory environment with decreased lighting, sounds, and activity. This modified environment enhances parents' experience and allows the parent–infant dyad to relax and spend quality time together. SSC supports the infant and parent to develop reciprocity or coregulation through synchronous interaction. It is essential that parents have a calm, soothing atmosphere while holding their infant to support bonding and for reciprocity to occur, ensuring the experience is positive for both participants. Nurses often attend to the demands of the environment at the infant's bedside and are aware of how the atmosphere influences SSC experiences for both parents and infants, making them the ideal health professional to facilitate the SSC process.

Safety can also be enhanced by making sure the right supports are available during SSC with the high-risk infant and family. This includes having comfortable chairs with arm supports that recline at the bedside. It also includes having supportive staff available to encourage and assist the mother during the transfer. Monitoring is essential, yet privacy for the mother–infant dyad also needs to be considered. There are also mother–baby wraps available to support the infant during SSC, but no evidence of the safety of these items during SSC exists. More research is needed to best understand how to use these items to support the mother and infant.

Evidence-Based Practice Recommendations

1. Infants with labile physiologic responses to environmental disturbances need to be closely monitored during transfer into and out of SSC and throughout SSC, especially with the first and/or during extended hours of continuous provision of SSC.

2. Infants need to be positioned prone during SSC, with flexed extremities, to promote motor development.

3. Infants need to be positioned during SSC with their heads in very slight extension to prevent neck flexion and airway occlusion.

4. For both the mother and the infant, standing transfer is much less stressful than sitting transfer. Be sure that infant arms are in midline and that legs are contained so they cannot flail and that the infant is covered during transfer to prevent physiologic, especially temperature, compromise. Monitor the infant closely for 5 to 15 minutes post transfer to be sure all vital signs have returned to baseline after transfer. It has been documented that peripheral oxygen saturation and cerebral oxygen saturation take approximately 3 minutes to recover from transfer (Schultz et al., 2019).

5. Ask mothers not to smoke or wear strong perfumes prior to coming to SSC and not to wear smoke-scented clothing as smoke is a noxious scent to infants and jeopardizes olfactory learning during SSC (Kostandy & Ludington-Hoe, 2019).

6. Infants ≤28 weeks PMA will need a heating unit over them during SSC to prevent cold stress (WHO immediate KMC study group).

7. Be sure infants are securely positioned in SSC; there are many products available to secure the infant to the parent's chest, such as the Zaky Zak™ by Nurtured by Design, to assure the infant does not fall off the parent's chest during SSC. A comfortable chair that reclines with side arms is also recommended to support the mother and infant during SSC.

8. To best promote breast milk production and let down reflex leave the infant in SSC for at least 20 minutes within the first hour of delivery and promote the regular implementation of SSC during each postpartum day (Karimi et al., 2019).

9. To promote swift delivery of hind milk to the suckling preterm infant, facilitate SSC for at least 20 minutes before anticipated feeding time (Johnson, 2007).

10. To avoid picking up extra systoles and abnormal heart rate patterns from the mother's cardiac system, place the premature infant's heart rate monitoring leads in the axilla (Barnes & Roberts, 2005).

11. Mothers may fall asleep during SSC, and although this has benefits to the mother such as increased prolactin secretion and respite from the stressful experience of having an infant in intensive care (Discenza, 2009), sleeping mothers are less vigilant in maintaining the infant's position in SSC and, if doing SSC in a bed, mothers can potentially roll over onto the infant, so let the mother sleep when staff are available to monitor the infant's position.

12. Position infant on the chest at a 20- to 30-degree incline to assist prone positioning influences on respiratory muscles and optimize outward recoil of the infant's chest and to facilitate expression of primitive neonatal reflexes that facilitate breastfeeding.

13. SSC sessions should ideally last for at least 1 hour. One hour is needed to allow for one complete sleep cycle; completion of sleep cycles fosters brain maturation (Kostandy & Ludington-Hoe, 2019). Some benefits are derived from less SSC time, especially benefits to maternal feelings of competence, attachment (Feldman et al., 2014), and confidence, and to breastfeeding. However, longer SSC events are recommended. In addition, it has been demonstrated that state and brain benefits require at least 1 hour of SSC for benefits to be apparent (Kaffashi et al., 2013; Scher et al., 2009).

14. Infants with chronic lung disease need to be monitored closely throughout SSC because the prone position and increased warmth may compromise oxygen saturation during hospitalization and as infants mature.

15. Mothers who are providing mother's own milk should be encouraged to provide SSC every day for as long as possible because SSC promotes human milk production (Oras et al., 2016), replaces foremilk with energy-rich hind milk when provided for 20 minutes or longer. SSC independently predicts breastfeeding initiation in preterm and in full-term infants (Mekonnen et al., 2019) and also predicts exclusivity of breast milk feedings (Mekonnen et al., 2019). SSC also increases duration of breastfeeding (Moore et al., 2016).

16. Mothers of preterm infants are at risk of depression, yet SSC prevents depression and minimizes the severity of existing depression (Agudelo et al., 2020). Thus, preterm birth mothers and mothers with symptoms of PPD should be supported and encouraged to provide SSC.

Overcoming Barriers to SSC Implementation

Nurses report that, although knowledge about SSC has improved, confusion still exists among them with regard to safety and appropriate use of SSC that create barriers to SSC implementation. A recent qualitative synthesis of nurses' experiences surrounding implementation of SSC revealed four key themes that influenced nurse SSC implementation decision making: (1) varying thresholds for getting started; (2) difficulty identifying adequate resources; (3) infant complexity; and (4) balanced with parental readiness (Vittner et al., 2015). In addition, nurses have reported that the support from leadership, education on SSC, and adequate staffing levels are all factors that influence their decision to facilitate SSC. Often there are inadequate resources limiting physical space as constraints associated with inadequate institutional support hindering SSC (Gontijo et al., 2012; Kymre & Bondas, 2013). When there were adequate infrastructure and sufficient human resources within a nursery as well as ample physical space for chairs, although the staff acknowledged the advantages of SSC, daily practice was not considered.

Nurses often navigate competing demands in the NICU, which influence when or if SSC is initiated. Nurses at the bedside need to plan accordingly, using critical thinking skills for various components of how best to support and facilitate SSC with high-risk infants. It is not only the physical resources of comfortable reclining chairs or adequate staffing that influences SSC practices but also the nurse's emotional competence and wherewithal to prioritize caregiving tasks that also affect the SSC process for infants and families (Vittner et al., 2015). A priority of most healthcare professionals is for safe implementation of SSC to ensure a positive experience for the parent and infant. Demographic characteristics appear to influence nurses' implementation of SSC (Vittner et al., 2016).

Persistent yet invalid barriers to SSC implementation include fear of infant physiologic instability, decreases in infant temperature, and challenges with meeting the complexity of the infant's care needs within the provision of SSC (Bergman et al., 2019; Ludington-Hoe, 2011; Moore et al., 2016). Skin-to-skin care needs to be a mutually cohesive experience for both the parent and the infant supporting their developing relationship. It is imperative to consider the infant's needs as well as parental readiness when facilitating SSC. Parental support in the form of encouragement as well as SSC education is necessary for success.

CONCLUSION

In summary, SSC provides the ideal neurobiologic sensory environment for infants and is an integral developmental care intervention for infants and their families and has been acknowledged as such (Conde-Agudelo & Díaz-Rossello, 2016; Karimi et al., 2019; Kostandy & Ludington-Hoe, 2019; Mekonnen et al., 2019; Scime et al., 2019). Around the world SSC is offered as a standard intervention in 92% of hospital intensive care settings (Litmanovitz et al., 2021). The evidence to support SSC implementation is compelling and uncontestable; thus, opportunities for daily SSC for hospitalized infants must be considered by healthcare professionals for infants in all hospital settings.

TABLE 16-5 Research Questions Related to SSC Implementation Yet to Be Answered

Prevention	How can SSC be encouraged to begin in the delivery room and/or in the first 24 hours after birth for the vulnerable and fragile extremely early born infant and family in the NICU?
	Given the degree of potential infection in the NICU, how can families best be supported to continue to provide SSC even in the face of this adversity?
Confirmation	What educational strategies best support families in the successful delivery of SSC?
	What strategies can be used to decrease the inherent barriers to SSC in the NICU environment?
	What intervention strategies need to be further developed and studied to facilitate safety during SSC?
	How does SSC affect physiologic biomarkers such as those in the inflammatory response (cytokines, erythrocyte sediment levels, C-reactive proteins) and growth factors to facilitate brain development?
Treatment	SSC decreases the pain response and as such use of SSC as an intervention strategy needs to be further explored.
	SSC effect on mothering has been explored, but more needs to be understood about how SSC facilitates attachment and bonding in mother–infant dyads.

Thus, because the normal milieu of newborn care is to be in SSC with their mother (Bergman et al., 2019; Klaus, 2009), separating the infant from the mother and placing the infant in an incubator/radiant warmer and retaining the incubator/radiant warmer as principal domicile of the infant is an *aversive* alteration of the natural skin-to-skin milieu (Bentley Waddoups et al., 2019). The negative consequences of separation have been clearly enumerated in all studies comparing physiologic status during SSC to incubator periods reviewed above and elsewhere (Kostandy & Ludington-Hoe, 2019). Supporting parents for immediate and prolonged nonseparation through SSC enhances containment, skin, scent, and milk that modulate infant physiology and behavior toward physiologic homeostasis and optimal growth and development (Feldman, 2015b; WHO Immediate KMC Study Group, 2020). Most directly, separation limits development of the brain (all three levels of brain development, brainstem, limbic, and cortex) and the sympathetic nervous system, which are two major pathophysiologic pathways strongly influenced by the newborn environment. Limiting maternal–infant SSC can also disrupt the emerging maternal–infant relationship (Feldman, 2015b), and a maternal–infant relationship marked by limited or lack of maternal touch is associated with impairments in stress responsivity and impairments in maternal behavior in adult offspring (Carter et al., 2020). The ideal newborn environment is the parent's chest with prolonged opportunities for SSC (Bergman et al., 2019). In addition, developmental care practices should routinely use interventions like SSC that include the mothers and fathers because positive effects of parental touch are sustained into adulthood by these influences on gene expression in the offspring. Thus, SSC as soon as possible, as often as possible, for as long as possible, and as continuously (uninterrupted) as possible is indicated for immediate and long-term developmental effects. Kangaroo Mother Care (KMC) units, units in which the mother is the preterm (beginning at 25 to 26 weeks PMA) infant's bed 24 hours/day, 7 days per week, are common throughout Sweden, Germany, Belgium, and South Africa (WHO Immediate KMC Study Group, 2020) and are the recommended environment for preterm infants starting yesterday and continuing throughout the future. Research questions yet to be answered about SSC are found in Table 16-5.

REFERENCES

Abdulghani, N., Edvardsson, K., & Amir, L. (2018). Worldwide prevalence of mother-infant skin-to-skin contact after vaginal birth: A systematic review. *PLoS One, 13*(10), e0205696. https://doi.org/10.1371/journal.pone.0205696

Abdulkader, H. M., Freer, Y., Garry, E. M., Fleetwood-Walker, S. M. & McIntosh, N. (2008). Prematurity and neonatal noxious events exert lasting effects on infant pain behavior. *Early Human Development, 84*(6), 351–355.

Agudelo, S., Díaz, D., Maldonado, M., Acuña, E., Mainero, D., Pérez, O., Pérez, L., & Molina, C. (2020). Effect of skin-to-skin contact at birth on early neonatal hospitalization. *Early Human Development, 144*, 105020. https://doi.org/10.1016/j.earlhumdev.2020.105020

Akbari, E., Binnoon-Erez, N., Rodrigues, M., Ricci, A., Schneider, J., Madigan, S., & Jenkins, J. (2018). Kangaroo mother care and infant biopsychosocial outcomes in the first year: A meta-analysis. *Early Human Development, 122*, 22–31. https://doi.org/10.1016/j.earlhumdev.2018.05.004

Anand, K. J. (2008). Analgesia for skin breaking procedures in newborns and children: What works best? *Canadian Medical Association Journal, 179*(1), 11–12.

Als, H., & McAnulty, G. (2011), The newborn individualized developmental care and assessment program (NIDCAP) with kangaroo mother care: Comprehensive care for preterm infants. *Current Women's Health Reviews, 7*, 288–301.

Athanasopoulou, E., & Fox, J. (2014). Effects of kangaroo mother care on maternal mood and interaction patterns between parents and their preterm, low birth weight infants: A systematic review. *Infant Mental Health Journal, 35*, 245–262. https://doi.org/10.1002/imhj.21444

Baley, J. (2015). Skin-to-skin care for term and preterm infants in the neonatal ICU. *Pediatrics, 136*, 596. https://doi.org/10.1542/peds.2015-2335

Barnes, N. P., & Roberts, P. (2005). "Extrasystoles" during Kangaroo Care. *Pediatric Critical Care Medicine, 6*(2), 230.

Begum, E. A., Bonno, M., Ohtani, N., Yamashita, S., Tanaka, S., Yamamoto, H., Kawai, M., & Komada, Y. (2009). Cerebral oxygenation responses during kangaroo care in low birth weight infants. *Neonatal Intensive Care, 2*(2), 2–25.

Bentley Waddoups, A., Yoshikawa, H., & Strouf, K. (2019). Developmental effects of parent—child separation. *Annual Reviews Developmental Psychology, 1,* 387–410.

Bergman, N., Ludwig, R., Westrup, B., & Welch, M. (2019). Nurturescience versus neuroscience: A case for rethinking perinatal mother—infant behaviors and relationship. *Birth Defects Research, 111*(15), 1110–1127. https://doi.org/10.1002/bdr2.1529

Bigelow, A., Power, M., MacLellan-Peters, J., Alex, M., & McDonald, C. (2012). Effect of mother/infant skin-to-skin contact on postpartum depressive symptoms and maternal physiological stress. *Journal of Obstetric, Gynecologic and Neonatal Nursing, 41,* 369–382.

Boundy, E., Dastjerdi, R., SpiegelmanFawzi, W.,, Missmer, S., Lieberman, E., Kajeepeta, S., Wall, S., & Chan, G. (2016). Kangaroo mother care and neonatal outcomes. A meta-analysis. *Pediatrics, 137*(1), e20152238.

Bracht, M., O'Leary, L., Lee, S. K., & O'Brien, K. (2013). Implementing family-integrated care in the NICU: A parent education and support program. *Advances in Neonatal Care, 13*(2), 115–126.

Brazelton, T. B. (1978. The brazelton neonatal behavior assessment Scale: Introduction. *Monogram Social Resources Child Development, 43*(5–6), 1–13.

Campbell-Yeo, M., Disher, T., Benoit, B., & Johnston, C. (2015). Understanding kangaroo care and its benefits to preterm infants. *Pediatric Health Medicine and Therapeutics, 6,* 15–32.

Carter, C. (2014). Oxytocin pathways and the evolution of human behavior. *Annual Reviews Psychology, 65,* 17–39. https://doi.org/10.1146/annurev-psych-010213-115110

Carter, C., Kenkel, W., MacLean, E., Wilson, S., Perkeybile, A., Yee, F. C., Nazarloo, H., Porges, S., Davis, M., Connelly, J., & Kingsbury, M. (2020). Is oxytocin "nature's medicine"? *Pharmacological Reviews, 72*(4), 829–861. https://doi.org/10.1124/pr.120.019398

Champagne, F. A. & Curley, J. P. (2009). Epigenetic mechanisms mediating the long-term effects of maternal care on development. *Neuroscience and Biobehavioral Reviews, 33,* 593–600.

Chan, G., Valsangkar, B., Kajeepeta, S., Boundy, E. O., & Wall, S. (2016). What is kangaroo mother care: Systematic review of the literature. *Journal of Global Health, 6*(1), 10701. https://doi.org/10.7189/jogh.06.010701

Chen, E. M., Gau, M. L., Liu, C. Y., & Lee, T. Y. (2017). Effects of father-neonate skin-to-skin contact on attachment: A randomized controlled trial. *Nursing Research and Practice, 2017,* 8612024. https://doi.org/10.1155/2017/8612024

Chi Luong, K., Long Nguyen, T., Huynh Thi, D., Carrara, H., & Bergman, N. (2016). Newly born low birthweight infants stabilise better in skin-to-skin contact than when separated from their mothers: A randomised controlled trial. *Acta Paediatrica, 105*(4), 381–390.

Conde-Agudelo, A., & Díaz-Rossello, J. (2016). Kangaroo mother care to reduce morbidity and mortality in low birthweight infants. *Cochrane Database of Systematic Reviews,* (8), CD002771. https://doi.org/10.1002/14651858.CD002771.pub4

Cong, X., Ludington-Hoe, S., & Walsh, S. (2011). Randomized crossover trial of kangaroo care to reduce biobehavioral pain responses in preterm infants: A pilot study. *Biological Research for Nursing, 13*(2), 204–216. https://doi.org/10.1177/1099800410385839

Cong, X., Ludingtong-Hoe, S., Hussain, N., Cusson, R., Walsh, S., Vasquez, V., Bierre, C. E., & Vittner, D. (2015). Parental oxytocin responses during skin to skin contact in preterm infants. *Early Human Development, 91,* 401–406. http://doi.org/10.1016/j.earlhumdev.2015.04.012

Crespi, B. J. (2016). Oxytocin, testosterone, and human social cognition. *Biological Reviews, 91*(2), 390–408.

D'Agata, A., Sanders, M., Grasso, D., Young, E., Cong, X., & McGrath, J. (2017). Unpacking the burden of care for infants in the NICU. *Infant Mental Health Journal, 38*(2), 306–317. https://doi.org/10.1002/imhj.21636

D'Agata, A., Young, E., Cong, X., Grasso, D., & McGrath, J. (2016). Infant medical trauma in the neonatal intensive care unit (IMTN): A proposed

concept for science and practice. *Advances in Neonatal Care, 16*(4), 289–297. https://doi.org/10.1097/ANC.0000000000000309

Discenza, D. (2009). Taking care of the NICU mom. *Neonatal Network, 28*(5), 351–352.

Disher, T., Benoit, B., Johnston, C., & Campbell-Yeo, M. (2017). Skin-to-skin contact for procedural pain in neonates: Acceptability of novel systematic review synthesis methods and GRADEing of the evidence. *Journal of Advanced Nursing 73*(2), 504–519. https://doi.org/10.1111/jan.13182

Elhalik, M, & El-Atawi, K. (2016). Breast feeding and kangaroo care. *Journal of Pediatrics & Neonatal Care, 4*(6), 160.

Erlandsson, K., Dsilna, A., Fagerberg, I., & Christensson, K. (2007). Skin-to-skin care with father after cesarean birth and its effect on newborn crying and pre-feeding behavior. *Birth, 34*(2), 105–114.

Feldman, R. (2015a). Sensitive periods in human social development: New insights from research on oxytocin, synchrony and high-risk parenting. *Development and Psychopathology, 27,* 369–395. http://dx.doi.org/10.1017/S0954579415000048

Feldman, R. (2015b). The adaptive human parental brain: Implications for children's social development. *Trends in Neuroscience, 38*(6), 387–399. http://dx.doi.org/10.1016/j.tins.2015.04.004

Feldman-Winter, L., Douglass-Bright, A., Bartick, M. C., & Matranga, J. (2013). The new mandate from the joint commission on the perinatal care core measure of exclusive breast milk feeding: implications for practice and implementation in the United States. *Journal of Human Lactation, 29*(3):291–295. https://doi.org/10.1177/0890334413485641

Feldman-Winter, L., Goldsmith, J., & Committee on Fetus and Newborn, AAP Task Force on Sudden Infant Death Syndrome. (2016). Safe sleep and skin-to-skin care in the neonatal period for healthy term newborns. *Pediatrics, 138*(3), e20161889.

Feldman, R., Rosenthal, Z., & Eidelman, A. (2014). Maternal-preterm skin-to-skin contact enhances child physiologic organization and cognitive control across the first 10 years of life. *Biological Psychiatry, 75*(1):56–64.

Gettler, L., Kuo, P., Sarma, M., Trumble, B., Burke Lefever, J., & Braungart-Rieker, J. (2021). Fathers' oxytocin responses to first holding their newborns: Interactions with testosterone reactivity to predict later parenting behavior and father-infant bonds. *Developmental Psychobiology, 63*(5), 1384–1398. https://doi.org/10.1002/dev.22121

Geva, R., & Feldman, R. (2008). A neurobiological model for the effects of early brainstem functioning on the development of behavior and emotion regulation in infants: Implications for prenatal and perinatal risk. *Journal of Child Psychology and Psychiatry, 49*(10), 1031–1041.

Gontijo, T., Xavier, C., Freitas, M. (2012). Evaluation of implementation of kangaroo care for managers, professionals and mothers of newborns. *Journal of Public Health, 28*(5), 935–944. https://doi.org/10.1590/S0102-311x2012000500012

Gordon, I., Pratt, M., Bergunde, K., Zagoory-Sharon, O., & Feldman, R. (2017). Testosterone, oxytocin, and the development of human parental care. *Hormones and Behavior, 93,* 184–192.

Handlin, L., Jonas, W., Petersson, M., Ejdebäck, M., Ransjö-Arvidson, A., Nissen, E., & Uvnäs-Moberg, K. (2009). Effects of sucking and skin-to-skin contact on maternal ACTH and cortisol levels during the second day postpartum-influence of epidural analgesia and oxytocin in the perinatal period. *Breastfeeding Medicine, 4*(4), 207–220. https://doi.org/10.1089/bfm.2009.0001

Hardin, J., Jones, N., Mize, K., & Platt, M. (2020). Parent-training with kangaroo care impacts infant neurophysiological development & mother-infant neuroendocrine activity. *Infant Behavior & Development, 58,* 101416. https://doi.org/10.1016/j.infbeh.2019.101416

Johnston, C., Campbell-Yeo, M., Disher, T., Benoit, B., Fernandes, A., Streiner, D., Inglis, D., & Zee, R. (2017). Skin-to-skin care for procedural pain in neonates. *Cochrane Database of Systematic Reviews, 2*(2), CD008435. https://doi.org/10.1002/14651858.CD008435.pub3

Joshi, R., Kommers, D., Guo, C., Bikker, J., Feijs, L., van Pul, C., & Andriessen, P. (2019). Statistical modeling of heart rate variability to unravel the factors affecting autonomic regulation in preterm infants. *Scientific Reports, 9*(1), 7691. https://doi.org/10.1038/s41598-019-44209-z

Kaffashi, F., Scher, M., Ludington-Hoe, S., & Loparo, K. (2013). An analysis of the kangaroo care intervention using neonatal EEG complexity: A preliminary study. *Clinical Neurophysiology, 124*(2), 238–246. https://doi.org/10.1016/j.clinph.2012.06.021

Karimi, F., Sadeghi, R., Maleki-Saghooni, N., & Khadivzadeh, T. (2019). The effect of mother–infant skin to skin contact on success and duration of first breastfeeding: A systematic review and meta-analysis. *Taiwan Journal of Obstetrics and Gynecology, 58*(1), 1–9. https://doi.org/10.1016/j.tjog.2018.11.002

Kirca, N., & Adibelli, D. (2021). Effects of mother–infant skin-to-skin contact on postpartum depression: A systematic review. *Perspectives Psychiatric Care.* https://doi.org/10.1111/ppc.12727

Klaus. M. H. (2009). Commentary: An early, short, and useful sensitive period in the human infant. *Birth, 36*(2), 110–112.

Kommers, D., Joshi, R., Pul, C., Feijs, L., Oei, G., Oetomo, S., & Andriessen, P. (2018). Unlike kangaroo care, mechanically simulated kangaroo care does not change heart rate variability in preterm neonates. *Early Human Development, 121*, 27–32. https://doi.org/10.1016/j.earlhumdev.2018.04.031

Kommers, D., Joshi, R., van Pul, C., Atallah, L., Feijs, L., Oei, G., Bambang Oetomo, S., & Andriessen, P. (2017). Features of heart rate variability capture regulatory changes during kangaroo care in preterm infants, *Journal of Pediatrics, 182*, 92–98.

Kostandy, R., & Ludington-Hoe, S. M. (2019). The evolution and the science of kangaroo mother care (skin-to-skin contact). *Birth Defects Research, 111*(15), 1032–1043. https://doi.org/10.1002/bdr2.1565

Kristoffersen, L., Stoen, R., Rygh, H., Sognnaes, M., Follestad, T., Mohn, H., Nissen, I., & Bergeng, H. (2016). Skin-to-skin care after birth for moderately preterm infants. *Journal of Obstetric, Gynecologic and Neonatal Nursing, 45*, 339–345.

Kymre, I., & Bondas, T. (2013). Balancing premature infant's developmental needs with parents' readiness for skin to skin care: A phenomenological study. *International Journal of Qualitative Studies Health Well-Being, 8*(1), 21370. http://dx.doi.org/10.3402/qhw.v8i0.21370

Lee, J., & Bang, K. (2011). The effect of kangaroo care on maternal self-esteem and premature infant's physiologic stability. *Korean Journal of Women Health Nursing, 17*(5), 454–462. http://dx.doi.org/10.4069/kjwhn.2011.17.5.454

Lee, H. J., Macbeth, A. H., Pagani, J. H., & Young, W. S. (2009). Oxytocin: The great facilitator of life. *Progressive Neurobiology, 88*(2), 127–151.

Linnér, A., Westrup, B., Lode-Kolz, K., Klemming, S., Lillieskold, S., Markhus Pike, H., Morgan, B., Bergman, N., Rettedal, S., & Jonas, W. (2020). Immediate parent-infant skin-to-skin study (IPISTOSS): Study protocol of a randomised controlled trial on very preterm infants cared for in skin-to-skin contact immediately after birth and potential physiological, epigenetic, psychological and neurodevelopmental consequences. *BMJ Open, 10*(7), e038938. https://doi.org/10.1136/bmjopen-2020-038938

Litmanovitz, I., Silberstein, D., Butler, S., Vittner, D. (2021). Care of hospitalized infants and their families during the COVID-19 pandemic: An international survey. *Journal of Perinatology, 41*, 981–987. https://doi.org/10.1038/s41372-021-00960-8

Lorenz, L., Dawson, J., Jones, H., Jacobs, S. E., Cheong, J. L., Donath, S. M., Davis, P. G., & Kamlin, C. O. F. (2017). Skin-to-skin care in preterm infants receiving respiratory support does not lead to physiological instability. *Archives of Disease in Childhood Fetal Neonatal Education, 102*(4), F339–F344.

Ludington-Hoe, S. (2011). Evidence-based review of physiologic effects of kangaroo care. *Current Women Health Reviews*, 243–253.

Mallet, I., Bomy, H., Govaert, N., Goudal, I., Brasme, C., Dubois, A., Boudringhien, S., & Pierrat, V. (2007). Skin- to-skin contact in neonatal care: Knowledge and expectations of health professionals in 2 neonatal intensive care units. *Archives de Pediatrie, 14*(7), 881–886.

Mekonnen, A., Yehualashet, S., & Bayleyegn, A. (2019). The effects of kangaroo mother care on the time to breastfeeding initiation among preterm and LBW infants: A meta-analysis of published studies. *International Breastfeeding Journal, 14*(12). https://doi.org/10.1186/s13006-019-0206-0

Moon, R. (2016). Task force on sudden infant death syndrome. SIDS and other sleep-related infant deaths: Evidence base for 2016 updated recommendations for a safe infant sleeping environment. *Pediatrics, 138*(5), e20162940. https://doi.org/10.1542/peds.2016-2940

Moore, E., Bergman, N., Anderson, G., & Medley, N. (2016). Early skin-to-skin contact for mothers and their healthy newborn infants. *Cochrane Database of Systematic Reviews, 11*(11), CD003519. https://doi.org/10.1002/14651858.CD003519.pub4

Mörelius, E., Örtenstrand, A., Theodorsson, E., & Frostell, A. (2015). A randomised trial of continuous skin-to-skin contact after preterm birth and the effects on salivary cortisol, parental stress, depression, and breastfeeding. *Early Human Development, 91*(1), 63–70. https://doi.org/10.1016/j.earlhumdev.2014.12.005

Mori, R., Khanna, R., Pledge, D, & Nakayama, T. (2010). Meta analysis of physiologic effects of skin to skin contact for newborns and mothers. *Pediatrics International, 52*, 161–170. http://dx.doi.org/10.1111/j.1442-200x.2009.02909.x

Nuyt, M. A. (2008). Mechanisms underlying developmental programming of elevated blood pressure and vascular dysfunction: evidence from human studies and experimental animal models. *Clinical Science, 114*, 1–17.

Oras, P., Thernström Blomqvist, Y., Hedberg Nyqvist, K., Gradin, M., Rubertsson, C., Hellström-Westas, L., & Funkquist, E. (2016). Skin-to-skin contact is associated with earlier breastfeeding attainment in preterm infants. *Acta Paediatrica, 105*(7), 783–789. https://doi.org/10.1111/apa.13431

O'Reilly, H., Johnson, S., Ni, Y., Wolke, D., & Marlow, N. (2020). Neuropsychological outcomes at 19 years of age following extreme preterm birth. *Pediatrics, 145*(2), e20192087. https://doi.org/10.1542/peds.2019-2087

Quigley, M., & McGuire, W. (2014). Formula versus donor breast milk for feeding preterm or low birth weight infants. *Cochrane Database of Systematic Reviews, 4*, CD002971.

Rajendra Acharya, U., Joseph, P., Kannathal, N., Lim, C., & Suri, J. (2006). Heartrate variability: A review. *Medical and Biological Engineering and Computing, 44*, 1031–1051.

Roque, A., Lasiuk, G., Radünz, V., & Hegadoren, K. (2017). Scoping review of the mental health of parents of infants in the NICU. *Journal of Obstetric, Gynecologic & Neonatal Nursing, 46*, 576–587. https://doi.org/10.1016/j.jogn.2017.02.005

Ross, H. E., & Young, L. J. (2009). Oxytocin and the neural mechanisms regulating social cognition and afflictive behavior. *Frontal Neuroendocrinology, 30*(4), 534–547.

Sampaio, Á., Bousquat, A., & Barros, C. (2016). Skin-to-skin contact at birth: A challenge for promoting breastfeeding in a "baby friendly" public maternity hospital in northeast Brazil. *Epidemiologia e Serviços de Saúde, 25*(2), 281–290.

Scatliffe, N., Casavant, S., Vittner, D., & Cong, X. (2019). Oxytocin and early parent-infant interactions: A systematic review. *International Journal of Nursing Sciences, 6*(4), 445–453. https://doi.org/10.1016/j.ijnss.2019.09.009

Scher, M., Ludington-Hoe, S., Kaffashi, F., Johnson, M., Holditch-Davis, D., & Loparo, K. (2009). Neurophysiologic assessment of brain maturation after an 8-week trial of skin-to-skin contact on preterm infants. *Clinical Neurophysiology, 120*(10), 1812–1818. https://doi.org/10.1016/j.clinph.2009.08.004

Schultz, D., Shindruk, C., Gigolyk, S., Ludington-Hoe, S., & Kostandy, R. (2019). A standardized transfer procedure for fragile and intubated infants in the NICU. *Birth Defects Research, 111*(15), 1073–1080. https://doi.org/10.1002/bdr2.1525

Scime, N., Gavarkovs, A., & Chaput, K. (2019). The effect of skin-to-skin care on postpartum depression among mothers of preterm or low birth-weight infants: A systematic review and meta-analysis. *Journal of Affective Disorders, 253*, 376–384. https://doi.org/10.1016/j.jad.2019.04.101

Sharma, A. (2016). Efficacy of early skin-to-skin contact on the rate of exclusive breastfeeding in term neonates: A randomized controlled trial. *African Health Sciences, 16*(3), 790–797.

Shattnawi, K., & Al-Ali, N. (2019). The effect of short duration skin to skin contact on premature infants' physiological and behavioral outcomes: A quasi-experimental study. *Journal of Pediatric Nursing, 46*, e24–e28. https://doi.org/10.1016/j.pedn.2019.02.005

Shorey, S., He, H., & Morelius, E. (2016). Skin-to-skin contact by fathers and the impact on infant and paternal outcomes: An integrative review. *Midwifery, 40*, 207–217. https://doi.org/10.1016/j.midw.2016.07.007

Srivastava, S., Gupta, A., Bhatnagar, A., & Dutta, S. (2014). Effect of very early skin to skin contact on success at breastfeeding and preventing early hypothermia in neonates. *Indian Journal of Public Health, 58*(1), 22–26.

Tully, K., Holditch-Davis, D., White-Traut, R., David, R., O'Shea, T., & Geraldo, V. (2016). A test of kangaroo care on preterm infant breastfeeding. *Journal of Obstetric, Gynecologic and Neonatal Nursing, 45*(1), 45–61.

Uvnäs Moberg, K., Ekström, A., Buckley, S., Massarotti, C., Pajalic, Z., Luegmair, K., Kotlowska, A., Lengler, L., Olza, I., & Grylka-Baeschlin, S. (2020a). Maternal plasma levels of oxytocin during breastfeeding—a systematic review. *PLoS One, 15*, e0235806.

Uvnäs Moberg, K., Gross, M., Agius, A., Downe, S., & Calleja-Agius, J. (2020b). Are there epigenetic oxytocin-mediated effects on the mother and infant during physiological childbirth? *Molecular Science, 21*, 9503. https://doi.org/10.3390/ijms21249503

van Sleuwen, B. E., Engelberts, A. C., Boere-Boonekamp, M. M., Kuis, W., Schulpen, T. W. J., & L'Hoir, M. P. (2007). Swaddling: A systematic review. *Pediatrics, 120*, e1097–1106.

Vittner, D., Butler, S., Smith, K., Makris, N., Brownell, E., Samra, H., & McGrath, J. (2019). Parent engagement correlates with parent and preterm infant oxytocin release during skin-to-skin contact, *Advances in Neonatal Care, 19*(1), 73–79. http://doi.org/10.1097/ANC.0000000000000558

Vittner, D., Casavant, S., & McGrath, J. (2015). A meta-ethnography: Skin-to-skin holding from the caregiver's perspective. *Advances in Neonatal Care, 15*(3), 191–200. http://doi.org/10.1097/ANC.0000000000000169

Vittner, D., Cong, X., Ludington-Hoe, S., & McGrath, J. M. (2016). A skin-to-skin contact survey of perinatal nurses. *Applied Nursing Research, 33*, 19–23. http://doi.org/10.1016/j.apnr.2016.09.006

Vittner, D., McGrath, J. M., Robinson, J., Lawhon, G., Cusson, R., Eisenfeld, L., Walsh, S., Young, E., & Cong, X. (2018). Increases in oxytocin from skin-to-skin contact enhances development of parent–infant relationships. *Biological Research for Nursing, 20*(1), 54–62. http://doi.org/10.1177/1099800417735633

Vogl, J., Dunne, E., Liu, C., Bradley, A., Rwei, A. Lonergan, E., Hopkins, B., Kwak, S., Simon, C., Rand, C., Rogers, J., Weese-Mayer, D., & Garfield, C. (2021). Kangaroo father care: A pilot feasibility study of physiologic and psychosocial measures to capture the effects of father-infant and mother-infant skin to skin contact in neonatal intensive care. *Developmental Psychobiology, 63*(5), 1521–1533. https://doi.org/10.1002/dev.22100

Wang, C., Li, X., Zhang, L., Wu, L., Tan, L., Yuan, F., Guo, Y., Williams, S., & Xu, T. (2020). Early essential newborn care is associated with increased breastfeeding: A quasi-experimental study from sichuan province of western China. *International Breastfeeding Journal, 15*(1), 99. https://doi.org/10.1186/s13006-020-00343-3

WHO Immediate KMC Study Group. (2020). Impact of continuous kangaroo mother care initiated immediately after birth (iKMC) on survival of newborns with birth weight between 1.0 to <1.8 kg: Study protocol for a randomized controlled trial. *Trials, 21*(1), 280. https://doi.org/10.1186/s13063-020-4101-1

Young, E., D'Agata, A. L., Vittner, D., & Baumbauer, K. (2017). Neurobiological consequences of early painful experience: Basic science findings and implications for evidence-based practice. *Journal of Perinatal and Neonatal Nursing, 31*(2), 178–185. http://doi.org/10.1097/JPN.0000000000000258

CHAPTER 17

Sensory Interventions for the High-Risk Infant

Rosemary White-Traut, Brenna Hogan, Christina Rigby-McCotter, and Jacqueline M. McGrath

---

IFCDC Standard for Systems Thinking in Collaborative Practice

Standard 1: Systems Thinking
- The intensive care unit (ICU) shall exhibit an infrastructure of leadership, mission, and a governance framework to guide the performance of the collaborative practice of IFCDC.

Standard 2: Positioning and Touch
- Babies in intensive care settings shall be positioned to support musculoskeletal, physiological, and behavioral stability.

Standard 3: Pain and Stress, Families
- The interprofessional team shall document increased parent/caregiver well-being and decreased emotional distress during the intensive care hospital (ICU) stay. Distress levels of baby's siblings and extended family should also be considered.

INTRODUCTION

Multisensory interventions that include touch, massage, voice, rocking, and eye-to-eye contact for preterm infants are caregiving interventions that have been explored by many investigators. The sense of touch is the most developed of the senses during the neonatal period. However, preterm infant touch and massage research results are ongoing. The Physical Environment Exploratory Group endorses the use of sensory interventions including massage as the standard of care after 30 to 31 weeks postmenstrual age (PMA). Some touch is "good" providing pleasure and support. Some touch is "bad" causing pain and damage to tissues. Every high-risk infant who enters the environment of the neonatal intensive care unit (NICU) will experience both good and bad touch (White-Traut et al., 2021). Much of that touch will be noxious touch related to the medical interventions required to sustain the infant's life. Some of it will be gentle loving touch provided by caregivers and family members to support and comfort the infant during this vulnerable time of recovery. Massage is a therapeutic intervention with many uses that has existed since ancient times. It is a common practice that has been used in many cultures and for different purposes. Infant touch in conjunction with other sensory input such as eye-to-eye contact, voice, stimulation, and rocking engages the caregiver with the infant and supports the development of patterns of interaction between the infant, parents, and

caregivers. Implementation of such behavioral interventions is vital to advancing developmental care of the high-risk infant. This chapter will provide guidance to caregivers about the application of touch and other sensory modalities when provided as a behavioral intervention with high-risk infants.

SENSORY EXPERIENCES IN THE NICU

The sensation of touch is frequently the first positive connection between parents and their infants. Yet, for infants born preterm, the initial sensations of touch are often noxious, medically related, and not contingent on the infant's cues (Zeiner et al., 2016). Researchers have found that social nurturing touch in conjunction with other social interaction, such as gently stroking to comfort the infant, may be less than 5% of the touch preterm infants receive routinely (Slevin et al., 2000). Adverse effects of the touch associated with medical and nursing procedures include hypoxia, bradycardia, sleep disruptions, and increased intracranial pressure (ICP) (Zeiner et al., 2016). Repeated episodes of hypoxia and increased ICP may place preterm infants at increased risk of complications such as intraventricular hemorrhage (IVH) and subsequent neurodevelopmental delays. Because of the concerns over adverse effects of handling associated with medical and nursing procedures, many NICUs have instituted minimal handling guidelines for the most vulnerable infants. These guidelines often pertain to all handling, thereby also limiting potential positive tactile experiences for the infant (Harrison, 2004; Latini et al., 2003; Stack, 2001; Vandenberg, 2007a). Algorithms to reduce infant stress have been developed to guide clinicians as they provide care (Burns et al., 1994). These algorithms include assessment of autonomic and behavioral response during medical and nursing procedures and sensory interventions.

Thus, engagement between the parent and child in the NICU may be delayed or altered by the infant's illness, distress, immaturity, and inability to manage stimulation within the already stressful environment. Touch is one of the first senses to develop in the fetus, emerging at about 7.5 weeks of gestation, whereas the development of other senses follows during gestation (Burns et al., 1994; White-Traut et al., 2009). The last sense to develop is the visual pathway, which is why nurses protect the infants from light. In the past it was believed to be more beneficial for preterm infants to be left undisturbed since they were overstimulated in the NICU. Parents were told not to touch so the infant could rest more quietly between the necessary medical interventions and procedures. Parents were often delayed in their ability to engage and interact with their infants, potentially altering the infant's normal growth and development and decreasing parent satisfaction with the NICU experience. Parents who provide sensory interventions in the NICU report satisfaction with this practice (Holditch-Davis et al., 2013).

Touch can be both positive and negative for these high-risk infants. Some studies have been done showing evidence that light gentle human touch (GHT) may provide immediate comforting affects others have not (Harrison et al., 1996; Harrison et al., 2000; Jay, 1982; Modcrin-McCarthy et al., 1997; Modcrin-Talbott et al., 2003). Adverse effects of GHT include apnea, bradycardia, decreased oxygen saturation levels, excessive energy expenditure through increased activity (Modcrin-McCarthy et al., 1997), and avoidance behaviors, tachycardia, tachypnea, and hypoxemia (Bijari et al., 2013; Modcrin-Talbott et al., 2003). In addition, no long-term benefits have been noted with GHT in any of the studies mentioned above, whereas those involving massage with stroking and deeper pressure have demonstrated both short- and long-term benefits with fewer costs to the infants (Fathollahzadeh, 2020).

GHT has been defined as placing one hand on the head and one on the trunk without stroking or massage (Harrison et al., 2000). This intervention has been studied by several researchers with physiologically fragile preterm infants in the NICU. Harrison et al. (1996) first examined the effects of GHT provided for 15 minutes a day with preterm infants in the NICU from day 7 to day 12 of life. Thirty preterm infants were randomly assigned to the treatment or control group. Baseline data included heart rate and oxygen saturation levels every 6 seconds for 10 minutes before and after the treatment. Videotape recordings during the treatment were used to gather data related to behavioral state, signs of distress, and activity levels. The treatment group demonstrated no significant differences in oxygen saturation or heart rate

levels before, during, or after GHT. There was also no significant difference in the percentage of quiet sleep comparing baseline, touch, and posttouch periods. There was, however, significantly less active sleep during the GHT compared with baseline data. There was also significantly less motor activity and behavioral distress during GHT sessions than during baseline or posttouch periods. There was no difference between the groups on morbidity scores, numbers of days spent on supplemental oxygen, weight gain, or Brazelton Neonatal Behavioral Assessment Scale scores. These results suggest that a 15-minute GHT intervention has no adverse effect on the heart rate or oxygen saturation levels of small preterm infants. One surprising finding was that infants in the treatment group spent more days under phototherapy than the controls. No explanation was found for this difference. GHT appears to have immediate soothing effect on fragile preterm infants, as evidenced by decreased levels of active sleep, motor activity, and behavioral distress; however, no long-term effects were noted. These results are exemplary of results of research with this intervention across the seven studies found. Since more negative than positive results were found in these studies, the practice of GHT has not been widely implemented.

MULTISENSORY INTERVENTIONS THAT INCLUDE MASSAGE

Infant massage has been included in the care of infants for centuries throughout the world (Mainous, 2002). Infant massage has profound influences on the health and development of premature and full-term infants (Acolet et al., 1993; Feijó et al., 2006; Guzzetta et al., 2009; Hernandez-Reif et al., 2007; Lee, 2006; O'Higgins et al., 2008; Onozawa et al., 2001; Underdown et al., 2006). Infants who receive massage therapy have shown a reduction in stress response (Acolet et al., 1993; Guzzetta et al., 2009; Hernandez-Reif et al., 2007; O'Higgins et al., 2008) and an improvement in mother and infant interactions (Feijó et al., 2006; Lee, 2006; Onozawa et al., 2001). Furthermore, infant massage improves infant growth, neurobehavior, and development (Guzzetta et al., 2009; Kim et al., 2003; Mathai et al., 2001; Vaivre-Douret et al., 2009). However, despite current research supporting infant massage, a recent survey of neonatology staff members revealed that only 38% of respondents utilized infant massage in the NICU, whereas 86% of respondents continued to incorporate on their units a "minimal touch approach," thereby supporting the philosophy that touching the infant should be limited as much as possible (Field et al., 2006). Also, research shows that less than 5% of touch received by preterm infants is for comforting or soothing the infant (McGrath et al., 2007). These reports are concerning. Preterm infants are at increased risk of unstable fluctuations in autonomic function such as heat loss (Soll, 2008), elevated levels in stress hormones (White-Traut et al., 2009), central nervous system disorganization (Foreman et al., 2008), poor mother–infant interaction (Feeley et al., 2005), delayed weight gain (Euser et al., 2008), and longer hospital stays (Khashu et al., 2009; Ringborg et al., 2006). Implementing a noninvasive developmental approach such as infant massage could greatly reduce adverse sequelae and improve clinical outcomes for these at-risk preterm infants.

Multisensory behavioral intervention that includes voice via infant-directed speech, massage, eye-to-eye contact, and rocking yields positive behavioral and physiological infant responses. This intervention termed ATVV (Auditory, Tactile, Visual, and Vestibular) results in increased alertness and improved sleep–wake patterns (White-Traut & Pate, 1987; White-Traut et al., 2002a; White-Traut et al., 2002b), a reduction in stress response (White-Traut & Pate, 1987; White-Traut et al., 2009), and an improvement in mother and infant interactions (White-Traut & Nelson, 1988). In addition, ATVV improves hospital progress by significantly increasing feeding behaviors and infant weight gain and by reducing number of hospital days (White-Traut et al., 2002b). Furthermore, the ATVV intervention improves infant growth, neurobehavior, and development (Kim et al., 2003; Nelson et al., 2001). The ATVV intervention also improves hospital progress by significantly increasing feeding readiness behaviors and infant weight gain and by reducing number of hospital days (Nelson et al., 2001).

Two forms of infant massage dominate the research presented here. The ATVV multisensory intervention incorporates systematic moderate pressure massage with behaviors naturally employed by mothers with their infants (Burns et al., 1994; White-Traut, 2004). A second method of massage combines moderate pressure massage and kinesthetic stimulation without human social interaction (Massaro et al., 2009). Of note, when massage only was compared with the ATVV intervention in healthy full-term infants, stress reactivity was significantly increased in the massage-only group, whereas it was significantly reduced in the ATVV group. These data provide strong evidence that massage in conjunction with human social interaction reduces stress reactivity. Reduction of stress reactivity is a goal of intervention, and thus, the ATVV is superior to massage only. The ATVV improved infant oral feeding and social interactive skills prior to and during feeding, improved in-hospital growth (weight gain) and development, and reduced length of hospital stay (Nelson et al., 2001; White-Traut & Goldman, 1988; White-Traut & Nelson, 1988; White-Traut & Tubeszewski, 1986; White-Traut et al., 1993; White-Traut et al., 1997; White-Traut et al., 1999; White-Traut et al., 2002a; White-Traut et al., 2002b; White-Traut et al., 2002c).

Although the ATVV improved infant outcomes and mother–infant interaction, parents continued to report high stress while interacting with their premature infants and their need for extra social support. Thus, the ATVV intervention was enhanced with the addition of participatory guidance for parents to help them engage with their infants despite their immature behaviors. In addition, social support was offered by the nurse. The enhanced intervention is called H-HOPE (Hospital-Home Transition: Optimizing Prematures' Environment) (White-Traut et al., 2009; White-Traut et al., 2021).

H-HOPE simultaneously addresses the needs of both preterm infants and their parents, especially their need for mutual engagement, and is uniquely suited as an early developmental/behavioral intervention for preterm infants in NICUs. The parent-directed component of H-HOPE consists of four participatory guidance sessions for parents, two during the NICU stay and two post discharge. Mothers in the H-HOPE program expressed growing understanding of their infants; as one said, *"I learned to listen to my child. Even though she couldn't speak, I can read her body language and facial expressions."* H-HOPE's efficacy was documented by improved developmental maturation (more mature behavioral states, increased frequency of orally directed behaviors, faster transition from gavage to oral feeding, improved sucking organization and motor development), greater in-hospital growth (weight gain and length), reduced initial in-hospital costs (net savings of $13,976 per infant after adjusting for the mean intervention cost of $680), and reduced illness at 6 weeks chronological age (CA) (Griffith et al., 2017; Medoff-Cooper et al., 2015; Vonderheid et al., 2016; Vonderheid et al., 2020; White-Traut, 2015; White-Traut et al., 2014a; White-Traut et al., 2015). Mothers and infants exhibited enhanced engagement, social interactive behaviors, and improved infant responsivity at 6 weeks CA (White-Traut et al., 2013; White-Traut et al., 2014a, 2014b). The addition of the participatory guidance and the social support enhanced engagement between mother and infant.

DEFINING INFANT MASSAGE

The broad definition of massage encompasses any form of tactile (stroking) stimulation performed systematically by human hands; however, in the NICU environment, massage is often incorporated with additional methods of stimulation such as human social contact (talking, eye contact), rocking, or kinesthetic stimulation (passive extension and flexion of arms and legs) (Vickers et al., 2007). For example, infant stroking and massage has been defined as the manipulation of tissues systematically with the hands to produce effects that help to restore and improve the body's function and health (Agarwal et al., 2000; Beider & Moyer, 2007). There is some confusion about the different methods of touch, such as what is considered massage, stroking, or rubbing. Massage implies kneading, whereas rubbing implies friction. Stroking is defined as passing the hand or fingertips softly in one direction (Harrison, 2004; Vickers et al., 2004). Unfortunately, some of this confusion exists because each researcher has used a different set of definitions and massage and stroking protocols, making it difficult to compare outcomes across studies or build a cohesive body of knowledge that helps us better understand what kind of touch or massage is best for infants.

In general, infant massage is a type of massage that flows from the baby's head to the trunk and legs. Using soft, gentle touches, the infant massage starts at the head, moves to the arms, back, chest, and stomach and then finishes with the legs. Overall, infant massage includes moderate touch. Massage with preterm infants is somewhat different; it begins with moderate touch stroking and involves only one extremity at a time.

OBJECTIVES

Upon completion of this chapter, the clinician will gain evidence-based knowledge on the influence of infant massage on key indicators of infant growth and development. These indicators include (1) autonomic function; (2) behavioral state; (3) hospital progress, including length of hospital stay, feeding progression, and weight gain; (4) stress reduction; (5) mother–infant interaction; and (6) infant health, growth, and development. The clinician will understand the components of infant massage and incorporate these into their caregiving. Evidence will be provided to support all recommendations made (see Table 17-1).

EVIDENCE TO SUPPORT INTEGRATION OF INFANT MASSAGE INTO ROUTINE PRACTICE IN THE NICU

Autonomic Function

Safety of infant massage, specifically for healthy preterm and medically unstable infants, has been a topic of debate; however, recent research confirms that infant massage in preterm infants is not only safe but also regulates preterm infant autonomic function (see Table 17-1). Among full-term cocaine-exposed infants, a correlation was found between pulse rate and infant behavioral state, thereby supporting the hypothesis that ATVV regulates short-term autonomic function (White-Traut et al., 2002a). Following ATVV, preterm infants of varying ages and health status have maintained pulse and respiratory rates, body temperature, and oxygen saturation within normal ranges (White-Traut, 2004; White-Traut & Goldman, 1988; White-Traut et al., 1993; White-Traut et al., 1997). Healthy preterm infants at 35 weeks PMA and born at a mean 31 weeks' gestational age who received ATVV revealed a normal heart and respiratory rate and body temperature (White-Traut & Nelson, 1988). Similar results were found

among 33- to 34-week-old healthy PMA preterm infants, who maintained a normal pulse rate and oxygen saturation during and after ATVV (White-Traut et al., 1993). The safety of infant massage following ATVV was further extended to stable very-low-birth-weight preterm infants born at 23 to 26 weeks' gestational age and infants with IVH born at 24 to 32 weeks' gestational age (White-Traut et al., 2004). These infants maintained stable oxygen hemoglobin saturation and heart and respiratory rates following ATVV (White-Traut et al., 2004). ATVV also was found to be safe in very-low-birth-weight preterm infants and premature infants with grades III and IV IVH and periventricular leukomalacia (PVL) (White-Traut et al., 1999; White-Traut et al., 2004). Among preterm infants at 33 weeks PMA with an average gestational age at birth of 29 weeks and a diagnosis of PVL, respiratory rates and oxygen saturation remained within stable limits, although heart rates remained elevated after ATVV completion (White-Traut et al., 1999). In this particular study, however, heart rates of control group infants with PVL were higher than infants of the same PMA who were not diagnosed with PVL.

Infant massage has not only been deemed safe based on preservation of normal autonomic measures but has also been found to mitigate preterm infant autonomic response to pain (Arditi et al., 2006; Diego et al., 2009). For preterm infants with a mean gestational age of 34.7 weeks undergoing a procedural painful stimulus (extraction of surgical tape on the infant's outer calf), administration of moderate pressure massage and kinesthetic stimulation prior to the painful stimulus significantly modulated infant heart rate (Diego et al., 2009). Although all infants in the study had a marked increase in heart rate within the 5 seconds following the stimulus, infants who received the massage intervention 15 minutes prior to the painful stimulus exhibited (1) a smaller increase in heart rate during the 2-minute period immediately following tape removal ($p < .05$), (2) a lower maximum heart rate following tape removal ($p < .05$), and (3) a faster recovery time to baseline (95% confidence interval [CI]; $p < .05$).

Behavioral State

Infant behavioral state is an important indicator of the infant's neurobehavioral organization and thus central nervous system functioning. Examining infant behavioral state

TABLE 17-1	Rating System for the Hierarchy of Evidence
Level I	Evidence from a systematic review or meta-analysis of all relevant randomized controlled trials [RCTs], or evidence-based clinical practice guidelines based on systematic reviews of RCTs
Level II	Evidence obtained from at least one well-designed RCT
Level III	Evidence obtained from well-designed controlled trials without randomization
Level IV	Evidence from well-designed case–control and cohort studies
Level V	Evidence from systematic reviews of descriptive and qualitative studies
Level VI	Evidence from a single descriptive or qualitative study
Level VII	Evidence from the opinion of authorities and/or reports of expert committees

provides the clinician with an understanding of the infant's neurologic and behavioral proficiency (Bell et al., 2008, 2013; Halpern et al., 1995; VandenBerg, 2007b; White-Traut et al., 2014a, 2014b). Furthermore, assessing infant behavior state and the ways in which each infant regulates their behavioral states allows clinicians to understand an infant's ability to respond to the environment (VandenBerg, 2007b).

Researchers have shown that infant massage modulates infant behavioral state by influencing infant alertness and sleep-wake behaviors (Kelmanson & Adulas, 2006; White-Traut & Pate, 1987; White-Traut et al., 1993; White-Traut et al., 1999; White-Traut et al., 2014a, 2014b; White-Traut et al., 2002b, 2002c). Among healthy preterm infants aged 35 weeks' gestational age, nearly 60% of those receiving the ATVV intervention (provided after feeding) experienced a quiet, alert state immediately after the intervention (White-Traut & Pate, 1987). Following ATVV, researchers found a significant increase in the quiet alert state among preterm infants aged 33.6 weeks PMA and diagnosed with PVL when the ATVV was administered after feeding (White-Traut et al., 1999). The benefits of ATVV on infant behavioral state extend to drug-exposed full-term infants as well. ATVV was found to modulate the behavioral state of drug-exposed infants so that their behavioral state was similar to the non-drug-exposed infants (White-Traut et al., 2002c). In examining the effects of ATVV on both drug-exposed and non-drug-exposed infants aged 35 to 41 weeks' gestational age, researchers found that the non-drug-exposed infants and drug-exposed infants who received the ATVV intervention expressed more alertness and less quiet sleep than infants in the control groups ($p < .05$) (White-Traut et al., 2002c). When mothers administered the H-HOPE intervention similar findings were reported (White-Traut et al., 2014a).

Hospital Progression: Feeding, Weight Gain, and Length of Hospital Stay

An important indicator of an infant's hospital progression is the infant's ability to feed and gain weight. ATVV and infant massage have been found to improve infant feeding behaviors and promote infant weight gain, leading to shorter hospital stay (Chen et al., 2008; Dieter et al., 2003; Ferber et al., 2002; Lahat et al., 2007; Mathai et al., 2001; Medoff-Cooper et al., 2015; Nelson et al., 2001; Vaivre-Douret et al., 2009; White-Traut et al., 2002b; White-Traut et al., 2002c; White-Traut et al., 2005; White-Traut et al., 2014b; White-Traut et al., 2015).

Infant Feeding. Premature infants experience feeding-related difficulties when compared with infants at term equivalent age, suggesting feeding interventions are needed (Pineda, 2020). ATVV produces a transition from a sleep to alert state and thereby is believed to result in improved feeding efficiency (Medoff-Cooper et al., 2015; White-Traut et al., 2002b; White-Traut et al., 2002c; White-Traut et al., 2014b; White-Traut et al., 2015). An examination of ATVV's influence prior to feeding among infants aged 33 to 35 weeks PMA revealed a significant increase in the active alert state,

which correlated with a trend in greater feeding efficiency (White-Traut et al., 2002c). In addition, preterm infants aged 33 to 34 weeks PMA and born between 32 and 33 weeks' gestational age receiving ATVV 1 hour prior to the scheduled feeding showed a significant increase in alertness (quiet and active alert states combined) at both 1 and 30 minutes post intervention (White-Traut et al., 1993). This same study revealed a sustained significant increase in alertness over the 4-day study period. Healthy preterm infants aged 29 to 33 weeks' gestational age who received the ATVV intervention 20 minutes prior to their next scheduled feeding showed more alertness following the intervention, which led to increased feeding efficiency (Griffith et al., 2017; Medoff-Cooper et al., 2015; White-Traut et al., 1993; White-Traut et al., 2014b). In addition, the multisensory ATVV intervention significantly increased the frequency of feeding readiness behaviors (mouthing, hand to mouth, tonguing, rooting, and yawning) while simultaneously increasing the frequency of alert behavioral states immediately prior to feeding (White-Traut et al., 2002c). Of note, orally directed behavioral cues (also called feeding readiness behaviors) may be more valid than behavioral states for assessment of feeding readiness (Bell et al., 2008). Research results indicate that the alert behavioral state is related to the increase in orally directed behaviors and improved sucking organization (Griffith et al., 2017). Furthermore, among medically stable very-low-birth-weight infants and low-birth-weight preterm infants with PVL, IVH, or both PVL and IVH, implementation of the ATVV intervention led to a significantly faster progression from gavage-only feeding to complete nipple feeding (White-Traut et al., 2002c). Study group infants progressed to gavage-only feeding by an average of 12 days compared with 16 days among the control group (White-Traut et al., 2002c). The results of these studies suggest that ATVV administered before feeding modulates infant behavior by increasing active alertness, which then contributes to improved feeding (Griffith et al., 2017; White-Traut et al., 1993; White-Traut et al., 1999; White-Traut et al., 2002c). Additional data support these findings. Recent analysis evaluated the relationship between prefeeding behavioral state and feeding efficiency. A ratio of oral volume intake to length of feeding (mL/min) was calculated to determine feeding efficiency. Compared with infants in a sleepy behavioral state, infants in the alert state revealed significant differences in the amount of oral intake (*mean* = 0.55 mL/min vs. 1.22 mL/min, consecutively; $t = -2.20, p = .039$). It was thus concluded that an association exists between alert behavioral states immediately prior to oral feeding and improved feeding efficiency (White-Traut et al., 2009) (see Figures 17-1).

Growth. Infant massage has also led to a significant increase in weight gain among preterm infants. Healthy preterm infants with a mean gestational age of 35.5 weeks for the control and 35.3 weeks for the treatment group who received ATVV revealed an increased weight gain of 2 pounds compared with controls (White-Traut et al., 2015; White-Traut & Tubeszewski, 1986). In addition, healthy

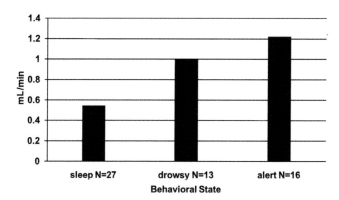

FIGURE 17-1. Average volume intake (mL/min) by the infants in the three behavioral state categories.

preterm infants (mean gestational age of 34 weeks) showed a significantly increased weight gain of 4.24 g/day (Mathai et al., 2001) or 21.92% more per day as compared with controls (Scafidi et al., 1990). These earlier studies (with the exception of Mathai et al.) used nonelectronic infant scales; thus, the reliability of these findings is questioned. Researchers have also found that the use of oil in massage can enhance weight gain among preterm infants aged 32 to 34 weeks' gestation (Ahmed et al., 2007; Janci, 2008). Infants who received multisensory massage with ISIO4 blended oil (rich in essential fatty acids) twice daily for 10 days experienced an increased weight gain of 301 g compared with 192 g by the control group (Vaivre-Douret et al., 2009). The use of oil and massage was also found to improve weight gain among infants aged 33 to 35 weeks' gestation (Arora et al., 2005). After removing from the analysis infants for whom the intervention was interrupted for >20% of the intervention period, a significant increase in weight gain was found among infants receiving massage with sunflower oil. Among infants with a mean gestational age of 30.1 weeks who received moderate-pressure massage therapy with kinesthetic stimulation 3 days a week for 5 weeks, there was an average 26-g greater weight gain per day compared with the control group (Dieter et al., 2003). Similar results were found among infants (mean gestational age of 30 to 32 weeks) who received moderate pressure massage by either staff or the infants' mothers three times daily for 10 days. The results of this study revealed an increased weight gain of 26.4 g/day (massage by mothers) and 28.3 g/day (massage by staff) compared with 20.5 g/day by the control group and confirmed the benefit of infant massage administered by the infant's mother (Ferber et al., 2002). When integrating ATVV with H-HOPE for an intervention with hospitalized preterm infants, the study found an increase in growth and weight gain when massage was used (White-Traut et al., 2015).

Current research has sought to understand the relationship between infant massage, weight gain, stooling patterns, and jaundice. Based on correlational analyses, a significant relationship between both relative weight gain and changes in vagal tone ($p < .01$), and relative weight gain and changes

in gastric motility following massage has been identified ($p < .01$) (Diego et al., 2005). Infant massage also increased serum insulin and insulin-like growth factor-1 (IGF-1; Field et al., 2008). Insulin and IGF-1 play an important role in improving growth (Guzzetta et al., 2009). Furthermore, researchers examined the influence of kinesthetic stimulation with massage by comparing the weight gain of stable preterm infants who received no intervention, massage therapy only, or massage therapy with kinesthetic stimulation (Massaro et al., 2009). The researchers revealed that infants weighing >1,000 g who received both massage and kinesthetic stimulation had a significant increase in weight gain, whereas control group infants and infants receiving massage alone did not. The researchers attributed the weight gain to kinesthetic stimulation. The relationship between bilirubin levels and stool frequency has also been evaluated. In response to massage, bilirubin levels decreased and stool frequency was higher (Ahmadipour et al., 2019; Chen et al., 2011; Dalili et al., 2016).

In addition to the benefits of infant massage on infant feeding, weight gain, stooling patterns, and jaundice, massage has also resulted in a reduced hospital stay. Among infants with a mean gestational age of 35.5 weeks, ATVV administered once a day for 10 days led to a 2-day decrease in length of hospitalization (White-Traut & Tubeszewski, 1986). Recently, researchers confirmed this trend. Utilizing a multisensory infant massage and sweet almond oil, ISIO4 blended oil, or placebo twice daily for 10 days the researchers found a mean decrease in hospital stay of 15 days among infants aged 31 to 34 weeks' gestation ($p = .005$) (Vaivre-Douret et al., 2009). Among infants with a mean gestational age of 29 weeks, those receiving maternal infant massage with kinesthetic stimulation four times daily had a chance of early discharge 1.85 (95% CI: 1.09 to 3.13; $p = .023$) times greater than the control group (Mendes & Procianoy, 2008). In addition, infant massage was associated with a reduction in sepsis and, thus, improved hospital progression and decreased hospital stay (Mendes & Procianoy, 2008). Furthermore, for preterm infants diagnosed with PVL, receiving ATVV twice per day reduced the infants' average hospital stay by 9 days (White-Traut et al., 1999). Similarly, among medically stable very-low-birth-weight infants and low-birth-weight preterm infants with PVL, IVH, or both PVL and IVH, the use of ATVV twice per day led to a hospital stay 1.6 weeks shorter than control group infants ($p < .05$) (White-Traut et al., 2002c) (Table 17-2).

Infant Stress Reduction

During times of stress, maternal or caregiver behaviors of talking, touching, eye-to-eye contact, and rocking have been found to soothe the infant and foster infant self-regulation (Braarud & Stormark, 2006; Jahromi et al., 2004). A common, although methodologically challenging, measure of infant stress reactivity is elevated cortisol (White-Traut et al., 1998). Researchers have found that

TABLE 17-2 Benefits of Massage for Infants

Recommended Benefits	Level of Evidence	References
Enhances behavioral development	Level II	White-Traut et al. (2018) White-Traut et al. (2017) Griffith et al. (2017) White-Traut et al. (2014b) White-Traut et al. (2012) White-Traut et al. (2009) White-Traut and Pate (1987)
Enhances neurological development	Level II Level III	Field et al. (1996) Guzzetta et al. (2009) Nelson et al. (2001) Kim et al. (2003) Mathai et al. (2001) Vaivre-Douret et al. (2009)
Enhances control of muscle tone	Level II Level III	Braarud and Stormark (2006) Vaivre-Douret et al. (2009)
Enhances bone development	Level I Level II	Schulze (2008) Aly et al. (2004) Elmoneim et al. (2021) Litmanovitz et al. (2007) Moyer-Mileur et al. (2008) Vignochi et al. (2008)
Improves sensory awareness	Level II	White-Traut et al. (2002a) Vandenberg (2007) Dieter et al. (2003) White-Traut and Pate (1987) White-Traut et al. (1993) White-Traut et al. (1999) White-Traut et al. (2002b)
Enhances deep sleep	Level II Level III	White-Traut et al. (2002a) White-Traut and Pate (1987) White-Traut et al. (1993) White-Traut et al. (1999) White-Traut et al. (2002b) Dieter et al. (2003) Kelmanson and Adulas (2006)
Improved temperature stability	Level II	Diego et al. (2009) White-Traut et al. (1999) White-Traut (2004)
Increases oxygen saturation and nutrient flow to cells	Level II	White-Traut et al. (1997) White-Traut (2004) White-Traut and Goldman (1988) White-Traut et al. (1993)
Improves circulation, heart rate	Level II	White-Traut et al. (2002a) White-Traut et al. (1999) White-Traut (2004) Diego et al. (2009) Field et al. (2004)
Reduces stress	Level II	White-Traut et al. (2009) Acolet et al. (1993) Field et al. (1996) Guzzetta et al. (2009) Hernandez-Reif et al. (2007) Yoo (2005)

TABLE 17-2 Benefits of Massage for Infants (Continued)

Recommended Benefits	Level of Evidence	References
Reduces levels of cortisol in plasma and saliva	Level II	Acolet et al. (1993) Guzzetta et al. (2009) Hernandez-Reif et al. (2007) White-Traut et al. (2009) Yoo (2005)
Enhances the immune system	Level II	Hernandez-Reif et al. (2007)
Enhances release of hormones in the body including growth hormone	Level II Level III	Guzzetta et al. (2009) Hernandez-Reif et al. (2007) Diego et al. (2005) Yoo (2005)
Improves functioning of the digestion system, growth	Level I Level II	Arora et al. (2005) Chen et al. (2008) Diego et al. (2005) Field et al. (2008) Mendes and Procianoy (2008) White-Traut et al. (2002b) Dieter et al. (2003) Ferber et al. (2002) Field et al. (2006) Lahat et al. (2007) Mathai et al. (2001) Nelson et al. (2001) Scafidi et al. (1990) Vaivre-Douret et al. (2009) White-Traut et al. (2002c) White-Traut et al. (2005) White-Traut et al. (2002c) White-Traut and Tubeszewski (1986) White-Traut (2015) Dalili et al. (2016) Chen et al. (2011) Ahmadipour et al. (2019)
Enhances feeding outcomes	Level II	Diego et al. (2005) Field et al. (2008) Medoff-Cooper et al. (2015) Mendes and Procianoy (2008) White-Traut (2002) White-Traut et al. (2009) White-Traut et al. (2002b) White-Traut et al. (2002c) Griffith et al. (2017), p. 2862 White-Traut et al. (2005), p. 284
Skin stimulation–all the physiological systems are stimulated	Level II	Diego et al. (2009)
Decrease response to painful stimulus	Level II	Arditi et al. (2006) Diego et al. (2009)

elevated cortisol levels have a damaging effect on brain development (Chugani et al., 2001). In contrast, reducing infant stress correlates with improved infant learning and memory (Bonnier, 2008). The ATVV intervention has been found to reduce salivary cortisol levels and stress behaviors among healthy infants born between 36 and 41 weeks' gestation (White-Traut et al., 2009). However, it is important to properly implement the intervention as research on infant

touch and stress has revealed that healthy full-term infants experienced a steady decline in salivary cortisol, whereas a group of comparable infants who received tactile-only stimulation with no additional human interaction showed an increase in stress reactivity (White-Traut et al., 2009). Based on this research, it is recommended that massage intervention should be offered in conjunction with human social interaction.

Stress reduction following infant massage also has been found among infants born to mothers with depression. Full-term infants with depressed mothers who received 15 minutes of massage with kinesthetic activity for 2 days a week for 6 weeks showed a decrease in urinary epinephrine and norepinephrine and salivary cortisol, as well as an increase in serotonin (Field et al., 1996). Research on preterm infants revealed similar results. Preterm infants aged 30 to 33 weeks' gestation who received massage with kinesthetic activity for 2 blocks of 5 days (with an interim 2-day break) showed a significant decrease in serum cortisol levels compared with controls (Asadollahi et al., 2016; Guzzetta et al., 2009). In addition, following the use of gentle massage with arachis oil, preterm infants (mean age 29 weeks' gestational age) showed a consistent decrease in plasma cortisol, although no change was found in adrenaline and noradrenaline levels (Acolet et al., 1993). Healthy preterm infants (mean age 29.5 weeks' gestational age) have also expressed fewer stress behaviors (Hernandez-Reif et al., 2007). Massage therapy administered three times per day for 5 days revealed a decrease in stress behaviors from the first day to the last. Following massage, the infants also showed less active behaviors (Hernandez-Reif et al., 2007).

Maternal and Infant Interaction

For preterm infants hospitalized in the NICU and separated from their mothers, or for infants of depressed mothers, fostering positive mother and infant interaction is imperative (see Table 17-3 for a summary of research to support benefits for mothers from infant massage). Infant massage, the ATVV intervention, and H-HOPE have been found to improve the interaction between mothers and infants. Researchers revealed that the ATVV intervention performed by the mother improved maternal sensitivity toward her infant's cues and cognitive-growth-fostering behaviors (White-Traut & Nelson, 1988). Infants receiving routine nursing care or verbal-only stimulation did not gain the same benefit as those receiving ATVV. Similar results were found when infant massage enhanced with auditory and visual interaction was extended to infants aged 2, 4, 5, and 6 months (Lee, 2006). In this study, following a 4-week-long auditory, tactile/kinesthetic, and visual multisensory intervention performed by the mother, mother–infant interaction scores were significantly increased. Compared with mothers who did not participate in the intervention, mothers who performed the multisensory intervention showed a significant difference in eight maternal behaviors: expression of affect, visual interaction, style of play interaction, vocalization styles, attempts at smile elicitation, and kinesthetic quality of interaction. The behaviors of infants who received the intervention showed a significant change in the three areas evaluated: expressed affect, response, and visual interaction. Furthermore, compared with controls, mother–infant dyads receiving the intervention showed significant

differences in the two dyadic behaviors measured: dyadic quality of interaction and synchrony of affect. Thus, the multisensory intervention improved infant behavior and maternal response to her infant and these benefits extend to infants aged 2 to 6 months. H-HOPE revealed similar findings. Mothers and infants assigned to H-HOPE showed improved interaction during feeding. Specifically, mothers had higher maternal social–emotional growth fostering behaviors and infants had more clarity of cues and responsivity to the mother. In addition, mothers and infants were more responsive toward each other during play at 6 weeks CA (White-Traut et al., 2013). Massage intervention that engages with both mother and infant is a sure approach to help premature infants achieve the social interaction patterns essential for optimal development (White-Traut et al., 2018).

An infant's ability to regulate emotion has been deemed a necessary component for the infant's capacity to learn, manage stress, and develop coping abilities (Weller & Feldman, 2003). It is within the confines of the mother–infant relationship that the infant's ability to regulate emotions is born; however, certain factors can hinder the development of emotion regulation, including maternal depression (Weller & Feldman, 2003). To counteract the influence of depression on the mother–infant relationship, researchers have examined the influence of infant massage on mother–infant interaction, specifically with depressed mothers. Among postnatally depressed mothers, massaging their preterm infants reduced maternal anxiety (Fujita et al., 2006; Field et al., 2006; Mathai et al., 2001). For postnatally depressed mothers participating in a mother–infant massage class (which included instruction on how to recognize infant behavioral cues), there was a significant improvement in maternal attitude toward her full-term infant, in the infant's responses to their mother, and in the overall mother–infant interaction (Glover et al., 2002; Lai et al., 2016; Mathai et al., 2001; Onozawa et al., 2001). Also, after participating in a massage class, postnatally depressed mothers had a significantly reduced score on the Edinburgh Postnatal Depression Scale (EPDS) (Glover et al., 2002; O'Higgins et al., 2008), and, after 1 year, compared with nondepressed mothers, in maternal sensitivity (Kim, 2005; O'Higgins et al., 2008). Furthermore, preterm infants receiving massage with kinesthetic activity showed greater improvement in emotionality, and they appeared more sociable and more able to soothe (Kim, 2005; Lai et al., 2016).

Health and Development

Infant massage has also improved infant health and development. Researchers examined the responses of Korean full-term infants housed in an orphanage to the ATVV intervention (Kim, 2005). The infants were stimulated 1 hour prior to feeding twice daily, 5 days per week for

TABLE 17-3 Benefits of Massage for Parents

Documented Benefits	Level of Evidence	References
Increases mother–infant interaction	Level II Level III	White-Traut and Goldman (1988) White-Traut et al. (2013) Onozawa et al. (2001) Feijó et al. (2006) Kim (2005) Lee (2006) Fujita et al. (2006) Jean et al. (2009) O'Higgins et al. (2008)
Increases closeness to the infant	Level II Level III	O'Higgins et al. (2008) Fujita et al. (2006) Jahromi et al. (2004) Braarud and Stormark (2006)
Eases stress about separation from infant	Level II	O'Higgins et al. (2008) Jean et al. (2009)
Increases opportunity for eye contact with infant	Level II Level III	Braarud and Stormark (2006) White-Traut and Goldman (1988) White-Traut et al. (2013) Onozawa et al. (2001) Feijó et al. (2006) Lee (2006) O'Higgins et al. (2008) White-Traut (2012)
Allows parent alone and quiet time with their infant	Level II	Fujita et al. (2006) O'Higgins et al. (2008)
Increases bonding/attachment	Level II Level III	White-Traut and Goldman (1988) White-Traut et al. (2013) Onozawa et al. (2001) Feijó et al. (2006) Lee (2006) O'Higgins et al. (2008) White-Traut (2012)
Decreases maternal depression	Level II Level III	O'Higgins et al. (2008) Onozawa et al. (2001) Glover et al. (2002) Feijó et al. (2006)
Increases sense of maternal competence	Level II Level III	White-Traut and Goldman (1988) Onozawa et al. (2001) Feijó et al. (2006) Lee (2006) O'Higgins et al. (2008) Mathai et al. (2001)
Provides an active role in caregiving for parent in the NICU	Level II Level III	Onozawa et al. (2001) White-Traut et al. (2013) Fujita et al. (2006)
Increases parent self-esteem about caregiving	Level II Level III	Fujita et al. (2006) White-Traut and Goldman (1988) Onozawa et al. (2001) Feijó et al. (2006) Lee (2006) Jean et al. (2009) Kim (2005) Onozawa et al. (2001) White-Traut (2012) White-Traut and Goldman (1988)

(Continued)

TABLE 17-3 Benefits of Massage for Parents (Continued)		
Documented Benefits	Level of Evidence	References
Provides parent with opportunity to better understand behaviors and cues of their infant	Level II	

Note: Level II, evidence obtained from at least one well-designed RCT; level III, evidence obtained from well-designed controlled trials without randomization.

4 weeks. The intervention significantly improved infant growth. For the infants receiving ATVV stimulation there was a significant increase in weight gain each week, with infants receiving the intervention gaining 60.86 g in the fourth week compared with 21.62 g for the control group. The infants receiving ATVV had a significant increase in body length ($p < .01$) and an increase in average head circumference (HC; $p < .01$). The significant difference in infant weight, height, and HC held true at both 4 weeks and 6 months. Furthermore, at 6 months, the orphaned infants receiving ATVV had fewer illnesses and subsequent visits compared with the control group infants. During hospitalization, the smaller, sicker infants used less hospital resources if they were assigned to the H-HOPE group (Vonderheid et al., 2020). In addition, infants assigned to the H-HOPE intervention had fewer illnesses after hospital discharge (Vonderheid et al., 2016). Massage or massage in conjunction with human social interaction improves infant development. Among preterm infants at a mean 33.1 weeks' gestational age, infant massage with ISIO4 oil significantly improved infant oculomotor and sensorimotor skills, psychomotor scores, as well as visual-auditory orientation scores (Vaivre-Douret et al., 2009). For infants at 34.5 weeks' gestational age, massage also resulted in a significant improvement in neurobehavioral measures (based on the Brazelton Neuro-Behavioral Assessment Scale), such as *orientation, range of state, regulation of state,* and *autonomic stability* (Mathai et al., 2001). Interestingly, the findings by Mathai et al. contradict results by Arora et al. (2005), who did not find a significant difference in neurobehavioral measures on the Brazelton scale following massage with oil or massage alone. However, the conflicting results could be due to the difference in study duration, as Mathai et al. examined infants for 8 to 10 weeks, whereas the neurobehavior of infants was evaluated by Arora et al. after 10 days of treatment. Furthermore, following ATVV intervention, very-low-birth-weight preterm infants and preterm infants with IVH revealed improved motor and mental capabilities and, at 1 year, cerebral palsy diagnoses were decreased by 23% (Nelson et al., 2001). The H-HOPE intervention was designed to improve mutual dyadic responsiveness of mothers and preterm infants and contributes to better infant language development (White-Traut, 2018).

More recently, researchers examined the influence of massage on brain development and, more specifically,

on the development of the visual system among preterm infants aged 30-33 weeks and, simultaneously, on early postnatal rat pups (Guzzetta et al., 2009). Infants received the massage intervention three times per day for 5 days followed by a 2-day break and then an additional 5 days of massage. One marker used to measure development was IGF-1, a molecule known to provide multiple benefits in development, including visual development. Plasma IGF-1 was measured at both 1 and 4 weeks. Although there was a decrease in IGF-1 for all infants, infants who received the massage maintained a significantly higher serum level of IGF-1 compared with controls. By incorporating analysis with rat pups, the researchers revealed that IGF-1 is significantly increased by massage and this increase in IGF-1 influences brain growth and, more specifically, accelerates the development of visual function.

Bone development is another important consideration among preterm infants because they are at risk of osteopenia of prematurity, thus increasing their risk of bone deformities and fractures (Aly et al., 2004). Researchers have shown that physical therapy reduces the risk of osteopenia of prematurity (Litmanovitz et al., 2007; Moyer-Mileur et al., 2008; Vignochi et al., 2008). Of interest, combining infant massage with physical therapy has also been shown to improve the formation of bone, thereby reducing the risk of osteopenia of prematurity and its sequelae (Aly et al., 2004; Schulzke et al., 2014). Other investigators have examined bone growth and body composition in preterm infants following massage. In addition to an increase in daily weight gain and growth velocity, total body mass and bone mineral density significantly increased when compared with a routine care group (Elmoneim et al., 2021). Additional research is warranted to confirm findings on bone growth and development.

Administration of Multisensory Stimulation and Infant Massage Therapy

The ATVV intervention incorporates normal maternal, social interactive behavior (White-Traut et al., 2004). Provided in 15-minute intervals, the ATVV intervention starts with auditory stimulation via infant-directed talk by a soothing female voice. The infant-directed talk is performed using a higher-pitched voice with pauses, offering the infant the opportunity to respond. Following at least 30 seconds of talk, the infant is then placed in a supine position for moderate pressure massage. First the head is massaged, followed by strokes on the chest and abdomen, the legs from thigh to ankle, and the arms. The infant is placed in prone position and the back is massaged using straight continuous strokes and circular strokes directly over the spine. The head is then massaged from the hairline to the nape of the neck. Massage should take place for 10 minutes. Following massage, the infant is swaddled. Swaddling provides the infant a feeling of security. However, this act can be performed by simply holding the infant with arms and legs flexed. The infant is then rocked for the final 5 minutes. Horizontal rocking is commonly used for preterm infants, although vertical rocking appears to be the preferred method for term infants. Throughout the entire 15-minute intervention, the provider attempts eye contact with the infant. Furthermore, the intervention is designed to be contingent on infant behavior (Burns et al., 1994). As a result, if the infant expresses disengagement cues during a particular component of the intervention, the intervener pauses, allowing the infant to disengage and then re-engage. When the infant is re-engaged, the massage continues. Infant individuality is continually assessed, e.g., some infants prefer different components of the massage. When the intervener has determined which tactile components receive a positive response from the infant, these tactile components are repeated, and the tactile components that elicit disengagement cues are discontinued.

With ATVV stimulation, the intervener provides social interaction (auditory and visual cues) based on the infant's engagement cues (White-Traut et al., 2004). This provides the infant the opportunity to learn social interaction skills. As the mother/intervener responds to the infant's engagement and disengagement cues, the premature infant begins to learn about social interaction. The mother also learns about her infant's response capabilities and engagement and disengagement cues. Furthermore, the mother learns how to respond to her infant to promote optimal behavior.

Although the ATVV improved infant outcomes and mother–infant interaction, parents continued to report high stress while interacting with their premature infants and their need for extra social support. Thus, the ATVV intervention was enhanced with the addition of participatory guidance for parents to help them engage with their infants despite their immature behaviors. In addition, social support is offered by the nurse. The enhanced intervention is called H-HOPE (Hospital-Home Transition: Optimizing Prematures' Environment) (White-Traut et al., 2009). The ATVV component is now considered the infant-directed component of H-HOPE. The parent-directed component includes the participatory guidance while the parents learn the ATVV intervention and receive social support from the nurse (White-Traut et al., 2009). The parent-directed component of H-HOPE consists of four participatory guidance sessions for parents, two during the NICU stay and two post discharge. Therefore, H-HOPE simultaneously addresses the needs of both preterm infants and their parents, especially their need for mutual engagement, and is uniquely suited as an early developmental/behavioral intervention for preterm infants in NICUs. An important consideration when administering any sensory intervention is the infant's physiological and behavioral response. Burns et al. (1994) published a decision tree that guides clinicians through an intervention offering how to modify the intervention based on the infant's responses. Others recommend using moderate-pressure massage instead of light-pressure massage. In addition, a multisensory behavioral approach that includes massage versus massage only is recommended to reduce infant stress.

Parent-Administered Infant Massage

Determining who administers infant massage is another important consideration. Parents who are trained to administer interventions provide a safe and effective alternative to interventions offered by trained staff and clinicians (Burns et al., 1994; Medoff-Cooper et al., 2015; Moyer-Mileur et al., 2008; White-Traut et al., 2013). Parent-trained interventions for premature infants have been found to improve infant neurodevelopment, with results lasting up to 36 months of age (Vanderveen et al., 2009). Although much research has examined the implementation of infant massage by a trained clinician and/or researcher, research has examined and confirmed the benefits of infant massage by the infant's parent (Jean et al., 2009; McGrath et al., 2007; Medoff-Cooper et al., 2015; White-Traut et al., 2012; White-Traut et al., 2013) (see Table 17-3 for benefits to parents). Parent-administered massage by first-time parents of full-term infants led to the parent's perceived decrease in stress, an improved perception in parenting ability, and an improved ability to recognize infant cues and calm the infant (Jean et al., 2009). As previously noted, infant massage by the mother or caregiver improves mother–infant interaction (Jahromi et al., 2004; Lee, 2006; White-Traut & Nelson, 1988; White-Traut et al., 2013), thereby modulating mother and infant behavior and improving the mother–infant relationship. Incorporating parent-administered massage is especially important among infants of depressed mothers. As mentioned, mother-administered massage among depressed mothers not only improves the mother's interaction with her infant but also reduces maternal anxiety and depression scores (Feijó et al., 2006; Glover et al., 2002; O'Higgins et al., 2008; Onozawa et al., 2001). Considering the benefits of infant massage for both mother and infant, it is recommended that infant massage programs incorporate the mother/care provider in the massage protocol. See Table 17-4 for a list of recommendations to use when teaching and working with parents about the implementation of massage with their high-risk infant. See Table 17-5 for examples of how to deliver massage to vulnerable preterm infants. These pictures show how massage can be delivered and tolerated in this high-risk population.

TABLE 17-4 Areas to Address When Teaching Parents About Preterm Infant Massage

- Help the parents to respond to the infant's physiological needs before considering massage: Is the infant hungry or tired? Consider the infant's sleep/wake cycle.
- Decrease extraneous visual or auditory stimuli before beginning the session.
- Assess infant's readiness and reactivity. Are they in a state where they are easily overstimulated?
- Place the infant in a comfortable position prior to beginning the massage.
- Fragile or ill preterm infants can be potentially hypersensitive to tactile input so proceed cautiously.
- Has the infant had a stressful day and does massage needs to be considered at a different time or day? Consider infant state before handling.
- Check in with parent. Are they relaxed? Stressed? Infants will respond to these emotions.
- Use a unimodal approach to begin with: sensory processing can be limited in the preterm infant; progress to multimodal as the infant demonstrates increased tolerance for touch and handling.
- Offer comforting pressure by laying the relaxed hand on the child's forehead or abdomen or other part while waiting for the infant to become less distressed.
- Provide swaddling for natural warmth especially if the infant is fragile or easily overstimulated.
- Initial reactivity to touch is common among sensitive infants: proceed slowly. Touch should begin gradually and be rhythmical in nature.
- Duration of the massage should depend on the infant's cues, responses, and developmental maturity.
- Reassess the infant with each movement.
- Talk to the infant using a predictable approach, but watch for tolerance.
- If the infant seems distressed, consider decreasing or increasing the pressure being used during the massage.
- If the infant seems distressed, change the location of the tactile input, consider going back to a location that has been comfortable for the infant in the past.
- Use different types of strokes such as long sweeping strokes instead of wringing motions; avoid light stroking, this can be irritating to the infant.
- Discontinue the massage and use an alternative calming technique, such as vestibular input (slow rocking), proprioceptive input, or rhythmical music if the infant is distressed.
- Provide skin-to-skin holding (kangaroo care) for the more preterm infant who is fragile and easily overstimulated.
- If the infant has high tone, consider firm, soft, gentle movement, clockwise for relaxation.
- Discontinue the massage until a later time if the infant becomes distressed or unstable.
- Tactile stimulation such as massage should not be just another task but should be administered when and if the infant's cues are indicative of the infant's availability for stimulation.
- After the massage make sure the infant is repositioned and supported, assess organization of the infant, continue to reassess for delayed reactivity to the massage.
- If facial masks or shields are needed to prevent transfer of disease, it is important to consider voice (tone) and types of touch to facilitate interaction. Facial shields are recommended rather than a mask to allow the infant to see the parent's entire face. Touch may be considered after good hand washing; however, touch should also be only cautiously considered if there is a risk for transfer of disease. Placing the infant in an infant seat and interacting with them from 6 feet away without a mask may also be considered but should be done with caution. Parental vaccination (when available) is highly recommended to increase the potential for more optimal parent–infant interactions.

TABLE 17-5 Recommendations for Implementation Into Practice: Evidence to Support Integration of Massage Into Caregiving With High-Risk Infants

Type	Recommendation	Level of Evidence	References
Intervention	Utilize infant massage to maintain temperature stability and modulate autonomic regulation	Level II	White-Traut (2004) White-Traut et al. (2002a) White-Traut et al. (1997) White-Traut et al. (1993) White-Traut and Goldman (1988)
Intervention	Implement infant massage to modulate neurobehavioral organization	Level II Level IV	Dieter et al. (2003) White-Traut et al. (2002a) White-Traut et al. (2002b) White-Traut et al. (1999) White-Traut et al. (1993) White-Traut and Pate (1987) Kelmanson and Adulas (2006)

TABLE 17-5 Recommendations for Implementation Into Practice: Evidence to Support Integration of Massage Into Caregiving With High-Risk Infants (Continued)

Type	Recommendation	Level of Evidence	References
Intervention	Implement infant massage to modify sensory development	Level II	Vaivre-Douret et al. (2009)
Intervention	Utilize infant massage to improve infant feeding	Level II	White-Traut et al. (2002b) White-Traut et al. (2002c)
Intervention	Increase infant weight gain by utilizing infant massage	Level II Level IV	Dieter et al. (2003) Massaro et al. (2009) Vaivre-Douret et al. (2009) Ferber et al. (2002) Diego et al. (2005) Field et al. (2006) Mathai et al. (2001) Scafidi et al. (1990)
Intervention	Perform infant massage to reduce preterm infant hospital length of stay	Level II Level IV	Mendes and Procianoy (2008) Vaivre-Douret et al. (2009) White-Traut et al. (2002b) White-Traut et al. (1999) Scafidi et al. (1990)
Intervention	Implement infant massage to reduce infant stress	Level II Level IV	Field et al. (1996) Hernandez-Reif et al. (2007) White-Traut et al. (2009) Acolet et al. (1993)
Intervention	Perform infant massage to enhance parent–infant interaction	Level II Level IV	Feijó et al. (2006) Field et al. (1996) Onozawa et al. (2001) White-Traut and Goldman (1988) Lee (2006)
Intervention	Utilize infant massage to modify infant altered growth	Level II	Kim et al. (2003)
Intervention	Perform infant massage to modify neurodevelopment	Level II Level III	Nelson et al. (2001) Vaivre-Douret et al. (2009) Mathai et al. (2001) Guzzetta et al. (2009)

CONCLUSION

Infant massage is a form of massage that is often incorporated with additional methods of stimulation such as human social contact (talking, eye contact), rocking, and kinesthetic stimulation (passive extension and flexion of arms and legs) (Vickers et al., 2004). Although infant massage is an intervention used throughout the world, it has not been used fully in the United States. Based on research, infant massage improves infant autonomic stability and modifies infant hospital progress by improving infant feeding efficiency, increasing infant weight gain, and reducing length of hospital stay.

Furthermore, infant massage modulates infant behavioral state thereby modifying neurobehavioral organization. Infant massage has also been implicated in reducing infant stress, enhancing mother and infant interaction, and improving infant neurodevelopment. Further research is needed in understanding the relationship between infant massage and stress reduction, recognizing what mediates infant and maternal response to massage, how infant massage reduces maternal anxiety, the hormones involved in infant neurohormonal response to massage, how infant massage increases infant weight gain, and, finally, the best approach of infant massage based on infant age and health status.

Potential Research Questions

Prevention

How can the implementation of touch and massage reduce stress and promote more normal neurobehavioral development?

What mediates infant and maternal response to massage?

What are the best approaches to massage based on infant age and health status?

Confirmation

Neurohormonal responses—what hormones are involved in and mediated by massage?

Is there a dose–response for infant massage, and if so, is there a dose that is too little or too much?

Treatment

What are the mechanisms that make weight gain an outcome of massage?

How does parent participation in infant massage reduce anxiety for parents/caregiver?

REFERENCES

Acolet, D., Modi, N., Giannakoulopoulos, X., Bond, C., Weg, W., Clow, A., & Glover, V. (1993). Changes in plasma cortisol and catecholamine concentrations in response to massage in preterm infants. *Archives of Disease in Childhood, 68*, 29–31.

Agarwal, K., Gupta, A., Pushkarna, R., Bhargava, S., Faridi, M., & Prabhu, M. (2000). Effects of massage & use of oil on growth, blood flow & sleep pattern in infants. *Indian Journal of Medical Research, 112*, 212–217.

Ahmadipour, S., Mardani, M., Mohsenzadeh, A., Baharvand, P., & Nazeri, M. G. (2019). The lowering of bilirubin levels in full-term newborns by the effect of combined massage therapy and phototherapy practice. *American Journal of Perinatology.* https://doi.org/10.1055/s-0039-1685493. PMID: 30999382.

Ahmed, A. S., Saha, S. K., Chowdhury, M. A., Law, P. A., Black, R. E., Santosham, M., & Darmstadt, G. L. (2007). Acceptability of massage with skin barrier-enhancing emollients in young neonates in Bangladesh. *Journal of Health Population and Nutrition, 25*, 236–240.

Aly, H., Moustafa, M. F., & Hassanein, S. M. (2004). Physical activity combined with massage improves bone mineralization in premature infant: A randomized trial. *Journal of Perinatology, 24*, 305–309.

Arditi, H., Feldman, R., & Eidelman, A. I. (2006). Effects of human contact and vagal regulation on pain reactivity and visual attention in newborns. *Developmental Psychobiology, 48*(7), 561–573.

Arora, J., Kumar, A., & Ramji, S. (2005). Effect of oil massage on growth and neurobehavior in very low birth weight preterm neonates. *Indian Pediatrics, 42*, 1092–1100.

Asadollahi, M., Jabraeili, M., Mahallei, M., Jafarabadi, M. A., & Ebrahimi, S. (2016). Effects of gentle human touch and field massage on urine cortisol level in premature infants? A randomized, controlled clinical trial. *Journal of Caring Science, 5*(30), 187–194.

Beider, S., & Moyer, C. (2007). Randomized controlled trials of pediatric massage: A review. *Evidence-Based Complementary and Alternative Medicine, 4*(1), 23–34. https://doi.org/10.1093/ecam/nel068

Bell, A. F., Lucas, R., & White-Traut, R. (2008). Concept clarification of neonatal neurobehavioural organization. *Journal of Advanced Nursing, 61*(5), 570–581. https://doi:10.1111/j.1365-2648.2007.04561.x

Bell, A. F., White-Traut, R., & Rankin, K. (2013). Fetal exposure to synthetic oxytocin and the relationship with prefeeding cues within one hour post-birth. *Early Human Development, 89*(3), 137–143.

Bijari, B. B., Iranmanesh, S., Eshghi, F., & Baneshi, M. R. (2013). Gentle human touch and Yakson: The effect on preterm's behavioral reactions.

ISRN Nursing, 2012, 750363. https://doi.org/10.5402/2012/750363. PMID: 22792482. PMCID: PMC3389696.

Bonnier, C. (2008). Evaluation of early stimulation programs for enhancing brain development. *Acta Paediatrica, 97*, 853–858.

Braarud, H. C., & Stormark, K. M. (2006). Maternal soothing and infant stress responses: Soothing, crying and adrenocortical activity during inoculation. *Infant Behavior & Development, 29*, 70–79.

Burns, K., Cunningham, N., White-Traut, R., Silvestri, J., & Nelson, M. N. (1994). Infant stimulation: Modification of an intervention based on physiologic and behavioral cues. *Journal of Obstetrical Gynecological and Neonatal Nursing, 23*, 581–589.

Chen, J., Sadakata, M., Ishida, M., Sekizuka, N., & Sayama, M. (2011). Baby massage ameliorates neonatal jaundice in full-term newborn infants. *Tohoku Journal of Experimental Medicine, 223*, 97–102.

Chen, L., Su, Y., Su, C., Lin, H., & Kuo, H. (2008). Acupressure and meridian massage: Combined effects on increasing body weight in premature infants. *Journal of Clinical Nursing, 17*, 1174–1181.

Chugani, H. T., Behen, M. E., Muzik, O., Juhasz, C., Nagy, F., & Chugani, D. C. (2001). Local brain functional activity following early deprivation: A study of postinstitutionalised Romanian orphans. *NeuroImage, 14*, 1290–1301.

Dalili, H., Sheikhi, S., Shariat, M., & Haghnazarian, E. (2016). Effects of baby massage on neonatal jaundice in healthy Iranian infants: A pilot study. *Infant Behavior & Development, 42*, 22–26.

Diego, M. A., Field, T., & Hernandez-Reif, M. (2005). Vagal activity, gastric motility, and weight gain in massaged preterm neonates. *Journal of Pediatrics, 147*, 50–55.

Diego, M. A., Field, T., & Hernandez-Reif, M. (2009). Procedural pain heart rate responses in massaged preterm infants. *Infant Behavior Development, 32*, 226–229.

Dieter, J. N., Field, T., Hernandez-Reif, M., Emory, E. K., & Redzepi, M. (2003). Stable preterm infants gain more weight and sleep less after five days of massage therapy. *Journal of Pediatric Psychology, 28*, 403–411.

Elmoneim, M. A., Mohamed, H. A., Awad, A., Elp-Hawary, A., Salem, N., El Helaly, R., Nasef, N., & Abdel-Hady, H. (2021). Effect of tactile/kinesthetic massage therapy on growth and body composition of preterm infants. *European Journal of Pediatrics, 180*(1), 207–215. https://doi.org/10.1007/s00431-020-03738-w. PMID: 32666281.

Euser, A. M., de Wit, C. C., Finken, M. J., Rijken, M., & Wit, J. M. (2008). Growth of preterm born children. *Hormone Research, 70*, 319–328.

Fathollahzadeh, M. H. (2020). *Co-simulation environments for integrated energy modeling, demand, and resource optimization.* Presented at 2020 ASHRAE Virtual Conference.

Feeley, N., Gottlieb, L., & Zelkowitz, P. (2005). Infant, mother, and contextual predictors of mother-very low birth weight infant interaction at 9 months of age. *Journal of Developmental and Behavioral Pediatrics, 26*, 24–33.

Feijó, L., Hernandez-Reif, M., Field, T., Burns, W., Valley-Gray, S., & Simco, E. (2006). Mothers' depressed mood and anxiety levels are reduced after massaging their preterm infants. *Infant Behavior Development, 29*, 476–480.

Ferber, S. G., Kuint, J., Weller, A., Feldman, R., Dollberg, S., Arbel, E., & Kohelet, D. (2002). Massage therapy by mothers and trained professionals enhances weight gain in preterm infants. *Early Human Development, 67*, 37–45.

Field, T., Diego, M., Dieter, J., Hernandez-Reif, M., Schanberg, S., Kuhn, C., Yando, R., & Bendell, D. (2004). Prenatal depression effects on the fetus and the newborn. *Infant Behavior and Development, 27*, 216–229. https://doi.org/https://doi.org/10.1016/j.infbeh.2003.09.010

Field, T., Diego, M., Hernandez-Reif, M., Dieter, J. N., Kumar, A. M., Schanberg, S., & Kuhn, C. (2008). Insulin and insulin-like growth factor-1 increased in preterm neonates following massage therapy. *Journal of Developmental and Behavioral Pediatrics, 29*, 463–466.

Field, T., Grizzle, N., Scafidi, F., Abrams, S., & Richardson, S. (1996). Massage therapy for infants of depressed mothers. *Infant Behavior and Development, 19*, 107–112.

Field, T., Hernandez-Reif, M., Feijo, L., & Freedman, J. (2006). Prenatal, perinatal and neonatal stimulation: A survey of neonatal nurseries. *Infant Behavior Development, 29*, 24–31.

Foreman, S. W., Thomas, K. A., & Blackburn, S. T. (2008). Individual and gender differences matter in preterm infant state development. *Journal of Obstetrical Gynecological and Neonatal Nursing, 37*, 657–665.

Fujita, M., Endoh, Y., Saimon, N., & Yamaguchi, S. (2006). Effect of massaging babies on mothers: Pilot study on the changes in mood states and salivary cortisol level. *Complementary Therapies in Clinical Practice, 12*, 181–185.

Glover, V., Onozawa, K., & Hodgkinson, A. (2002). Benefits of infant massage for mothers with postnatal depression. *Seminars in Neonatology, 7*, 495–500.

Griffith, T., Rankin, K., & White-Traut, R. (2017). The relationship between behavioral states and oral feeding efficiency in preterm infants. *Advances in Neonatal Care, 17*(1), E12–E19. https://doi.org/10.1097/ANC.0000000000000318

Guzzetta, A., Baldini, S., Bancale, A., Baroncelli, L, Ciucci, F, Ghirri, P., Putignano, E., Sale, A., Viegi, A., Berardi, N., Boldrini, A., Cioni, G., & Maffei, L. (2009). Massage accelerates brain development and the maturation of visual function. *Journal of Neuroscience, 29*(18), 6042–6051.

Halpern, L. F., MacLean, W. E., & Baumeister, A. A. (1995). Infant sleep-wake characteristics: Relation to neurological status and the prediction of developmental outcome. *Developmental Review, 15*, 255–291.

Harrison, L. (2004). Tactile stimulation of neonatal intensive care unit preterm infants. In Field, T. (Ed.), *Touch and massage in early child development* (pp. 139–162). Johnson & Johnson Pediatric Institutive L.L.C.

Harrison, L., Olivet, L., Cunningham, K., Bodin, M., & Hicks, C. (1996). Effects of gentle human touch on preterm infants: Pilot study results. *Neonatal Network, 15*(2), 35–42.

Harrison, L. L., Williams, A. K., Leeper, J., Stein, J. T., & Wang, L. (2000). Factors associated with vagal tone responses in preterm infants. *Western Journal of Nursing Research, 22*(7), 776–792.

Hernandez-Reif, M., Diego, M., & Field, T. (2007). Preterm infants show reduced stress behaviors and activity after 5 days of massage therapy. *Infant Behavior Development, 30*, 557–561.

Holditch-Davis, D., White-Traut, R., Levy, J., Williams, K. L., Ryan, D., & Vonderheid, S. (2013). Maternal satisfaction with administering infant interventions in the neonatal intensive care unit. *Journal of Obstetric, Gynecologic, and Neonatal Nursing, 42*(6), 641–654.

Jahromi, L. B., Putnam, S. P., & Stifter, C. A. (2004). Maternal regulation of infant reactivity from 2 to 6 months. *Developmental Psychology, 40*, 477–487.

Janci, L. B. R. (2008). Effect of oil massage on changes in weight and neurobehavioural response of low birth weight babies. *Nursing Journal of India, 99*, 256–258.

Jay, S. S. (1982). The effects of gentle human touch on mechanically ventilated very short gestation infants. *Maternal-Child Nursing Journal, 11*, 199–256.

Jean, A. D. L., Stack, D. M., & Fogel, A. (2009). A longitudinal investigation of maternal touching across the first 6 months of life: Age and context effects. *Infant Behavior and Development, 32*, 344–349.

Kelmanson, I. A., & Adulas, E. I. (2006). Massage therapy and sleep behaviour in infants born with low birth weight. *Complementary Therapies in Clinical Practice, 12*, 200–205.

Khashu, M., Narayanan, M., Bhargava, S., & Osiovich, H. (2009). Perinatal outcomes associated with preterm birth at 33 to 36 weeks' gestation: A population-based cohort study. *Pediatrics, 123*, 109–113.

Kim, J. (2005). Effects of a massage program on growth of premature infants and on confidence and satisfaction in the mothering role. *Korean Journal of Child Health Nursing, 11*, 381–389.

Kim, T. I., Shin, Y. H., & White-Traut, R. C. (2003). Multisensory intervention improves physical growth and illness rates in Korean orphaned newborn infants. *Research in Nursing & Health, 26*, 424–433.

Lahat, S., Mimouni, F., Ashbel, G., & Dollberg, S. (2007). Energy expenditure in growing preterm infants receiving massage therapy. *Journal of the American College of Nutrition, 26*, 356–359.

Lai, M. M., D'Acunto, G., Guzzetta, A., Boyd, R. N., Rose, S. E., Fripp, J., Finnigan, S., Ngenda, N., Love, P., Whittingham, K., Pannek, K., Ware, R. S., & Colditz, P. B. (2016). PREMM: Preterm early massage by the mother. Protocol of a randomised controlled trial of massage therapy in very preterm infants. *BMC Pediatrics, 16*, 146. https://doi.org/10.1186/s12887-016-0678-7

Latini, G., DeFelice, C., Presta, E., Rosati, E., & Vacca, P. (2003). Minimal handling and bronchopulmonary dysplasia in extremely low-birth-weight infants. *European Journal of Pediatrics, 2*(4), 227–229.

Lee, H. K. (2006). The effects of infant massage on weight, height, and mother-infant interaction. *Journal of Korean Academy of Nursing, 36*, 1331–1339.

Litmanovitz, I., Dolfin, T., Arnon, S., Regev, R., Nemet, D., & Eliakim, A. (2007). Assisted exercise and bone strength in preterm infants. *Calcified Tissue International, 80*, 39–43.

Mainous, R. O. (2002). Infant massage as a component of developmental care: Past, present, and future. *Holistic Nursing Practice, 16*, 1–7.

Massaro, A. N., Hammad, T. A., Jazzo, B., & Aly, H. (2009). Massage with kinesthetic stimulation improves weight gain in preterm infants. *Journal of Perinatology, 29*, 352–357.

Mathai, S., Fernandez, A., Mondkar, J., & Kanbur, W. (2001). Effects of tactile-kinesthetic stimulation in preterms: A controlled trial. *Indian Pediatrics, 38*, 1091–1098.

McGrath, J. M., Thillet, M., & Van Cleave, L. (2007). Parent delivered infant massage: Are we truly ready for implementation? *Newborn and Infant Nursing Reviews, 7*, 39–46.

Medoff-Cooper, B., Rankin, K., Li, Z., Liu, L., & White-Traut, R. (2015). Multi-sensory intervention for preterm infants improves sucking organization. *Advances in Neonatal Care, 15*(2), 142–149.

Mendes, E. W., & Procianoy, R. S. (2008). Massage therapy reduces hospital stay and occurrence of late-onset sepsis in very preterm neonates. *Journal of Perinatology, 28*, 815–820.

Modcrin-McCarthy, M., Harris, M., & Marlar, C. (1997). Touch and the fragile infant: Comparison of touch techniques with implications for nursing practice. *Mother Baby Journal, 2*(4), 12–19.

Modcrin-Talbott, M., Harrison, L., Groer, M., & Younger, M. (2003). The biobehavioral effects of gentle human touch on preterm infants. *Nursing Science Quarterly, 16*(1), 60–67.

Moyer-Mileur, L. J., Ball, S. D., Brunstetter, V. L., & Chan, G. M. (2008). Maternal-administered physical activity enhances bone mineral acquisition in premature very low birth weight infants. *Journal of Perinatology, 28*, 432–437.

Nelson, M. N., White-Traut, R. C., Vasan, U., Silvestri, J., Comiskey, E., Meleedy-Rey, P., Littau, S., Gu, G., & Patel, M. (2001). One-year outcome of auditory-tactile-visual-vestibular intervention in the neonatal intensive care unit: Effects of severe prematurity and central nervous system injury. *Journal of Child Neurology, 16*, 493–498.

O'Higgins, M., Roberts, S. J., & Glover, V. (2008). Postnatal depression and mother and infant outcomes after infant massage. *Journal of Affective Disorders, 109*, 189–192.

Onozawa, K., Glover, V., Adams, D., Modi, N., & Kumar, R. C. (2001). Infant massage improves mother-infant interaction for mothers with postnatal depression. *Journal of Affective Disorders, 63*, 201–207.

Pineda, B. (2020). The neonatal eating outcome (NEO) assessment: A new developmental feeding assessment for preterm infants in the NICU. *The American Journal of Occupational Therapy, 73*, 7311500065. https://doi.org/10.5014/ajot.2019.73S1-RP304C

Ringborg, A., Berg, J., Norman, M., Westgren, M., & Jonsson, B. (2006). Preterm birth in Sweden: What are the average lengths of hospital stay and the associated inpatient costs? *Acta Paediatics, 95*, 1550–1555.

Scafidi, F. A., Field, T. M., Schanberg, S. M., Bauer, C. R., Tucci, K., Roberts, J., Morrow, C., & Kuhn, C. M. (1990). Massage stimulates growth in preterm infants: A replication. *Infant Behavior & Development, 13*, 167–188.

Schulze, K. J., Christian, P., Ruczinski, I., Ray, A. L., Nath, A., Wu, L. S. F., & Semba, R. D. (2008). Hepcidin and iron status among pregnant women in Bangladesh [Article]. *Asia Pacific Journal of Clinical Nutrition, 17*(3), 451–455. http://search.ebscohost.com/login.aspx?direct=true&db=aph&AN=35157418&site=ehost-live

Schulzke, S., Kaempfen, S., Trachsel, D., & Patole, S. (2014). Physical activity programs for promotion bone mineralization and growth in preterm infants. *Cochrane Database Systematic Review*, (4), CD005387. https://doi.org/10.1002/14651858.CD005387.pub3

Slevin, M., Farrington, N., Duffy, G., Daly, L., & Murphy, J. F. (2000). Altering the NICU and measuring infants' responses. *Acta Paediatrics, 89*(5), 577–581.

Soll, R. F. (2008). Heat loss prevention in neonates. *Journal of Perinatology, 28*(Suppl. 1), S57–S59.

Stack, D. (2001). The saliency of touch and physical contact during infancy: Unraveling some of the mysteries of the somesthetic sense. In Bremner, G., & Fogel, G. (Eds.), *Blackwell handbook of infant development* (pp. 351–378). Blackwell Publishers.

Underdown, A., Barlow, J., Chung, V., & Stewart-Brown, S. (2006). Massage intervention for promoting mental and physical health in infants aged under six months. *Cochrane Database of Systematic Reviews*, (4), CD005038.

Vaivre-Douret, L., Oriot, D., Blossier, P., Py, A., Kasolter-Pere, M., & Zwang, J. (2009). The effect of multimodal stimulation and cutaneous application of vegetable oils on neonatal development in preterm infants: A randomized controlled trial. *Child Care Health and Development, 35*(1), 96–105.

VandenBerg, K. A. (2007a) Individualized developmental care for high risk newborns in the NICU: A practice guideline. *Early Human Development, 83*(7), 433–442.

VandenBerg, K. A. (2007b). State systems development in high-risk newborns in the neonatal intensive care unit: Identification and management of sleep, alertness, and crying. *Journal of Perinatal and Neonatal Nursing, 21*, 130–139.

Vanderveen, J. A., Bassler, D., Robertson, C. M., & Kirpalani, H. (2009). Early interventions involving parents to improve neurodevelopmental outcomes of premature infants: A meta-analysis. *Journal of Perinatology, 29*, 343–351.

Vickers, A., Ohlsson, A., Lacy, J. B., & Horsley, A. (2004). Massage for promoting growth and development of preterm and/or low birth-weight infants. *Cochrane Database Systematic Reviews, 2004*(2), CD000390. https://doi.org/10.1002/14651858.CD000390.pub2

Vickers, A., Ohlsson, A., Lacy, J. B., & Horsley, A. (2007). Massage for promoting growth and development of preterm and/or low birth-weight infants. *Cochrane Database of Systematic Reviews*, (4), CD000390. https://doi.org/10.1002/14651858.CD000390.pub2

Vignochi, C. M., Miura, E., & Canani, L. H. (2008). Effects of motor physical therapy on bone mineralization in premature infants: A randomized controlled study. *Journal of Perinatology, 28*(9):624–631. https://doi.org/10.1038/jp.2008.60

Vonderheid, S. C., Park, C., Rankin, K., Norr, K. F., & White-Traut, R. (2020). Impact of an integrated mother-preterm infant intervention on birth hospitalization charges. *Journal of Perinatology, 40*(60), 1–9.

Vonderheid, S. C., Rankin, K., Norr, K., Vasa, R., Hill, S., & White-Traut, R. (2016). Health care use outcomes of an integrated hospital-to-home mother-preterm infant intervention. *Journal of Obstetric, Gynecologic, and Neonatal Nursing, 45*(5), 625–638.

Weller, A., & Feldman, R. (2003). Emotion regulation and touch in infants: The role of cholecystokinin and opioids. *Peptides, 24*, 779–788.

White-Traut, R. C., & Goldman, M. B. (1988). Premature infant massage: Is it safe? *Pediatric Nursing, 14*, 285–289.

White-Traut, R. C., & Nelson, M. N. (1988). Maternally administered tactile, auditory, visual, and vestibular stimulation: Relationship to later interactions between mothers and premature infants. *Research in Nursing & Health, 11*, 31–39.

White-Traut, R. C., & Pate, C. M. H. (1987). Modulating infant state in premature infants. *Journal of Pediatric Nursing, 2*, 96–101.

White-Traut, R. C., & Tubeszewski, K. A. (1986). Multimodal stimulation of the premature infant. *Journal of Pediatric Nursing, 1*, 90–95.

White-Traut, R. C., Nelson, M. N., Silvestri, J. M., Patel, M. K., & Kilgallon, D. (1993). Patterns of physiologic and behavioral response of intermediate care preterm infants to intervention. *Pediatric Nursing, 19*, 625–629.

White-Traut, R. C., Nelson, M. N., Silvestri, J. M., Cunningham, N., & Patel, M. (1997). Responses of preterm infants to unimodal and multimodal sensory intervention. *Pediatric Nursing, 23*, 169–175.

White-Traut, R., Powlesland, J., Gelhar, D., Chatterton, R., & Morris, M. (1998). Methodologic issues in the measurement of oxytocin in human neonates. *Journal of Nursing Measurement, 6*, 155–174.

White-Traut, R. C., Nelson, M. N., Silvestri, J. M., Patel, M., Vasan, U., Han, B. K., Cunningham, N., Burns, K., Kopischke, K., & Bradford, L. (1999). Developmental intervention for preterm infants diagnosed with periventricular leukomalacia. *Research in Nursing & Health, 22*, 131–143.

White-Traut, R., Studer, T., Meleedy-Rey, P., Murray, P., Labovsky, S., & Kahn, J. (2002a). Pulse rate and behavioral state correlates after auditory, tactile, visual, and vestibular intervention in drug-exposed neonates. *Journal of Perinatology, 22*, 291–299.

White-Traut, R. C., Nelson, M. N., Silvestri, J. M., Vasan, U., Littau, S., Meleedy-Rey, P., Gu, G., & Patel, M. (2002b). Effect of auditory, tactile, visual, and vestibular intervention on length of stay, alertness, and feeding progression in preterm infants. *Developmental Medicine and Child Neurology, 44*, 91–97.

White-Traut, R. C., Nelson, M. N., Silvestri, J. M., Vasan, U., Patel, M., & Cardenas, L. (2002c). Feeding readiness behaviors and feeding efficiency in response to ATVV intervention. *Newborn and Infant Nursing Reviews, 2*, 166–173.

White-Traut, R. C., Nelson, M. N., Silvestri, J. M., Patel, M., Berbaum, M., Gu, G. G., & Rey, P. M. (2004). Developmental patterns of physiological response to a multisensory intervention in extremely premature and high-risk infants. *Journal of Obstetrical Gynecological and Neonatal Nursing, 33*, 266–275.

White-Traut, R. C., Berbaum, M. L., Lessen, B., McFarlin, B., & Cardenas, L. (2005). Feeding readiness in preterm infants: The relationship between preterm behavioral state and feeding readiness behaviors and efficiency during transition from gavage to oral feeding. *Maternal-Child Nursing Journal, 30*, 52–59.

White-Traut, R. C., Schwertz, D., McFarlin, B., & Kogan, J. (2009). Salivary cortisol and behavioral state responses of healthy newborn infants to tactile-only and multisensory interventions. *Journal of Obstetrical, Gynecological and Neonatal Nursing, 38*, 22–34.

White-Traut, R. C., Wink, T., Minehart, T., & Holditch-Davis, D. (2012). Frequency of premature infant engagement and disengagement behaviors during two maternally administered interventions. *Newborn and Infant Nursing Reviews, 12*(3), 124–131. https://doi.org/10.1053/j.nainr.2012.06.005

White-Traut, R., Norr, K. F., Fabiyi, C., Rankin, K. M., Li, Z., & Liu, L. (2013). Mother-infant interaction improves with a developmental intervention for mother-preterm infant dyads. *Infant Behavior & Development, 36*(4), 694–706. https://doi.org/10.1016/j.infbeh.2013.07.004

White-Traut, R., Rankin, K. M., Pham, T., Li, Z., & Liu, L. (2014a). Preterm infants' orally directed behaviors and behavioral state responses to integrated H-Hope intervention. *Infant Behavior & Development, 37*(40), 583–596.

White-Traut, R., Rankin, K. M., Pham, T., Li, Z., & Liu, L. (2014b). Premature infants' orally directed behavioral cues and behavioral state responses to a pre-feeding multisensory intervention. *Infant Behavior & Development, 37*, 583–596.

White-Traut, R., Rankin, K. M., Yoder, J. C., Liu, L., Vasa, R., Gerald, V., & Norr, K. F. (2015). Influence of H-HOPE intervention for premature infants on growth, feeding progression and length of stay during initial hospitalization. *Journal of Perinatology, 35*(8), 636–651.

White-Traut, R., Liu, L., Norr, K., Rankin, K., Campbell, S. K., Griffith, T., Vasa, R., Geraldo, V., & Medoff-Cooper, B. (2017). Do orally-directed behaviors mediate the relationship between behavioral state and nutritive sucking in preterm infants? *Early Human Development, 109*, 26–31. https://doi.org/10.1016/j.earlhumdev.2017.04.007

White-Traut, R. C., Rankin, K. M., Yoder, J., Zawacki, L., Campbell, S., Censullo, M., Kavanaugh, K., Brandon, D., & Norr, K. F. (2018). Relationship between mother-infant mutual dyadic responsiveness and premature infant development as measured by the Bayley III at 6 weeks corrected age. *Early Human Development, 121*, 21–26. https://doi.org/10.1016/j.earlhumdev.2018.04.018. PMID: 29730131.

White-Traut, R., Brandon, D., Kavanaugh, K., Gralton, K., Pan, W., Myers, E. R., Andrews, B., Msall, M., & Norr, K. F. (2021). Protocol for implementation of an evidence based parentally administered intervention for preterm infants. *BMC Pediatrics, 142*(2021). https://doi.org/10.1186/s12887-021-02596-1

White-Traut, R. (2004). Providing a nurturing environment for infants in adverse situations: Multisensory strategies for newborn care. *Journal of Midwifery & Women's Health, 49*, 36–41.

White-Traut, R. (2015). Nurse management of the NICU environment is critical to optimal infant development. *Journal of Obstetric, Gynecologic, and Neonatal Nursing, 44*(2), 169–170.

Yoo, K. (2005). The effects of massage on stress hormone in premature infants. *Korean Journal of Child Health Nursing, 11*, 25–31.

Zeiner, V., Storm, H., & Koheny, K. K. (2016). Preterm infants' behaviors and skin conductance responses to nurse handling in the NICU. *Journal of Maternal, Fetal, & Neonatal Medicine, 29*(15), 2531–2536.

CHAPTER 18

Pain Assessment and Nonpharmacologic Management

Robin Clifton-Koeppel

Standards in Pain Assessment and Management

Standard 1: Infant

- The interprofessional team shall develop care practices that prioritizes multiple methods to optimize baby outcomes by minimizing the impact of stressful and painful stimuli.
- A flexible and individualized approach is taken toward all hands-on caregiving interactions, with continual responsiveness to each infant's competencies, vulnerabilities, and thresholds.
- Recognizes and assesses pain during all procedures, assessments, and caregiving tasks.
- Provides appropriate pain management when noxious procedures are necessary.

INTRODUCTION

Standards of Practice

Standards of practice for pain assessment and management are based on scientific literature and clinical recommendations from professional and accrediting organizations such as the National Association of Neonatal Nurses (Walden & Gibbins, 2012), the Joint Commission (2017), and the American Academy of Pediatrics/Canadian Pediatric Society (AAP/CPS, 2006; AAP, 2016). There is considerable consistency in the recommendations set by these professional and accrediting organizations (a summary of these organizations' guidelines and standards is provided in Table 18-1). The various guidelines have provided momentum for institutions to reexamine their pain management philosophies and practices. Clinical challenges remain regarding ways in which to implement these standards in institutional settings based on patient types, clinical procedures performed, and current staffing patterns. This chapter will discuss pain assessment and management from a nonpharmacologic perspective.

PHYSIOLOGY OF PAIN

The theory of nociception divides the pain system into three components: peripheral nervous system, spinal cord, and supraspinal/integrative level. This brief explanation of pain physiology introduces the basics of pain.

Peripheral Nervous System (Evans, 2001)

The peripheral nervous system is responsible for registering initial noxious stimuli; initiating local pain reactions through the release of biochemical mediators such as substance P and prostaglandins, which results in hyperalgesia (increased sensitivity to painful stimuli), allodynia (pain caused by a stimulus that ordinarily does not cause pain), or dendritic sprouting and hyperinnervation (which results in hypersensitivity and a lower pain threshold that may persist into adulthood); and conducting nociceptive input to the spinal cord and central nervous system. Transmission of nociceptive impulses occurs along two types of afferent sensory fibers. A-delta fibers are thinly myelinated, rapid-conducting fibers associated with acute pain or "first pain" (e.g., sharp, localized, pricking). C fibers are polymodal, unmyelinated, slow-conducting fibers associated with aching, burning, throbbing, poorly localized, chronic, or "second pain." It is notable that nociceptive impulses are carried through unmyelinated and thinly myelinated fibers even in adult peripheral nerves, as well.

Spinal Cord (Evans, 2001)

The dorsal horns of the spinal cord integrate pain and other sensory stimuli and modulate pain perception. Afferent fiber neurotransmitters stimulate *N*-methyl-d-aspartate and tachykinin receptors in the dorsal horns, producing central sensitization (increased excitability of dorsal horn neurons

TABLE 18-1 Summary of Pain Recommendations From Professional and Accrediting Organizations

Type	Recommendation	Level of Evidence	References
Assessment/ Treatment	Education and competency in pain assessment and management should be conducted during orientation and at regularly defined intervals throughout employment for all nurses who deliver care to neonates and young infants.	VII	AAP/CPS (2006); AAP (2016); Joint Commission (2017); Walden & Gibbins (2012)
Assessment	Pain is assessed and reassessed at regular intervals throughout an infant's hospitalization. A valid and reliable multidimensional pain assessment instrument should be used.	VII	AAP/CPS (2006), AAP (2016); Joint Commission (2017); Walden & Gibbins (2008)
Prevention/ Treatment	Use both nonpharmacologic and pharmacologic therapies to control and/or prevent pain.	VII	AAP/CPS (2006); AAP (2016); Joint Commission (2017); Walden & Gibbins (2012)
	A collaborative, interdisciplinary approach to pain control should be used, including soliciting input from the entire healthcare team and the infant's family, when appropriate.	VII	
Assessment/ Treatment	Pain assessment and management practices should be documented in a manner that facilitates regular reassessment and follow-up intervention.	VII	Joint Commission (2017)
Policy	Institutions should establish policies and procedures that support and promote optimal pain assessment and management practices.	VII	AAP/CPS (2006); AAP (2016); Joint Commission (2017)
Evaluation	Institutions should collect data to monitor the appropriateness and effectiveness of pain-management practices.	VII	Joint Commission (2017)

Note: Level I = evidence from a systematic review or meta-analysis of all relevant randomized controlled trials (RCTs) or evidence-based clinical practice guidelines based on systematic reviews of RCTs; Level II = evidence obtained from at least one well-designed RCT; Level III = evidence obtained from well-designed controlled trials without randomization; Level IV = evidence from well-designed case-control and cohort studies; Level V = evidence from systematic reviews of descriptive and qualitative studies; Level VI = evidence from a single descriptive or qualitative study; Level VII = evidence from the opinion of authorities and/or reports of expert committees.
Modified from Carrier, C. T., & Walden, M. (2001). Integrating research and standards to improve pain management practices for newborns and infants. *Newborn and Infant Nursing Reviews, 1*(2), 122–131.

that spreads to several adjacent segments of the spinal cord), "wind-up" (perceived increase in intensity or duration of painful stimuli), or secondary hyperalgesia (hypersensitivity elicited by both painful and nonpainful stimuli that extends to areas beyond the site of injury).

A characteristic pattern of pain behavior such as increases in heart and respiratory rate and facial responses such as brow bulge, eye squeeze, and nasolabial furrow occurs when the capacities of neural mechanisms are exceeded by nerve impulses arriving in the dorsal horns (Melzack & Wall, 1965). Local spinal cord response to pain impulses from peripheral afferent fibers also stimulates efferent somatomotor neurons in the anterior horn and produces reflex withdrawal.

Modulation of nociceptive transmission occurs through the release of met-enkephalin from local interneurons as well as dopamine, norepinephrine, and serotonin from descending inhibitory axons. Preterm infants, however, have limited ability to modulate pain. Dopamine and norepinephrine are not available to modulate pain before 36 to 40 weeks' gestation, and serotonin is not released until approximately 6 to 8 weeks after birth.

Supraspinal/integrative level (Evans, 2001) Supraspinal centers (thalamus, cerebral cortex) integrate and process pain information, elaborately modifying the cascade of neurochemical events triggered by nociception. Supraspinal centers also are involved in memory and learning from nociceptive experiences and produce systemic responses to pain including cardiovascular, respiratory, hormonal, metabolic, and immune adaptations and alterations.

This basic understanding of pain has been expanded to recognize that pain also has a response component. This component actually changes the nervous system and the way in which it responds to pain (Anand, 2000; Anand et al., 2007; Bartocci et al., 2006). The physiologic response and its significance will be discussed in the next sections.

SIGNIFICANCE OF PAIN RESPONSE IN NEONATES

Repetitive, unrelieved pain can lead to serious and adverse consequences for neonates. Short-term consequences of painful procedures include decreased oxygen saturations and increased heart rates and blood pressure that can place increased demands on the cardiorespiratory system. In addition, pain can cause elevation in intracranial pressure, increasing risk for intraventricular hemorrhage in preterm neonates.

The long-term effects of pain in animals are clear, with changes observed in pain thresholds, social behaviors, stress responses, and pain responses to nonpainful stimuli (Goldschneider & Anand, 2003). Preliminary human data suggest that early pain experiences may alter future pain responses. Johnston and Stevens (1996) reported that neonates who were born at 28 weeks' gestation and were hospitalized in a neonatal intensive care unit (NICU) for 4 weeks (32 weeks postmenstrual age [PMA]) had decreased behavioral response and significantly higher heart rate and lower oxygen saturation during a heel-stick procedure compared with newly born neonates at 32 weeks' gestation. In another study, Taddio et al. (1995) reported that males circumcised within 2 days of birth had significantly longer crying bouts and higher pain intensity scores at immunization at 4 or 6 months of age than males who were not circumcised.

For preterm infants, cumulative effects of stress and pain cannot be underestimated. Cong et al. (2017) demonstrated that infants with more painful/stressful procedures demonstrated more stress signs and adverse neurobehavioral outcomes. Alternatively, increased daily skin-to-skin contact and direct breastfeeding assisted to reduce stress/pain response and was associated with better neurodevelopmental outcome (Cong et al., 2017). More studies are needed evaluating the relationship of early stress/pain and neurodevelopmental outcomes in preterm infants.

DEFINITION OF PAIN

Pain is a multidimensional phenomenon that is dependent on a person's sensory and emotional perception of its existence (Melzack & Wall, 1965). The International Association for the Study of Pain (IASP), with member specialists in anesthesia, dentistry, neurology, neurosurgery, neurophysiology, psychiatry, and psychology, previously defined pain as an "unpleasant sensory and emotional experience associated with actual or potential tissue damage or described in terms of such damage" (IASP, 1979, p. 250). The IASP recently published an updated pain definition to include six additional qualifiers or "notes" that further detail the pain definition. One of the six qualifiers include, "Verbal description is only one of several behaviors to express pain; inability to communicate does not negate the possibility that a human or a nonhuman animal experiences pain" (Raja et al., 2020, p. 1997). This is an important addition to the IASP pain definition clarifying that lack of verbalization of pain does not mean lack of pain.

In neonates, responses to painful stimuli include immediate physiological, behavioral, and hormonal indicators that provide objective and quantifiable information about the location, intensity, and duration of painful stimuli. Although these responses are not specific to pain, they can be used in conjunction with other contextual indicators to infer the existence of pain. Furthermore, because pain is a multidimensional phenomenon, a composite measure that incorporates both physiologic and behavioral indicators should be used for its assessment.

PAIN ASSESSMENT

Pain research on neonates has produced several instruments with acceptable measurement properties. However, most tools assess acute pain in response to procedures or to postoperative pain; tools assessing prolonged or chronic pain have not been developed or not completely validated. Prolonged pain may be common for infants in the NICU (Anand, 2007). The four most commonly published multidimensional instruments include the CRIES (Crying, Requires oxygen saturation, Increased vital signs, Expression, Sleepless) Neonatal Postoperative Pain Measurement Score (Krechel & Bildner, 1995); the Premature Infant Pain Profile and its revision, PIPP-R (PIPP; Stevens et al., 1996; PIPP-R; Stevens et al., 2014); the Neonatal Pain, Agitation, and Sedation Scale (N-PASS; Hummel et al., 2008; Hummel et al., 2010); and the Neonatal Infant Pain Scale (NIPS; Lawrence et al., 1993).

The CRIES (Table 18-2) is a pain measure originally validated to assess postoperative pain in infants 32 to 60 weeks gestational age. Recent studies have documented its clinical

TABLE 18-2 CRIES: Neonatal Postoperative Pain Assessment Score

Indicator	0	1	2
Crying	No	High-pitched	Inconsolable
Requires oxygen for saturation >95%	No	<30%	>30%
Increased vital signs	Heart rate and blood pressure within 10% of preoperative value	Heart rate and blood pressure 11%–20% higher than preoperative value	Heart rate and blood pressure at least 21% higher than preoperative value
Expression	None	Grimace	Grimace/grunt
Sleepless	No	Wakes at frequent intervals	Constantly awake

From Krechel, S. W., & Bildner, J. (1995). CRIES: A new neonatal post-operative pain measurement score. Initial testing of validity and reliability. *Pediatric Anesthesia, 5*(1), 53–61.

utility in assessing procedural pain in preterm and term neo-nates (Ahn, 2006; Belda et al., 2004; Herrington et al., 2004). The CRIES is an acronym for the five parameters it measures: *C*rying, *R*equires oxygen to maintain saturation greater than 95%, *I*ncreased vital signs, *E*xpression, and *S*leepless. Total scores for the CRIES range from 0 to 10, with scores lower than 4 indicating mild pain requiring nonpharmacologic pain relief measures and scores higher than or equal to 5 consistent with moderate to severe pain requiring pharma-cologic intervention in conjunction with comfort measures.

The PIPP (Table 18-3) has been used routinely with infants between 28 and 40 weeks' gestational age and is the most stud-ied pain assessment tool for infants. Although the PIPP origi-nally was developed to measure procedural pain (Stevens et al., 1996), it recently has been used in term and preterm infants to assess postoperative pain (El Sayed et al., 2007; McNair et al., 2004). A critical evaluation of the PIPP over 13 years since its inception (1996 to 2009) demonstrated a high degree of reliabil-ity and validity across multiple studies (Stevens et al., 2010). The PIPP includes a recommended scoring adjustment for use with neonates of varying gestational ages and behavioral states, two contextual factors that are known to modify pain expression in preterm neonates. The PIPP contains two physiologic indica-tors (heart rate and oxygen saturation) and three facial indica-tors (brow bulge, eye squeeze, and nasolabial furrow). Although total scores vary between 18 and 21 depending on an infant's gestational age, scores between 7 and 12 usually signify mild to moderate pain requiring nonpharmacologic comfort measures and scores higher than 12 indicate moderate to severe pain requiring pharmacologic intervention in addition to comfort measures (Stevens et al. 2014).

Recently, the PIPP has been revised (PIPP-R) to simplify scoring and improve usability with initial construct validity and feasibility demonstrated (Gibbons et al., 2014; Stevens et al., 2014).

Similar to the PIPP, the N-PASS (Table 18-4) also includes a recommended scoring adjustment for use with neonates of varying gestational ages. Total pain scores vary depending on the infant's gestational age but scores higher than 3 usually sig-nify pain requiring nonpharmacologic comfort measures and/or pharmacologic pain intervention. The N-PASS is clinically useful, easily applied at the bedside across a large gestational age

TABLE 18-3 PIPP: The Premature Infant Pain Profile: Revised

Infant Indicator	Indicator Score				Infant Indicator Score
	0	+1	+2	+3	
Change in heart rate (bpm) Baseline:_____	0–4	5–14	15–24	>24	
Decrease in oxygen saturation (%) Baseline: _____	0–2	3–5	6–8	>8 or increase in O$_2$	
Brow bulge (Seconds)	None (<3)	Minimal (3–10)	Moderate (11–20)	Maximal (>20)	
Eye squeeze (Seconds)	None (<3)	Minimal (3–10)	Moderate (11–20)	Maximal (>20)	
Naso-Labial furrow (Seconds)	None (<3)	Minimal (3–10)	Moderate (11–20)	Maximal (>20)	
				* Sub-total Score:	
Gestational age (Weeks + Days)	>36 weeks	32 –35 weeks, 6 days	28 –31 weeks, 6 days	<28 weeks	
Baseline behavioral state	Active and awake	Quiet and awake	Active and asleep	Quiet and asleep	
				** Total Score:	

Scoring instructions

Step 1: Observe infant for **15 seconds at rest** and assess vital sign indicators [highest heart rate (HR) and lowest O$_2$ Saturation (O$_2$SAT)] and behavioural state.

Step 2: Observe infant for **30 seconds after procedure** and assess **change** in vital sign indicators [maximal HR, lowest O$_2$ SAT and duration of facial actions observed].
* If infant requires an increase in oxygen at any point before or during procedure, they receive a score of 3 for the O$_2$ SAT indicator

Step 3: Score for corrected gestational age (GA) and behavioural state (BS) if the sub-total score >0.

Step 4: Calculate total score by adding **Sub-total Score + BS Score.**

Premature Infant Pain Profile-Revised (PIPP-R). *Subtotal for physiological and facial indicators. If subtotal score >0, add GA and BS indicator scores. **Total score: subtotal score+ GA score+ BS score. BS indicates behavioral state; GA, gestational age.
Used with permission from Stevens, B., Gibbins, S., Yamada, J., Dionne, K., Lee, G., Johnston, C., & Taddio, A. (2014). The premature infant pain profile-revised (PIPP-R): initial validation and feasibility. *The Clinical Journal of Pain, 30*(3), 238–243, Wolters Kluwer.

TABLE 18-4 N-PASS: Neonatal Pain Agitation and Sedation Scale

Assessment Criteria	Sedation		Normal	Pain/Agitation	
	−2	−1	0	1	2
Crying, irritability	No cry with painful stimuli	Moans or cries minimally with painful stimuli	Appropriate crying, not irritable	Irritable or crying at intervals, consolable	High-pitched or silent-continuous cry, inconsolable
Behavior state	No arousal to any stimuli, no spontaneous movement	Arouses minimally to stimuli, little spontaneous movement	Appropriate for gestational age	Restless, squirming, awakens frequently	Arching, kicking, constantly awake, or arouses minimally/no movement (not sedated)
Facial expression	Mouth is lax, no expression	Minimal expression with stimuli	Relaxed, appropriate	Any pain expression intermittent	Any pain expression continual
Extremities, tone	No grasp reflex, flaccid tone	Weak grasp reflex, muscle tone	Relaxed hands and feet, normal tone	Intermittent clenched toes, fists, or finger splay; body is not tense	Continual clenched toes, fists, or finger splay; body is tense
Vital signs (HR, RR, BP, SaO$_2$)	No variability with stimuli, hypoventilation, or apnea	<10% variability from baseline with stimuli	Within baseline or normal for gestational age	10%–20% from baseline; SaO$_2$ 76%–85% with stimulation–quick	>20% from baseline; SaO$_2$ < 75% with stimulation– slow, out of sync with vent

Points are added to the premature infant's pain score based on gestational age:

+3 if <28 weeks gestation/corrected age.

+2 if 28–31 weeks gestation/corrected age.

+1 if 32–35 weeks gestation/corrected age Sedation assessment requires an assessment of response to stimuli.

Notes: Pain and sedation scores are recorded separately. HR = heart rate, RR = respiratory rate, BP = blood pressure, SaO$_2$ = oxygen saturation.

From Hummel, P., Puchalski, M., Creech, S. D., & Weiss, M. G. (2008). Clinical reliability and validity of the N-PASS: Neonatal pain, agitation and sedation scale with prolonged pain. *Journal of Perinatology*, *28*(1), 55–60.

TABLE 18-5 NIPS: Neonatal Infant Pain Scale

	Before Time		During Time					After Time		
	1	2	1	2	3	4	5	1	2	3
Facial expression 0 = Relaxed 1 = Grimace										
Cry 0 = No cry 1 = Whimper 2 = Vigorous										
Breathing patterns 0 = Relaxed 1 = Change in breathing										
Arms 0 = Relaxed/restrained 1 = Flexed/extended										
Legs 0 = Relaxed/restrained 1 = Flexed/extended										
State of arousal 0 = Sleeping/awake 1 = Fussy										
Total										

Note: Time is measured in 1-minute intervals. Thus, this table demonstrates data collection for 2 minutes before a procedure, 5 minutes during and 3 minutes after.

From Lawrence, J., Alcock, D., McGrath, P., Kay, J., MacMurray, S., & Dulberg, C. (1993). The development of a tool to assess neonatal pain. *Neonatal Network*, *12*(6), 59–66.

group (Hillman et al., 2015). The N-PASS is unique in that the instrument also incorporates a separate scoring system to assess level of sedation, a useful adjunct for infants receiving opioid therapy. Following an assessment of response to stimuli, sedation is scored between 0 and −2 for each behavioral and physiological criteria, then summed and noted as a negative score (0 to −10). Scores of −10 to −5 are considered deep sedation, while light-sedation scores range from −5 to −2 (Hummel et al., 2008). However, validity and reliability of the sedation component of the N-PASS has not been demonstrated (Giordano et al., 2014).

The NIPS (Table 18-5) has been used with both preterm and term infants. Although originally developed to assess procedural pain, recent literature also validates its utility with postoperative pain (Rouss et al., 2007; Suraseranivongse et al., 2006). This instrument provides clinical utility in monitoring pain in healthy newborns, as the instrument does not require an infant to be attached to a cardiac monitor or pulse oximeter as assessment parameters. Total score ranges from 0 to 7. Although guidelines for pain interventions based on total score are not provided by NIPS researchers, all pain instruments in neonates are based on the premise of increasing pain intensity. In tools without scoring guidelines for pain management, when pain scores reach the mid-range of the total possible points for that tool (approximately 4 or higher with the NIPS), nurses may infer an infant is experiencing moderate to severe pain and that pharmacologic intervention for that pain is warranted.

CONTEXTUAL FACTORS MODIFYING NEONATAL PAIN RESPONSES

Developmental maturity, health status, and environmental factors all may contribute to an inconsistent, less robust pattern of pain responses between infants and within the same infant over time and situations. Consequently, contextual factors that have been demonstrated to modify the pain experience must be considered when assessing for the presence of pain in neonates. Behavioral state has been shown to moderate behavioral pain response in both full-term and preterm infants. Infants in awake or alert states demonstrate a more robust reaction to painful stimuli than infants in sleep states.

Research examining facial and body activity has demonstrated that the magnitude of infants' observable behavioral response to pain is less vigorous and less robust when the infant is of a less mature PMA. Craig et al. (1993) suggested the less vigorous behavioral responses demonstrated by younger preterm infants "should be interpreted in the context of the energy resources available to respond and the relative immaturity of the musculoskeletal system" (p. 296). In addition, many preterm infants do not cry in response to a noxious stimulus. The absence of response may only indicate the depletion of response capability and not a lack of pain perception (Walden & Franck, 2003). Furthermore, when a pain stimuli or pain persists for hours or days without intervention, an infant may exhibit a decompensatory response. The sympathetic nervous system or the fight-or-flight

TABLE 18-6 Pain Assessment Recommendations

Type	Recommendation	Level of Evidence	References
Assessment	Frequency of pain assessments for postoperative, procedural, and disease-related pain in hospitalized infants should be based on the expected intensity and duration of pain. Pain should be assessed upon admission and at regularly defined intervals throughout an infant's hospitalization. Pain assessment should occur before, during, and after painful procedures.	II VII VII, VII, VII VII, V	AAP (2016); Joint Commission (2017); Walden & Gibbins (2012) Walden & Franck (2003) AAP/CPS (2006); AAP (2016); Walden & Gibbins (2012)
	A high index of suspicion should be used when assessing infants for the presence, absence, or intensity of pain. Pain's presence should be presumed in all situations considered to cause pain in adults and children, even in the absence of behavioral or physiologic signs. Reliable and valid multidimensional instruments should be used to assess pain in infants.	VII, V V VII, IV	Grunau & Craig (1987); Duhn & Medves (2004) Duhn & Medves (2004) NANN (2012)
	In choosing an instrument to use in assessing pain in infants, caregivers should take into consideration all published psychometric data, including the aspects of validity, reliability, and clinical utility. Caregivers also should consider infant population, setting, and type of pain experienced when choosing a pain instrument. Contextual factors that have been demonstrated to modify the pain experience must be considered when assessing for the presence of pain in neonates.	V VII, IV	Duhn & Medves (2004) NANN (2012) Craig et al. (1993); Gibbins & Stevens (2003); Grunau et al. (2004); Johnston et al. (1993); Shapiro (1993)

Note: Level I = evidence from a systematic review or meta-analysis of all relevant randomized controlled trials (RCTs), or evidence-based clinical practice guidelines based on systematic reviews of RCTs; Level II = evidence obtained from at least one well-designed RCT; Level III = evidence obtained from well-designed controlled trials without randomization; Level IV = evidence from well-designed case-control and cohort studies; Level V = evidence from systematic reviews of descriptive and qualitative studies; Level VI = evidence from a single descriptive or qualitative study; Level VII = evidence from the opinion of authorities and/or reports of expert committees.

mechanism can no longer compensate. As a result, physiologic parameters return to baseline, but this does not indicate that the pain is no longer felt or tolerated; it only makes pain assessment more difficult (Hummel & van Dijk, 2006).

Finally, less mature behavioral responses to noxious stimuli are noted with an increased number of painful procedures to which an infant is exposed, increased postnatal age at time of observation, and shorter length of time since the last painful procedure (Ranger et al., 2007). Specific recommendations related to pain assessment can be found in Table 18-6.

NONPHARMACOLOGIC INTERVENTIONS FOR CLINICAL PROCEDURES CAUSING MINOR PAIN

Painful procedures in the NICU are unavoidable; therefore, it is vital that caregivers investigate strategies to help infants cope with and recover from necessary painful clinical procedures. Nonpharmacologic strategies have been shown to be important accompaniments to clinical procedures to help minimize neonatal pain and stress while maximizing the infant's regulatory and coping abilities.

This particularly is true for preterm infants who have less capacity for recovery after acute procedure-induced pain than do term, healthy infants (AAP/CPS, 2006; Sharek et al., 2006; Walden et al., 2001).

Although it is beyond the scope of this chapter to discuss the pharmacologic management of pain in neonates, it is important to be able to recognize when pharmacologic interventions are indicated for relief of pain in the NICU. Analgesics should be used when severe or prolonged pain is assessed or anticipated (Anand et al., 2006; Anand, 2007). Although sedatives may have an adjunctive role to opioids in managing pain, sedatives blunt behavioral responses to noxious stimuli without providing pain relief and should only be used when pain has been ruled out (Hartley et al., 1989). Franck and Miaskowski (1998) performed an excellent research critique on the use of opioids to provide analgesia in critically ill, premature neonates.

The evidence base for pain management is presented within a developmentally supportive care framework. Components of developmental care can be divided into those related to the total nursery environment (macroenvironment) and those related to an individual infant's environment or care experiences (microenvironment).

TABLE 18-7 Recommendations for the Macro- and Micro-Environments

Type	Recommendation	Level of Evidence	References
Prevention (Macro)	Reduce the number of procedures when possible.	VII	AAP [2016]; Sharek et al. [2006]
	Cluster care and procedures based on behavioral cues.	II, VII	Sizun et al. [2002]; AAP/CPS [2006]
	Recognize sleep states and minimize interruptions.	II, VII, II, VII	Sizun et al. [2002]; AAP/CPS [2006]
	Reduce environmental sources of stress by lowering light and sound levels in the NICU.	III	Sizun et al. [2002]; AAP/CPS [2006]
	Use automated incision devices when doing heel sticks.	I	McIntosh et al. [1994]
	Consider performing venipuncture vs. heel sticks to minimize pain from blood collection.		Shah and Ohlsson [2011]
Prevention (Micro)	Recognize infant's stress cues to determine timing of painful procedures and periods of recovery.	II	Sizun et al. [2002]
	Decrease physiologic/behavioral destabilization associated with procedural handling.	II	Sizun et al. [2002]
	Ensure that developmentally supportive techniques are used to position infants before painful clinical procedures.	II	Sizun et al. [2002]
	Limit unnecessary handling.	II	Sizun et al. [2002]
Treatment (Micro)	Provide containment strategies before, during, and after procedures until the infant returns to baseline as determined by behavioral and physiological cues.	II	Corff et al. [1995]; Gomes Neto et al. [2020]; Pillai Riddell et al. [2011]
	Promote skin-to-skin contact as a nonpharmacologic intervention during painful procedures.	II	Johnston et al. [2014]
	Support the use of nonnutritive sucking as a nonpharmacologic pain intervention.	II	AAP [2016]; Pillai Riddell et al. [2011]
	Use sucrose with or without an accompanying pacifier as a nonpharmacologic pain intervention.	I	Stevens et al. [2013]
	Use breastfeeding or supplemental breast milk to alleviate pain during single procedures.	I	Shah et al. [2012]
	Involve parents in the recognition and treatment of pain.	III	Franck et al. [2004]

Note: Level I = evidence from a systematic review or meta-analysis of all relevant randomized controlled trials (RCTs), or evidence-based clinical practice guidelines based on systematic reviews of RCTs; Level II = evidence obtained from at least one well-designed RCT; Level III = evidence obtained from well-designed controlled trials without randomization; Level IV = evidence from well-designed case-control and cohort studies; Level V = evidence from systematic reviews of descriptive and qualitative studies; Level VI = evidence from a single descriptive or qualitative study; Level VII = evidence from the opinion of authorities and/or reports of expert committees.

Macroenvironment

Components of the macroenvironment that address pain management include reducing the total noxious load to which the infant is exposed, streamlining procedural techniques, and restructuring the physical environment to reduce light and noise levels. Table 18-7 provides recommendations and evidence to support the infant's macro- and micro-environments.

Prevention is the first step to reducing an infant's exposure to noxious stimuli, so strategies to prevent pain should be employed whenever possible. Over the past decade, practice patterns reveal a reduction of the numbers of painful procedures in the NICU and increased use of pharmacologic and nonpharmacologic measures; however, pain is still undertreated in the NICU (Lago et al., 2013; Roofthooft et al., 2014). To reduce painful procedures, all diagnostic and therapeutic procedures should be examined daily in caregiver rounds to determine medical necessity (AAP, 2016; Sharek et al., 2006). Laboratory studies that will not be acted upon should be discontinued. Care procedures also should be examined, such as frequency of endotracheal suctioning (ETS). Routine orders for ETS should be avoided and instead be performed only when clinically indicated by physical examination findings or deteriorating blood-gas values. Other examples of caregiving strategies to prevent or limit the noxious load to which an infant might be exposed include grouping blood draws to minimize the number of venipunctures per day and limiting adhesive tape and gentle removal of tape to minimize epidermal stripping.

The pain experienced by hospitalized patients often is affected by the manner in which procedures are approached. A multipronged pain-prevention approach is recommended for NICU patient including reducing painful procedures, routine assessment of pain, using both pharmacologic and nonpharmacologic approach to prevent and reduce pain associated with minor bedside procedures, and medications to manage postoperative pain (AAP, 2016). Guidelines for treatment of pain have been published and are useful in guiding practice (Lago et al., 2009; Spence et al., 2010). The Vermont Oxford Network Collaborative (Anand et al., 2004; Neonatal Intensive Care Quality Improvement Collaborative, 2002) developed potentially better practices to reduce pain in NICU infants that encompass all aspects ranging from prevention to assessment and treatment (Sharek et al., 2006). Further, Anand (2008) detailed a stepwise approach to anticipate, prevent, and manage pain from commonly performed bedside procedures.

Facilitated tucking, skin-to-skin contact, and the use of sucrose pacifiers decrease the pain responses associated with the heel-stick procedure (Corff et al., 1995; Ramenghi et al., 1996; Skogsdal et al., 1997; Stevens et al., 1997). A meta-analysis on venipuncture vs. heel lance for blood sampling in term neonates reported that venipuncture, when performed by a trained phlebotomist, was associated with less pain and appears to be the method of choice for blood sampling in term neonates (Larsson et al., 1998; Shah & Ohlsson, 2011; Shah et al., 1997).

Little research has been conducted to systematically document the effects of sound and ambient light levels on pain responses in preterm infants. Preliminary and emerging research suggests that playing a recording of maternal voice, white noise, or lullabies during heel-lance procedure reduced the pain responses of infants (Azarmnejad et al., 2017; Chirico et al., 2017; Johnston et al., 2007; Kahraman et al., 2020; Krueger, 2010; Küçükoğˇlu et al., 2016; Kurdahi Badr et al., 2017; Sajjadian et al., 2017). A systemic review of music as a nonpharmacologic intervention to reduce pain found inconsistent results (Hartling et al., 2009). More research is needed in this area to validate these findings across gestational ages and with a variety of bedside procedures.

Microenvironment

Microenvironmental components include organization of caregiving, containment/positioning strategies, nonnutritive sucking (NNS) with or without sucrose, and integration of the infant's family. Table 18-7 provides recommendations and evidence to support the infant's macro- micro- environments.

Caregiving activities should be organized to provide periods of rest and recovery. Emerging evidence suggests that after exposure to a painful stimulus, preterm infants' pain sensitivity is accentuated by increased excitability of nociceptive neurons in the dorsal horn of the spinal cord. This sensory hypersensitivity, referred to as the wind-up phenomenon, has been documented in immature rat pups that were compared with adult rats (Fitzgerald et al., 1989; Fitzgerald et al., 1988). This finding suggests that for prolonged periods after a painful stimulus, other nonnoxious stimuli (handling, physical examination, nursing procedures, etc.) may cause heightened activity in nociceptive pathways, leading to systemic physiologic responses to stress in preterm infants. Consequently, it is reasonable to recommend that adequate rest periods be provided after painful clinical procedures. It also is reasonable to consider introducing the least noxious stimuli first in a caregiving cluster and the most noxious stimuli last so the stress of caregiving is not unnecessarily heightened for an infant.

Porter et al. (1991) demonstrated that preterm neonates observed before and during lumbar punctures showed as much heightened arousal from the time they were positioned at the start of the lumbar puncture as they did during the lumbar puncture itself. In a subsequent study, Porter et al. (1998) reported that healthy, preterm, and full-term newborns who experienced a series of handling and immobilization manipulations before a routine heel stick exhibited significantly more physiologic responses and behavioral arousal to the heel stick compared with infants who had not been handled. *Hand swaddling* is a broad term that describes the use of hands to encompass or position infants to provide a "nest." These positioning procedures facilitate the infant's self-regulatory development. Containment is thought to reduce pain by providing gentle stimulation across the proprioceptive, thermal, and tactile sensory systems (Mackenna & Callander, 1990). Studies have been conducted in the preterm population using two different methods of swaddling. A hand swaddling technique known as "facilitated tucking" (holding the infant's extremities flexed and contained close to the trunk), implemented before the heel-stick procedure, was shown to reduce pain responses in preterm neonates as young as 25 weeks' gestational age (Corff et al., 1995). In that study, preterm infants in the post–heel-stick recovery phase demonstrated significantly reduced heart rates and crying and more stability in sleep-wake cycles in the hand-swaddled position.

A similar containment study conducted by Fearon et al. (1997) used blanket swaddling for nesting. The researchers examined the effectiveness of blanket swaddling after a heel stick in younger (younger than 31 weeks PMA) and older (or older than 31 weeks PMA) preterm infants. Swaddling was effective in reducing heart rate and negative facial displays in the post–heel-stick phase for the older infants, and oxygen saturation levels were higher for younger infants in the swaddled condition.

A systematic review and meta-analysis of the use of facilitated tucking during painful procedures as a pain management technique analyzed 15 studies including over 600 preterm infants. Facilitated tucking was shown to reduce the pain expression during painful procedures (heel stick and endotracheal tube suctioning) when compared to routine care (Gomes Neto et al., 2020). Although NNS has been used for generations, it has only recently been examined rigorously as a nonpharmacologic intervention. NNS is thought to produce analgesia through stimulation of orotactile and mechanoreceptors when a pacifier is introduced into an infant's mouth. NNS is hypothesized to modulate transmission or processing of nociception through mediation by the endogenous nonopioid system (Blass et al., 1987; Gunnar et al., 1988).

NNS has been shown to reduce behavioral pain responses in term infants during immunizations (Blass, 1997) and heel lances in term and preterm infants (Blass & Shide, 1994; Miller & Anderson, 1993).

However, pain relief was greater in infants who received both NNS and sucrose. Compared with blanket swaddling (Campos, 1989) or rocking (Campos, 1994) during painful procedures, NNS reduced duration of cry and soothed infants more rapidly. NNS with sucrose or breastfeeding during a minor painful procedure is more effective than using NNS alone (Shann, 2007). Unlike blanket swaddling, however, there was a rebound in distress when an NNS pacifier was removed from an infant's mouth. The efficacy of NNS is immediate but appears to terminate almost immediately upon sucking cessation.

Oral sucrose is commonly used to provide pain relief to infants undergoing mild painful procedures, such as heel sticks. Sucrose is a disaccharide consisting of fructose and glucose. A meta-analysis of 57 studies demonstrated sucrose both safe and effective in reducing pain from minor procedures (Stevens et al., 2013). However, sucrose appears most effective for brief, intermittent procedural pain and less effective for pain from procedures of longer duration. Sucrose used in conjunction with other nonpharmacologic interventions including NNS and swaddling provides pain relief when the procedure is prolonged, such as ophthalmologic examinations (Stevens et al., 2013).

A critical role for NICU care providers is to support family integration into care from admission to discharge. Families often do not receive the information they need regarding pain assessment and management. This limits parental involvement, and the situation may lead to increased parental stress (Franck et al., 2004). To watch or to know that a child is in pain is among the most difficult experiences for a parent. It is important that parents and caregivers work together to help minimize pain and support infants so they can cope with commonly performed painful clinical procedures.

CONCLUSION

Nurses play an important role in ensuring that optimal pain assessment and management practices are employed in the NICU. Nurses are positioned to observe infant responses to painful procedures and clinical conditions using valid and reliable pain instruments. They can use this assessment data to effectively implement nonpharmacologic approaches to caregiving that will minimize the deleterious effects of pain on neonates.

Potential Research Questions

Prevention

- How can the NICU caregiving environment be structured to reduce the number of painful procedures that infants experience?

Assessment

- How can researchers optimally assess pain in infants who have dampened behavioral responses to pain due to immaturity, illness, neurologic impairment, or end-of-life status?

- How does the macroenvironment of sound and light influence a preterm neonate's ability to cope with and respond to painful clinical procedures?

Treatment

- How long should nursing care be delayed after a painful procedure to minimize the potential for wind-up pain?

REFERENCES

Ahn, Y. (2006). The relationship between behavioral states and pain responses to various NICU procedures in premature infants. *Journal of Tropical Pediatrics, 52*(3), 201–205.

American Academy of Pediatrics Committee on Fetus and Newborn and Section on Anesthesiology and Pain Medicine. (2016). Prevention and management of procedural pain in the neonate: An update. *Pediatrics, 105*, 454–461.

American Academy of Pediatrics/Canadian Paediatric Society. (2006). Prevention and management of pain and stress in the neonate: An update. *Pediatrics, 118*, 2231–2241.

Anand, K. J. S. (2000). Pain, plasticity, and premature birth: A prescription for permanent suffering? *Nature Medicine, 6*, 971–973.

Anand, K. J. S. (2007). Pharmacological approaches to the management of pain in the neonatal intensive care unit. *Journal of Perinatology, 27*, S4–S11.

Anand, K. J. (2008). Analgesia for skin-breaking procedures in newborns and children: What works best? *Canadian Medical Association Journal. 179*(1), 11.

Anand, K. J. S., Aranda, J. V., Berbe, C. B., Buckman, S., Capparelli, E. V., Carlo, W., Hummel, P., Johnston, C. C., Lantos, J., Tutag-Lehr, V., Lynn, A. M., Maxwell, L. G., Oberlander, T. F., Raju, T. N., Soriano, S. G., Taddio, A., & Walco, G. A. (2006). Summary proceedings from the neonatal pain-control group. *Pediatrics, 117*(3), S9–S22.

Anand, K. S., Johnson, C., Handyside, J., & Members of the Pain and Sedation Exploratory Group. (2004). *NICQ 2002: Reducing pain in infants in the NICU resource kit.* Vermont Oxford Network.

Anand, K. J. S., Stevens, B. J., & McGrath, P. J. (2007). *Pain in neonates: Pain research and clinical management series* (3rd ed.). Elsevier Health Sciences.

Azarmnejad, E., Sarhangi, F., Javadi, M., Rejeh, N., Amirsalari, S., Tadrisi, S. D. (2017). The effectiveness of familiar auditory stimulus on hospitalized neonates' physiologic responses to procedural pain. *International Journal of Nursing Practice, 23*(3), e12527. https://doi.org/10.1111/ijn.12527

Bartocci, M., Bergqvist, H., Lagercrantz, H., & Anand, K. (2006). Pain activates cortical areas in the preterm newborn brain. *Pain, 122*(1), 109–117.

Belda, S., Pallas, C. R., De la Cruz, J., & Tejada, P. (2004). Screening for retinopathy of prematurity: Is it painful? *Biology of the Neonate, 86*(3), 195–200.

Blass, E. (1997). Milk-induced hypoalgesia in human newborns. *Pediatrics, 99*(6), 825–829.

Blass, E., Fitzgerald, E., & Kehoe, P. (1987). Interactions between sucrose, pain, and isolation distress. *Pharmacology, Biochemistry & Behavior, 26*(3), 483–489.

Blass, E., & Shide, D. (1994). Some comparisons among the calming and pain relieving effects of sucrose, glucose, fructose and lactose in infant rats. *Chemical Senses, 19*(3), 239–249.

Campos, R. (1989). Soothing-pain-elicited distress in infants with swaddling and pacifiers. *Child Development, 60*(4), 781–792.

Campos, R. G. (1994). Rocking and pacifiers: Two comforting interventions for heelstick pain. *Research in Nursing & Health, 17*(5), 321–331.

Carrier, C. T., & Walden, M. (2001). Integrating research and standards to improve pain management practices for newborns and infants. *Newborn and Infant Nursing Reviews, 1*(2), 122–131.

Chirico, G., Cabano, R., Villa, G., Bigogno, A., Ardesi, M., & Dioni, E. (2017). Randomised study showed that recorded maternal voices reduced pain in preterm infants undergoing heel lance procedures in a neonatal intensive care unit. *Acta Paediatrica, 106*, 1564–1568. https://doi.org/10.1111/apa.13944

Cong, X., Wu, J., Vittner, D., Xu, W., Hussain, N., Galvin, S., Fitzsimons, M., McGrath, J. M., & Henderson, W. A. (2017). The impact of cumulative pain/stress on neurobehavioral development of preterm infants in the NICU. *Early Human Development, 108*, 9–16. https://doi.org/10.1016/j.earlhumdev.2017.03.003. PMID: 28343092. PMCID: PMC5444300.

Corff, K., Seideman, R., Venkataraman, P., Lutes, L., & Yates, B. (1995). Facilitated tucking: A nonpharmaco-logic comfort measure for pain in preterm neonates. *Journal of Obstetric, Gynecologic, & Neonatal Nursing, 24*(2), 143–147.

Craig, K., Whitfield, M., Grunau, R., Linton, J., & Hadjistavropoulos, H. D. (1993). Pain in the preterm neonate: Behavioral and physiological indices. *Pain, 52*(3), 287–299.

Duhn, L., & Medves, J. (2004). A systematic integrative review of infant pain assessment tools. *Advances in Neonatal Care, 4*(3), 126–140.

El Sayed, M. F., Taddio, A., Fallah, S., De Silva, N., & Moore, A. M. (2007). Safety profile of morphine following surgery in neonates. *Journal of Perinatology, 27*(7), 444–447.

Evans, J. C. (2001). Physiology of acute pain in preterm infants. *Newborn and Infant Nursing Reviews, 1*(2), 75–84.

Fearon, I., Kisilevsky, B. S., Hains, S. M., Muir, D. W., & Tranmer, J. (1997). Swaddling after heel lance: Age-specific effects on behavioral recovery in preterm infants. *Journal of Developmental and Behavioral Pediatrics, 18*(4), 222–232.

Fitzgerald, M., Millard, C., & McIntosh, N. (1989). Cutaneous hypersensitivity following peripheral tissue damage in newborn infants and its reversal with topical anaesthesia. *Pain, 39*(1), 31–36.

Fitzgerald, M., Shaw, A., & MacIntosh, N. (1988). Post-natal development of the cutaneous flexor reflex: A comparative study in premature infants and newborn rat pups. *Developmental Medicine and Child Neurology, 30*(4), 520–526.

Franck, L. S., Cox, S., Allen, A., & Winter, I. (2004). Parental concern and distress about infant pain. *Archives of Diseases in Childhood Fetal & Neonatal Edition, 89*, F71–F75.

Franck, L., & Miaskowski, C. (1998). The use of intravenous opioids to provide analgesia in critically ill, premature neonates: A research critique. *Journal of Pain and Symptom Management, 15*(1), 41–69.

Gibbins, S., & Stevens, B. (2003). The influence of gestational age on the efficacy and short-term safety of sucrose for procedural pain relief. *Advances in Neonatal Care, 3*(5), 241–249.

Gibbons, S., Stevens, B., Yamada, J., Dionne, K., Campbell-Yeo, M., Lee, G., Caddell, K., Johnstond, C., & Taddio, A. (2014). Validation of the premature infant pain profile-revised. *Early Human Development, 90*, 189–193.

Giordano, V., Deindl, P., Kuttner, S., Waldhor, T., Berger, A., & Olischar, M. (2014). The neonatal pain, agitation and sedation scale reliably detected oversedation but failed to differentiate between other sedation levels. *Acta Paediatrica, 103*(12), e515–e521.

Goldschneider, K. R., & Anand, K. S. (2003). Long-term consequences of pain in neonates. In Schechter, N. L., Berde, C. B., & Yaster, M. (Eds.), *Pain in infants, children, and adolescents* (2nd ed., pp. 58–70). Lippincott Williams & Wilkins.

Gomes Neto, M., da Silva Lopes, I. A., Araujo, A. C. C. L. M., Oliveira, L. S., & Saquetto, M. B. (2020). The effect of facilitated tucking position during painful procedure in pain management of preterm infants in neonatal intensive care unit: A systematic review and meta-analysis. *European Journal of Pediatrics, 179*(5), 699.

Grunau, R., & Craig, K. (1987). Pain expression in neonates: Facial action and cry. *Pain, 28*(3), 395–410.

Grunau, R., Linhares, M. B., Holsti, L., Oberlander, T. F., & Whitfield, M. F. (2004). Does prone or supine position influence pain responses in preterm infants at 32 weeks gestational age? *Clinical Journal of Pain, 20*(2), 76–82.

Gunnar, M., Connors, J., Isensee, J., & Wall, L. (1988). Adrenocortical activity and behavioral distress in human newborns. *Developmental Psychobiology, 21*(4), 297–310.

Hartley, S., Franck, L., & Lundergan, R. (1989). Maintenance sedation of agitated infants in the NICU with chloral hydrate: New concerns. *Journal of Perinatology, 2*(2), 162–164.

Hartling, L., Shaik, M. S., Tjosvold, L., Leicht, R., Liang, Y., Kumar, M. (2009). Music for medical indications in the neonatal period: A systematic review of randomised controlled trials. *Archives of Disease in Childhood Fetal and Neonatal Edition, 94*(5), F349.

Herrington, C. J., Olomu, I. N., & Geller, S. M. (2004). Salivary cortisol as indicators of pain in preterm infants: A pilot study. *Clinical Nursing Research, 13*(1), 53–68.

Hillman, B. A., Tabrizi1, M. N., Gauda, E. B., Carson, K. A., & Aucott, S. W. (2015). The neonatal pain, agitation and sedation scale and the bedside nurse's assessment of neonates. *Journal of Perinatology, 35*(2), 128–131. https://doi.org/10.1038/jp.2014.154

Hummel, P., Lawlor-Klean, P., & Weiss, M. (2010). Validity and reliability of the N-PASS assessment tool with acute pain. *Journal of Perinatology, 30*, 474–478.

Hummel, P., Puchalski, M., Creech, S. D., & Weiss, M. G. (2008). Clinical reliability and validity of the N-PASS: Neonatal pain, agitation and sedation scale with prolonged pain. *Journal of Perinatology, 28*(1), 55–60.

Hummel, P., & van Dijk, M. (2006). Pain assessment: Current status and challenges. *Seminars in Fetal & Neonatal Medicine, 11*, 237–245.

International Association for the Study of Pain Subcom-mittee on Taxonomy. (1979). Pain terms: A list with definitions and notes on usage. *Pain, 6*(3), 249–252.

Johnston, C., Campbell-Yeo, M., Fernandes, A., Inglis, D., Streiner, D., & Zee, R. (2014) Skin-to-skin care for procedural pain in neonates. *Cochrane Database of Systematic Reviews*, (1), CD008435. Update in: Cochrane Database of Systematic Reviews, 2017, (2), CD008435. PMID: 24459000. https://doi.org/10.1002/14651858.CD008435.pub2

Johnston, C. C., Filion, F., & Nuyt, A. M. (2007). Recorded maternal voice for preterm neonates undergoing heel lance. *Advances in Neonatal Care, 7*(5), 258–266. https://doi.org/10.1097/01.ANC.0000296634.26669.13

Johnston, C., & Stevens, B. (1996). Experience in a neona-tal intensive care unit affects pain response. *Pediatrics, 98*(5), 925–930.

Johnston, C., Stevens, B., Craig, K., & Grunau, R. (1993). Developmental changes in pain expression in premature, full-term, two-and four-month-old infants. *Pain, 52*, 201–208.

Joint Commission. (2017). *Pain assessment and management standards for hospitals*. https://www.jointcommission.org/-/media/tjc/documents/standards/r3-reports/r3_report_issue_11_2_11_19_rev.pdf

Kahraman, A., Gümüs, M., Akar, M., Sipahi, M., Yılmaz, H., Zümrüt, B. (2020). The effects of auditory interventions on pain and comfort in premature newborns in the neonatal intensive care unit; a randomised controlled trial. *Intensive & Critical Care Nursing, 61*, 1–7.

Krechel, S., & Bildner, J. (1995). Cries: A new neonatal post-operative pain measurement score. Initial testing of validity and reliability. *Paediatric Anaesthesia, 5*(1), 53–61.

Krueger, C. (2010). Exposure to maternal voice in preterm infants: A review. *Advances in Neonatal Care, 10*(1), 13–20. https://doi.org/10.1097/ANC.0b013e3181cc3c69

Kurdahi Badr, L., Demerjian, T., Daaboul, T., Abbas, H., Hasan Zeineddine, M., & Charafeddine, L. (2017). Preterm infants exhibited less pain during a heel stick when they were played the same music their mothers listened to during pregnancy. *Acta Paediatrica, 106*(3), 438–445. https://doi.org/10.1111/apa.13666

Küçukog˘lu, S., Aytekin, A., Celebioglu, A., Celebi, A., Caner, I., & Maden, R. (2016). Effect of white noise in relieving vaccination pain in premature infants. *Pain Management Nursing, 17*(6), 392–400. https://doi.org/10.1016/j.pmn.2016.08.006

Lago, P., Boccuzzo, G., Garetti, E., Pirelli, A., Pieragostini, L., Merazzi, D., & Ancora, G. (2013). Pain management during invasive procedures at Italian NICUs: Has anything changed in the last five years? *Journal of Maternal-Fetal and Neonatal Medicie, 26*(3), 303–305.

Lago, P., Garetti, E., Merazzi, D., Pieragostini, L., Ancora, G., Pirelli, A., & Bellieni, C. V. (2009). Pain study group of the Italian society of neonatology. Guidelines for procedural pain in the newborn. *Acta Paediatrica, 98*(6), 932–939. https://doi.org/10.1111/j.1651-2227.2009.01291.x. PMID: 19484828. PMCID: PMC2688676.

Larsson, B., Tannefeldt, G., Lagercrantz, H., & Olsson, G. L. (1998). Venipuncture is more effective and less painful than heel lancing for blood tests in neonates. *Pediatrics, 101*(5), 882–886.

Lawrence, J., Alcock, D., McGrath, P., Kay, J., MacMur-ray, S. B., & Dulberg, C. (1993). The development of a tool to assess neonatal pain. *Neonatal Network, 12*(6), 59–66.

Mackenna, B. R., & Callander, R. (1990). *Central nervous system locomotor system*. In *Illustrated physiology* (5th ed., pp. 220–284). Churchill Livingstone.

McIntosh, N., Van Veen, L., & Brameyer, H. (1994). Alleviation of the pain of heel prick in preterm infants. *Archives of Disease in Childhood, 70*, F177–F181.

McNair, C., Ballantyne, M., Dionne, K., Stephens, D., & Stevens, B. (2004). Postoperative pain assessment in the neonatal intensive care unit. *Archives of Disease in Childhood Fetal & Neonatal Edition, 89*(6), F537–F541.

Melzack, R., & Wall, P. (1965). Pain mechanisms: A new theory. *Science, 150*(699), 971–978.

Miller, H., & Anderson, G. (1993). Nonnutritive sucking: Effects on crying and heart rate in intubated infants requiring assisted mechanical ventilation. *Nursing Research, 42*(5), 305–307.

Pillai Riddell, R., Racine, N. M., Turcotte, K., Uman, L., Horton, R., Din Osmun, L., Ahola Kohut, S, Stevens, B., & Gerqitz-Stern, A., (2011). Non-pharmacological management of infant and young child procedural pain. *Cochrane Database of Systematic Reviews*, (10), CD006275.

Porter, F., Miller, J., Cole, F., & Marshall, R. W. (1991). A controlled clinical trial of local anesthesia for lumbar puncture in newborns. *Pediatrics, 88*(4), 663–669.

Porter, F., Wolf, C., & Miller, J. (1998). The effect of han-dling and immobilization on the response to acute pain in newborn infants. *Pediatrics, 102*(6), 1383–1389.

Raja, S. N., Carr, D. B., Cohen, M., Finnerup, N., Flor, H., Gibson, S., Keefe, J., Mogil, J., Ringkamp, M., Sluka, K., Song, X., Stevens, B., Sullivan, M.,Tutelman, P., Ushida, T., & Vader, K. (2020). The revised international association for the study of pain definition of pain: Concepts, challenges, and compromises. *Pain, 161*, 1976–1982.

Ramenghi, L., Griffith, G., Wood, C., & Levene, M. I. (1996). Effect of non-sucrose sweet-tasting solution on neonatal heel prick responses. *Archives of Disease in Childhood Fetal & Neonatal Edition, 74*, F129–F131.

Ranger, M., Johnston, C., & Anand, K. (2007). Current controversies regarding pain assessment in neonates. *Seminars in Perinatology, 31*, 283–288.

Roofthooft, D. W., Simons, S. H., Anand, K. J., Tibboel, D., & van Dijk, M. (2014). Eight years later, are we still hurting newborn infants? *Neonatology, 105*(3), 218–226.

Rouss, K., Gerber, A., Albisetti, M., Hug, M., & Bernet, V. (2007). Long-term subcutaneous morphine administration after surgery in newborns. *Journal of Perinatal Medicine, 35*(1), 79–81.

Sajjadian, N., Mohammadzadeh, M., Alizadeh, , Taheri, P., & Shariat, M. (2017). Positive effects of low intensity recorded maternal voice on physiologic reactions in premature infants. *Infant Behavior and Development, 46*:59–66. https://doi.org/10.1016/j.infbeh.2016.11.009

Shah, P. S., Herbozo, C., Aliwalas, L. L., & Shah, V. S. (2012). Breastfeeding or breast milk for procedural pain in neonates. *Cochrane Database of Systematic Reviews, 12*:CD004950. https://doi.org/10.1002/14651858.CD004950.pub3. PMID: 23235618.

Shah, V. S., & Ohlsson, A. (2011). Venepuncture versus heel lance for blood sampling in term neonates. *The Cochrane Database Of Systematic Reviews, 2011*(10):1–30, CD001452. https://doi.org/10.1002/14651858.CD001452.pub4

Shah, V., Taddio, A., Bennett, S., & Speidel, B. D. (1997). Neonatal pain response to heel stick vs. venipuncture for routine blood sampling. *Archives of Disease in Childhood, 77*(2), 143–144.

Shann, F. (2007). Suckling and sugar reduce pain in babies. *Lancet, 369*(9563), 721.

Shapiro, C. (1993). Nurses' judgments of pain in term and preterm newborns. *Journal of Obstetric, Gynecologic, & Neonatal Nursing, 22*(1), 41–47.

Sharek, P. J., Powers, R., Koehn, A., & Anand, K. J. S. (2006). Evaluation and development of potentially bet-ter practices to improve pain management of neonates. *Pediatrics, 118*(Suppl. 2), S78–S86.

Sizun, J., Ansquer, H., Browne, J., Tordjman, S., & Morin, J. F. (2002). Developmental care decreases physiologic and behavioral pain expression in preterm neonates. *Journal of Pain, 3*(6), 446–450.

Skogsdal, Y., Eriksson, M., & Schollin, J. (1997). Analgesia in newborns given oral glucose. *Acta Paediatrica, 86*(2), 217–220.

Spence, K., Henderson-Smart, D., New, K., Evans, C, Whitelaw, J., Woolnough, R., & Australian and New Zealand Neonatal Network, . (2010). Evidenced-based clinical practice guideline for management of newborn pain. *Journal of Paediatrics and Child Health, 46*(4), 184–192. https://doi.org/10.1111/j.1440-1754.2009.01659.x. PMID: 20105248.

Stevens, B., Gibbins, S., Yamada, J., Dionne, K., Lee, G., Johnston, C., & Taddio, A. (2014). The Premature infant pain profile-revised (PIPP-R): Initial validation and feasibility. *Clinical Journal of Pain, 30*(3), 238–243.

Stevens, B., Johnston, C., Petryshen, P., & Taddio, A. (1996). Premature infant pain profile: Development and initial validation. *Clinical Journal of Pain, 12*(1), 13–22.

Stevens, B., Johnston, C., Taddio, A., Gibbons, S., & Yamada, J. (2010). The premature infant pain profile: Evaluation 13 years after development. *Clinical Journal of Pain, 26,* (9), 813–830.

Stevens, B., Taddio, A., Ohlsson, A., & Einarson, T. (1997). The efficacy of sucrose for relieving procedural pain in neonates: A systematic review and meta-analysis. *Acta Paediatrica, 86*(8), 837–842.

Stevens, B., Yamada, J., Lee, G. Y., Ohlsson, A. (2013). Sucrose for analgesia in newborn infants undergoing painful procedures. *Cochrane Database of Systematic Reviews, 1*(1), CD001069.

Suraseranivongse, S., Kaosaard, R., Intakong, P., Pornsirip-rasert, S., Karnchana, Y., Kaopinpruck, J., & Sangjeen, K. (2006). A comparison of postoperative pain scales in neonates. *British Journal of Anaesthesia, 97*(4), 540–544.

Taddio, A., Goldbach, M., Ipp, M., Stevens, B., & Koren, G. (1995). Effect of neonatal circumcision on pain responses during vaccination in boys. *Lancet, 345*(8945), 291–292.

Walden, M., & Franck, L. (2003). Identification, manage-ment, and pre-vention of newborn/infant pain. In Kenner, C. & Lott, J. W. (Eds.), *Comprehensive neonatal nursing: A physiologic perspective* (3rd ed., pp. 843–856). W. B. Saunders.

Walden, M., & Gibbins, S. (2012). *Pain assessment and management: Guideline for practice.* National Association of Neonatal Nurses.

Walden, M., & Gibbins, S. (2012). *Newborn pain assessment and man-agement guideline for practice.* NANN. https://apps.nann.org/store/product-details?productId=545

Walden, M., Penticuff, J. H., Stevens, B., Lotas, M. J., Kozinetz, C. A., & Clark, A. (2001). Maturational changes in physiological and behavioral responses of preterm neonates to pain. *Advances in Neonatal Care, 1*(2), 94–106.

CHAPTER 19

Palliative Care

Tanya Sudia

Standards in Developmental Care

Standard 1: Infant
- The individualized developmental care plan is identified and reviewed before care is provided.
- Caregiving is guided by an infant's developmental background and behavior cues.
- The caregiver recognizes and assesses pain during all procedures, assessments, and caregiving tasks for signs of infant distress.

Standard 2: Family
- The health professional shows respect and is welcoming toward families.
- The caregiver is flexible regarding family needs and encourages family participation in decision-making regarding the needs of their infant.
- The caregiver is supportive and includes families in caring for the infant in a meaningful way from the time of birth throughout the infant's hospitalization and until death if that is the outcome.
- The health professional explores opportunities for siblings and extended family members to be involved with the care of the infant.

INTRODUCTION

Developmental care is implemented for the benefit of all infants regardless of their life expectancy. Whether infants are in the active dying phase or at some point on a trajectory that is incompatible with long-term survival, they and their families deserve comprehensive developmental and palliative care.

The best approach is to provide individualized care based on the holistic needs of infants and families. Care should foster positive growth and development and prevent further complications. This approach is just as important to a child and family with a poor prognosis as it is to those for whom the outcome is bright. Palliative care in many respects incorporates the essence of developmental care, which is a highly individualized, collaborative, culturally sensitive, and family-centered philosophy of care delivery.

NEONATAL AND PEDIATRIC PALLIATIVE CARE BACKGROUND

This chapter describes palliative care for infants within a developmental care framework. It also offers evidence-based guidelines for practice and identifies areas for further research.

Pediatric palliative care incorporates pain and symptom management for children while attending to the psychological, social, and spiritual needs of children and families (American Academy of Pediatrics [AAP], 2000). Palliative care measures should be implemented as an essential aspect of the treatment plan at the time of diagnosis and must continually evolve as a child's condition changes (Institute of Medicine [IOM], 2003).

Palliative care programs for newborns and infants and their families have evolved since their early stages; however, they continue to be underused in many neonatal intensive care units (NICUs) in the United States and abroad (Baker et al., 2007; Brandon et al., 2007; Catlin & Carter, 2002; Hutton, 2002; Kyc et al., 2020; Malcolm et al., 2008; Pierucci et al., 2001; Sudia-Robinson, 2003). Comprehensive palliative care cannot be provided if infants and parents do not have fully supportive intervention programs from the moment of birth to the moment of death and beyond. For an infant's parents and siblings, support and bereavement services must continue for as long as needed as they progress through the grieving process at their own pace and in their own unique way. Finally, if these programs are to be self-sustaining, the supportive needs of healthcare providers must routinely be incorporated into NICU palliative care programs (Jones et al., 2007; Mackenzie & MacCallam, 2009; Morgan, 2009; Rushton et al., 2006).

NORMALIZATION OF DYING

Dying occurs along a continuum. The time from diagnosis of a terminal condition to the moment of death can be as brief as minutes or hours. In other cases, an infant might live for a year or more. Consequently, it is recommended that palliative care measures be incorporated into every existing plan of care at the time of diagnosis (AAP, 2000; Milstein, 2003; Sahler, 2000; Wolfe et al., 2000; Wolfe et al., 2002). However, palliative care measures can be added at any point along this continuum and still provide some benefit for infants and families (Table 19-1).

The newborn and infant care team can initiate the palliative care process by evaluating an infant's need for comfort and supportive measures. Just as parents are involved in other aspects of the overall care plan for their infant, NICU professionals must affirm their parenting role by seeking their input for this aspect of care (Dzau et al., 2017). A comprehensive palliative care plan will reflect measures adapted to the infant's needs while simultaneously reflecting parental preferences. This plan of care cannot be static and must change as an infant's condition warrants and as the family progresses through anticipatory grieving phases.

ALLEVIATING PAIN AND SUFFERING

Adequate pain management is an important component of optimal care throughout the dying phase. Continued, aggressive support until the moment of death often is experienced by many infants and children (Docherty et al., 2007; Kane,

TABLE 19-1 Practice Recommendations for Palliative Care

Type	Recommendation	Level of Evidence	References
Comfort Care	Palliative care is initiated at the time of diagnosis and should reflect an individualized plan of care.	V	AAP, 2000; Catlin & Carter, 2002; IOM, 2003; Pierucci et al., 2001
	Infants' pain routinely is assessed and adequately managed.	I	Anand, 2007; Anand et al., 2004; Ferrell et al., 2020; Walden & Carrier, 2009
	Skin-to-skin holding is incorporated into the infant's palliative care plan.	I	Ferber & Makhoul, 2008; Kashaninia et al., 2008
	Music therapy is used based on parental preferences and individual NICU considerations.	VI	Arnon et al., 2006
	Soft lighting from lamps is used in individual infant rooms or dimmed lighting is used when individual rooms are not available to promote a calm, relaxed environment.	VII	Joshi, 2005
	Aromatherapy may produce a calming effect for infants or family members and should be considered within the NICU setting.	VII	Buckle, 2007; Butje et al., 2008
	Gentle massage by a parent or caregiver may be implemented and assessed for its potential soothing effect on the infant.	VII	Beachy, 2003; Kassity-Krich & Jones, 2007
Family Care	Parents' choices and requests are respected to the fullest possible extent.	VII	AAP, 2000; IOM, 2003; Dzau et al., 2017
	Supportive services are routinely provided to parents.	VII	AAP, 2000; IOM, 2003
	Sibling support needs are assessed and interventions provided.	V	AAP, 2000; Himelstein, 2006; IOM, 2003
NICU Team Care	NICU professionals must have appropriate training to provide comprehensive palliative care.	V	AAP, 2000; Rushton et al., 2006; Jones et al., 2007; Fortney & Steward, 2017
	Support services must be available to NICU professionals.	V	AAP, 2000; Kain et al., 2009; Rushton et al., 2006; Sudia & Catlin, 2019.

Note: Level I = evidence from a systematic review or meta-analysis of all relevant randomized controlled trials (RCTs) or evidence-based clinical practice guidelines based on systematic reviews of RCTs. Level II = evidence obtained from at least one well-designed RCT. Level III = evidence obtained from well-designed controlled trials without randomization. Level IV = evidence from well-designed case-control and cohort studies. Level V = evidence from systematic reviews of descriptive and qualitative studies. Level VI = evidence from a single descriptive or qualitative study. Level VII = evidence from the opinion of authorities and/or reports of expert committees.

2006; Kopelman, 2006; Pierucci et al., 2001; Rebagliato et al., 2000). This phenomenon raises questions about whether infants suffer needlessly during their last moments of life (Sudia-Robinson, 2003). Ensuring that adequate pain and supportive palliative medication is provided is an initial step to providing comprehensive, developmentally appropriate NICU care (Anand, 2007; Anand et al., 2004; Ferrell et al., 2020; Walden & Carrier, 2009) and promoting a more peaceful death for infants (Abe et al., 2001; Catlin & Carter, 2002; Himelstein, 2006; IOM, 2003). NICU interprofessional team members also have an obligation to continue to explore additional supportive measures to further ease infant suffering. Such measures include providing comfort positioning, alleviating noxious stimuli, and eliminating noncurative tests and procedures.

INCORPORATING DEVELOPMENTAL CARE MEASURES

Although most aspects of developmental care can benefit infants who need palliative care, the measures highlighted in this section include skin-to-skin holding (kangaroo care), music therapy, ambient lighting, aromatherapy, and infant massage.

Kangaroo Care

Researchers have demonstrated the effectiveness of skin-to-skin holding or kangaroo care for preterm infants (Ferber & Makhoul, 2008; Kashaninia et al., 2008; Ludington-Hoe et al., 2006) and parents (Anderson, 1991; Chia et al., 2006; Gale et al., 1993). Among the most positive aspects of kangaroo care as a component of palliative care is that it provides parents precious moments, without interference, that they will treasure after their infant has died. Memories of how their infant felt when held skin-to-skin will linger forever in their minds.

It is important to note, however, that upon initially seeing their infant in a NICU, some parents may not be ready to participate when first approached about skin-to-skin holding during kangaroo care. This hesitancy must be respected, and great care should be taken to avoid causing any guilt for such a decision. Sometimes parents need personal space and time to process the overwhelming feelings that accompany the birth of a baby who is not likely to survive (Lundqvist et al., 2002). They might fear that holding their infant will cause his or her death to come more quickly. Most parents who initially distance themselves from their baby eventually begin to touch and then hold their child. Allowing parents to progress at their own pace respects their role as parents and as decision-makers for this new child. Acknowledging to parents that they can always make this decision later leaves the door open for this intervention when they are ready. (For more information about skin-to-skin holding, see Chapter 16.)

Music Therapy

Music therapy is among the interventions that is easiest to incorporate into a NICU, and it can be continued if an infant is discharged to be cared for at home. In addition to its soothing aspects for infants and parents, music therapy provides parents with another opportunity to enact their preferences for their infant's care.

The NICU team should provide initial guidance for families in the selection of music for their infant. Suggest a calming instrumental piece and place the volume indicator at the lowest setting. It is helpful if NICUs have a selection of appropriate CDs or audiotapes from which parents can choose. This especially is important when the active dying phase occurs shortly after birth. If an infant is hospitalized for a long time, parents may wish to bring in their own music selections.

Researchers have found that live music can have even greater positive calming effects than recorded music for some preterm infants (Arnon et al., 2006). Further, researchers have demonstrated the effectiveness of music therapy over the use of chloral hydrate for selected infants and young children undergoing electroencephalogram testing (Loewy et al., 2006). Soothing, live music provided by a parent, family member, or music therapist is an option that should be offered whenever feasible.

Ambient Lighting

Adjustable ambient lighting at an infant's bedside can help to maintain day-night and sleep-wake cycles (Blackburn, 1996). There are various inexpensive ways to modify bedside lighting (Joshi, 2005), including the use of individual adjustable lamps and shielding light with blankets or cloth. When infants are in private rooms, the options for altered lighting are more varied. Lamps with soft, pastel blue light bulbs can help create a calming environment and are relatively inexpensive and easy to implement. Parents can be invited to share their preferences for adjustable lighting whenever possible in the NICU and encouraged to use this intervention if their infant is discharged home.

Aromatherapy

Aromatherapy can encompass a variety of measures ranging from exposing infants to maternal scent to pleasantly modifying full-room scents. Although there is little research focused on the potential benefits of aromatherapy for critically ill infants and their families, indicators suggest that such measures may prove beneficial (Buckle, 2007; Butje et al., 2008; Kassity et al., 2003).

Some of the few studies in this area focus on infants' apparent recognition of the scent of their own mother's milk (Mizuno et al., 2004; Raimbault et al., 2007). When a mother cannot be present at the bedside, placing a cloth with the mother's scent near the infant may have a calming effect.

Eradicating typical hospital smells and replacing them with a soothing, mild vanilla or lavender scent can help parents relax and help engrain a more pleasant memory of the environment. Providing scents is inexpensive and, along with other measures, can help transform the NICU into a more calming environment.

Infant Massage

In most cases, massage can be soothing to an infant and has been associated with increased weight gain in preterm infants (Diego et al., 2007). As with any additional care measures, an infant's physiologic and behavioral responses must be evaluated and further plans for incorporation should be modified accordingly. Infant massage also provides an opportunity for parents to become involved in their infant's care if they feel comfortable doing so. The neonatal care team can use this parent-infant interaction to praise parents on their caregiving skills (Beachy, 2003). Comments such as "He relaxes when you gently massage his back like that" and "She recognizes your gentle touch" provide powerful positive feedback to parents. Parents of critically ill infants need to feel they can do something that all parents want to do—provide love and comfort to their child. (See Chapter 12 for more information about touch and massage.)

PROVIDING PARENTING OPPORTUNITIES

One of the most endearing gifts the NICU team can give to parents is the opportunity to engage in parenting activities for their infant. For some parents, interaction with their infant may be extremely limited by quantitative measurement—hours or days. However, their experience can be memorable if planned from a qualitative perspective. It only takes a few moments to create memories that parents will hold onto forever. This approach is aligned with the two standards found at the beginning of this chapter. These standards focus on individualization of care on both the infant and family.

NICU staff can provide parents with the opportunity to assist with most of their infant's personal care activities, such as cutting a lock of hair (instead of the nurse cutting it, ask parents if one or both of them would like to do so). For parents who prefer to not engage in such activities, offer to do these things in their presence. Recognize that while they might not be comfortable engaging in an initially offered activity, they may express a desire to do so in the future. Regardless of the activity, try to focus on a task the parents feel comfortable doing and something that will create a pleasant memory for the family, whether it is holding, touching, singing, or journaling.

Both timing and type of engagement activity can vary over time. Thus, if parents choose to not participate in one care measure, this does not mean they will not want to participate in other caregiving activities. For example, a parent might find it difficult to cut a lock of hair yet might desire to help dress their child. Another parent might consider the

child too fragile to dress, yet they may welcome the opportunity to gently brush his or her hair. With sensitivity to preferences, continue to extend opportunities for involvement. Respect that some parents might not desire to touch or photograph a dying child. Pictures that are taken can be placed in a file in case the parents request them at a future point in their grief and coping process. However, cultural values must be considered as some cultures do not believe that pictures of a dying baby should be taken. This type of care must be a family-centered integrative, culturally sensitive care (Kenner et al., 2015).

Timing of Involvement Opportunities

Parents will be on an emotional roller coaster. Some days they will cope better than others, and their level of energy for even the smallest task will vary. They might be involved in their infant's care 1 day but return the next day and prefer to stand at the bedside and watch. Again, an increased sensitivity to their needs and emotions is key to promoting further parenting opportunities.

First-Time Parents Versus Parents With Other Children

Parents come with different personal experiences upon which they draw as well as different parenting skills if they already are parents. Initial interventions to involve parents must consider these differences.

First-time parents will not have any direct parenting experience to draw upon. Their thoughts about what they can do and what others might expect them to do might conflict. They may desire to be more involved in their infant's care but feel uncomfortable verbalizing this to the staff. Their uncertainty may be more pronounced if they are very young or if they need additional support services. Or cultural preferences may dictate that another family member participates in select care aspects.

Parents with other children bring a wide range of experiences and have varying degrees of expectations about their role. To assist staff in assessing potential parental expectations, it may be helpful to broadly categorize parents by the ages of their other children (Himelstein, 2006). Generally, experiences for parents with children younger than 2 years will focus on direct caretaking activities. These parents may feel comfortable participating in care such as grooming.

Parents of preschool-age children may primarily be concerned about how to help their other children understand what is happening to their new baby brother or sister. Parents of young school-age children may also seek guidance regarding explaining a sibling's pending death. Parents may benefit from help exploring the reactions and feelings of the infant's siblings. In some cases, a sibling may harbor feelings such as guilt or other fears. Parents of older children might need help deciding how to involve these children in the visitation and care of their critically ill sibling. When available, age-appropriate sibling support groups (Himelstein, 2006; Pearson, 1997) and other psychosocial support measures should be offered to these families (Dighe et al., 2008; IOM, 2003; Malcolm et al., 2008).

Parents with children from previous marriages for whom the dying infant is a stepbrother or stepsister can have unique concerns. A stepsibling might experience guilt, particularly if they were not happy about the pending birth of this child or about their parent's divorce or remarriage. They may fear that their thoughts about not wanting a new baby brother or sister actually caused the infant's illness. Appropriate support services for these children should be explored.

Virtual Visitation and Engagement

For varying reasons, it may not be possible or practical for parents, siblings, or other family members to visit the infant in person. Many of the aforementioned practices of engagement can be replicated and, in some cases, even further enhanced in a virtual environment. Technology opens additional opportunities for participating in or engaging with the infant while in the NICU.

Virtual visits can be calming to the parents who may otherwise feel guilt or sadness when they are not able to be present at the bedside. Virtual visits also permit an extended window to reaffirm that NICU professionals are providing expert and comforting care for their infant. They can also provide an opportunity for grandparents and other family members to see and further understand what the infant and parents are enduring. This can be of benefit if family members or significant others can then offer additional support to the parents. More research is needed to better understand how the virtual world can be used to enhance closeness for families.

OPENNESS TO INNOVATIVE PRACTICES

Parents should be encouraged to suggest measures to the NICU staff that are unique to their cultural background or share interventions they would like to implement. It is important that their suggested practices are evaluated in the same manner they would be for any other infant. The most important question to consider is whether the proposed practice would cause any direct harm to the infant. Parents should not have to provide any evidence beyond their belief that a therapy might be beneficial for the team to consider their request. The ensuing evaluation for potential harm should come from the neonatal team directly caring for the infant in collaboration with the NICU leadership team. While remaining sensitive to the gravity of the infant's condition, it is unethical to dismiss potential harmful effects (Beauchamp & Childress, 2009; Penticuff, 1995). The NICU staff is obligated to continue to weigh the risks and benefits of their actions throughout the dying process.

When an infant's death is imminent and the risk of harm seems unlikely, NICU staff need to consider waiving a formal review of the parents' request to implement a culture-based practice. To meet their ethical obligation of weighing risks and benefits, the NICU staff directly involved in an infant's care and present at the bedside can discuss the parents' request, and when deemed permissible, allow them to immediately proceed. For example, parents may request to rub an herbal ointment onto their infant's skin. Unless it is known that this substance will be painful once placed on the skin or cause an adverse physiologic response, the NICU staff can allow the parents to apply it as they desire. However, if something is known to potentially cause the infant further pain or unintended harm, the practice should be avoided. Additional pain must never be inflicted or rationalized as acceptable simply because an infant is in the active dying phase. The ethical obligation to avoid causing intentional harm to infants is just as important during the dying process as it is during the curative phase of care.

In cases in which an infant's death is not likely to occur in the next few days or weeks, NICU staff can take the time needed to evaluate the parents' request. However, proceeding with the evaluation as quickly as possible is in everyone's best interest, as the infant might, indeed, benefit. Parents will feel a sense of control in aiding their infant, and the parent-staff relationship will have an additional degree of mutual respect.

NICU TEAM CARE

Comprehensive palliative care programs must include sufficient training sessions and support measures for the entire NICU team. These measures need to be implemented and evaluated in a systematic, ongoing manner. In addition, as NICU palliative care programs evolve, incorporating innovative training and support enhancements are necessary.

Education and Support

Palliative care training for NICU team members is essential for the delivery of optimal care (Ferrell et al., 2020; Fortney & Steward, 2017; Gale & Brooks, 2006; Kain, 2006; Mackenzie & MacCallam, 2009; Morgan, 2009). This training must incorporate all areas of practice recommendations for palliative care, including comfort care measures for infants and the provision of supportive family care. Additionally, staff must be knowledgeable of the support measures available to them as care providers. Access to palliative care consultation services is also beneficial when available (McLaughlin et al., 2020).

Support measures for the NICU team encompass the creation of an engaging environment conducive to integrated teamwork. Staff-supportive palliative care environments provide opportunities for open dialogue about care issues as well as forums for grief-based discussion. Among the most important facilitators for effective NICU, palliative practice is maintaining an environment in which the values and opinions of NICU health professionals can be respectfully shared (Kain et al., 2009). With the diversity of care providers and the range of circumstances that can arise in a NICU, it is inevitable that care providers will experience differing beliefs and values. It is imperative that all members of the NICU team feel supported and encouraged to discuss concerns as they arise.

The availability of supportive counseling services for NICU staff also fosters effective palliative care programs (Gale & Brooks, 2006; Kain et al., 2009). Measures such as bereavement debriefing sessions (Rushton et al., 2006) provide physicians and nurses with an opportunity to discuss and manage their grief. In addition, access to professional counseling services is essential. Staff attendance at patient funerals and memorials can be supportive for both the infant's family and the NICU team. Further, allowing NICU nurses and all staff members as appropriate to schedule time off following a particularly difficult patient care situation can facilitate the grief and self-renewal process. These collective measures foster the supportive teamwork necessary for the delivery of optimal palliative care.

CONCLUSION

Palliative care is a critical aspect of comprehensive newborn/infant and family-centered developmental care. A variety of measures can be instituted to help alleviate infant pain and suffering while simultaneously involving parents as valued primary caretakers for their infant. The neonatal care team must continue to explore existing and novel interventions that can help meet these goals and incorporate them into the plan of care. Implementing such practices can provide positive outcomes not only for the infant but also for the parents and the neonatal care team. Parents feel less like bystanders when they can suggest or participate in supplemental care practices. The neonatal care team benefits if they

see an improvement in an infant's comfort level, and they may develop a more positive relationship with parents. More research about ways to better support infants and families is needed in this area of caregiving. The following box features a listing of palliative care resources.

Palliative Care Resources

American Academy of Pediatrics
www.aap.org

Center to Advance Palliative Care
www.capc.org

Children's International Project on Palliative and Hospice Services
www.nhpco.org

American Association of Colleges of Nursing (AACN) and City of Hope End-of-Life Nursing Education Consortium (ELNEC)
https://www.aacnnursing.org/ELNEC

The Initiative for Pediatric Palliative Care
www.ippcweb.org

National Academy of Sciences: Institute of Medicine
www.IOM.org

The Robert Wood Johnson Foundation
www.promotingexcellence.org

Potential Research Questions

There are many unanswered questions and opportunities for research in neonatal and infant palliative care. Some of the most pertinent questions that can further improve NICU palliative care pertain to specific types of care and professionals.

Comfort care

- Is there a synergistic effect of combined comfort care measures?
- What are the positive physiologic effects of live music therapy for critically ill infants?
- Are their benefits of aromatherapy for critically ill infants?
- Does infant massage effect positive physiologic change in critically ill infants?
- What is the most comprehensive pharmacologic means to prevent infant suffering throughout the trajectory of the dying process?

Family Care

- What comfort care measures do parents consider most meaningful for their infant?
- What are the unmet needs of parents?
- Are the needs of siblings adequately assessed and addressed?
- What are the needs of extended family members?
- What are best practices for virtual visitation in the NICU?

NICU Professionals

- What self-caretaking and other supportive measures do NICU professionals need?
- Which palliative care measures are most and least likely to be implemented? What are the associated facilitators and barriers?
- What additional support do NICU professionals need for virtual visitation?

REFERENCES

Abe, N., Catlin, A. J., & Mihara, D. (2001). End of life in the NICU: A study of ventilator withdrawal. *MCN. The American Journal of Maternal Child Care, 28*(3), 141–146.

American Academy of Pediatrics. (2000). Palliative care for children. *Pediatrics, 106*(2), 351–357.

Anand, K. J. S. (2007). Pharmacological approaches to the management of pain in the neonatal intensive care unit. *Journal of Perinatology, 27,* S4–S11.

Anand, K. J. S., Hall, R. W., Desai, N., Shephard, B., Bergqvist, L. L., Young, T. E., Boyle, E. M., Carbajal, R., Bhutani, V. K., Moore, M. B., Kronsberg, S. S., Barton, B. A., & NEOPAIN Trial Investigators Group. (2004). Effects of morphine analgesia in ventilated preterm neonates: Primary outcomes from the NEOPAIN randomised trial. *The Lancet, 363,* 1673–1682.

Anderson, G. C. (1991). Current knowledge about skin-to-skin (kangaroo) care for preterm infants. *Journal of Perinatology, 11*(3), 216–226.

Arnon, S., Shapsa, A., Forman, L., Regev, R., Bauer, S., Litmanovitz, I., & Dolfin, T. (2006). Live music is beneficial to preterm infants in the neonatal intensive care unit environment. *Birth, 33*(2), 131–136.

Baker, J. N., Torkildson, C., Baillargeon, J. G., Olney, C. A., & Kane, J. R. (2007). National survey of pediatric residency program directors and residents regarding education in palliative medicine and end-of-life care. *Journal of Palliative Medicine, 10*(2), 420–429.

Beachy, J. M. (2003). Premature infants massage in the NICU. *Neonatal Network, 22*(3), 39–45.

Beauchamp, T. L., & Childress, J. F. (2009). *Principles of biomedical ethics* (6th ed.). Oxford University Press.

Blackburn, S. T. (1996). Research utilization: Modifying the NICU light environment. *Neonatal Network, 15*(4), 63–66.

Brandon, D., Docherty, S., & Thorpe, J. (2007). Infant and child deaths in acute care settings: Implications for palliative care. *Journal of Palliative Medicine, 10*(4), 910–918.

Buckle, J. (2007). Literature review: Should nursing take aromatherpy more seriously? *British Journal of Nursing, 16*(2), 116–120.

Butje, A., Repede, E., & Shattell, M. M. (2008). Healing scents: An overview of clinical aromatherpay for emotional distress. *Journal of Psychosocial Nursing and Mental Health Services, 46*(10), 47–52.

Catlin, A., & Carter, B. (2002). Creation of a neonatal end-of-life palliative care protocol. *Journal of Perinatology, 22*(3), 184–195.

Chia, P., Sellick, K., & Gan, S. (2006). The attitudes and practices of neonatal nurses in the use of kangaroo care. *Australian Journal of Advanced Nursing, 23*(4), 20–27.

Diego, M. A., Field, T., Hernandez-Reif, M., Deeds, O., Ascencio, A., & Begert, G. (2007). Preterm infant mas-sage elicits consistent increases in vagal activity and gastric motility that are associated with greater weight gain. *Acta Paediatrica, 96,* 1588–1591.

Dighe, M., Jadhav, S., Muckaden, M. A., & Socani, A. (2008). Parental concerns in children requiring palliative care. *Indian Journal of Palliative Care, 14*(1), 16–22.

Docherty, S. L., Miles, M. S., & Brandon, D. (2007). Search for "The Dying Point": Providers' experiences with palliative care in pediatric acute care. *Pediatric Nursing, 33*(4), 335–341.

Dzau, V. J., McClellan, M., Burke, S., Coye, M. J., Daschle, T. A., Diaz, A., Frist, W. H., Gaines, M. E., Hamburg, M. A., Henney, J. E., Kumamyika, S., Leavitt, M. O., McGinnis, J. M., Parker, R., Sandy, L. G., Schaeffer, L. D., Steele, G. D., Thompson, P., & Zerhouni, E. (2017). *Vital directions for health and health care: Priorities from a National Academy of Medicine Initiative.* NIAM Perspectives. Discussion Paper. National Academy of Medicine. https://doi.org/10.31478/201703e

Ferber, S. G., & Makhoul, I. R. (2008). Neurobehavioural assessment of skin-to-skin effects on reaction to pain in preterm infants: A randomized controlled within-subject trial. *Acta Paediatrica, 97,* 171–176.

Ferrell, B., Thaxton, C. A., & Murphy, H. (2020). Preparing nurses for palliative care in the NICU. *Advances in Neonatal Care, 20*(2), 142–150. https://doi.org/10.1097/ANC.0000000000000705

Fortney, C. A., & Steward, D. K. (2017). A qualitative study of nurse observations of symptoms in infants at end-of-life in the neonatal intensive care unit. *Intensive and Critical Care Nursing, 40,* 57–63. https://doi.org/10.1016/j.iccn.2016.10.004

Gale, G., & Brooks, A. (2006). Implementing a palliative care program in a newborn intensive care unit. *Advances in Neonatal Care, 6*(1), 37–53.

Gale, G., Franck, L., & Lund, C. (1993). Skin-to-skin (kangaroo) holding of the intubated premature infant. *Neonatal Network, 12*(6), 49–57.

Himelstein, B. P. (2006). Palliative care for infants, children, adolescents, and their families. *Journal of Palliative Medicine, 9*(1), 163–181.

Hutton, N. (2002). Pediatric palliative care: The time has come. *Archives of Pediatrics & Adolescent Medicine, 156*(1), 9–10.

Institute of Medicine. (2003). *When children die: Improving palliative and end-of-life care for children and their families.* National Academies Press.

Jones, B. L., McClain, S., Greathouse, J., Legett, S., Hig-gerson, R. A., & Christie, L. A. (2007). Comfort and confidence levels of health care professionals providing pediatric palliative care in the intensive care unit. *Journal of Social Work in End-of-Life & Palliative Care, 3*(3), 39–58.

Joshi, D. (2005). "Virtual" pediatric palliative care: A novel concept for small pediatric programs. *Journal of Palliative Medicine, 8*(6), 1089–1090.

Kain, V. J. (2006). Palliative care delivery in the NICU: What barriers do neonatal nurses face? *Neonatal Network, 25*(6), 387–392.

Kain, V., Gardner, G., & Yates, P. (2009). Neonatal pallia-tive care attitude scale: Development of an instrument to measure the barriers to and facilitators of palliative care in neonatal nursing. *Pediatrics, 123*(2), e207–e211.

Kane, J. R. (2006). Pediatric palliative care moving for-ward: Empathy, competence, quality, and the need for systematic change. *Journal of Palliative Medicine, 9*(4), 847–849.

Kashaninia, Z., Sajedi, F., Rahgozar, M., & Noghabi, F. A. (2008). The effect of kangaroo care on behavioral responses to pain of an intramuscular injection in neonates. *Journal for Specialists in Pediatric Nursing, 13*(4), 275–280.

Kassity-Krich, N., & Jones, J. (2007). Complementary and integrative therapies. In Kenner, C. & Lott, J. W. (Eds.), *Comprehensive neonatal nursing: A physiologic perspective* (4th ed., pp. 543–550). W. Saunders.

Kassity, N. A., Jones, J., Kenner, C., Turner, A., & Hayes, M. J. (2003). Complementary therapies. In Kenner, C. & Lott, J. W. (Eds.), *Comprehensive neonatal nursing: A physiologic perspective* (3rd ed., pp. 868–875). W. B. Saunders.

Kenner, C., Press, J., & Ryan, D. (2015). Recommendations for palliative and bereavement care in the NICU: A family-centered integrative approach. *Journal of Perinatology, 35,* S19-S23.

Kopelman, A. E. (2006). Understanding, avoiding, and resolving end-of-life conflicts in the NICU. *The Mount Sinai Journal of Medicine, 73*(3), 580–586.

Kyc, S. J., Bruno, C. J., Shabanova, V., & Montgomery, A. M. (2020). Perceptions of neonatal palliative care: Similarities and differences between medical and nursing staff in a level IV neonatal intensive care unit. *Journal of Palliative Medicine, 23*(5), 662–660. https://doi.org/10.1089/jpm.2019.0523

Loewy, J., Hallan, C., Psych, L., Friedman, E., & Martinez, C. (2006). Sleep/sedation in children undergoing EEG testing: A comparison of chloral hydrate and music therapy. *American Journal of Electroneurodiagnostic Technology, 46*(4), 343–355.

Ludington-Hoe, S. M., Lewis, T., Morgan, K., Cong, X., Anderson, L., & Reese, S. (2006). Breast and infant temperatures with twins during shared kangaroo care. *Journal of Obstetric, Gynecologic, and Neonatal Nursing, 35*(2), 223–231.

Lundqvist, A., Nilstun, T., & Dykes, A. K. (2002) Experiencing neonatal death: An ambivalent transition to motherhood. *Pediatric Nursing, 28*(6), 621–625, 610.

Mackenzie, J., & MacCallam, J. (2009). Preparing staff to provide bereavement support. *Paediatric Nursing, 21*(3), 22–24.

Malcolm, C., Forbat, L. Knighting, K., & Kearney, N. (2008). Exploring the experiences and perspectives of families using a children's hospice and professionals providing hospice care to identify future research priorities for children's hospice care. *Palliative Medicine, 22,* 921–928.

McLaughlin, S. N., Song, M., Hertzberg, V., & Piazza, A. J. (2020). Use of palliative care consultation services for infants with life-threatening conditions in a metropolitan hospital. *Advances in Neonatal Care, 20*(2), 136–141. https://doi.org/10.1097/ANC.0000000000000698

Milstein, J. M. (2003). Detoxifying death in the neonate: In search of meaningfulness at the end of life. *Journal of Perinatology, 23,* 333–336.

Mizuno, K., Mizuno, N., Shinohara, T., & Noda, M. (2004). Mother-infant skin-to-skin contact after delivery results in early recognition of own mother's milk odour. *Acta Paediatrica, 93,* 1640–1645.

Morgan, D. (2009). Caring for dying children: Assessing the needs of the pediatric palliative care nurse. *Pediatric Nursing, 35*(2), 86–90.

Pearson, L. (1997). Family-centered care and the anticipated death of a newborn. *Pediatric Nursing, 23,* 178–182.

Penticuff, J. H. (1995). Nursing ethics in perinatal care. In Goldworth, A., Silverman, W., Stevenson, D. K., &Young, E. W. D. (Eds.), *Ethics and perinatology* (pp. 405–426). Oxford University Press.

Pierucci, R. L., Kirby, R. S., & Leuthner, S. R. (2001). End-of-life care for neonates and infants: The experience and effects of a palliative care consultation service. *Pediatrics, 108*(3), 653–660.

Raimbault, C., Saliba, E., & Porter, R. H. (2007). The effect of the odour of mother's milk on breastfeeding behaviour of premature neonates. *Acta Paediatrica, 96,* 368–371.

Rebagliato, M., Cuttini, M., Broggin, L., Berbik, I., de Vonderweid, U., Hansen, G., Kaminski, M., Kollée, L. A., Kucinskas, A., Lenoir, S., Levin, A., Persson, J., Reid, M., Saracci, R., & EURONIC Study Group (European Project on Parents' Information and Ethical Decision Making in Neonatal Intensive Care Units). (2000). Neonatal end-of-life decision making: Physicians' attitudes and relationship with self-reported practices in 10 European countries. *Journal of the American Medical Association, 284*(19), 2451–2459.

Rushton, C. H., Reder, E., Hall, B., Comello, K. Sellers, D. E., & Hutton, M. D. (2006). Interdisciplinary interventions to improve pediatric palliative care and reduce health care professional suffering. *Journal of Palliative Medicine, 9*(4), 922–933.

Sahler, O. J. (2000). Medical education about end-of-life care in the pediatric setting: Principles, challenges, and opportunities. *Pediatrics, 105*(3, Pt. 1), 575–584.

Sudia-Robinson, T. (2003). Hospice and palliative care. In Kenner, C. & Lott, J. W. (Eds.), *Comprehensive neonatal nursing: A physiologic perspective* (3rd ed., pp. 127–131). W. B. Saunders.

Sudia, T., & Catlin, A. (2019). Ethical issues. In Verklan, M. T. & Walden, M. (Eds.). *AWHONN: Core curriculum for neonatal intensive care nursing* (6th ed.). Elsevier Saunders.

Walden, M., & Carrier, C. (2009). The ten commandments of pain assessment and management in preterm neonates. *Critical Care Nursing Clinics of North America, 21*(2), 235–252.

Wolfe, J., Friebert, S., & Hilden, J. (2002). Caring for children with advanced cancer integrating palliative care. *Pediatric Clinics North of America, 49*(5), 1043–1062.

Wolfe, J., Klar, N., Grier, H. E., Duncan, J., Salem-Schatz, S., Emanuel, E. J., & Weeks, J. C. (2000). Understanding of prognosis among parents of children who died of cancer: Impact on treatment goals and integration of palliative care. *Journal of the American Medical Association, 284*(19), 2469–2475.

CHAPTER 20

Beyond the NICU: Measurable Outcomes of Developmental Care

Barbara A. Reyna, Nicole Cistone, and Rita H. Pickler

Standards in Systems Thinking

Standard 3: Systems thinking

- The practice of infant- and family-centered developmental care (IFCDC) in the intensive care unit (ICU) shall be based on evidence that is ethical, safe, timely, quality-driven, efficient, equitable, and cost-effective.

Standard 4: Systems thinking

- The ICU practice and outcomes will provide evidence that demonstrates the continuous monitoring of information relative to IFCDC practice.

Standard 6: Systems thinking

- The interprofessional collaborative team should provide IFCDC through transition to home and continuing care for the baby and family to support the optimal physiologic and psychosocial health needs of the baby and family.

Standards in Positioning and Touch

Standard 1: Positioning and touch

- Babies in intensive care settings shall be positioned to support musculoskeletal, physiological, and behavioral stability.

Standard 2: Positioning and touch

- Collaborative efforts among parents and ICU interprofessionals shall support optimal cranial shaping and prevent torticollis and skull deformity.

Standard 4: Positioning and touch

- Babies in ICU settings shall experience human touch by family and caregivers.

Standards in Sleep and Arousal

Standard 1: Sleep and arousal

- ICUs shall promote developmentally appropriate sleep and arousal states and sleep-wake cycles.

Standard 2: Sleep and arousal

- ICU shall provide modifications to the physical environment and to caregiving routines that are specifically focused on optimization of sleep and arousal of ICU babies.

Standard 3: Sleep and arousal

- The ICU shall encourage family presence at the baby's bedside and family participation in the care of their baby.

Standard 5: Sleep and arousal

- Families shall be provided multiple opportunities to observe and interpret their baby's state of arousal and sleep, and to practice safe sleep positioning, to support successful parent–infant participation in care routines during the transition home.

Standards in Skin-to-Skin Contact With Intimate Family Members

Standard 1: Skin-to-skin contact

- Parents shall be encouraged and supported in early, frequent, and prolonged skin-to-skin contact (SSC) with their babies.

Standard 4: Skin-to-skin contact

- Parents shall be provided information about the benefits of SSC that continue for babies and parents after discharge.

Standards in Reducing and Managing Pain and Stress in Newborns and Families

Standard 1: Pain and stress, Families

- The interprofessional team shall document increased parental/caregiver well-being and decreased emotional distress (WB/D) during the ICU stay. Distress levels of baby's siblings and extended family should also be considered.

Standard 2: Pain and stress, Babies

- The interprofessional collaborative team shall develop care practices that prioritize multiple methods to optimize baby outcomes by minimizing the impact of stressful and painful stimuli.

Standards in Feeding, Eating, and Nutrition Delivery

Standard 1: Feeding

- Feeding experiences in the ICU shall be behavior-based and baby-led. Baby-led principles are similar whether applied to enteral, breast, or bottle-feeding experience.

Standard 2: Feeding

- Every mother shall be encouraged and supported to breastfeed and/or provide human milk for her baby.

Standard 3: Feeding

- Nutrition shall be optimized during the ICU period.

Standard 5: Feeding

- Caregiving activities shall consider baby's response to input, especially around face/mouth, and aversive noncritical care oral experiences shall be minimized.

Standard 6: Feeding

- Professional staff shall consider smell and taste experiences that are biologically expected.

Standard 8: Feeding

- Environments shall be supportive of an attuned feeding for both the feeder and the baby.

Standard 11: Feeding

- Feeding management shall consider short- and long-term growth and feeding outcomes.

INTRODUCTION

Individualized, family-centered, developmental care (IFDC) for preterm and sick infants has resulted in both revolutionary and evolutionary change in neonatal care practices. For the purpose of this chapter, developmental care refers to strategies used to modify the neonatal intensive care unit (NICU) environment and approaches to care taken to reduce the effect of stressors on infant's developing brain. The concept of "developmental care" is derived from Als' work based on the Synactive Theory of Infant Development (Als, 1986), which provides a framework to understand the behavior of preterm and sick infants (Milette et al., 2017), although other frameworks for neonatal developmental care exist (Altimier & Phillips, 2013). IFDC incorporates many interventions, some of which have not been fully tested through well-designed research studies (Griffiths et al., 2019). Developmental care programs are designed primarily to bring about change in the NICU to mediate the effects of too much, too little, or inappropriate forms of stimulation. Some of these programs and their associated interventions may influence outcomes at discharge and beyond. However, the long-term effects of developmental interventions or programs have not been well studied, and when studied, long-term effects tend to be highly variable (Ohlsson & Jacobs, 2013).

When interpreting research for developmental care practices, it is important to consider the design limitations of studies (Spittle & Treyvaud, 2016). Although it is not possible to fully control for variations in care provided in the NICU, researchers should clearly describe aspects of care that were controlled. Additionally, variations in developmental care

practices themselves complicate interpretation of research reports. Challenges to research design also need to be identified and, to the extent possible, controlled. For example, it is difficult in studies conducted in open bay units to isolate control infants from all aspects of developmental care and to completely blind caregivers to treatment group assignment. In addition, maintaining developmental care interventions throughout the period required for studies measuring long-term outcomes poses a challenge. Many randomized control trials (RCTs) testing developmental care practices tend to use small samples, and although multicenter trials may result in a more adequate sample size, it is difficult to control for variations in nursing and clinical practice among centers (Burke, 2018; Soleimani et al., 2020).

Outcomes associated with developmental care in the NICU can be organized in several ways. Figure 20-1 illustrates one organizational approach. As seen in the figure, many factors may place an infant at risk for poor neurobehavioral development, which may be compounded by preterm birth. Although discussion of these risk factors is beyond the scope of this chapter, such risks include genetic predisposition, maternal infection or illness, and sociodemographic factors such as poverty (Pickler et al., 2010). These factors, along with preterm birth and postbirth conditions, may further compound an infant's risk for poor neurobehavioral outcomes (Crilly et al., 2021). A NICU hospitalization further potentiates an infant's risk for poor neurobehavioral outcomes, especially if those experiences do not support the infant's developing neurological system (Soleimani et al., 2020). Practices that support optimal development have the potential to improve outcomes. These practices may be

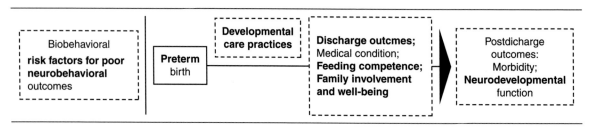

FIGURE 20-1. Model of discharge and postdischarge outcomes.

considered neuroprotective, especially if they take advantage of a preterm infant's neuroplasticity (Pickler et al., 2010). The improvements resulting from these practices often are seen at discharge, particularly improvements in medical condition, feeding competence, and parental involvement. Improved long-term outcomes of developmental care practices are more difficult to demonstrate; however, some evidence supports the effects of developmental care interventions and programs on long-term morbidity, neurodevelopmental function, and family well-being (Griffiths et al., 2019).

EVIDENCE TO SUPPORT INTEGRATING DEVELOPMENTAL CARE INTO ROUTINE PRACTICE OUTCOMES AT DISCHARGE

Despite the difficulties in studying developmental care practice outcomes, some research has focused on short-term outcomes and benefits at discharge that have been realized as the result of programs that fall under the developmental care umbrella. Although the methodologic quality of this research is mixed (Burke, 2018; Griffiths et al., 2019), some findings warrant consideration. See Table 20-1 for a summary of practice recommendations.

Reduced Morbidity

Improved medical outcomes during initial hospitalization have been associated with NICU care that is based on developmental care models. In particular, there is documentation from early research that use of individualized developmentally supportive practices results in fewer days during which mechanical ventilation and oxygen therapy are required (Als et al., 1986, 1994) and an associated decrease in severe lung disease and intraventricular hemorrhage (IVH), improved

self-regulatory abilities, and improved mental and psychomotor developmental at 9 months of age (Als et al., 1986, 1996; Als & Gilkerson, 1997; Buehler et al., 1995; Cardin et al., 2015). Additionally, developmental care practices have been shown to decrease length of hospital stay and cost, improved weight gain, decrease time to full enteral feeds, and improved neurodevelopmental outcomes at 9 to 12 months of age and up to 8 years of life (Cardin et al., 2015). Improved medical outcomes during initial hospitalization including reduction in severity of chronic lung disease and the incidence of IVH are also associated with NICU care that is based on developmental care models such as "small baby programs" and "IVH bundles" (de Bijl-Marcus et al., 2020). However, with limited evidence supporting individual interventions, the establishment of evidence-based protocols using an interdisciplinary team-based approach may be critical to improving both short- and long-term outcomes (Altimier & Phillips, 2018).

Despite these findings, there is conflicting evidence about the positive effects (Legendre et al., 2011; Symington & Pinelli, 2009). For example, in a study examining the effects of massage therapy on short- and long-term outcomes, only pain scores were significantly lower after treatment (Abdallah et al., 2013); there was no effect on weight gain, length of stay (LOS), motor scores, or breastfeeding duration. Moreover, in a recent study involving developmental care education, training, and intervention implementation, LOS increased after program implementation (Painter et al., 2019). A systematic review of the effects of developmental care on short-term medical outcomes and neurodevelopmental outcomes of preterm infants also found mixed results. Of the nine studies reviewed, four reported a decrease in oxygen support, fewer days on external feeds, better weight gain, better overall growth, and fewer days in the NICU for those infants who received developmental care compared to standard care (Legendre et al., 2011). However, results of the other five

TABLE 20-1 Practice Recommendations

Type	Recommendation	Level of Evidence	References
Morbidity	Formal, individualized developmental care programs Neuroprotective standardized care practices	II V	Als et al., 1986, Als & McAnulty, 2011 Altimier & Phillips, 2018
Neurodevelopmental function	Formal, individualized developmental care programs	II	Als et al., 1986, 1994, 2003
Feeding	Self-regulated feeding protocols Feeding experience	VI II	Pickler et al., 2009 Pickler et al., 2015, 2020
Family	Education for families about infant and child behaviors Target interventions to reduce stress and promote positive caring in the NICU	II II III II	Melnyk et al., 2006, 2008 Heo & Oh, 2019 Holditch-Davis et al., 2015 O'Brien et al., 2015

Note: Level I = evidence from a systematic review or meta-analysis of all relevant randomized controlled trials (RCTs) or evidence-based clinical practice guidelines based on systematic reviews of RCTs. Level II = evidence from at least one well-designed RCT. Level III = evidence from well-designed controlled trials without randomization. Level IV = evidence from well-designed case-control and cohort studies. Level V = evidence from systematic reviews of descriptive and qualitative studies. Level VI = evidence from a single descriptive or qualitative study. Level VII = evidence from the opinion of authorities and/or reports of expert committees.

studies showed no difference in respiratory support, days in the NICU, and overall growth for infants receiving developmental care.

When examining basic developmental care practices such as the use of incubator covers and nesting or swaddling devices, the effects are even less evident and the effect of these practices beyond the NICU has not been demonstrated. In addition, studies involving less intensive developmental care programs or individual interventions are limited in number and design (Symington & Pinelli, 2009).

Feeding Outcomes

Although beyond the scope of this chapter, we must acknowledge the overwhelming evidence of improved morbidity, including improved brain and neurocognitive development, in infants who receive mother's own milk (MOM) (Belfort et al., 2016; Smith et al., 2017). Please see Chapter 15 for more information on oral feedings. Beyond the substance of preterm infant feeding, however, there are a myriad of feeding practices that remain unresolved. For example, how and when oral feeds are initiated continues to be controversial, and feeding practices are highly variable among centers although several large centers have published guidelines with research support (Dutta et al., 2015). Assessing for oral feeding readiness is important to promote successful oral feeding as is managing the feeding environment (Pickler et al., 2013). Clinical pathways for advancing oral feedings that are cue-based or have indicators that rely on an infant's self-regulatory capacity have been touted as important for earlier achievement of full oral feeding (Shaker, 2013) and LOS. However, evidence supporting cue-based feeding is not based on well-designed research and is complicated by the inconsistent definition of "cues" or other infant behaviors suggesting readiness for oral feeding (Settle & Francis, 2019). Sucking behaviors are thought to be a barometer of central nervous system maturation as well as overall organization of behaviors and have been used as a measure for neurodevelopment outcomes (Alberts & Pickler, 2012; Lau, 2015). However, little research that involves IFDC interventions has measured sucking outcomes.

Providing more opportunities to oral feed and maximizing an infant's experience may result in more rapid maturation of sucking characteristics and promote a quicker transition to full oral feedings (Pickler et al., 2006, 2009). Additionally, a multisensory intervention showed improved sucking organization, suggesting the potential to improve maturation of oral feeding (Medoff-Cooper et al., 2015). Although there is only minimal evidence, patterned feeding experiences such as these that are designed to take advantage of neurobehavioral organization have shown promise in reducing the transition time from gavage to oral feeding and start of oral feeding to full oral feeding (Pickler et al., 2015, 2020). Of particular importance, the data are quite clear that once oral feedings have begun, infants who "miss" those feedings achieve full oral feedings much later and stay in the hospital much longer than those infants who have are offered the opportunity to oral feed at each scheduled feeding (Tubbs Cooley et al., 2015).

One feeding-related intervention often found within developmental care protocols that has demonstrated positive outcomes is nonnutritive sucking (NNS). Shortened LOS, secondary to shortened transition from all gavage feeding to oral feeding, is the primary beneficial effect of providing NNS during intermittent gavage feeding for low-birth-weight preterm infants (Say et al., 2018). NNS also appears to improve oral feeding performance (Foster et al., 2016) and may decrease the time to full oral feeds including infants who are breastfeeding (Grassi et al., 2019; Kaya & Aytekin, 2017). Offering NNS before feeding has not been shown to have a direct effect on nutritive suck, breathing, or behavior state during bottle feedings (Pickler & Reyna, 2004). Data on outcome measures with respect to offering NNS during gavage feeding are inconclusive, and further study is needed. No published studies have reported adverse outcomes associated with NNS when safe pacifiers are used (Foster et al., 2016).

POSTDISCHARGE OUTCOMES

Morbidity After Discharge

Despite substantial improvements in overall survival for preterm infants, there continues to be a high incidence of morbidity related to ongoing medical problems (Rogers & Hintz, 2016). Increased morbidity can result from complications of chronic lung disease, necrotizing enterocolitis (NEC), and IVH, which are themselves morbidities of prematurity. Follow-up studies have revealed high rates of neurobehavioral disability among very preterm infants born before 28 weeks postmenstrual age with the highest risk group being those born at 22 to 25 weeks and surviving (Anderson et al., 2016). Motor delays are common in preterm infants, with rates of cerebral palsy increasing for infants born at younger gestational ages (Spittle et al., 2020). Although it can be reassuring when an infant does not experience an IVH, more subtle neurologic findings can become apparent throughout childhood, manifesting as difficulties with coordination, completing activities of daily living, and atypical fine motor abilities (Romeo et al., 2021).

Determining specific developmental care practices that influence longer term outcomes remain elusive. However, in a longitudinal, multicenter study, very preterm infants hospitalized in NICUs with lower quality of developmental care practices had lower levels of neurobehavioral adaptability at 18 months of age. In addition, mothers whose infants were hospitalized in NICUs assessed to have lower quality developmental care practices demonstrated greater postnatal depressive symptoms at infant discharge and when infants were 6 months (Montirosso et al., 2018).

Efforts have specifically examined the effects of developmental care practices on long-term morbidity outcomes, including those related to respiratory function. However, the data are conflicting with some studies showing no significant differences in short-term medical outcomes or long-term neurodevelopment, and no specific developmental care program appears to have an advantage over general developmentally supportive care (Ohlsson et al., 2013).

Perhaps more promising, a Cochrane review of the effects of early-intervention programs for preterm infants after NICU discharge showed favorable effects on cognitive and motor outcomes during infancy with some of the cognitive benefits evident at preschool age. However, just like NICU developmental care practices, there is variability in postdischarge intervention programs that makes it difficult to draw substantial conclusions (Spittle et al., 2015). Nevertheless, having parents participate in developmental care interventions has been shown to help them acquire the capacity to provide developmentally supportive care after discharge, which can bridge the gap with early intervention services (Dusing et al., 2018; Spittle & Treyvaud, 2016).

The risk of rehospitalization after NICU discharge increases with decreasing gestational age at birth. Infants with chronic conditions such as bronchopulmonary dysplasia and short bowel syndrome may require rehospitalization for exacerbation of their chronic disease. Children with complex medical needs at discharge including those with genetic or congenital abnormalities are more likely to require emergency department visits and inpatient admissions (Kieran et al., 2019). Other infants may require rehospitalization or emergency department care for acute respiratory illness, gastrointestinal or growth problems, infection other than respiratory illness, and surgery (Luu et al., 2010). The most vulnerable infants appear to be those with prolonged NICU hospitalizations, those born <28 weeks gestation, and those infants with more than one major morbidity at discharge (Ambalavanan et al., 2011; Kuint et al., 2017; Luu et al., 2010).

Despite these statistics, there are no data correlating developmental care practices to either acute-care visits or rehospitalization rates. For example, although there are published data that detail rates of readmission after NICU discharge, these data have not kept up with changing trends in either preterm infant care (such as new ventilator treatments) or healthcare trends. Moreover, while comparisons to current rates of readmission may be useful as developmental care becomes more widely practiced, it will be difficult to distinguish the independent effects of developmental care versus those related to other changes in NICU care. Research that accounts for the interactions of all these variables should be developed so that long-term implications of developmental care practices in the NICU can be better assessed and recommendations for future practices can be made.

Neurobehavioral Function

Preterm birth places a child at a higher risk for poor developmental outcomes of long-term duration (Blencowe et al., 2013; Harmon et al., 2015). Infants born preterm historically have a high incidence of poor neurodevelopmental outcome, including low intelligence quotient, cerebral palsy, visual impairment, hearing impairment, and learning disabilities (Blencowe et al., 2013; Jarjour, 2015). Nearly 20% of preterm infants develop major cognitive disabilities by middle-school age. Consequently, although survival of preterm infants has improved dramatically over the past 3 decades, the incidence of major disability in these children remains high depending upon year of birth, birth weight, and birth gestation (Jarjour, 2015). In addition, although the incidence of major motor, sensory, and intellectual handicaps in preterm infants who do not have significant medical complications has declined, there is continuing concern that the physical and social characteristics of the NICU environment may delay or distort optimal developmental patterns. In fact, improved survival rates of the gestationally youngest preterm infants may place these children at higher developmental risk because they typically remain hospitalized for extended periods when their neurologic and behavioral systems are immature and unstable (Legendre et al., 2011).

Individualized developmental care during hospitalization has been found to have positive short-term effects on autonomic, motor, behavioral, and attentional organization in preterm infants (Cardin et al., 2015). Neurobehavioral improvements in the period immediately after discharge also have been documented (Buehler et al., 1995; Feldman & Eidelman, 1998; Ohgi et al., 2002). Assessing the longer term benefits of developmental care has proven more difficult, especially in such areas as cognition and motor outcomes although some researchers have reported continuation of improvements in the immediate postdischarge period (Als et al., 2004; Legendre et al., 2011; Peters et al., 2009).

Cognitive development is an important outcome to consider when evaluating the benefits of interventions based on models of developmental care. Although intelligence quotations (IQs) may be normal for many children who were born preterm, many children born preterm will have lower cognitive scores on standardized tests with lower scores for motor skills, behavior, reading, mathematics, and spelling (Allotey et al., 2018). Most cognitive deficits persist at least through high school with gestational age at birth accounted for well over a third of the variable in IQ. Moreover, "behavior" disorders including attention-deficit/hyperactivity disorder (0 and autism spectrum disorders) are more common in children who were born preterm, making learning more difficult (Altimier & Phillips, 2016; Arpi & Ferrari, 2013).

Intervention studies designed to improve neurodevelopmental outcomes of premature infants in the NICU are limited in number and quality (Burke, 2018). Developmental care in the NICU appears to have some positive effects on the neurodevelopment of preterm infants in the short-term, but there is no systematic review of long-term outcomes of individualized developmental care. However, despite the paucity of research findings demonstrating clear effects of developmental care on long-term neurodevelopmental outcomes, some studies suggest important benefits to more contingently patterned caregiving. For example, research involving a small sample has shown that preterm infants who receive individualized developmental care during hospitalization have more differentiation of brain tissue than full-term peers (Pickler et al., 2017). This differentiation shows particularly interesting changes in frontal lobe functioning, an area associated with attention and memory, although further research is needed to substantiate these findings. Long-term studies of Newborn Individualized Developmental Care and Assessment Program (NIDCAP®) (Boston, MA) have also shown that improved neurobehavior and morbidity in the newborn period predict the beneficial brain function effects at age eight, again in a small sample (McAnulty et al., 2010).

Another area of major concern for infants born preterm is motor function. Birth weight is a major predictor of motor development; the lower the birth weight, the greater the likelihood of delays in motor development. As the survival rates have increased for extremely premature infants, 40% to 60% of survivors born less than 28 weeks gestation may develop moderate to severe impairments including cerebral palsy, intellectual disabilities, deafness, and blindness (Parikh & Juul, 2019).

Parental Involvement and Family Well-Being

Lengthy hospital stays in NICUs can jeopardize the development of maternal/parental-infant attachment by impeding close contact between mothers, fathers, and their babies (Woodward et al., 2014). It is well established that prolonged hospitalization of preterm infants has detrimental effects on family functioning and parent–child interaction. In particular, disruptions of the parent–child relationship and the inability to feel like a parent are significant sources of stress for parents of hospitalized preterm infants (Griffin & Pickler, 2011; Provenzi et al., 2016). In addition, parenting can be affected by global concern regarding the health and well-being of their infant. The anxiety and worry over whether an infant will survive and thrive after discharge may continue to influence parents long after discharge from the NICU (Holditch-Davis et al., 2015; Schappin et al., 2013).

There is evidence supporting the ongoing psychological distress experienced by mothers of preterm infants. Mothers report the event itself of delivering preterm is traumatic and the feelings are reexperienced on their child's first birthday. Other posttraumatic symptoms reported at 1 year include fatigue, depressive mood, and anxiety (Garel et al., 2006; Jubinville et al., 2012). Hence, the psychological distress experienced by mothers of preterm infants is a complex combination of depressive symptoms, stress, anxiety, and posttraumatic stress symptoms. Mothers who experience very high distress and those with high depressive and anxiety symptoms remain at high risk of significant psychological distress for up to 1 year after discharge and also have less positive perceptions of their infants (Holditch-Davis et al., 2015). Identifying mothers in the NICU at increased risk

for ongoing psychological distress after discharge can help with targeting interventions to reduce or alleviate distress and promote positive coping mechanisms. Implementing a "buddy" program to provide support from trained peers can help mothers deal with the stress of a preterm birth (Hall et al., 2015; Preyde & Ardal, 2003). NICU follow-up programs should include psychological screening and support services. Further studies are needed to understand the influence of developmental care interventions on long-term psychological well-being.

Providing care that recognizes the family as an active member of the care team positively influences family functioning and parental well-being. Interventions and strategies that support parental presence and participation can reduce parental stress and support infant development. For example, the more an infant is held has been associated with better reflex development and better gross and fine motor development. In addition, whereas both being held by a parent in their arms and held skin-to-skin have been associated with better short-term developmental outcomes, only skin-to-skin holding has been associated with better long-term developmental outcomes (Pineda et al., 2018). Practices such as early skin-to-skin holding and 24-hour visitation encourage parental involvement. Creating family-friendly spaces, reducing environmental noise, and providing parents with details about procedures and prognoses are opportunities that can facilitate maternal engagement and parenting confidence (Klawetter et al., 2019). Thus, parental visitation and holding are important interventions for healthy attachment and may influence early developmental outcomes (Reynolds et al., 2013). Identifying barriers to parental visitation and implementing interventions that promote engagement are critical.

The family integrated care (FIC) model is a program that promotes parents as the lead providers of all care (except for advanced care) for their infants while nurses provide education and support. Four pillars comprise the program; parent education, nursing staff education and support, psychosocial support, and NICU environment (Cheng et al., 2019). Improved breastfeeding rates and reduced stress and anxiety prior to discharge have been reported with parents participating in this program (O'Brien et al., 2015; Verma et al., 2017). Strategies such as parental participation in daily rounds, NICU tours by other parents, a parent buddy program, and involving parents in major milestones such as the first gavage feed are recommended for parents to promote involvement (Cheng et al., 2019).

Intervention programs initiated in the NICU such as NIDCAP facilitates a mother's feeling of closeness to her infant (Kleberg et al., 2007). The NIDCAP framework embraces skin-to-skin or kangaroo mother care as an integral intervention for supporting the parent-infant dyad by promoting physical and emotional closeness (Als & McAnulty, 2011). However, there have been mixed results on the impact of NIDCAP on parenting stress and on enhancing parents' perceptions of their infants (Kleberg et al., 2007; van der Pal et al., 2007). For some mothers, there was a perceived greater level of nursing support, increased confidence in their caregiving abilities, and greater satisfaction with NICU nursing care (Sannino et al., 2016). Programs that provide parent education also have been shown to reduce parental stress, enhance coping during hospitalization, and reduce depressive symptoms after discharge (Heo & Oh, 2019; Melnyk et al., 2006, 2008).

There are a limited number of reliable tools that specifically measure parent satisfaction with NICU care and the outcomes of IFDC. Institutions frequently assess parental satisfaction after discharge with generalized questionnaires that are designed to measure parental satisfaction with overall hospitalization; these questionnaires seldom include items related to NICU practices or IFDC. A systematic review of available instruments measuring parent satisfaction with family-centered care (FCC) in the NICU found 11 studies published from 2006 to 2016 meeting this criterion. Only two of the instruments included all six of the FCC principles with the other studies including most of the principles. Psychometric analysis of the instruments was limited (Dall'Oglio et al., 2018). The two validated instruments available to assess parent satisfaction with FCC were the empowerment of parents in the intensive care neonatology (EMPATHIC-N) and the Neonatal Satisfaction Survey (NSS)-13 (Dall'Oglio et al., 2018).

The empowerment of parents in the intensive care (EMPATHIC) instrument was developed in the Netherlands to measure parent satisfaction in pediatric ICUs (Latour et al., 2012). Shorter versions have been introduced and the EMPATHIC-N was developed to measure NICU parent satisfaction. The tools contain five domains that address care provider performance and include parental satisfaction and a domain for parental participation. They have been translated into other languages and psychometric properties established (Lake et al., 2020). The EMPATHIC-NICU-USA Questionnaire has recently been adapted from the EMPATHIC-30 instrument for English and Spanish speaking parents in the United States. Additional items were added from the EMPATHIC-N instrument in order to capture the distinctive aspects of NICU nursing care of infants and parents. Thus, the tool has been linguistically adapted and demonstrates satisfactory psychometric properties and for use with the diverse racial and ethnic backgrounds of NICU parents in the United States (Lake et al., 2020).

The NSS-13 was developed through literature reviews, focus groups conducted with health personnel and parents of children in the NICU, and then tested with parents in a pilot study and further refined. The survey consists of 13 categories and 69 items exploring areas of care in which parents were dissatisfied. A drawback of the instrument is it has only been tested in Norway and not in an English-speaking population (Hagen et al., 2015).

Tools measuring parent satisfaction with NICU care hold promise for providing valuable information to better refine care practices that meet their needs. However, parents are not aware of the spectrum of developmental care options that might be available for their infant. Surveys targeting specific developmental care practices and evaluating how they contribute to parental feelings of competence and well-being during hospitalization and after discharge need to be tested and validated.

CONCLUSION

Research on the outcomes of individualized developmental care has demonstrated modest improvement in both short- and long-term outcomes for preterm infants. Although NIDCAP and similar programs have been used in the NICU setting for more than 30 years, little research has been done outside of major NIDCAP centers to demonstrate the long-term effect of these programs or of specific interventions included in the programs. The lack of rigorously conducted research and the limited number of interventions that have been developed and studied contributes to a paucity of data about effectiveness.

Long-term follow-up studies of children who were born preterm and hospitalized in NICUs before the widespread use of developmental care programs clearly demonstrate the serious, enduring sequelae to preterm birth and lengthy stays in NICUs (Sullivan et al., 2012a, 2012b). In addition, new theoretical frameworks and new basic science research about brain and neurologic development suggest a need to revisit some conceptual ideas, assumptions, and outcome expectations (Nist et al., 2019).

As research continues on the effects of developmental care on both short- and long-term outcomes for preterm infants, investigators and clinicians should be aware of the mediation of the home environment on these outcomes. The effects of the early social environment and parent-infant interactions over time can influence later development and must be considered when examining the long-term benefits of developmental care practices (Spittle & Treyvaud, 2016). In addition, the neuroplasticity of the human brain allows for at least some mediation of the adverse effects of the NICU environment (DeMaster et al., 2019).

As research continues to improve our understanding of the effect of neonatal intensive care on short- and long-term outcomes, attention will need to be given to ensuring adequately sized and diverse samples from many settings. In addition, clinicians and researchers will need to clarify language regarding the type and character of developmental care being provided and studied. Environmental and individually directed interventions that reduce or modify the adverse characteristics of the NICU based on developmental care models require further study before recommendations can be made for universal adoption. Research about these interventions must be methodologically sound, and measures of effectiveness should incorporate short- and long-term biologic and behavioral outcomes. As research in this area proceeds, the underlying mechanisms by which developmental care interventions result in improved outcomes will be revealed and incorporated into routine caregiving in the NICU.

Potential Research Questions

Neurodevelopmental Function

- What are the long-term benefits of specific or programmatic developmental practices beyond the first 2 years of life? Are there measurable effects at school age or beyond?
- What are the effects of developmental care practices on sensory disorders?
- What is the influence of developmental care practice bundles on short- and long-term neurodevelopmental outcomes?
- What interventions postdischarge optimize long-term neurodevelopmental outcomes?

Morbidity

- What are the effects of developmental care practices on rehospitalization rates?
- Do developmental practice models influence the morbidities associated with NICU hospitalization?

Feeding Outcomes

- Do developmental care practices improve feeding skill development and nutritional outcomes in both the short and long term?

Family Outcomes

- What developmental care practices are most likely to improve parent involvement during hospitalization and family well-being in the postdischarge period?
- What markers of parent distress in the NICU predict maternal psychological well-being postdischarge?
- Which developmental care interventions or practices do parents find most meaningful?
- Do socioeconomic, race, and cultural differences influence the outcomes of developmental care practices?

Cost-of-Care

- What is the cost-effectiveness of developmental care practice models?

REFERENCES

Abdallah, B., Badr, L. K., & Hawwari, M. (2013). The efficacy of massage on short and long term outcomes in preterm infants. *Infant Behavior & Development, 36*, 662–669. https://doi.org/10.1016/j.infbeh.2013.06.009

Alberts, J. R., & Pickler, R. H. (2012). Evolution and development of dual ingestion systems in mammals: Notes on a new thesis and its clinical implications. *International Journal of Pediatrics, 2012*, 730673. https://doi.org/10.1155/2012/730673

Allotey, J., Zamora, J., Cheong-See, F., Kalidindi, M., Arroyo-Manzano, D., Asztalos, E., van der Post, J. A. M., Mol, B. W., Moore, D., Birtles, D., Khan, K. S., & Thangaratinam, S. (2018). Cognitive, motor, behavioural and academic performances of children born preterm: A meta-analysis and systematic review involving 64061 children. *British Journal of Obstetrics and Gynecology, 125*, 16–25. https://doi.org/10.1111/1471-0528.14832

Als, H. (1986). A synactive model of neonatal behavioral organization: Framework for the assessment of neurobehavioral development in the premature infant and for support of infants and parents in the neonatal intensive care environment. *Physical & Occupational Therapy in Pediatrics, 6*(3–4), 3–53. https://doi.org/10.1080/J006v06n03_02

Als, H., Duffy, F. H., & McAnulty, G. B. (1996). Effectiveness of individualized developmental care in the newborn intensive care unit (NICU). *Acta Pediatrics Supplement, 416*, 21–30.

Als, H., Duffy, F. H., McAnulty, G. B., Rivkin, M. J., Vajapeyam, S., Mulkern, R. V., Warfield, S. K., Huppi, P. S., Butler, S. C., Conneman, N., Fischer, C., & Eichenwald, E. C. (2004). Early experience alters brain function and structure. *Pediatrics, 113*, 846–857. https://doi-org.proxy.lib.ohio-state.edu/10.1542/peds.113.4.846

Als, H., & Gilkerson, L. (1997). The role of relationship-based developmentally supportive newborn intensive care in strengthening outcome of preterm infants. *Seminars in Perinatology, 21*, 178–189. https://doi.org/10.1016/S0146-0005(97)80062-6

Als, H., Gilkerson, L., Duffy, F. H., McAnulty, G. B., Buehler, D. M., Vandenberg, K., Sweet, N., Sell, E., Parad, R. B., Ringer, S. A., Butler, S. C., Blickman, J. G., & Jones, K. J. (2003). A three-center, randomized, controlled trial of individualized developmental care for very low birth weight preterm infants: Medical, neurodevelopmental, parenting, and caregiving effects. *Journal of Developmental and Behavioral Pediatrics, 24*, 399–408. https://doi-org.proxy.lib.ohio-state.edu/10.1097/00004703-200312000-00001

Als, H., Lawhon, G., Duffy, F. H., McAnulty, G. B., Gibes-Grossman, R., & Blickman, J. G. (1994). Individualized developmental care for the very low-birth-weight preterm infant: Medical and neurofunctional effects. *Journal of the American Medical Association, 272*, 853–858. https://doi.org/10.1001/jama.1994.03520110033025

Als, H., & McAnulty, G. B. (2011). The Newborn Individualized Developmental Care and Assessment Program (NIDCAP) with Kangaroo Mother Care (KMC): Comprehensive care for preterm infants. *Current Women's Health Reviews, 7*, 288–301. https://doi.org/10.2174/157340411796355216

Altimier, L., & Phillips, R. M. (2013). The neonatal integrative developmental care model: Seven neuroprotective care measures for family-centered developmental care. *Newborn & Infant Nursing Reviews, 13*, 9–22. https://doi.org/10.1053/j.nainr.2012.12.002

Altimier, L., & Phillips, R. (2016). The neonatal integrative developmental care model: Advanced clinical applications of the seven core measures for neuroprotective family-centered developmental care. *Newborn and Infant Nursing Reviews, 16*, 230–244. https://doi.org/10.1053/j.nainr.2016.09.030

Altimier, L., & Phillips, R. (2018). Neuroprotective care of extremely preterm infants in the first 72 hours after birth. *Critical Care Nursing Clinics of North America, 30*, 563–583. https://doi.org/10.1016/j.cnc.2018.07.010

Ambalavanan, N., Carlo, W. A., McDonald, S. A., Yao, Q., Das, A., Higgins, R. D., & Generic Database and Follow-up Subcommittees of the Eunice Kennedy Shriver National Institute of Child Health and Human Development Neonatal Research Network. (2011). Identification of extremely premature infants at high risk of rehospitalization. *Pediatrics, 128*(5), e1216–e1225. https://doi.org/10.1542/peds.2011-1142

Anderson, J. G., Baer, R. J., Partridge, J. C., Kuppermann, M., Franck, L. S., Rand, L., Jelliffe-Pawlowski, L. L., & Rogers, E. E. (2016). Survival and major morbidity of extremely preterm infants: A population-based study. *Pediatrics, 138*(1), e20154434. https://doi.org/10.1542/peds.2015-4434

Arpi, E., & Ferrari, F. (2013). Preterm birth and behaviour problems in infants and preschool-age children: A review of the recent literature. *Developmental Medicine and Child Neurology, 55*, 788–796. https://doi.org/10.1111/dmcn.12142

Belfort, M. B., Anderson, P. J., Nowak, V. A., Lee, K. J., Molesworth, C., Thompson, D. K., Doyle, L. W., & Inder, T. E. (2016). Breast milk feeding, brain development, and neurocognitive outcomes: A 7-year longitudinal study in infants born <30 weeks' gestation. *Journal of Pediatrics, 177*, 133–139. https://doi.org/10.1016/j.jpeds.2016.06.045

de Bijl-Marcus, K., Brouwer, A. J., De Vries, L. S., Groenendaal, F., & Wezel-Meijler, G. V. (2020). Neonatal care bundles are associated with a reduction in the incidence of intraventricular haemorrhage in preterm infants: A multicentre cohort study. *Archives of Disease in Childhood. Fetal and Neonatal Edition, 105*, 419–424. https://doi.org/10.1136/archdischild-2018-316692

Blencowe, H., Lee, A. C. C., Cousens, S., Bahalim, A., Narwal, R., Zhong, N., Chou, D., Say, L., Modi, N., Katz, J., Vos, T., Marlow, N., & Lawn, J. E. (2013). Preterm birth-associated neurodevelopmental impairment estimates at regional and global levels for 2010. *Pediatric Research, 74*(Suppl. 1), 17–34. https://doi.org/10.1038/pr.2013.204

Buehler, D. M., Als, H., Duffy, F. H., McAnulty, G. B., & Liederman, J. (1995). Effectiveness of individualized developmental care for low-risk preterm infants: Behavioral and electrophysiologic evidence. *Pediatrics, 96*, 923–932.

Burke, S. (2018). Systematic review of developmental care interventions in the neonatal intensive care unit since 2006. *Journal of Child Health Care, 22*, 269–286. https://journals.sagepub.com/doi/10.1177/1367493517753085

Cardin, A. D., Rens, L., Stewart, S., Danner-Bowman, K., McCarley, R., & Kopsas, R. (2015). Neuroprotective core measures 1–7: A developmental care journey. Transformations in NICU design and caregiving attitudes. *Newborn and Infant Nursing Reviews, 15*, 132–141. https://doi.org/10.1053/j.nainr.2015.06.007

Cheng, C., Franck, L. S., Ye, X. Y., Hutchinson, S. A., Lee, S. K., & O'Brien, K. (2019). Evaluating the effect of family integrated care on maternal stress and anxiety in neonatal intensive care units. *Journal of Reproductive and Infant Psychology, 39*, 166–179. https://doi.org/10.1080/02646838.2019.1659940

Crilly, C. J., Haneuse, S., & Litt, J. S. (2021). Predicting the outcomes of preterm neonates beyond the neonatal intensive care unit: What are we missing? *Pediatric Research, 89*(3), 426–445. https://doi.org/10.1038/s41390-020-0968-5

Dall'Oglio, I., Mascolo, R., Gawronski, O., Tiozzo, E., Portanova, A., Ragni, A., Alvaro, R., Rocco, G., & Latour, J. M. (2018). A systematic review of instruments for assessing parent satisfaction with family-centred care in neonatal intensive care units. *Acta Paediatrica, 107*, 391–402. https://doi.org/10.1111/apa.14186

DeMaster, D., Bick, J., Johnson, U., Montroy, J. J., Landry, S., & Duncan, A. F. (2019). Nurturing the preterm infant brain: Leveraging neuroplasticity to improve neurobehavioral outcomes. *Pediatric Research, 85*, 166–175. https://doi.org/10.1038/s41390-018-0203-9

Dusing, S. C., Tripathi, T., Marcinowski, E. C., Thacker, L. R., Brown, L. F., & Hendricks-Munoz, K. D. (2018). Supporting play exploration and early developmental intervention versus usual care to enhance development outcomes during the transition from the neonatal intensive care unit to home: A pilot randomized controlled trial. *BMC Pediatrics, 18*, 46. https://doi.org/10.1186/s12887-018-1011-4

Dutta, S., Singh, B., Chessell, L., Wilson, L., Janes, M., McDonald, K., Shahid, S., Gardner, V. A., Hjartarson, A., Purcha, M., Watson, J., de Boer, C., Gaal, B., & Fusch, C. (2015). Guidelines for feeding very low birth weight infants. *Nutrients, 7*, 423–442. https://doi.org/10.3390/nu7010423

Feldman, R., & Eidelman, A. I. (1998). Intervention programs for premature infants: How and do they affect development? *Clinics in Perinatology, 25*, 613–625. https://doi.org/10.1016/S0095-5108(18)30101-5

Foster, J. P., Psaila, K., & Patterson, T. (2016). Non-nutritive sucking for increasing physiologic stability and nutrition in preterm infants. *Cochrane Database of Systematic Reviews, 2016*(10), CD001071. https://doi.org/10.1002/14651858.CD001071.pub3

Garel, M., Dardennes, M., & Blondel, B. (2006). Mothers' psychological distress 1 year after very preterm childbirth: Results of the EPIPAGE qualitative study. *Child: Care, Health and Development, 33*, 137–143. https://doi.org/10.1111/j.1365-2214.2006.00663.x

Grassi, A., Sgherri, G., Chorna, O., Marchi, V., Gagliardi, L., Cecchi, F., Laschi, C., & Guzzetta, A. (2019). Early intervention to improve sucking in preterm newborns: A systematic review of quantitative studies. *Advances in Neonatal Care, 19*, 97–109. https://doi.org/10.1097/ANC.0000000000000543

Griffin, J. B., & Pickler, R. H. (2011). Hospital-to-home: Transition of mothers of preterm infants. *The American Journal of Maternal Child Nursing, 36*(4), 252–257. https://doi.org/10.1097/NMC.0b013e31821770b8

Griffiths, N., Spence, K., Loughran-Fowlds, A., & Westrupef, B. (2019). Individualised developmental care for babies and parents in the NICU: Evidence-based best practice guideline recommendations. *Early Human Development, 139*, 104840. https://doi.org/10.1016/j.earlhumdev.2019.104840

Hagen, I. H., Vadset, T. B., Barstad, J., & Svindseth, M. F. (2015). Development and validation of Neonatal Satisfaction Survey—NSS-13. *Scandinavian Journal of Caring Sciences, 29*, 395–406. https://doi.org/10.1111/scs.12156

Hall, S. L., Ryan, D. J., Beatty, J., & Grubbs, L. (2015). Recommendations for peer-to-peer support for NICU parents. *Journal of Perinatology, 35*, S9-S13. https://doi.org/10.1038/jp.2015.143

Harmon, H. M., Taylor, H. G., Minich, N., Wilson-Costello, D., & Hack, M. (2015). Early school outcomes for extremely preterm infants with transient neurological abnormalities. *Developmental Medicine and Child Neurology, 57*, 865–871. https://doi.org/10.1111/dmcn.12811

Heo, Y. J., & Oh, W. O. (2019). The effectiveness of a parent participation improvement program for parents on partnership, attachment infant growth in a neonatal intensive care unit: A randomized controlled trial. *International Journal of Nursing Studies, 95*, 19–27. https://doi.org/10.1016/j.ijnurstu.2019.03.018

Holditch-Davis, D., Hudson, S., Levy, J., White-Traut, R., O'Shea, M., Geraldo, V., & David, R. (2015). Patterns of psychological distress in mothers of preterm infants. *Infant Behavior and Development, 41*, 154–163. https://doi.org/10.1016/j.infbeh.2015.10.004

Jarjour, I. T. (2015). Neurodevelopmental outcome after extreme prematurity: A review of the literature. *Pediatric Neurology, 52*, 143–152. https://doi.org/10.1016/j.pediatrneurol.2014.10.027

Jubinville, J., Newburn-Cook, C., Hegadoren, K., & Lacaze-Masmonteil, T. (2012). Symptoms of acute stress disorder in mothers of premature infants. *Advances in Neonatal Care, 12*, 246–253. https://doi.org/10.1097/ANC.0b013e31826090ac

Kaya, V., & Aytekin, A. (2017). Effects of pacifier use on transition to full breastfeeding and sucking skills in preterm infants: A randomised controlled trial. *Journal of Clinical Nursing, 26*(13–14), 2055–2063. https://doi.org/10.1111/jocn.13617

Kieran, E., Sara, R., Claydon, J., Hait, V., de Salaberry, J., Osiovich, H., & Shivananda, S. (2019). Outcomes of neonates with complex medical needs. *Advances in Neonatal Care, 19*, 275–284. https://doi.org/10.1097/ANC.0000000000000639

Klawetter, S., Neu, M., Roybal, K. L., Greenfield, J. C., Scott, J., & Hwang, S. (2019). Mothering in the NICU: A qualitative exploration maternal engagement. *Social Work in Health Care, 58*, 746–763. https://doi.org/10.1080/00981389.2019.1629152

Kleberg, A., Hellström-Westas, L., & Widström, A. (2007). Mothers' perception of newborn individualized developmental care and assessment program (NIDCAP) as compared to conventional care. *Early Human Development, 83*, 403–411. https://doi.org/10.1016/j.earlhumdev.2006.05.024

Kuint, J., Lerner-Geva, L., Chodick, G., Boyko, V., Shalev, V., Reichman, B., & the Israel Neonatal Network. (2017). Rehospitalization through childhood and adolescence: Association with neonatal morbidities in infants of very low birth weight. *The Journal of Pediatrics, 188*, 135.e2-141.e2. https://doi.org/10.1016/j.jpeds.2017.05.078

Lake, E. T., Smith, J. G., Staiger, D. O., Schoenauer, K. M., & Rogowski, J. A. (2020). Measuring parent satisfaction with care in neonatal intensive care units: The EMPATHIC-NICU-USA questionnaire. *Frontiers in Pediatrics, 8*, 541573. https://doi.org/10.3389/fped.2020.541573

Latour, J. M., Duivenvoorden, H. J., Hazelzet, J. A., & van Goudoever, J. B. (2012). Development and validation of a neonatal intensive care parent satisfaction instrument. *Pediatric Critical Care Medicine, 13*, 554–559. https://doi.org/10.1097/PCC.0b013e318238b80a

Lau, C. (2015). Development of suck and swallow mechanisms in infants. *Annals of Nutrition & Metabolism, 66*(suppl 5), 7–14. https://doi.org/10.1159/000381361

Legendre, V., Burtner, P. A., Martinez, K. L., & Crowe, T. K. (2011). The evolving practice of developmental care in the neonatal unit: A systematic review. *Physical & Occupational Therapy in Pediatrics, 31*(3), 315–338. https://doi.org/10.3109/01942638.2011.556697

Luu, T. M., Lefebvre, F., Riley, P., & Infante-Rivard, C. (2010). Continuing utilisation of specialised health services in extremely preterm infants. *Archives of Disease in Childhood. Fetal and Neonatal Edition, 95*(5), F320–F325. https://doi.org/10.1136/adc.2009.173138

McAnulty, G. B., Duffy, F. H., Butler, S. C., Bernstein, J. H., Zurakowski, D., & Als, H. (2010). Effects of the Newborn Individualized Developmental Care and Assessment Program (NIDCAP) at age 8 years: Preliminary data. *Clinical Pediatrics, 49*, 258–270. https://doi.org/10.1177/0009922809335668

Medoff-Cooper, B., Rankin, K., Li, Z., Liu, L., & White-Traut, R. (2015). Multisensory intervention for preterm infants improves sucking organization. *Advances in Neonatal Care, 15*, 142–149. https://doi.org/10.1097/ANC.0000000000000166

Melnyk, B. M., Crean, H. F., Feinstein, N. F., & Fairbanks, E. (2008). Maternal anxiety and depression after a pre-mature infant's discharge from the neonatal intensive care unit: Explanatory effects of the creating opportunities for parent empowerment program. *Nursing Research, 57*, 383–394. https://doi.org/10.1097/NNR.0b013e3181906f59

Melnyk, B. M., Feinstein, N. F., Alpert-Gillis, L., Fairbanks, E., Crean, H. F., & Sinkin, R. A. (2006). Reducing premature infants' length of stay and improving parents' mental health outcomes with the Creating Opportunities for Parent Empowerment (COPE) neonatal intensive care unit program: A randomized, controlled trial. *Pediatrics, 118*(5), e1414–e1427. https://doi.org/10.1542/peds.2005-2580

Milette, I., Martel, M. J., Ribeiro da Silva, M., & Coughlin McNeil, M. (2017). Guidelines for the institutional implementation of developmental neuroprotective care in the neonatal intensive care unit. Part A: Background and rationale. A joint position statement from the CANN, CAPWHN, NANN, and COINN. *The Canadian Journal of Nursing Research, 49*(2), 46–62. https://doi.org/10.1177/0844562117706882

Montirosso, R., Giusti, L., De Carli, P., Tronick, E., Borgatti, R., & NEO-ACQUA Study Group. (2018). Developmental care, neonatal behavior and postnatal maternal depressive symptomatology predict internalizing problems at 18 months for very preterm children. *Journal of Perinatology, 38*, 191–195. https://doi.org/10.1038/jp.2017.148

Nist, M. D., Harrison, T. M., & Steward, D. K. (2019). The biological embedding of neonatal stress exposure: A conceptual model describing the mechanisms of stress-induced neurodevelopmental impairment in preterm infants. *Research in Nursing & Health, 42*, 61–71. https://doi.org/10.1002/nur.21923

O'Brien, K., Bracht, M., Robson, K., Ye, X. Y., Mirea, L., Cruz, M., Ng, E., Monterrosa, L., Soraisham, A., Alvaro, R., Narvey, M., Da Silva, O., Lui, K., Tarnow-Mordi, W., & Lee, S. K. (2015). Evaluation of the family integrated care model of neonatal intensive care: A cluster randomized controlled trial in Canada and Australia. *BMC Pediatrics, 15*, 210. https://doi.org/10.1186/s12887-015-0527-0

Ohlsson, A., & Jacobs, S. E. (2013). NIDCAP: A systematic review and meta-analyses of randomized controlled trials. *Pediatrics, 131*(3), e881–e893. https://doi.org/10.1542/peds.2012-2121

Ohgi, S., Fukuda, M., Moriuchi, H., Kusumoto, T., Akiyama, T., Nugent, J. K., Brazelton, T. B., Arisawa, K., Takahashi, T., & Saitoh, H. (2002). Comparison of kangaroo care and standard care: behavioral organization, development, and temperament in healthy, low-birth-weight infants through 1 year. *Journal of Perinatology, 22*, 374–379. https://doi-org.proxy.lib.ohio-state.edu/10.1038/sj.jp.7210749

Painter, L., Lewis, S., & Hamilton, B. K. (2019). Improving neurodevelopmental outcomes in NICU patients. *Advances in Neonatal Care, 19*, 236–243. https://doi.org/10.1542/peds.2012-2121

van der Pal, S. M., Maguire, C. M., le Cessie, S., Wit, J. M., Walther, F. J., & Bruil, J. (2007). Parental experiences during the first period at the neonatal unit after two developmental care interventions. *Acta Paediatrica, 96*, 1611–1616. https://doi.org/10.1111/j.1651-2227.2007.00487.x

Parikh, P., & Juul, S. E. (2019). Neuroprotection strategies in preterm encephalopathy. *Seminars in Pediatric Neurology, 32*, 100772. https://doi.org/10.1016/j.spen.2019.08.008

Peters, K. L., Rosychuk, R. J., Hendson, L., Cote, J. J., McPherson, C., & Tyebkhan, J. M. (2009). Improvement of short- and long-term outcomes for very low birth weight infants: Edmonton NIDCAP trial. *Pediatrics, 124*(4), 1009–1020. https://doi.org/10.1542/peds.2008-3808

Pickler, R. H., Best, A., & Crosson, D. (2009). The effect of feeding experience on clinical outcomes in preterm infants. *Journal of Perinatology, 29*, 124–129. https://doi.org/10.1038/jp.2008.140

Pickler, R. H., Best, A., Reyna, B. A., Gutcher, G., & Wetzel, P. A. (2006). Predictors of nutritive sucking in preterm infants. *Journal of Perinatology, 26*, 693–699. https://doi.org/10.1038/sj.jp.7211590

Pickler, R. H., McGrath, J. M., Reyna, B. A., McCain, N., Lewis, M., Cone, S., Wetzel, P., & Best, A. (2010). A model of neurodevelopmental risk and protection for preterm infants. *Journal of Perinatal and Neonatal Nursing, 24*, 356–365. https://doi.org:10.1097/JPN.0b013e3181fb1e70

Pickler, R. H., McGrath, J. M., Reyna, B. A., Tubbs Cooley, H. L., Best, A. M., Lewis, M., Cone, S., & Wetzel, P. A. (2013). Effects of the neonatal intensive care unit environment on preterm infant oral feeding. *Research and Reports in Neonatology, 2013*(3), 15–20. https://doi.org/10.2147/RRN.S41280

Pickler, R. H., Meinzen-Derr, J., Moore, M., Sealschott, S., & Tepe, K. (2020). Effect of tactile experience during preterm infant feeding on clinical outcomes. *Nursing Research, 69*(5S suppl 1), S21–S28. https://doi.org/10.1097/NNR.0000000000000453

Pickler, R. H., & Reyna, B. A. (2004). Effects of non-nutritive sucking on nutritive sucking, breathing, and behavior during bottle feedings of preterm infants. *Advances in Neonatal Care, 4*, 226–234. https://doi.org/10.1016/j.adnc.2004.05.005

Pickler, R. H., Reyna, B. A., Wetzel, P. A., & Lewis, M. (2015). Effect of four approaches to oral feeding progression on clinical outcomes in preterm infants. *Nursing Research and Practice, 2015*, 716828. https://doi.org/10.1155/2015/716828

Pickler, R., Sealschott, S., Moore, M., Merhar, S., Tkach, J., Salzwedel, A. P., Lin, W., & Gao, W. (2017). Using functional connectivity magnetic resonance imaging to measure brain connectivity in preterm infants. *Nursing Research, 66*, 490–495. https://doi.org/10.1097/NNR.0000000000000241

Pineda, R., Bender, J., Hall, B., Shabosky, L., Annecca, A., & Smith, J. (2018). Parent participation in the neonatal intensive care unit: Predictors and relationships to neurobehavior and developmental outcomes. *Early Human Development, 117*, 32–38. https://doi.org/10.1016/j.earlhumdev.2017.12.008

Preyde, M., & Ardal, F. (2003). Effectiveness of a parent "buddy" program for mothers of very preterm infants in a neonatal intensive care unit. *Canadian Medical Association Journal, 168*, 969–973.

Provenzi, L., Barello, S., Fumagalli, M., Graffigna, G., Sirgiovanni, I., Savarese, M., & Montirosso, R. (2016). Experiences of becoming parents of a very preterm infant. *Journal of Obstetric, Gynecologic, & Neonatal Nursing, 45*, 528–541. https://doi.org/10.1016/j.jogn.2016.04.004

Reynolds, L. C., Duncan, M. M., Smith, G. C., Mathur, A., Neil, J., Inder, T., & Pineda, R. G. (2013). Parental presence and holding in the neonatal intensive care unit and associations with early neurobehavior. *Journal of Perinatology, 33*, 636–641. https://doi.org/va10.1038/jp.2013.4

Rogers, E. E., & Hintz, S. R. (2016). Early neurodevelopmental outcomes of extremely preterm infants. *Seminars in Perinatology, 40*, 497–509. https://doi.org/10.1053/j.semperi.2016.09.002

Romeo, D. M., Cowan, F. M., Haataja, L., Ricci, D., Pede, E., Gallini, F., Cota, F., Brogna, C., Vento, G., Romeo, M. G., & Mercuri, E. (2021). Hammersmith Infant Neurological Examination for infants born preterm: Predicting outcomes other than cerebral palsy. *Developmental Medicine and Child Neurology, 63*(8), 939–946. https://doi.org/10.1111/dmcn.14768

Sannino, P., Gianni, M. L., De Bon, G., Fontana, C., Picciolini, O., Plevani, L. Fumagalli, M., Consonni, D., & Mosca, F. (2016). Support to mothers of premature babies using NIDCAP method: A non-randomized controlled trial. *Early Human Development, 95*, 15–20. https://doi.org/10.1016/j.earlhumdev.2016.01.016

Say, B., Simsek, G. K., Canpolat, F. E., & Oguz, S. S. (2018). Effects of pacifier use on transition time from gavage to breastfeeding in preterm infants: A randomized controlled trial. *Breastfeeding Medicine, 13*, 433–437. https://doi.org/10.1089/bfm.2018.0031

Schappin, R., Wijnroks, L., Uniken Venema, M. M., & Jongmans, M. J. (2013). Rethinking stress in parent of preterm infants: A meta-analysis. *PLoS ONE, 8*(2), e54992. https://doi.org/10.1371/journal.pone.0054992

Settle, M., & Francis, K. (2019). Does the infant-driven feeding method positively impact preterm infant feeding outcomes? *Advances in Neonatal Care, 19*, 51–55. https://doi.org/10.1097/ANC.0000000000000577

Shaker, C. S. (2013). Cue-based feeding in the NICU: Using the infant's communication as a guide. *Neonatal Network, 32*, 404–408. https://doi.org/10.1891/0730-0832.32.6.404

Smith, E. R., Hurt, L., Chowdhury, R., Sinha, B., Fawzi, W., Edmond, K. M., & Neovita Study Group. (2017). Delayed breastfeeding initiation and infant survival: A systematic review and metaanalysis. *PLoS One, 12*, 1–16. https://doi.org/10.1371/journal.pone.0180722

Soleimani, F., Azari, N., Ghiasvand, H., Shahrokhi, A., Rahmani, N., & Fatollahierad, S. (2020). Do NICU developmental care improve cognitive and motor outcomes for preterm infants? A systematic review and meta-analysis. *BMC Pediatrics, 20*(1), 67. https://doi.org/10.1186/s12887-020-1953-1

Spittle, A. J., Dewey, D., Nguyen, T. N., Ellis, R., Burnett, A., Kwong, A., Lee, K., Cheong, J. L., Doyle, L. W., & Anderson, P. J. (2020). Rates of developmental co-ordination disorder in children born very preterm. *The Journal of Pediatrics, 231*, 61–67. https://www.jpeds.com/article/S0022-3476(20)31504-3/fulltext

Spittle, A., Orton, J., Anderson, P. J., Boyd, R., & Doyle, L. W. (2015). Early developmental intervention programmes provided post hospital discharge to prevent motor and cognitive impairment in preterm infants (Review). *Cochrane Database of Systematic Reviews, 11*, CD005495. https://doi.org/10.1002/14651858.CD005495.pub4

Spittle, A., & Treyvaud, K. (2016). The role of early developmental intervention to influence neurobehavioral outcomes of children born preterm. *Seminars in Perinatology, 40*, 542–548. https://doi.org/10.1053/j.semperi.2016.09.006

Sullivan, M. C., Miller, R. J., & Msall, M. E. (2012a). 17-year outcome of preterm infants with diverse neonatal morbidities: Part 2, impact on activities & participation. *Journal for Specialists in Pediatric Nursing, 17*, 275–287. https://doi.org/10.1111/j.1744-6155.2012.00337.x

Sullivan, M. C., Msall, M. E., & Miller, R. J. (2012b). 17-year outcome of preterm infants with diverse neonatal morbidities: Part 1, impact on physical, neurological, and psychological health status. *Journal for Specialists in Pediatric Nursing, 17*, 226–241. https://doi.org/10.1111/j.1744-6155.2012.00337.x

Symington, A., & Pinelli, J. (2009). Developmental care for promoting development and preventing morbidity in preterm infants. *Cochrane Database of Systematic Reviews, 2*, CD001814. https://doi.org/10.1002/14651858.CD001814.pub2

Tubbs Cooley, H. L., Pickler, R. H., & Meinzen-Derr, J. K. (2015). Missed oral feeding opportunities and preterm infants' time to achieve full oral feedings and neonatal intensive care unit discharge. *American Journal of Perinatology, 32*, 1–8. https://doi.org/10.1055/s-0034-1372426

Verma, A., Maria, A., Mohan Pandey, R., Hans, C., Verma, A., & Sherwani, F. (2017). Family-centered care to complement care of sick newborns: A randomized controlled trial. *Indian Pediatrics, 54*, 455–459. https://doi.org/10.1007/s13312-017-1047-9

Woodward, L. J., Samudragupta, B., Clark, C. A. C., Montgomery-Hönger, A., Pritchard, V. E., Spencer, C., & Austin, N. C. (2014). Very preterm birth: Maternal experiences of the neonatal intensive care environment. *Journal of Perinatology, 34*, 555–561. https://doi.org/10.1038/jp.2014.43

CHAPTER 21

Interdisciplinary Competency Validation

Susan Orlando, Jana Pressler, and Jacqueline M. McGrath

Standards in Systems Thinking

Standard 2: Systems Thinking
- The intensive care unit shall provide a professionally competent interprofessional collaborative practice team to support the baby, parent, and family's holistic physical, developmental, and psychosocial needs from birth through the transition of hospital discharge to home and assure continuity to follow-up care.

INTRODUCTION

Competent caregivers in various healthcare disciplines are essential in providing patients with high-quality care. Competent practice in the healthcare environment is crucial for all aspects of the workforce given patients' increased acuity and the technology in use at the bedside. As a result, developing and maintaining a competent caregiver workforce, identifying caregivers who perform less than competently in their caregiving assignments, and reeducating those who are less competent are of utmost importance. Yet that also means we must more fully embrace what competence means.

Neonatal care providers must demonstrate the ability to meet standard skill and competency levels to care for their patients. One well-known interdisciplinary competency requirement for practice in the neonatal intensive care unit (NICU) and birthing areas is Neonatal Resuscitation Program (NRP) certification. After completing standardized online lessons and examinations, NRP learners must demonstrate integration of cognitive knowledge and psychomotor skills in hands-on case-based simulation/debriefing that focus on critical leadership, communication, and team-work skills performing neonatal resuscitation as a cohesive team (AAP, 2020). The provision of family-centered developmentally supportive care, commonly referred to as "developmental care" for high-risk infants, also can be considered a type of competency. This is true, even though developmental care continues to *not* be a universal neonatal practice throughout all NICUs (Peters, 1999; Phillips, 2015; Zhang et al., 2016). Most NICUs worldwide are evolving in their developmental competence. Common themes throughout the developmental care literature related to this evolution include infant neurodevelopment, neuroprotection, environmental control, and support of the family; however, there is wide variation in the application of developmentally appropriate practice (Atun-Einy & Scher, 2008).

Although there continues to be a lack of understanding, appreciation, and acceptance of the importance of developmental care practices across all staff levels in many NICUs worldwide (Hendricks-Munoz et al., 2002), developmental care has continued to expand with support from the Newborn Individualized Developmental Care and Assessment Program (NIDCAP®) (Boston, MA), Assessment of Preterm Infants' Behavior (APIB) evaluations, Phillips WeeCare® Developmental Care (Cambridge, MA), Supporting and Enhancing Sensory Experiences (SENSE) program developed by Roberta Pineda and colleagues (see Chapter 12 for more information), and Mary Coughlin's Trauma-Informed Professional Certification for working with small and sick newborns and their families. Please see Chapter 3 for more information on NIDCAP® and APIB and Chapter 4 for information on trauma informed care. The European Foundation for the Care of Newborn Infants developed the interdisciplinary *European Standards of the Care for Newborn Health* (https://www.efcni.org/activities/projects-2/escnh/) *and the Gravens Consensus Committee of the Standards, Competencies, and Best Practices for Infant and Family-Centered Developmental Care in the Intensive Care Unit* (https://nicudesign.nd.edu/nicu-care-standards/) that was presented in Chapters 1 and 2 now offer standards and competencies in infant and family-centered developmental care (IFCDC). It is highly apparent that developmental care has branched out in terms of the types of professional caregivers delivering developmental care. Some of this growth relates to infant follow-up demonstrating profoundly beneficial developmental benefits in infants who received developmental care during their hospitalization. Second, developmental care has expanded as a consequence of caregivers wanting to be sure that as many high-risk neonates as possible receive family-centered developmental care that has been individually tailored for the infant and their family, creating a need for the involvement of more individuals and sheer person-power to implement this goal. Third, developmental care has expanded due to allied health professions who make a significant positive impact becoming eligible to receive payment for their services. Finally, some of developmental care expansion appears to be a consequence of neonatal nurses not fully integrating the implementation of developmental care in the NICU, for one reason or another. This could be related to the way NICUs are staffed (focus on acuity) rather than the individual neonatal nurse's desire to fully integrate developmental care practice into routine practices. Subsequently other professionals have become more directly involved in implementing developmental care interventions with neonates to address this void. This chapter updates how such changes might have affected interdisciplinary competency validation in delivery of developmental care and also updates barriers to implementation.

DEVELOPMENTAL CARE PROVIDER WORKFORCE

Having sufficient numbers of trained professional caregivers has served as rationale for becoming involved in developmental care in the NICU (Clubbs et al., 2019; Dusing et al., 2012; Goldstein, 2013). According to a 2019 report from the American Academy of Pediatrics' (AAP) Committee on Fetus and Newborn (COFN), formal care providers working in NICUs need to demonstrate a triad of (1) behavioral competencies, (2) cognitive abilities, and (3) technical skills to safely and effectively practice in this high-risk infant setting (Keels et al., 2019). The 2019 report, *Neonatal Provider Workforce,* reviews the education, competency requirements, training, and scopes of practice for infant caregivers within the NICU. That report offers recommendations for establishing and monitoring quality and safety of care. It also addresses potential solutions for workforce shortages.

The major point of the *Neonatal Provider Workforce* report is that there should be a base of credentialing and training for personnel working independently in an NICU. That report states that the neonatologist is the head of the team, but they might have a hospitalist, nurse practitioners, physician assistants, and others working on that team. Furthermore, the neonatologist needs their team members to have specific educational and technical abilities in common. The *Neonatal Provider Workforce* report presents a table of NICU procedures that hospitalists, neonatal nurse practitioners, acute care pediatric nurse practitioners, and physician assistants should be able to perform. The report notes that increasing collaboration of the neonatal workforce will be required of neonatologists, other NICU providers, and physician trainees on an ongoing basis to meet the future needs there.

DISCIPLINES AND PROFESSIONS INVOLVED IN THE NICU

Even though advances in perinatal care have resulted in decreased mortality rates in high-risk neonates, morbidity rates have continued to remain significantly high and a cause for concern. Developmental care is used to individualize care to neonates with the objective of maximizing neurological development and reducing long-term cognitive and behavioral problems/morbidities. Today the NICU caregiver workforce consists of a variety of professionals in varied stages of their careers with a wide range of degrees, training, experience, skills, and competencies. A relatively new subgroup of the physical therapy (PT) profession is the "neonatal therapists" who have considerable expertise in providing PT to the small and sick newborn (Brown & Dusing, 2019; Byrne & Campbell, 2013; Craig & Smith, 2020; Khurana et al., 2020; Neel et al., 2019; Sweeney et al., 2010).

Neonatal Therapists

The National Association of Neonatal Therapists, or NANT, is an organization founded in 2009 by an occupational therapist and certified neonatal therapist. Its stated aim is to improve neurodevelopmental outcomes for preterm and ill infants. According to their website, NANT's mission is to support the professional development and growth of neonatal occupational therapists, physical therapists, and speech–language pathologists. NANT provides education, networking, resources, and products targeted to advance knowledge, skills, and practice specific to the care of neonates. NANT ascribes to seven core values, including excellence, resilience, connection, service, alignment, innovation, and presence. NANT serves neonatal occupational therapists, physical therapists, and speech–language pathologists. NANT's vision is to define, support, and lead the field of neonatal therapy by providing neonatal therapists a means for strengthening improvement in neonatal development. The NANT Professional Collaborative is a multidisciplinary group of nine individuals. This collaborative includes occupational therapists, physical therapists, and speech–language pathologists who advise and assist in defining, creating, and reviewing emerging standards, practices, and guidelines for the National Association of Neonatal Therapists.

As defined by the NANT Professional Collaborative, neonatal therapy is the art and science of integrating typical development of the infant and family into the environment of the NICU. Neonatal therapy incorporates theories and scopes of practice from occupational therapy, physical therapy, and speech–language pathology. It requires advanced knowledge of the diagnoses and medical interventions used in NICUs to provide safe and effective assessment, planning, and treatment. Neonatal therapy promotes optimal long-term developmental outcomes and nurtures infant–parent relationships by addressing the neurobehavioral, neuromotor, neuroendocrine, musculoskeletal, sensory, and psychosocial systems. As such, these systems are thought to provide the foundation for the infant's development of functional skills.

Through the provision of elemental risk-adjusted neuroprotective care services, neonatal therapists are becoming accepted and more widespread in the United States.

The three disciplines comprising neonatal therapists have aligned themselves with specific professional organization competency recommendations for NICUs. Recognizing the staffing budget as one of the more difficult challenges hospital department leaders face in the United States, neonatal therapists are doing their best to present a formula-based approach to address staff allocations for neonatal therapists to serve as regular employees in NICU settings.

Neonatal Nurses Not Fully Implementing Developmental Care in the NICU

Evidence from research on developmental care has positively influenced neonatal caregivers to believe that it directly affects neonates cared for in the NICU in significantly positive ways (Detmer & Whelan, 2017; Dusing et al., 2018; Emery et al., 2019; Loewy et al., 2013; Nair, Sunitha, et al., 2014). Increasingly, neonatal staff nurses are observing developmental advantages in infants who receive developmental care. Empiric evidence supporting developmental care benefits also is increasing. Developmentally focused care of infants is a major topic in the population-focused nursing literature. According to Beal (2005), the well-studied aspects of family-centered developmental care should be an integral aspect of every neonatal nurse's caregiving practices in the NICU. But despite the continuing debate over whether randomized controlled trial (RCT) findings support developmental care's benefits and warrant its use to justify evidence-based practice, few will argue that any negative sequelae result from its implementation (Bredemeyer et al., 2008; Jacobs et al., 2002; Symington & Pinelli, 2006; Wallin & Eriksson, 2009; Westrup et al., 2002). Others view family-centered developmental care from a holistic and humane perspective, citing a need to reduce stress and pain in vulnerable infants (Westrup et al., 2007).

The development and evaluation of NICU providers to help ensure safe, quality, and cost-effective care of infants in NICUs has been recognized as a pressing need for over a decade (Pressler et al., 2010). Hendricks-Munoz and Prendergast (2007) reported that 90% of neonatal nurses whose NICU did not use developmental multidisciplinary team meetings, developmental care champions, or advocates were significantly more likely to identify both nurse and physician colleagues as barriers to implementation.

Park and Kim (2019) found that professional efficacy and perception of developmental care influenced how nursing care is delivered in the NICU. They also found that the task-orientation organizational culture, nurses' involvement, and the overall effort of the organization influence whether or not nurses carry out developmental care. A study conducted in China in 2015 reported that Chinese NICU nurses were not found to consistently implement developmental care (Zhang et al., 2016). Higher patient caseloads, fewer work hours per day, higher level of education, and fewer years worked in NICUs were the significant predictors for lower degree of implementation of developmental care.

The NICU nursing staff's attitudes and beliefs greatly influence the culture within a unit and the value placed on developmentally supportive care (Liaw et al., 2004; Cardin et al., 2015). As the gatekeeper and team member most frequently present at the infant's bedside, the NICU nurse coordinates delivery of care based on the needs of each infant. However, neonatal nurses have identified their own nursing and physician colleagues as barriers in delivery of individualized developmentally supportive care (Hendricks-Munoz & Prendergast, 2007). As presented at the beginning of the chapter, the infant and family-centered developmental care (IFCDC) standard regarding systems thinking is critical to the implementation of this care. Unit and even institutional policies must reflect IFCDC.

COLLABORATION IN IMPLEMENTING A TEAM-BASED APPROACH TO DEVELOPMENTAL CARE

A major change in the approach to NICU caregiving requires support from the entire team to ensure a successful transition. Knowledge, collaboration, and administrative support are required elements. Several events must take place before developmental care can be the standard of care within most NICUs. One fundamental revision in practice that must occur on a continuing basis is a change in NICU caregiving expectations and possibly credentials. To set the groundwork, NICU caregivers first must expect that additional education and training on developmental care will be a prerequisite or coprerequisite for employment (a major theme in the orientation education and process). Next, concomitant administrative changes must occur, such as revised position descriptions, qualifications for bedside practice, NICU policies and procedures, orientation, annual evaluations for all providers, and continuing education priorities, skill evaluations to optimize health outcomes, and established credentials. (See IFCDC Standard 1 at the beginning of the chapter on systems thinking.) Administrators must acknowledge that the type and level of caregiver developmental care competencies will financially influence human resource planning. Once achieved, staff competencies and certifications must be maintained and intermittently reassessed and renewed using an appropriate method.

A Roadmap for Implementation

A viable starting point to more fully implementing developmental care could be as simplistic as using a trained nurse educator to provide NICU staff nurses with useful information on developmental care, encouraging them to keep an open mind, and encouraging them to have a positive attitude toward developmental care. The NICU nurse manager should create an organizational culture in which nurses perceive developmental care to be an essential nursing task in their unit. This includes annual and peer evaluations of developmental care practices for all staff. Professional efficacy was shown to have had the largest influence on developmental care practice, followed by perception of developmental care and a task-oriented NICU organizational culture. Clinical and educational experience regarding developmental care and working environment was not associated with developmental care practice among NICU nurses. To enhance nurses' practice of developmental care, enhancement of nurses' individual competency, positive perception of developmental care, and organizational efforts are required. Nurses need a practical training program to promote confidence in implementing developmental care for preterm infants (Painter et al., 2019). Training also needs to include hands-on participation as well as reinforcement through other unit policies such as inclusion in annual evaluations.

Several organizations in the United States and Canada have collaborated to produce a joint position statement and endorse guidelines for the institutional implementation of developmental neuroprotective care in the NICU (Milette, Martel, et al., 2017). Use of an evidence-based framework to standardize the product (developmental care) and the process (implementation of a practice change) will assist in reducing inconsistencies in practice that lead to difficulties in comparing outcomes. Although individual practice guidelines exist (NANN, 2011; Altimier & Phillips, 2016), many institutions are seeking guidance on standardizing implementation. Phillips (2015) summarized the work from an interdisciplinary collaboration to develop measurable goals, interventions, and educational modalities to implement seven core measures of neuroprotective developmental care

in the NICU. Most recently, an interprofessional consensus committee developed evidence-based standards and competencies for six key practice domains of infant and family-centered developmental care (IFCDC). Consensus process results included recommended best practices for IFCDC, specifically components of systems thinking, positioning and touch, sleep and arousal, skin-to-skin contact, reduction of pain and stress for infants and families, and feeding (Browne et al., 2020).

Education and Competency as a Foundation to Produce Better Outcomes

Positive outcomes of infants who received developmentally supportive family-centered care in NICUs are well documented throughout this text. Less attention has been given to the systematic examination of care providers—specifically, the actions of the nurses, physicians, and therapists who deliver care. The first and most pressing issue that must be addressed is the lack of agreement regarding what constitutes core knowledge in developmental care. There is no standard developmental care educational requirement for new nurses or other health professionals who touch a small and sick newborn entering practice in the NICU. Several resources provide a framework for educating new staff, including textbooks, self-learning modules, digital video disks (DVDs), online training videos, and orientation programs (Table 21-1). The orientation and mentoring process for new NICU nurses varies greatly within and across

TABLE 21-1 Sources for Recommended Competencies/Guidelines for Developmental Care

Title	Authors	Internet Site	Content Summary
Program Guide: Newborn Individualized Development Care Assessment Program (NIDCAP®) and Education and Training Program for Health Professionals (Rev. ed.)	Als, 2001	www.nidcap.com	Developmental education and training program with NIDCAP competency and reliability testing Goal: A shift from task-oriented, protocol-based caregiving to individualized, relationship-based care General topics: • theoretical framework: Synactive Theory of Development (Als, 1982) • assessment and documentation of infant behaviors • recommendations for care modifications • structure of a developmentally supportive environment • developmentally supportive care interventions and supports • education and support of parents in the caretaking of their infant • guidance for facilitation and implementation of developmental care in the NICU
"Age appropriate care of the critically ill and hospitalized infant: Guideline for practice"	NANN, 2011	www.nann.org	Evidence-based guideline for care of premature and critically ill infants in the hospital environment Age-appropriate practice recommendations • sleep • pain assessment and management • family-centered care • healing environment

(Continued)

TABLE 21-1 Sources for Recommended Competencies/Guidelines for Developmental Care (Continued)

Title	Authors	Internet Site	Content Summary
Neonatal Developmental Care Training Series	White et al., 2007	www.neonatal developmentalcare. com	A series of six training DVDs with pretests and post-tests. Topics include • observing, interpreting, and responding to preterm infant cues • positioning preterm infants • feeding preterm infants • diapering preterm infants • bathing preterm infants • using developmentally supportive practices during routine and emergency medical care for preterm infants
Core Curriculum for Neonatal Intensive Care Nursing: Developmental Support	Spruill, 2021	N/A	Barriers to infant development in the NICU developmental care standards: • individualized care based on infant cues • developmentally supportive environment for infant and family based on infant response • parent support and involvement • teamwork and continuity of care Didactic content on all the above, along with neuromotor, auditory, and feeding information
Neonatal Orientation and Education Program (NOEP) 4th ed.	AWHONN, 2019	www.awhonn.org	Fifteen fully narrated modules on knowledge needed to provide holistic, family-centered care to newborn infants and their families includes a module on developmental care and management of pain
Developmental care CNE modules	NANN, 2020	www.nann.org	Twenty-seven modules in online learning format with pretests and posttests for nurses, respiratory therapists, physical therapists, occupational therapists, and speech therapists Includes an overview of all aspects of developmental care and related care standards with learning activities and supplemental readings

geographic locations. More standardization is needed, and more inclusion of developmental care practices as "standard of care" are needed. However, competence in developmental care is multidisciplinary and not limited to the nursing profession. Other disciplines, for example, occupational therapy and physical therapy, have addressed the specialized knowledge and skills required to practice in the NICU in detail (American Occupational Therapy Association, 2006; Sweeney et al., 1999). Entry level therapists require additional training, skills, and mentoring to function as members of an NICU developmental care team.

Frequently multidisciplinary human resources are allocated according to an NICU's bed capacity and level of care provided. Not every NICU will have a full complement of multidisciplinary professionals to staff a developmental care team. Efforts should focus on exploring available resource options that will produce the best results for each NICU. A professional with expertise in developmental care might be designated as the developmental specialist and leader of the developmental care team. The developmental specialist role might be filled by members from various disciplines, such as nursing, education, medicine, psychology, social work, occupational or physical therapy, as well as speech and language pathologists. Neonatal therapists are another more recent role for consideration. The developmental specialist also should have specialized knowledge of fetal and newborn brain development, medical conditions of high-risk infants, development and behaviors of preterm and full-term infants, the NICU environment, staffing patterns and the culture of caregiving, and parenting in the NICU.

A multidisciplinary team approach might be a highly efficacious way to implement developmental care practices in the NICU. The required competencies will vary according to the role and educational preparation of each team member. Staff nurses, advanced practice neonatal nurses, occupational therapists, and physical therapists represent the majority of team members; however, there is much variation in the composition of developmental care teams in NICUs. A multidisciplinary team approach with regularly scheduled meetings for team interaction and sharing of perspectives is key to reducing developmental care implementation barriers (Hendricks-Munoz & Prendergast, 2007).

What Evidence Supports Competency in Developmental Care?

The major efforts in developmental care research have focused on the effects of caregiving and the NICU environment on infant outcomes or the impact of the NICU environment, light, sound, touch, on infant outcomes. A review of the current published literature produced no reports of large RCTs examining the impact of a standardized educational program on professional competency in delivering developmentally supportive, family-centered care. They do not focus on competencies of the workforce. However, several small studies have examined caregiver attitudes and behavior changes after a training session on one or more aspects of developmental care. Most studies involved small sample sizes and the use of a single group of nurses in a pretest/posttest design after an education-focused intervention.

Liaw (2003) developed and tested a theory-based developmental care training program to improve nurses' abilities to assess preterm infant behavior and provide appropriate supportive developmental care. Nurses' knowledge level and observational abilities improved after exposure to multimethod educational sessions that included directed readings, discussions, case studies, and videotapes. In addition, each nurse was videotaped while performing a self-selected infant caregiving activity. Videotapes then were used as teaching tools for self-reflection, feedback, and reinforcement of high-quality developmentally supportive care. Liaw concluded that developmental care education was the key to initiating a behavior change among nurses caring for preterm infants.

In a larger follow-up study 6 years later, Liaw et al. (2009) focused on a single aspect of caregiving to examine nurse behaviors while bathing preterm infants. Nurses who received developmental care training demonstrated the ability to effectively adjust their caregiving after recognizing stress signals in preterm infants during a bath. Infants demonstrated fewer stress signals after experiencing cue-based changes in caregiving.

Handling and positioning are critical aspects of developmental care that are controlled by individual nurses. Louw and Maree (2005) examined the effect of formal training on developmentally supportive handling and positioning of preterm infants by NICU nurses. Before receiving formal training, nurses based care on informal observation of developmental caregiving. After the formal training session, significant improvements were noted in nurses' abilities to handle and position infants using developmental care principles.

The preterm infant's environment is another critical aspect of care that nurses can modify to prevent sensory overload. Milette et al. (2005) measured changes in nurse attitudes, intentions, and behaviors after a formal education program about developmental care principles and the impact of environment. The researchers noted that the key variables known to influence successful implementation of developmental care can be positively changed through education and increased knowledge.

Although short-term improvements in delivering developmental care have been seen following formal education programs, there continues to be a shortage of information on the sustainability of the initial training's desired effects. One study conducted over a 5-year period demonstrated initial improvement in nurses' use of positioning devices and positioning practices after pediatric physical therapists provided formal and informal education. Over time, however, there was a decline in nurses' positioning effectiveness (Perkins et al., 2004). These findings highlighted the need for follow-up and ongoing evaluation to preserve the positive gains made in educating staff and implementing developmental care practices. Altimier et al. (2015) reported positive results from a quality improvement project that involved 81 NICU sites where an 18-month comprehensive neuroprotective developmental care training program was implemented. The Wee Care Neuroprotective NICU training program was effective in significantly improving practices and scores on neuroprotective core measures. Education and training of the entire healthcare team led to improvements in staff providing neuroprotective care for premature infants. Research is needed to determine the effectiveness of such training over time and sustainability. More research is definitely needed to further support integration of developmental care practices into all NICU education and job descriptions.

The Supporting and Enhancing NICU Sensory Experiences (SENSE) program developed by Pineda and colleagues focuses on the sensory experience of the infant in the NICU and the education needed for families to participate in the care. This program requires staff training for the team providing care. A federally funded clinical trial was conducted to examine the impact of the SENSE program on infants equal to or less than 32 weeks' gestation (https://clinicaltrials.gov/ct2/show/NCT03316547). Pineda et al., 2020 have conducted a study that explored the use of SENSE and the differences in maternal mental health and neurobehavioral outcomes between the control and experimental group. Those mothers in the intervention group demonstrated more confidence than those in the control. The infants also had better neurobehavioral outcomes if they participated in the SENSE program. (Please see Chapter 12 for more information on SENSE.) This is an area of further research.

Sanders and Hall (2018) described the need for a trauma informed approach in the NICU. They tied the physiologic changes that occur when undergoing stress. Much of the research has focused on adverse childhood experiences and the link with negative health outcomes (Sanders & Hall, 2018). This area of research along with concern of maternal and infant mental health is growing.

As the Gravens Consensus Committee on Infant and Family-Centered Developmental Care (IFCD) (Browne et al., 2020) has evolved over 1,000 articles have been identified along with the levels of evidence that look at the concepts of developmental care from the infant and family perspective. The next steps in this work will be to implement and test these standards and competencies in practice.

Certification Options

Making developmental care a basic competency requirement or "standard" of practice in the NICU is important. A national collaborative effort to develop and implement potentially better practices to support infant brain development highlighted the need for self-assessment of current practice in NICUs. Participating centers acknowledged the importance of creating educational strategies to help staff understand the evidence supporting developmental care practices (Laudert et al., 2007). Interprofessional collaboration among all neonatal care providers is required to effectively provide high-quality developmental care. Historically, each discipline has worked in isolation to determine what specialized knowledge and skills are required to deliver developmental care. There is a recent trend toward interprofessional collaboration as demonstrated by inclusion of nonnurses in the eligibility criteria for subspecialty certification examinations that include developmental care content. The National Association of Neonatal Nurses (NANN) and National Certification Corporation (NCC) do not limit their certification examination eligibility criteria to nurses. Other neonatal healthcare providers are eligible to apply for certification by the NANN and NCC examinations.

Another certification that has evolved is the Trauma-Informed Professional Certification developed by Mary Coughlin and colleagues (https://www.caringessentials.net/). This certification is open to those who provide NICU care. It builds on Coughlin's work to transform NICU care to be trauma informed (Coughlin, 2021). Please see Chapter 4 for more information. Although both of these certifications now exist, there is no current evidence to support outcomes—more research is needed to increase their integration into practice requirements.

NANN'S Developmental Care Specialist Designation

NANN's Developmental Care Specialist designation has been designed to recognize and advance excellence at the bedside for practicing neonatal nurses. The designation was developed out of the belief that excellent neonatal nursing care is rooted in a foundation of family-centered developmentally supportive caregiving and is a part of the continuum of novice to expert neonatal nursing. Most neonatal nurses profess a belief in developmental care practices and have acquired more expert knowledge in this area during the past several years as the evidence to support these practices has grown. Even so, integration at the bedside has not yet been achieved. Collaboration among caregivers is needed for full integration of developmental caregiving. The Developmental Care Specialist designation, although rooted to bedside practitioners, is applicable to all caregivers in the NICU. Nurses, advanced practice nurses, and interdisciplinary partners in the NICU who integrate this expert knowledge into their everyday collaborative caregiving interactions with infants, families, and every member of the caregiving team have the

beginning skills to complete the competency. Test takers are asked to demonstrate integration of family-centered developmental care into their routine decision making and collaborative caregiving practices through critical decision making and application to practice in knowledge-based vignettes. More than 60% of the online testing is scenario based; an infant/family scenario is presented, and the test taker is asked to explain how a developmentally sensitive caregiver would provide care in a particular situation.

The NANN Developmental Care Specialist designation is designed to measure expert integration of developmental caregiving and care-related education and training. Those who have studied or have experience in developmental care are most likely to successfully complete the Specialist designation test. It is important that those who provide developmental care be lifelong learners because what is known today about best provision of developmental supportive caregiving will change as more about the developing brain and the ways vulnerable infants and their families can best be supported in the NICU environment is understood.

National Certification Corporation Examinations

National Certification Corporation (NCC), Chicago, offers certification examinations in maternal–newborn, low-risk, and neonatal intensive care nursing. Developmental care content is covered on the NCC neonatal intensive care nursing examination. Developmental care is not listed as a content area for either the low-risk neonatal nursing or maternal–newborn nursing examinations; however, NCC offers an optional developmental care self-study module for continuing education to meet neonatal nurses' competency validation needs. The NCC introduced a Neonatal Neuro-Intensive Care Certification that contains a large percentage of content that is applicable to developmental care and also an extremely low birth weight neonatal subspecialty certification that includes developmental care. Both of these examinations take a multidisciplinary approach to caregiving. Physicians, registered nurses, advanced practice registered nurses, neonatal therapists (PT, OT, SLP-speech–language pathologist), neonatal dieticians, Pharm-Ds, respiratory therapists, and paramedics are eligible to take the extremely low birth weight (ELBW) certification.

Neonatal Therapy National Certification Board

The National Association of Neonatal Therapists (NANT) established a Neonatal Therapist program in 2009. A certification process has been established for neonatal therapists. Neonatal therapy certification, via the Neonatal Therapy National Certification Board or NTNCB, identifies individuals who have demonstrated the time, knowledge, and commitment to serve high-risk infants in the NICU. At this stage of development, the therapist who possesses the knowledge and experience in order to function independently as a neonatal therapist ought to consider becoming officially certified as a neonatal therapist. Certification requirements include:

- PT, OT, or SLP credentialing for a period of 3 years
- 3,500 hours of direct practice in the NICU
- 40 hours of education related to NICU practice within the past 3 years
- 40 hours of mentored experiences
- Passing score on the Neonatal Therapy National Certification examination

These credentialing activities have impacted the extent and depth of developmental care implementation across NICUs. They have also had a positive impact on assuring competency in developmental caregiving in that they have certifications. However, regardless of their profession, neonatal care providers require basic competency in developmental care before they can reach a level of advanced competency.

FOUR KEY CONSTRUCTS PERTINENT TO UNDERSTANDING DEVELOPMENTAL CARE COMPETENCIES

To more fully explain what is meant by *developmental care competencies,* or the substantive piece of an RCT, it is important to define and discuss selected key constructs or complex concepts (Figure 21-1). Knowledge of these constructs will provide the infrastructure needed for more precise consideration of the content contained within developmental care competencies.

Competency

What is competency? Merriam-Webster's Online Dictionary (2020) identifies competence and competency as nouns and defines these terms similarly as "the condition or quality of being competent; well-qualified; capable; fit; sufficient; adequate; ability; fitness." Two authorities on competence in the workforce refer to competence as underlying characteristics that are casually related to criterion-related performance shown to be effective in a job (Spencer & Spencer, 1993). The underlying characteristics are believed to exist as a deep and enduring part of a person's work habits that reflect that person's activities across a variety of job tasks and situations. In the field of nursing, competencies have become important considerations, especially in light of the nursing shortage (Institute of Medicine [IOM], 2003). Among other things, the IOM report states that a core set of competencies must be woven into health-profession education: patient-centered care, interdisciplinary teams, evidence-based practice, continuous quality improvement, and informatics. Although this report has been out for many years, competency-based education for baccalaureate and higher degree programs is just now being considered as part of the new American Association of Colleges of Nursing (AACN) essentials for nursing education (https://www.aacnnursing.org/About-AACN/AACN-Governance/Committees-and-Task-Forces/Essentials).

Neonatal nursing experts concurred with a premise that Spencer and Spencer (1993) made 15 years earlier—that competency and competence are different. According to Strodtbeck and Kenner (2007), *competency* is an ongoing process that requires an individual to demonstrate the knowledge and corresponding skills that meet the expectations of a specific professional role, whereas *competence* refers to the skills and abilities of an individual. Strodtbeck and Kenner's recommendations echo those contained in the 2003 IOM report—that health professionals must be required to demonstrate competence, not simply pay a license renewal fee, to maintain their authority to practice. Strodtbeck and Kenner's discussion of competency incorporated the

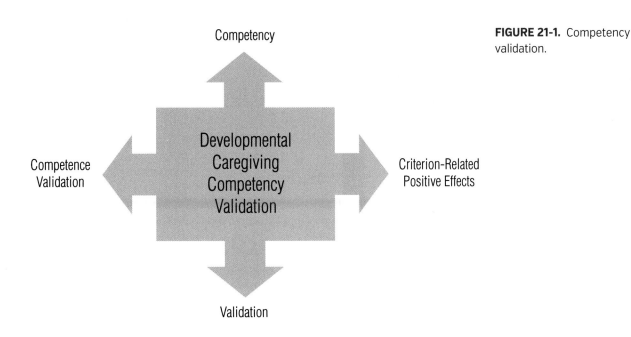

FIGURE 21-1. Competency validation.

American Nurses Association's (ANA) definitions of continuing competence and professional nursing (ANA, 2000). It is interesting to note that according to the ANA, professional nursing competence behavior is based not solely upon knowledge but also upon attitudes and beliefs.

In addition, Benner et al. (1996), authorities on levels of expertise in nursing practice reported that they derived their explanations of knowledge and skills that reflect competence from the Dreyfus Model of Skill Acquisition (Dreyfus, 1972; Dreyfus & Dreyfus, 1986). Benner et al. (1996) define competence as the increased clinical understanding, technical skills, organizational abilities, and ability to anticipate the likely course of events that typically emerges after 2 years of clinical nursing experience. To further clarify competency's meaning, it is worthwhile to consider a comment made by a renowned psychometric expert. Known for his development of the Cronbach alpha and recognized for his expertise on measurement and reliability, Cronbach (1971) stated, "Success on the job depends on nonverbal qualities that are hard to assess" (p. 487).

Cronbach's assertion about job success appears to have been correct. Certain tacit variables that are deeply embedded in a caregiver's personality (e.g., a caregiver's motives, attitudes, values, and self-confidence) can be assumed to significantly affect how caregivers' knowledge and skills are operationalized in clinical settings. However, because they are not outwardly visible, assessing and facilitating the development of those tacit, desirable variables (e.g., high motivation, positive attitudes, self-confidence) can be difficult. Spencer and Spencer (1993) recommended that, when a choice exists for ways in which to obtain specific caregiver qualities, it is more cost-effective to initially select for these qualities when hiring rather than trying to develop them after the fact.

Unfortunately, NICU managers are not in a position to hire all new personnel or even reassign staff members if they do not embody the desired combination of motives, attitudes, values, and self-confidence. Instead, NICU leaders must work on updating, reorienting, and reeducating staff. Those involved in continuing education are asked to help staff members achieve and maintain the desired levels of developmental care competencies while simultaneously, promptly, and courteously integrating reinforcement for the desired behaviors and their modifiers (e.g., high motivation, positive attitudes toward lifelong learning, self-confidence). It is crucial that these education activities be managed using a gentle and coregulatory process that is congruent with and sets an example for developmental care (Als & Gilkerson, 1997). These standards also need to be integrated into the annual staff evaluation process.

The Council of International Neonatal Nurses, Inc. developed neonatal nursing competencies for low-resourced countries (Jones, 2019). These are being used in global documents to describe the minimum level of competency that a nurse who cares for the small and sick newborn needs. These competencies help define the training needed for NICU personnel.

Criterion-Related Positive Effects

How can nurses be assured that their educative efforts have been successful and that they have gained reliable strategies worthy of endorsement? To answer these questions, one must refer to basic psychometric principles. Traditionally, psychometricians discuss the terms *criterion referenced* or *criterion related* when they discuss the reliability of something. *Criterion related* generally means that something has been measured according to a specific criterion or standard. To have criterion-related reliability or criterion-related positive effects, developmental care competencies should reflect and/or predict the work completed as measured according to a specific criterion or standard. Furthermore, one can technically distinguish between two types of criterion-related validity (Carmines & Zeller, 1979). If the criterion exists concurrently, correlating a measure and the criterion at the same point in time assesses *concurrent validity*. If the criterion exists in the future, then correlating the relevant measures with a future criterion assesses *predictive validity*. The logic for both types of criterion-related validity is the same; the only difference concerns the present or future existence of the criterion variable.

Criterion-related validity contains an intuitive meaning not shared by other types of validity. Also, because even under the best of circumstances performance can be challenging to measure, Cronbach (1971) has recommended that all validation reports include the warning, "insofar as the criterion is truly representative of the outcome we wish to maximize" (p. 488). It is important to emphasize that criterion-validation procedures cannot be applied to all measurement situations in all healthcare settings. As Symington and Pinelli (2006) have pointed out, it is critical that more high-quality RCTs be undertaken by different investigators in different settings to assess the true effects of developmental care on clinical outcomes. Criterion-related effects must be examined because the most relevant criterion variables might not have been identified. For example, it would be difficult to establish an accurate measure of some kinds of personality traits such as the self-confidence and contentedness sometimes associated with developmental care that could be generalized across populations. Specific types of behavior that people with high or low self-confidence or contentedness demonstrate are not understood to the extent that they can be used to validate measures of those personality traits.

Validation

Understanding the meaning of validation requires one important distinction: that "one validates not a test, but one's interpretation of data" arising from a certain evaluative process (Cronbach, 1971, p. 447). This distinction is central to any validation because when a person validates, they are validating the measuring tool in relation to the purpose for which it is being used, not the measuring tool in and of itself. To assess for and validate the existence of competencies, minimum entry-level criteria—or standards for practice effectiveness—must be established. The validation of achievement and maintenance of these standards then must be completed systematically. Some proposed developmental care competencies are summarized later in this chapter. At this time, however, the standards for developmental care practices are hypothetical and nonspecific in that they have yet to be formally validated using RCTs; the things that constitute the minimal data set for practice have not been tested.

Competence Validation

Competence validation must be a final consideration in establishing the knowledge infrastructure for developmental care. According to Loving (1991, 1993), competence validation within nursing is a special type of validation that refers to a process of identifying some type of competence, or to the overall competency of an individual nurse. Emanating from the ideas of Kuhn (1970) and Polanyi (1962) of "knowing that" and "knowing how," Simpson and Creehan (1998) claim two components are essential to any nursing competence validation: knowledge-based evaluation (knowing "that") and clinical skills verification (knowing "how"). Given that knowledge of that and how constantly is being revised based on the latest replicated research findings (a.k.a., evidence-based practice), competence validation in nursing exists as a dynamic process that requires thoughtful and intermittent evaluation on an ongoing and planned basis. If caregivers are to maintain current competencies, they must engage in continuing education programs of one sort or another and partake in regular reading or self-study to remain current on new information and ways in which to better perform particular clinical skills.

Lenburg (1999) advocated using a competency-based model for nursing education more than 20 years ago. Lenburg's Competency Outcomes and Performance Assessment (COPA) model may prove helpful in the ongoing creation and validation of competencies related to didactic and clinical aspects of developmental care. According to the COPA model, a competency performance system that is psychometrically sound incorporates the concepts of objectivity, acceptability, consistency, flexibility, and comparability. It is ideal to use theory and research to develop competencies in a competency-performance system. Burleson's (2001) findings from a study identifying the essential knowledge elements, skills, and competencies for newborn developmental specialists may provide insight into the things a developmental care competency system should include.

Designing Developmental Care Competencies

After examining the preceding constructs related to or constituting competency validation, readers might conclude it is premature to begin validating developmental care competencies in light of insufficient support by RCTs. However, it seems reasonable to speculate that developmental care is needed and will continue to be needed because preterm infants continue to require intensive care, important benefits

have been identified, no negative sequelae have been shown in recipients, and nurses and other caregivers do not want to lose the momentum that has been generated. Parents and families are requesting developmental care, and parents are forming support groups that endorse it on the Internet. Consequently, neonatal nurses, as well as others involved in care of NICU infants, must forge ahead and become competent developmental caregivers while concomitantly studying its effects.

Where do caregivers begin in their implementation of a developmental care competency system? From a logistical standpoint, it appears that, among the various clinicians involved in caring for newborns and infants, all disciplines should participate as team members in the implementation of developmental care competencies. If competency validation for developmental care achieves widespread acceptance, parents, other family members, other healthcare providers, and support service workers can be the next groups expected to demonstrate developmental care competencies (Figure 21-2) in addition to nurses, physicians, unlicensed nurses' aides, respiratory therapists, physical therapists, infant massage therapists, occupational therapists, clinical psychologists, speech–language therapists, radiology technicians, laboratory technicians, social workers, unit secretaries, housekeepers, nutritionists/dieticians, pharmacists, chaplains, child-life specialists, music therapists, and medical ethicists. Students of various disciplines (nurses, medical students, resident physicians, and neonatal fellows) also should be included. All of these groups need relevant information, demonstration of applied knowledge, and competency evaluation or validation as deemed appropriate. Each part of the education process requires effective learning materials, approaches, and evaluation tools. Administrators must be educated to understand the importance of developmental care and the resources required to implement it.

Continuing Nurse Education Professional Development

Nurses must acquire and maintain knowledge and competencies appropriate for their role and specialty practice area. Certification within a specialty is one way to demonstrate possession of specialty knowledge (Association of Women's Health, Obstetric, and Neonatal Nurses [AWHONN], 2019). Each NICU nurse must be accountable for their own competencies in the practice of neonatal nursing (ANA, 2013). The most practical first step in designing a workable system to validate caregiver competency in developmental care is to include the desired competencies in each NICU orientation program. Several resources are available to guide this process (selected resources are listed in Table 21-1). Basic neonatal orientation programs are available from two national nursing organizations. NANN offers the Foundations of Neonatal Care program, and AWHONN offers the Neonatal Orientation and Education program. NICU educators can augment the basic orientation programs with more detailed developmental care content delivered in a manner that best

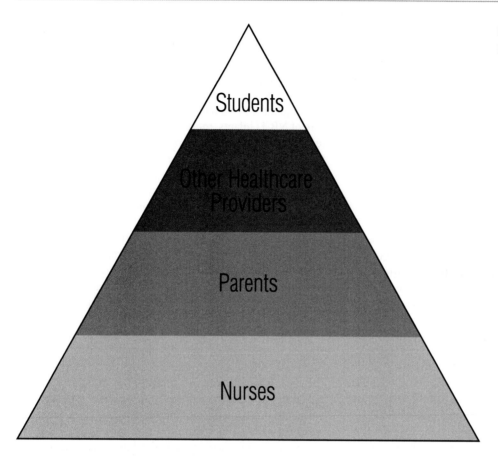

FIGURE 21-2. Prioritizing competency validation.

suits learners. Developmental care educational offerings can be delivered in various formats including DVDs, self-study modules, synchronous and asynchronous online learning, discussions, and demonstrations. Competencies appropriate to individual NICUs can be adopted from these resources and incorporated into each orientation program as a starting point. Many hospitals cross-train nurses to work in more than one clinical area, so orientation to a philosophy infant, family-centered, developmental care (IFCDC) must be available to these nurses, as well. Other hospitals employ agency nurses; consequently, it is critically important that all orientation programs on areas that provide care to newborns/infants and families include developmental care competencies.

In a joint venture, three national specialty nursing organizations, AWHONN, NANN, and the American Association of Critical Care Nurses, published *Core Curriculum for Neonatal Intensive Care Nursing* (Verklan et al., 2021). Developmental care content, categorized as a "cornerstone of clinical practice," has expanded significantly with each new edition. In the latest edition, Spruill (2021) presents an extensive discussion of developmental care with the objective of helping neonatal nurses apply standards of developmental care to guide NICU practice; assess physiologic and behavioral organization of preterm infants; design a developmental plan of care based on the unique needs of each infant in relation to environment, caregiving, parent support and consistency of caregiving; and practice pain management within a developmental framework (p. 172).

Individual institutions need to assume responsibility for mounting the first step toward establishing and requiring

competency validation of developmental care by neonatal nurses. Nursing leaders at each institution who have developmental care experience, confidence in the existing empiric evidence supporting developmental care practices, and belief in its benefits could oversee the competency validation. As these institutions enact competency requirements, their units could provide developmental care benchmarks for other neonatal care units around the country and internationally.

Specialty nursing organizations and other organizations such as the Joint Commission and the IOM can play a powerful role in promoting specialized competencies of nurses (Whittaker et al., 2000). NANN has taken a leading role in offering the Developmental Care Specialist designation. NCC has responded to neonatal nurses' desire to be recognized for their knowledge and competency in specialized areas within neonatal care by offering additional certifications in care of the ELBW infant and neonatal neurointensive care.

Additional Considerations Regarding Competency Education

Several approaches can be used to educate nonnurse caregivers in developmental care. It is the responsibility of each NICU to establish the level of knowledge and expertise desired by various caregivers and infant contacts and to designate qualified evaluators. Parents and family members should receive their basic instructions from the infant's bedside nurses, with opportunities given for return demonstrations of caregiving. If the institution employs a developmental care specialist, that individual can work with parents and family members to assess and validate their caregiving competencies. If the institution does not have a developmental care specialist, it may consider creating a developmental care team involving nurses and other health-related caregivers (e.g., occupational specialists, physical therapists, clinical psychologists) to fulfill these responsibilities. Members of the caregiving team should be knowledgeable about available educational resources so parents can learn about the developmental needs of their preterm infant.

It seems most appropriate for physicians and other nonnurse caregivers to receive their initial instructions and competency validation from a developmental care specialist or from developmental care team members who are familiar with the empiric literature on the subject and can substantiate the scientific basis for different techniques. Additional professional education can be obtained through virtual conferences and online learning modules.

Although the focus of this competency discussion has primarily centered on nurses, other disciplines are quickly moving forward on this issue as well. The roles of physical and occupational therapists and speech–language pathologists in the NICU and their discipline-specific competencies are evolving.

ASSESSING, VALIDATING, AND FURTHERING CAREGIVER DEVELOPMENTAL CARE COMPETENCIES

Standards of practice must guide caregivers in how they practice and what they do—not how they have been trained, think about practice, or discuss practice. Those who believe in such constraints are accustomed to hearing the common complaint that "science" does not provide sufficient information to practice. Although it is true that standards for competency do not yield knowledge of exactly what to do and when, caregivers have basic knowledge of providing care and follow basic principles for providing care (e.g., safety, asepsis, ethics).

THE REQUISITE OF CAREFUL PLANNING

The final yet crucial step in fostering developmental care competencies is to construct a plan for action. Planning involves thinking out and documenting acts and purposes in advance to effectively achieve goals (Scholnick, 1995). The very act of planning has been equated with problem solving because planning plays such a central role in problem solving (Friedman et al., 1987). When the costs and risks of making mistakes are high (e.g., the money involved in developmental care training and the money wasted by a lack of endorsement of developmental care by staff), efforts need to be devoted to internal cognitive processing to overcome the costs of recovering from making errors and inefficiency. The study of planning is central to explaining the interaction between motivation and cognition in intelligent behavior. Planning requires the ability to inhibit actions while thinking through the best way to achieve goals. Competency-based workforce planning involves addressing motivation, factual knowledge, intellectual/cognitive

levels, and interpersonal and psychomotor skills (Simpson & Creehan, 1998). Proven methods for teaching and maintaining competencies exist and have been documented extensively (Greiner & Knebel, 2003). Several examples include mastery learning (Block, 1971; Guskey, 1997; MacTurk & Morgan, 1995), discovery learning (Fujishin, 1997), interpersonal-skills training (Carcuff, 2000; Wondrak, 1998), cooperative learning (Kagan, 1994), adult education and training (Jarvis, 1995), apprenticeships (Summerfield & Cosgrove, 1994), and internships (Ciofalo, 1992).

Basic Rationale for Competency: Preventing Complications

Complications refer to sequelae resulting from the incomplete resolution of problems related to a primary diagnosis or from secondary problems related to one or more secondary diagnoses. As such, preventing complications may be associated with developmental care by lowering the rate of certain primary complications (e.g., intracranial hemorrhage, chronic respiratory problems) stemming from an initial diagnosis (primary prevention). By preventing primary complications, the rate of disabilities or complications resulting from an initial diagnosis in a nursery (secondary prevention; e.g., reflux and tube feeding because of uncoordinated oral motor movements) may be reduced, thereby reducing the rate of defective functioning or complications due to an existing disorder (tertiary prevention; e.g., spastic diplegia) and lessening a dying infant's pain and promoting personal contentment and social fulfillment to the extent possible of their family and friends (palliation). Although the sample sizes were small, developmental care was thought to have influenced some aspects of prevention in six clinical trials. Als et al. (1996) demonstrated shorter lengths of hospital stay and decreased healthcare costs in infants who received developmental care, suggesting that complications were fewer in those infants. Developmental interventions require technical skills, an awareness and understanding of evidence supporting their implementation, a special kind of art that involves connoisseurship, practice in performing developmental interventions, and education and mentoring to develop competency in performing these interventions.

CONCLUSION

This chapter reviews the issues of competency and the need for competency validation for health professionals committed to IFCDC. Issues surrounding developmental care as it relates to competency are discussed. We have come a long way toward full implementation of developmental care if our many disciplines are acknowledging the need for competencies in this area. Awareness and professional dialogues are the first step toward identifying developmental care competencies and the ways in which to measure them. This chapter has raised issues that nurses and multidisciplinary team members can propose at their institutions and within their professional disciplines.

Potential Research Questions

Prevention

- What developmental principles need to be better understood to meet the learning needs of neonatal nurses as technologies change in our world?
- What resources are needed to support competency validation and understanding of relationships with NICU outcomes?
- How often do competencies need to be validated and updated?

Confirmation

- What are the best ways to validate competencies? How will simulations change this process in the future?

- Does supporting neonatal nurses to complete competencies change practice and outcomes in the NICU?

Intervention/Education

- How do competencies and care bundles interface to support the best provision of caregiving? Or not?
- Do other competencies need to be developed for neonatal nurses to remain effective in their practice?

REFERENCES

Als, H. (1982). Toward a synactive theory of development: Promise for the assessment of infant individuality. *Infant Mental Health Journal, 3*, 229–243.

Als, H. (2001). *Program guide: Newborn Individualized Developmental Care Assessment Program (NIDCAP), an education and training program for health professionals* (Rev. ed.). Boston Children's Medical Center Corporation.

Als, H., Duffy, F. H., & McAnulty, G. B. (1996). Effectiveness of individualized neurodevelopmental care in the newborn intensive care unit (NICU). *Acta Paediatrica*, (Suppl. 416), 21–30. https://doi.org/10.1111/j.1651-2227.1996.tb14273.x

Als, H., & Gilkerson, L. (1997). The role of relationship-based developmentally supportive newborn intensive care in strengthening outcome of preterm infants. *Seminars in Perinatology, 21*(3), 178–189. https://doi.org/10.1016/s0146-0005(97)80062-6

Altimier, L., Kenner, C., & Damus, K. (2015). The WeeCare neuroprotective NICU program (WeeCare): The effect of a comprehensive developmental care training program on seven neuroprotective core measures for family-centered developmental care of premature neonates. *Newborn & Infant Nursing Reviews*, (15), 6–16. https://doi.org/10.1053/j.nainr.2015.01.006

Altimier, L., & Phillips, R. (2016). The neonatal integrative developmental care model: Advanced clinical applications of the seven core measures for neuroprotective family-centered developmental care. *Newborn & Infant Nursing Reviews, 16*, 230–244. https://doi.org/10.1053/j.nainr.2016.09.030

American Academy of Pediatrics (AAP). (2020). *Newborn Resuscitation Program: About NRP.* https://www.aap.org/en-us/continuing-medical-education/life-support/NRP/Pages/About-NRP.aspx

American Nurses Association. (2000). *Continued professional competence: Nursing's agenda for the 21st century (a working paper).* Author.

American Nurses Association. (2013). *Neonatal nursing: Scope and standards of practice* (2nd ed.). Author.

American Occupational Therapy Association. (2006). Specialized knowledge and skills for occupational therapy practice in the neonatal intensive care unit. *The American Journal of Occupational Therapy, 60*, 659–668. https://doi.org/10.5014/ajot.60.6.659

Association of Women's Health, Obstetric, and Neonatal Nurses. (2019). *Standards for professional nursing practice in the care of women and newborns* (8th ed.). Author.

Atun-Einy, O., & Scher, A. (2008). Measuring developmentally appropriate practice in neonatal intensive care units. *Journal of Perinatology, 28*, 218–225. https://doi.org/10.1038/sj.jp.7211908

AWHONN. (2019). *Neonatal orientation and education program (NOEP)* (4th ed.). www.awhonn.org

Beal, J. A. (2005). Evidence for best practices in the neonatal period. *MCN. The American Journal of Maternal/Child Nursing, 30*(6), 397–403. https://doi.org/10.1097/00005721-200511000-00008

Benner, P. A., Tanner, C. A., & Chesla, C. A. (1996). *Expertise in nursing practice: Caring, clinical judgment, and ethics.* Springer.

Block, J. H. (Ed.). (1971). *Mastery learning: Theory and practice.* Holt, Rinehart, & Winston.

Bredemeyer, S., Reid, S., Polverino, J., & Wocadlo, C. (2008). Implementation and evaluation of an individualized developmental care program in a neonatal intensive care unit. *Journal of Specialists in Pediatrics, 13*, 281–291. https://doi.org/10.1111/j.1744-6155.2008.00163.x

Brown, S. E., & Dusing, S. C. (2019). Knowledge translation lecture: Providing best practice in Neonatal Intensive Care and follow-up. A clinician-researcher collaboration. *Pediatric Physical Therapy, 31*(4), 308–314. https://doi.org/10.1097/PEP.0000000000000634

Browne, J. V., Jaeger, C. B., Kenner, C., & Gravens Consensus Committee on Infant and Family Centered Developmental Care. (2020). Executive summary: Standards, competencies, and recommended best practices for infant and family-centered developmental care in the intensive care unit. *Journal of Perinatology: Official Journal of the California Perinatal Association, 40*(Suppl. 1), 5–10. https://doi.org/10.1038/s41372-020-0767-1

Burleson, R. (2001). *Essential knowledge and skills of the newborn developmental specialist (Unpublished doctoral dissertation).* The University of Kentucky.

Byrne, E., & Campbell, S. K. (2013). Physical therapy observation and assessment in the neonatal intensive care unit. *Physical & Occupational Therapy in Pediatrics, 33*(1), 39–74. https://doi.org/10.3109/01942638.2012.754827

Carcuff, R. R. (2000). *The art of helping* (8th ed.). Human Resource Development Press.

Cardin, A. D., Rens, L., Stewart, S., Danner-Bowman, K., McCarley, R., & Kopsas, R. (2015). Neuroprotective core measures 1–7: A developmental care journey. Transformations in NICU design and caregiving attitudes. *Newborn & Infant Nursing Reviews, 15*, 132–141. http://dx.doi.org/10.1053/j.nainr.2015.06.007

Carmines, E. G., & Zeller, R. A. (1979). *Reliability and validity assessment (No. 07-017).* Sage Publications.

Ciofalo, A. (Ed.). (1992). *Internships: Perspectives on experiential learning. A guide to internship management for educators and professionals.* Krieger.

Clubbs, B. H., Barnette, A. R., Gray, N., Weiner, L., Bond, A., Harden, J., & Pineda, R. (2019). A community hospital NICU developmental care partner program: Feasibility and association with decreased nurse burnout without increased infant infection rates. *Advances in Neonatal Care, 19*(4), 311–320. https://doi.org/10.1097/ANC.0000000000000600

Coughlin, M. E. (2021). *Transformative nursing in the NICU: Trauma-informed, age-appropriate care* (2nd. ed.). Springer Publishing.

Craig, J. W., & Smith, C. R. (2020). Risk-adjusted/neuroprotective care services in the NICU: The elemental role of the neonatal therapist (OT, PT, SLP). *Journal of Perinatology, 40*(4), 549–559. https://doi.org/10.1038/s41372-020-0597-1

Cronbach, L. J. (1971). Test validation. In Thorndike, R. L. (Ed.), *Educational measurement* (2nd ed., pp. 443–507). American Council on Education.

Detmer, M. R., & Whelan, M. L. (2017). Music in the NICU: The role of nurses in neuroprotection. *Neonatal Network, 36*(4), 213–217. https://doi.org/10.1891/0730-0832.36.4.213

Dreyfus, H. L. (1972). What computers still can't do (Pt. II). *Creative Computing, 6*(1), 18–31. https://doi.org/10.2307/1575958

Dreyfus, H. L., & Dreyfus, S. E. (1986). *Skill acquisition model.* In *Mind over machine: The power of human intuitive expertise in the era of the computer.* Free Press.

Dusing, S. C., Tripathi, T., Marcinowski, E. C., Thacker, L. R., Brown, L. F., & Hendricks-Muñoz, K. D. (2018). Supporting play exploration and early developmental intervention versus usual care to enhance development outcomes during the transition from the neonatal intensive care unit to home: A pilot randomized controlled study. *BMC Pediatrics, 18*(1), 46. https://doi.org/10.1186/s12887-018-1011-4

Dusing, S. C., Van Drew, C. M., & Brown, S. E. (2012). Instituting parent education practices in the neonatal intensive care unit: An administrative case report of practice evaluation and statewide action. *Physical Therapy, 92*(7), 967–975. https://doi.org/10.2522/ptj.20110360

Emery, L., Hamm, E. L., Hague, K., Chorna, O. D., Moore-Clingenpeel, M., & Maitre, N. L. (2019). A randomised controlled trial of protocolised music therapy demonstrates milestone acquisition in hospitalized infants. *Acta Paediatrica, 108*(5), 828–834. https://doi.org/10.1111/apa.14628

Friedman, S. L., Scholnick, E. K., & Cocking, R. R. (1987). Reflections on reflections: What planning is and how it develops. In Friedman, S. L., Scholnick, E. K., & Cocking, R. R. (Eds.), *Blueprints for thinking* (pp. 515–534). Cambridge University Press.

Fujishin, R. (1997). *Discovering the leader within: Running small groups successfully.* Academy Books.

Goldstein, L. A. (2013). Family support and education. *Physical & Occupational Therapy in Pediatrics, 33*(1), 139–161. https://doi.org/10.3109/01942638.2012.754393

Greiner, A. C., & Knebel, E. (Eds.). (2003). *Health professions education: A bridge to quality.* The National Academies Press.

Guskey, T. R. (1997). *Implementing mastery learning* (2nd ed.). Wadsworth.

Hendricks-Munoz, K. D., & Prendergast, C. C. (2007). Barriers to provision of developmental are in the neonatal intensive care unit: Neonatal nursing perceptions. *American Journal of Perinatology, 24*(2), 71–77. https://doi.org/10.1055/s-2006-958156

Hendricks-Munoz, K. D., Prendergast, C. C., Caprio, M. C., & Wasserman, R. S. (2002). Developmental care: The impact of Wee Care developmental care training on short-term infant outcome and hospital costs. *Newborn & Infant Nursing Reviews, 2*(1), 39–45. https://doi.org/10.1053/nbin.2002.31492

Institute of Medicine. (2003). *Health professions education: A bridge to quality.* www.nap.edu/openbook.php?isbn=0309087236

Jacobs, S., Sokol, J., & Ohllsson, A. (2002). The newborn individualized developmental care and assessment program is not supported by meta-analyses of the data. *Journal of Pediatrics, 140*(6), 699–706. https://doi.org/10.1067/mpd.2002.123667

Jarvis, P. (1995). *Adult and continuing education: Theory and practice* (2nd ed.). Routledge.

Jones, T. (2019). International neonatal nursing competency framework. *Journal of Neonatal Nursing, 25*, 258–264.

Kagan, S. (1994). *Cooperative learning* (2nd ed.). Kagan Cooperative Learning.

Keels, E. L., Goldsmith, J. P., & Committee on Fetus and Newborn. (2019). Neonatal provider workforce, *Pediatrics, 144*(6), e20193147. https://doi.org/10.1542/peds.2019-3147

Khurana, S., Kane, A. E., Brown, S. E., Tarver, T., & Dusing, S. C. (2020). Effect of neonatal therapy on the motor, cognitive, and behavioral development of infants born preterm: A systematic review. *Developmental Medicine and Child Neurology, 62*(6), 684–692. https://doi.org/10.1111/dmcn.14485

Kuhn, T. S. (1970). *The structure of scientific revolutions* (2nd ed.). The University of Chicago Press.

Laudert, S., Liu, W. F., Blackington, S., Perkins, B., Martin, S., MacMillan-York, E., Graven, S., & Handyside, J. (2007) Implementing potentially better practices to support the neurodevelopment of infants in the NICU. *Journal of Perinatology, 27*, S75–S93. https://doi.org/10.1038/sj.jp.7211843

Lenburg, C. (1999, September 30). *The framework, concepts and methods of the competency outcomes and performance assessment (COPA) model.* https://ojin.nursingworld.org/MainMenuCategories/ANAMarketplace/ANAPeriodicals/OJIN/TableofContents/Volume41999/No2Sep1999/COPAModel.html

Liaw, J. (2003). Use of a training program to enhance NICU nurses' cognitive abilities for assessing preterm infant behaviors and offering supportive interventions. *Journal of Nursing Research, 11*, 82–91. https://doi.org/10.1097/01.jnr.0000347623.67531.78

Liaw, J., Chen, S., & Yin, T. (2004). Nurses' beliefs and values doing cue-based care in an NICU in Taiwan. *Journal of Nursing Research, 12*, 275–285. https://doi.org/10.1097/01.jnr.0000387512.36996.4c

Liaw, J., Yang, L., Chang, L., Chou, H., & Chao, S. (2009). Improving neonatal caregiving through a develop-mentally supportive care training program. *Applied Nursing Research, 22*, 86–93. https://doi.org/10.1016/j.apnr.2007.05.001

Loewy, J., Stewart, K., Dassler, A. M., Telsey, A., & Homel, P. (2013). The effects of music therapy on vital signs, feeding, and sleep in premature infants. *Pediatrics, 131*(5), 902–918. https://doi.org/10.1542/peds.2012-1367

Louw, R., & Maree, C. (2005). The effect of formal exposure to developmental care principles on the implementation of developmental care positioning and handling of preterm infants by neonatal nurses. *Health SA Gesondheid, 10*, 24–32.

Loving, G. L. (1991). *Nursing students' perceptions of learning clinical judgment in undergraduate nursing education* (Unpublished doctoral dissertation). The University of Texas at Austin.

Loving, G. L. (1993). Competence validation and cognitive flexibility: A theoretical model grounded in nursing education. *Journal of Nursing Education, 32*, 415–421. https://doi.org/10.3928/0148-4834-19931101-07

MacTurk, R. H., & Morgan, G. A. (Eds.). (1995). *Mastery motivation: Origins, conceptualizations and applications.* Ablex Publishing Corporation.

Merriam Webster's Online Dictionary. (2020). *Competency.* https://www.merriam-webster.com/dictionary/competency

Milette, I., Martel, M.-J., da Silva, M. R., & Coughlin McNeil, M. (2017). Guidelines for the institutional implementation of developmental neuroprotective care in the NICU. Part B: Recommendations and justification. A joint position statement from the CANN, CAPWHN, NANN, and COINN. *The Canadian Journal of Nursing Research, 49*(2), 63–74. https://doi.org/10.1177/0844562117708126

Milette, I., Richard, L., & Martel, M. (2005). Evaluation of a developmental training programme for neonatal nurses. *Journal of Child Health Care, 9*, 94–109. https://doi.org/10.1177/1367493505051400

Nair, M. K., Sunitha, R. M., Leena, M. L., George, B., Bhaskaran, D., & Russell, P. S. (2014). CDC Kerala 2: Developmental intervention package for babies <1,800 g—outcomes at 6 months using DASII. *The Indian Journal of Pediatrics, 81*(Suppl. 2), S73–S79. https://doi.org/10.1007/s12098-014-1624-z

National Association of Neonatal Nurses (NANN). (2011). *Age appropriate care* https://nann.org/uploads/Education/Age-Appropriate_Care-FINAL.pdf

National Association of Neonatal Nurses (NANN). (2020). *Developmental care CNE modules.* www.nann.org

Neel, M. L., Yoder, P., Matusz, P. J., Murray, M. M., Miller, A., Burkhardt, S., Emery, L., Hague, K., Pennington, C., Purnell, J., Lightfoot, M., & Maitre, N. L. (2019). Randomized controlled trial protocol to improve multisensory neural processing, language and motor outcomes in preterm infants. *BMC Pediatrics, 19*(81), 81–90. https://doi.org/10.1007/s12098-014-1551-z

Painter, L., Lewis, S., & Hamilton, B. K. (2019). Improving neurodevelopmental outcomes in NICU patients. *Advances in Neonatal Care, 19*(3), 236–243. https://doi.org/10.1097/ANC.0000000000000583

Park, J., & Kim, J.-S. (2019). Factors influencing developmental care practice among neonatal intensive care unit nurses. *Journal of Pediatric Nursing, 47*, E10–E15. https://doi.org/10.1016/j.pedn.2019.03.014

Perkins, E., Ginn, L., Fanning, J. K., & Bartlett, D. (2004). Effect of nursing education on positioning of infants in the neonatal intensive care unit. *Pediatric Physical Therapy, 16*(2), 2–12. https://doi.org/10.1097/01.PEP.0000112916.38869.5E

Peters, K. L. (1999). Infant handling in the NICU: Does developmental care make a difference? An evaluative review of the literature. *Journal of Perinatal and Neonatal Nursing, 13*(3), 83–109. https://doi.org/10.1097/00005237-199912000-00008

Phillips, R. M. (2015). Seven core measures of neuroprotective family-centered developmental care: Creating an infrastructure for implementation. *Newborn and Infant Nursing Reviews, 15*(3), 87–90. https://doi.org/10.1053/j.nainr.2015.06.004

Pineda, R., Wallendorf, M., & Smith, J. (2020). A pilot study demonstrating the impact of the supporting and enhancing NICU sensory experiences (SENSE) program on the mother and infant. *Early Human Development, 144*, https://doi.org/10.1016/j.earlhumdev.2020.105000

Polanyi, M. (1962). *Personal knowledge: Towards a post-critical philosophy.* The University of Chicago Press.

Pressler, J. L., Orlando, S. M., & McGrath, J. M. (2010). Interdisciplinary competency validation. In Kenner, C., & McGrath, J. (Eds.), *Developmental care of newborns and infants* (2nd ed., pp. 283–307).

Sanders, M. R., & Hall, S. L. (2018). Trauma-informed care in the newborn intensive care unit: Promoting safety, security and connectedness. *Journal of Perinatology, 38*(1), 3–10.

Scholnick, E. K. (1995). Direction I: Knowing and constructing plans. *SRCD Newsletter, Fall, 1–2,* 17.

Simpson, K. R., & Creehan, P. A. (1998). Introduction to competence validation for providers of perinatal care. In Simpson, K. R. & Creehan, P. A. (Eds.), *Competence validation for perinatal care providers: Orientation, continuing education, and evaluation* (pp. xiii–xv). Lippincott, Williams & Wilkins.

Spencer, L. M., & Spencer, S. M. (1993). *Competence at work: Models for superior performance.* John Wiley & Sons.

Spruill, C. T. (2021). Developmental support. In Verklan, M. T., Walden, M., & Forrest, S. (Eds.), *Core curriculum for neonatal intensive care nursing* (6th ed., pp. 172–190). Elsevier.

Strodtbeck, F., & Kenner, C. (2007). Competency-based education in neonatal nursing. In Kenner, C. & Lott, J. W. (Eds.), *Comprehensive neonatal care: An interdisciplinary approach* (4th ed., pp. 615–624). Saunders.

Summerfield, C. J., & Cosgrove, H. (Eds.). (1994). Jobs that let you earn while you learn, training programs by experts, combined classroom and on-the-job training. In Oakes, E. H. (Ed.), *Ferguson's guide to apprenticeship programs* (2nd ed.). Ferguson Publishing.

Sweeney, J. K., Heriza, C. B., Blanchard, Y., & Dusing, S. C. (2010). Neonatal physical therapy. Part II: Practice frameworks and evidence-based practice guidelines. *Pediatric Physical Therapy, 22*(1), 2–16. https://doi.org/10.1097/PEP.0b013e3181cdba43

Sweeney, J. K., Heriza, C. B., Reilly, M. A., Smith, C., & VanSant, A. F. (1999). Practice guidelines for the physical therapist in the neonatal intensive care unit (NICU). *Pediatric Physical Therapy, 11*, 119–132.

Symington, A. J., & Pinelli, J. (2006). Developmental care for promoting development and preventing morbidity in preterm infants. *Cochrane Database of Systematic Reviews, 2*, CD001814. https://www.cochranelibrary.com/cdsr/doi/10.1002/14651858.CD001814.pub2/full

Verklan, MT., Walden, M., & Forrest, S. (Eds.). (2021). *Core curriculum for neonatal intensive care nursing* (6th ed.). Elsevier.

Wallin, L., & Eriksson, M. (2009). Newborn individualized developmental care and assessment program (NIDCAP): A systematic review of the literature. *Worldviews on Evidence-Based Nursing, 2*, 54–69. https://doi.org/10.1111/j.1741-6787.2009.00150.x

Westrup, B., Kleberg, A., von Eichwald, K., Stjernqvist, K., & Lagercrantz, H. (2002). A randomized controlled trial to evaluate the effects of the newborn individualized developmental care and assessment program in a Sweden setting. *Pediatrics, 105*, 66–72. https://doi.org/10.1542/peds.105.1.66

Westrup, B., Sizan, J., & Lagercrantz, H. (2007). Family-centered developmental supportive care: A holistic and humane approach to reduce stress and pain in neonates. *Journal of Perinatology, 27*, S12–S18. https://doi.org/10.1038/sj.jp.7211724

White, C., Daniels, T., Philip, S. Prehn, J, Stewart, K. D., Henderson, R., Johnson, L., Browning, F., Glynn, E., Cahill, B., & Duncan, S. (2007). *Neonatal developmental care training series* (Vols. 1–6). www.neonataldevelopmentalcare.com/

Whittaker, S., Smolenski, M., & Carson, W. (2000, June 30). Assuring continued competence—policy questions and approaches: How should the profession respond? *Online Journal of Issues in Nursing.* https://ojin.nursingworld.org/MainMenuCategories/ANAMarketplace/ANAPeriodicals/OJIN/TableofContents/Volume52000/No3Sept00/ArticlePreviousTopic/ContinuedCompetence.html

Wondrak, R. F. (1998). *Interpersonal skills for nurses and health care professionals.* Blackwell Science.

Zhang, X., Lee, S.-Y., Chen, J., & Liu, H. (2016). Factors influencing implementation of developmental care among NICU nurses in China. *Clinical Nursing Research, 25*(3), 238–253. https://doi.org/10.1177/1054773814547229

CHAPTER 22

Developmental Care: Where Do We Go From Here?

Carole Kenner and Jacqueline M. McGrath

Standards in Systems Thinking

Standard 1: Systems Thinking
- The intensive care unit shall exhibit an infrastructure of leadership, mission, and a governance framework to guide the performance of the collaborative practice of Infant and Family-Centered Developmental Care (IFCDC).

Standard 2: Systems Thinking
- The intensive care unit shall provide a professionally competent interprofessional collaborative practice team to support the baby, parent, and family's holistic, developmental, and psychosocial needs from birth through the transition of hospital discharge to home and assure continuity to follow-up care.

INTRODUCTION

Despite the long history of developmental care, the impact of the neonatal intensive care unit (NICU) macro- and micro-environments on the physical development of infants and their families often is still not viewed as an essential aspect of care. This book is dedicated to integrating this essential care to its rightful position of importance in neonatal practice and education globally. We have provided the levels of evidence to support the integration of developmentally supportive, neuro-protective interventions and strategies. But a book can only do so much; words are not enough, actions must follow. We must together advocate within our discipline specific professional organization to continue to seek evidence to support infants and their families physically and emotionally during these critical early life experiences. Infant mental health is critical to the long-term outcomes for the family unit. It is no longer acceptable to just survive; each unique family unit needs to be supported to thrive and we must continue to see beyond the doors of the NICU and examine the long-term outcomes both in terms of the infant and the family unit.

Professional associations organize, motivate, educate, and advance a profession. The National Association of Neonatal Nurses (NANN) has done all of this and more for the neonatal nursing specialty. NANN has led the way in shaping neonatal nursing practice in a way that not only carves out the "niche" for the neonatal nurse role within the professional environment but also creates a role that acknowledges infants and families as partners in the NICU. NANN has taken the lead to bring several disciplines together to create a text that reflects the current thinking on

individualized, family-centered developmental care (IFDC) that is now evolving as presented in Chapters 1 and 2, Infant and Family-Centered Developmental Care (IFCDC). NANN adopted a blueprint for developmental competencies deemed necessary to promote positive growth and development for infants and their families. These recommendations are applicable to any member of the interdisciplinary team who might touch a small or sick infant or interact with a family. These competencies can be demonstrated through a portfolio review, education background, and practice and an examination (NANN, 2021). This is an exciting time for neonatal nurses, other health professionals, and families interested in promoting this philosophy of care. This chapter offers some "predictions" regarding the direction of developmental care in the future and raises questions that still need to be answered.

NANN'S DEVELOPMENTAL CARE SPECIALIST DESIGNATION REFLECTS FOUR STANDARDS

NANN's four standards are:

Standard 1: A flexible and individualized approach is taken toward all hands-on caregiving interactions with continual responsiveness to each infant's competencies, vulnerabilities, and thresholds.

Standard 2: Family-centered care is supported from birth.

Standard 3: All caregivers practice collaboratively.

Standard 4. A developmentally appropriate environment is provided for every infant and family.

PROFESSIONAL ASSOCIATIONS, PARENT GROUPS, AND INTERDISCIPLINARY WORKING GROUPS AND THEIR ROLE IN DEVELOPMENTAL CARE

Developmental care has attracted much professional and public attention, but it is important to remember that as recently as 2002, this aspect of care was listed as a useless therapy in a professional journal. To continue to change this mindset, professional associations, parent groups, and interdisciplinary working groups that support the full integration of developmental care into routine caregiving practices need to be vocal and visible on this subject. Family-centered developmental care is an essential element of ALL newborn care. Members include American Occupational Therapy Association (AOTA), Association of Physical and Natural Therapists (APNT), Council of International Neonatal Nurses, Inc. (COINN), European Foundation for the Care of Newborn Infants (EFCNI), PreemieWorld, NICU Parent Network, Gravens Consensus Committee for the Recommendation for NICU Design Standards, Gravens Consensus Committee on Standards, Competencies and Best Practices for Infant and Family-Centered Developmental Care in the Intensive Care Unit, NANN, National Perinatal Association (NPA), and World Health Organization. Such organizations must continue to take a stand on setting the pace and having the vision of advancing the future care needs of infants and families. These associations lend credibility to the work or standard of care. However, in the case of the developmental core, the support must be interdisciplinary. Integration of these practices require a team approach to foster developmental growth of the infant and family.

Each discipline and parent organization brings a rich history and perspective that is needed to deliver developmentally supportive care. We need a common language, however, to share the vision of the ultimate goal of developmental care. This foundational knowledge in this text represents a bridging across the languages of each of our disciplines and parents with the outcome being a product that will continue to influence practice in an interdisciplinary, integrative way. Such work requires putting aside turf issues and working together with families to promote positive growth and development of the family unit. This work requires, as noted from the standards listed at the beginning of this chapter, Systems Thinking—a unit culture shift and policies that support integrative infant and family-centered developmental care (IFCDC) (Kenner & Jaeger, 2019). To be effective, the competencies identified in the IFCDC framework must be integrated into every facet of care, professional development, and performance evaluation. As a consumer of this content, we ask that you think of ways that changes in systems thinking can occur. Recognize too, your discipline's unique contribution to the developmental care team but ultimately see how your views, including those of families, contribute to healthcare delivery.

DEMONSTRATION OF PROFESSIONAL COMPETENCE IN DEVELOPMENTAL CARE: IS IT NECESSARY?

Professional competence through certification or other tangible demonstration of competence, according to some experts, is just another artificial bureaucratic hoop to jump through. However, the more prevalent view is that certification is an outcome of the educational process. It provides tangible evidence of the degree to which the content has been integrated into one's knowledge. Health professionals are knowledge workers. We use the tools we acquire through practice, experiences, and education. A certification gives further proof that some level of knowledge has been acquired. However, it provides no assurance that the actual knowledge will be implemented at the bedside. That is the next step, where competency levels, checklists, or similar performance-outcome measures are used. These tools are nice but do nothing to ensure the actual integration of knowledge into practice without continued reflection and evaluation of the process. Nevertheless, the certification does demonstrate that there is a minimal level of comprehension of the content that a health professional providing developmental care has achieved. Certification also lends credence and credibility to the end product, in this case developmental care. If a group or groups have taken the time to create an examination to test the level of knowledge, then this content must be important. In this country, the passage of a certification examination is often a prerequisite of initial or continued employment. Is developmental certification necessary? The answer would seem to be "yes" if health professionals truly believe that developmental care is an essential part of neonatal/family-centered care. Competencies have been developed by NANN for the Developmental Care Specialist (NANN, 2021); the Neonatal Therapy Certification offered by Neonatal Therapy National Certification Board; Bobbi Pineda and Johanna Siemon are the current Co-Chairs (NTNCB, 2021); Mary Coughlin and her team have developed the Trauma-Informed Professional Certification Program (Coughlin, 2021); and Gravens Consensus Committee (Brown et al., 2019) has developed standards and competencies for IFCDC that are evidence based. However, until families, health professionals, licensure and certification examinations, and accreditors of healthcare delivery systems and educational programs adopt these standards and competencies, these will not be adopted as widely as needed to impact health outcomes.

NANN has embraced the use of competencies instead of mandating a credentialing process. This model follows the movement with end of life and genetics. The American Association of Colleges of Nursing (AACN) and the City of Hope created the End-of-Life Nursing Education Consortium (ELNEC) model to train the trainer and identify competencies for nurses. These competencies are now being incorporated into nursing curricula and licensure examinations throughout the country. The National Coalition for Health Professions Education in Genetics (NCPGEG) did the same thing. This group created the competencies in genetics that any health professional needs who touches patients and their families. In 2006, these competencies were then revised to be more specific for nursing thus leading the way to have them incorporated into nursing educational programs and regulatory examinations (Jenkins & Calzone, 2007). Thus, the impact of these competencies including developmental care will be greater than if they were tied to a specific credentialing examination.

Every aspect of this text's developmental care curriculum has set forth strategies for advancing the philosophy of IFCDC. The essence of the strategies for advancing the practice of developmental care is:

- Acceptance that developmental care is an essential part of individualized, infant/family-centered care.
- Commitment that developmental care reflects a change in philosophy of care and is interdisciplinary in nature.
- Acceptance that developmental care is a tool that all health professionals partnered with families can and should use with neonates/infants/children.
- Acceptance that an "elite group" of trained people will never move the masses forward toward recognition of developmental care as a standard of care.
- Change theory must be applied when contemplating the implementation of developmental care.
- Commitment to buy-in time: The hook (e.g., education, support, resources) must be provided to gather increasing support for developmental care; marketing the positives about developmental care to the masses before an attempt is made to fully implement this new approach to care delivery is essential.
- Provide evidence to support its use; evidence-based practice is essential.
- Acknowledge the gaps in evidence to support developmental care.
- Conduct well-designed, randomized, controlled clinical trials to demonstrate the effectiveness of developmental care.
- Do a cost versus benefits analysis (using an economic model) regarding use of developmental care.
- Share the vision with others; if the vision is not shared and the "policy" sits in a manual, developmental care will never be accepted.
- See one, do one, teach one; watch experts deliver developmental care, learn how and why to provide such care, practice the techniques, then share the knowledge with others.
- Encourage professional associations and parent groups to promote developmental care.

COVID-19 AND THE FUTURE

As COVID-19 turned the world upside down, separation of mothers/families and their babies occurred. Although some of this separation in the early stages of the pandemic was due to a lack of understanding of the virus and the transmission, as more knowledge was gained about COVID it appeared that an overabundance of caution continued the separation, or at least very limited hours the mother and/or family could be with their babies. Many healthcare organizations including the World Health Organization, European Foundation for Newborn Care of Infants, and Global Alliance for Newborn Care (GLANCE) all called for zero separation. The American Academy of Pediatrics (AAP) has issued guidelines that include how to safely keep the majority of mothers and babies together. These can be found at https://services.aap.org/en/pages/2019-novel-coronavirus-covid-19-infections/clinical-guidance/faqs-management-of-infants-born-to-covid-19-mothers/. Parents are an essential part of the healthcare team and promote infant mental health even during a pandemic (Behr et al., 2021; McGlothen-Bell et al., 2021).

The long-term ramifications of the pandemic are not known, but concerns center on the lack of socialization of babies once discharged with other children, family members, and friends as would usually occur. Will this affect positive growth and development in these infants? Will they develop speech–language skills as easily? Will they exhibit more problems socializing with others? Only time will tell. However, health professionals who are involved in follow-up should watch these babies carefully.

PREDICTIONS FOR DEVELOPMENTAL CARE IN THE FUTURE

Individualized, infant and family-centered developmental care is growing in importance as an essential part of the healthcare of infants and families. Where will it go in the future?

The predictions we make are:

1. Developmental care will be embraced as the driving philosophy of newborn, infant, and family-centered care.
2. Use of a "core curriculum" by health professionals and families will grow and foster its use as a standard for all neonatal care.
3. Developmental care will be a model for interdisciplinary education and healthcare management.
4. Developmental care will be integrated as an essential aspect of standard orientation and continued competency evaluation for health professionals who work with newborns, infants, children, and their families.
5. Developmental care that includes the family as an essential partner will become the framework from which all neonatal care is delivered.
6. Developmental care will be incorporated as an essential aspect of health professional education—integrated into basic and advanced education, no matter the discipline.
7. Developmental care teams will be an expectation in neonatal care delivery.

8. Evidence will mount to support positive healthy outcomes for newborns, infants, and their families when developmental care is the overarching philosophy of care.

9. Interdisciplinary research studies will increase to examine various aspects of developmental care.

10. More emphasis will be placed on maternal and infant mental health in the NICU and the transition home.

CONCLUSION

In summary, NANN is grateful for the opportunity to work with such dedicated professionals and parents on this project. Even though this text is entering its third edition, there is still much work to be done to truly see integration of IFCDC in all NICUs globally. The core knowledge on development found in these pages must be integrated and applied. More research needs to be conducted to demonstrate IFCDC's impact on outcomes for infants and their families. It must be embraced as a philosophical underpinning of neonatal care that is deemed an essential part of care.

REFERENCES

Behr, J. H., Brandon, D., & McGrath, J. (2021). Parents are "essential" caregivers. *Advanced in Neonatal Care, 21*(2), 93–94. https://doi.org/10.1097/ANC.0000000000000861

Browne, J. V., Jaeger, C. B., on behalf of the Gravens Consensus Committee, . (2019). *Report of the first Consensus Conference on standards, competencies and best practices for infant and family-centered developmental care in the intensive care unit.* https://nicudesign.nd.edu/nicu-care-standards/

Coughlin, M. (2021). *Trauma-informed professional certification program.* https://www.caringessentials.net/portrait

Jenkins, J., & Calzone, K. (2007). Establishing the essential nursing competencies for genetics and genomics. *Journal of Nursing Scholarship, 39*(1), 10–16. https://doi.org/10.1111/j.1547-5069.2007.00137.x. PMID: 17393960.

Kenner, C., & Jaeger, C. B. (2019). *IFCDC-recommendation for best practices in systems thinking.* https://nicudesign.nd.edu/nicu-care-standards/ifcdc--recommendation-for-best-practices-in-systems-thinking/

McGlothen-Bell, K., Browne, J. V., Jaeger, C. B., & Kenner, C. (2021). Promoting infant mental health in the newborn intensive care unit: Considerations in the time of COVID-19. *Advances in Neonatal Care, 21*(3), 169–170. https://doi.org/10.1097/ANC.00000000000008

NANN developmental care products. (2021). http://nann.org/education/educational-products/developmental-care-product-suite

Neonatal therapy certification board (2021). https://neonataltherapycertification.com/

Index

Note: Page numbers followed by "*f*" indicate figures and "*t*" indicate tables.